AF587954

METAL IONS IN BIOLOGY AND MEDICINE

LES IONS MÉTALLIQUES EN BIOLOGIE ET EN MÉDECINE

Volume 9

ORGANIZERS AND CONTRIBUTORS

ORGANIZERS

Instituto de Ambiante e Vida
Faculdade de Ciências e Tecnologia da Universidade de Coimbra
Insituto Superior Técnico, Universidade Técnica de Lisboa
Armed Forces Institute of Pathology
Universidade Técnica de Lisboa

CONTRIBUTORS

Conseil Général de la Haute Corse
Nickel Producers Environmental Research Association (NIPERA)
Jackson State University
Sciedade Portugesa de Bioqimica
Fundaçao Oriente
BPI
Storaenso
Caixa Geral de Depositos
Somincor
Delta Cafés
Universidade de Coimbra

METAL IONS IN BIOLOGY AND MEDICINE

LES IONS MÉTALLIQUES EN BIOLOGIE ET EN MÉDECINE

Volume 9

Proceedings of
the 9th International Symposium
on Metal Ions in Biology and Medicine
Held in Lisboa, Portugal, Europe
on May 21-24, 2006.

9e Symposium International sur les Ions
Métalliques en Biologie et en Médecine,
Lisbonne, Portugal, Europe, 21-24 mai 2006.

Edited by
Maria Carmen Alpoim
Paula Vasconcellos Morais
Maria Amelia Santos
Armando J. Cristóvão
José A. Centeno
Philippe Collery

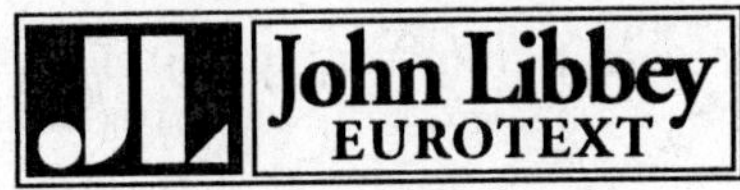

Historical Perspective

The International Symposia on Metal Ions in Biology and Medicine have been organized since 1990, chaired and co-chaired by the distinguished colleagues:

1st: Ph. Collery & J. C. Etienne (Reims, France, 1990)

2nd: J. Anastassopoulou & T. Theophanides (Loutraki, Greece, 1992)

3rd: N. A. Littlefield & L. Poirier (Montreal, Canada, 1994)

4th: J. L. Domingo, J. M. Llobet & J. Corbella (Barcelona, Spain, 1996)

5th: P. Bratter, V. Negretti de Bratter & P. Schramel (Münich, Germany, 1998)

6th: J. A. Centeno (San Juan, Puerto Rico, USA, 2000)

7th: L. A. Khassanova (Saint Petersburg, Russia, 2002)

8th: M. Á. Cser, I. S. László (Budapest, Hungary, 2004)

The first volume of the series was published in May 1990
Eds. Ph. Collery, L.A. Poirier, M. Manfait, J.-C. Étienne

The second volume of this series was published in May 1992
Eds. J. Anatassopoulou, Ph. Collery, J.-C. Étienne, T. Theophanides

The third volume of this series was published in May 1994
Eds. Ph. Collery, L.A. Poirier, N.A. Littlefield, J.-C. Étienne

The fourth volume of this series was published in May 1996
Eds. Ph. Collery, J. Corbella, J.L. Domingo, J.-C. Étienne, J.M. Llobet

The fifth volume of this series was published in May 1998
Eds. Ph. Collery, P. Brätter, V. Negretti de Brätter, L. Khassanova, J.-C. Étienne

The sixth volume of this series was published in May 2000
Eds. J.A. Centeno, Ph. Collery, G. Vernet, R.B. Finkelman, H. Gibb, J.-C. Étienne

The seventh volume of this series was published in May 2002
Eds. L.A. Khassanova, Ph. Collery, I. Maymard, Z. Khassanova, J.-C. Étienne

The eighth volume of this serjes was published in May 2004
Eds. A. Cser, I. Lászlo, J.-C. Étienne, Y. Maymard, J.A. Centeno, L. Khassanova, Ph. Collery

Editor-in-Chief
Philippe Collery
Service de Cancérologie
Polyclinique Maymard
20200 Bastia, France
Philippe.Collery20220@wanadoo.fr

Éditions John Libbey Eurotext
127, avenue de la République, 92120 Montrouge, France
Tél. : (1) 46.73.06.60 – Fax : (1) 40.84.09.99
e-mail : contact@jle.com
Website : http://www.jle.com

© Avril 2006, Paris

ISBN 2-7420-0629-X

Il est interdit de reproduire intégralement ou partiellement le présent ouvrage sans autorisation de l'éditeur ou du Centre Français d'Exploitation du Droit de copie (CFC), 20, rue des Grands-Augustins, 75006 Paris.

List and addresses of Editors

Armando Jorge Cristóvão, Center for Neuroscience and Cell Biology, Dept of Zoology, University of Coimbra, 3004-517 Coimbra, Portugal

Paula Vasconcellos Morais: Instituto Ambiente e Vida, 3004-517 Coimbra, Portugal.

Maria Amélia Santos: Centro de Quimica Estrutural, Instituto Superior Tecnico, Av. Rovisca Pais, 1049-001, Lisboa, Portugal

Maria Carmen Alpoim, Departamento de Bioquimica, Universidade de Coimbra, Apartado 3126, 3001-401, Coimbra, Portugal.

José A. Centeno, U.S Armed forces, Insitute of Pathology, Washington DC 20306 6000, United-States

Philippe Collery, Polyclinique Maymard, Service de Cancérologie Médicale, 20200 Bastia, France

Chair Person

Maria Carmen Alpoim

Co chairpersons

Paula Vasconcellos Morais
Maria Amelia Santos
Armando J. Cristóvão
José A. Centeno

Organizing Committee

M. C. Alpoim (Portugal)
P. V. Morais (Portugal)
M. A. Santos (Portugal)
A. J. Cristóvão (Portugal)
J. A. Centeno (USA)

National Scientific Committee:

L. Almeida (FFUC)
M. Castro (FCTUC)
M. Costa (FCTUC)
J. Fraústo da Silva (IST, UTL)
C. Geraldes (FCTUC)
M.L. Gonçalves (IST, UTL)
M. J. Laires (FMH, UTL)
J. Matos Dias (FCTUC)
J. Moura (FCT, UNL)
C. Oliveira (FMUC)
R. Ribeiro (FCTUC)
E. Silva (UA)
A. Soares (UA)
J. P. Sousa (FCTUC)
A. Xavier (IQTB, UNL)

International Scientific Committee:

J. Anastassopoulou (Greece)
A. Balla (USA)
S. Caroli (Italy)
G.F. Combs (USA)
J. Corbella (Spain)
M. Costa (USA)
R.B. Finkelman (USA)
S. de Flora (Italy)
B. Fowler (USA)
M. Hofmann (Switzerland)
R. G. Kuperman (USA)
N.A. Littlefield (USA)
B. Michalke (Germany)
A.K. Mohamed (USA)
F. G. Mullick (USA)
J.B. Nielsen (Dennmark)
G. Nowak (Poland)
A.R. Oller (USA)
S. Patierno (USA)
T. Rossman (USA)
A.M. Roussell (France)
E. Sabbioni (Italy)
O. Selenius (Sweden)
D. Slaney (New Zealand)
S. J. Sørensen (Denmark)
C. Supuran (Italy)
P. Tchounwou (USA)
C.-H. Tseng (Taiwan, PRC)
G. Vivoli (Italy)
P. Weinstein (Australia)
G. Zaray (Hungary)
P. Zatta (Italy)

CONTENTS/SOMMAIRE

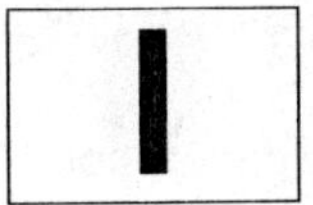

METAL-BASED DRUGS

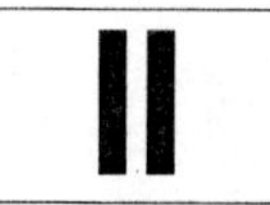

ANALYTICAL METHODS

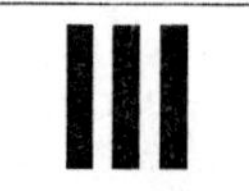

MOLECULAR STUDIES

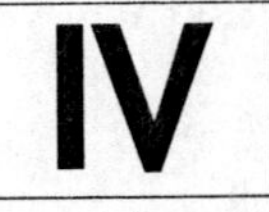

SOILS AND PLANTS

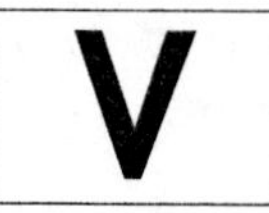

MICROORGANISMS

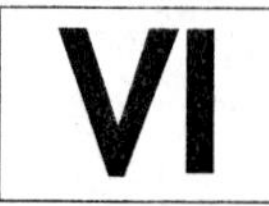

CELL STUDIES

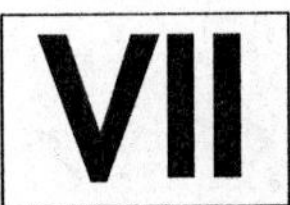

VII *EXPERIMENTAL STUDIES*

Anatomopathological studies

Distribution

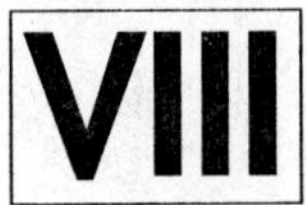

ECOLOGICAL STUDIES

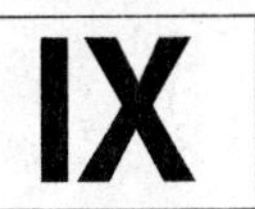

NUTRITION

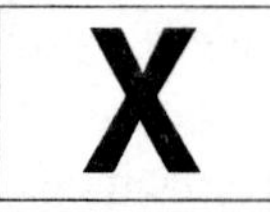

REVIEWS

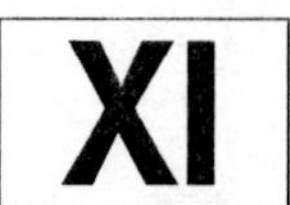

HUMAN STUDIES

I METAL-BASED DRUGS

Metal Ions in Biology and Medicine: vol. 9. Eds Maria Carmen Alpoim, Paula Vasconcellos Morais, Maria Amélia Santos, Armando J. Cristóvão, José A. Centeno, Philippe Collery.
John Libbey Eurotext, Paris © 2006 pp. 3-1.

Metal-Based Drugs for Diagnosis and Therapy

Susana Alves, Rute Vitor, Paula D. Raposinho, Fernanda Marques, João D. G. Correia, António Paulo, Isabel Santos

Departamento de Química, Instituto Tecnológico e Nuclear, Estrada Nacional 10, 2686-953 Sacavém, Portugal

The compound 3,5Me-pz$(CH_2)_2$NH$(CH_2)_2$$NH_2$ (**L^1**) is a very effective chelator for the *fac*-$[M(CO)_3(H_2O)_3]^+$ (M = Re (**1**) ^{99m}Tc (**1a**)) moieties, yielding the building blocks *fac*-$[M(CO)_3(k^3\text{-}\mathbf{L^1})]^+$ (M = Re (**2**) ^{99m}Tc (**2a**)). The evaluation of the *in vitro* and *in vivo* behaviour of **2a** has shown that this stable building block displays a favourable biological profile for labelling biomolecules with ^{99m}Tc, namely biologically active peptides. Due to its versatility, **L^1** was integrated through its secondary amine into a peptide with affinity for MC1 receptors (**L^2**), and derivatized with an anthracenyl group at the C(4) position of the pyrazolyl ring (**L^3**). The resulting bifunctional chelators react with **1a** yielding the well defined *fac*-$[^{99m}Tc(CO)_3(k^3\text{-}\mathbf{L})]^+$ (L = **L^2** (**3a**), **L^3** (**4a**)) complexes with excellent stability *in vitro* and *in vivo*. Complex **3a** presents a significant internalization in B16F1 melanoma cells, showing *in vivo* a significant overall excretion and a reasonable tumour uptake, with a fast clearance from most organs and tissues. For complex **4a**, *in vitro* studies using B16F1 melanoma cells showed significant nuclear internalization and an enhanced radiotoxicity for this compound, most probably due to the presence of the anthracenyl group which is a well known DNA intercalator. The results obtained for complexes **3a** and **4a** indicate that this family of compounds is potentially useful to develop novel *specific* ^{99m}Tc radiopharmaceuticals directed for both detection and therapy of melanoma.

INTRODUCTION

Many metal ions and/or metal complexes are essential nutrients for life, but many others became increasingly important as diagnostic or therapeutic agents to study or treat a wide variety of diseases and metabolic disorders. Rapid growth stems from the great success achieved, namely in the development of contrast agents for magnetic resonance imaging and in radiopharmaceuticals for nuclear medicine diagnosis and therapy [1-4].

In the radiopharmaceutical field most of the research work focused on compounds with high sensitivity for diagnosis and selectivity for targeted therapy [2-4].

Among the *d*-transition metals, ^{99m}Tc is the most important radionuclide for diagnosis in nuclear medicine. The main reasons for this importance are its decay characteristics (6-hour half-life, 140 keV gamma photons with 89% abundance), availability from ^{99}Mo/^{99m}Tc generators, the cost and also the widespread availability of single-photon-emission tomography (SPECT) facilities, in comparison with positron emission tomography (PET) [5-8]. Based on this radiometal, significant efforts are being made to develop radiopharmaceuticals for a specific biological target. This means, for example, to target receptors expressed on tumour cells of a given type of cancer (i.e. breast and prostate cancers, melanoma, etc.) which are selective for specific peptides [8-10]. To achieve this goal, one possibility is to use the so called *bifunctional approach*, which means to put together a *bioactive peptide* and a ^{99m}Tc complex through a linker *scheme 1(a)*. In terms of therapy, most type of tumours are treated using conventional methodologies, such as surgery, external radiotherapy and chemotherapy. However, these methods have limited success in the eradication of disseminated small tumours and metastasis. This motivate the finding of new and more effective therapeutic strategies, such as targeted anti-tumour therapy with radiometals [11, 12]. Until now, most of the efforts have been made with beta emitters, which are particularly adequate for targeting large tumour clusters, due to the longer range of the energetic beta particle. However, beta emitters can lead to more or less severe side effects, like bone-marrow suppression. Auger-emitters are expected to minimise such side effects, since their low-energy Auger electrons have short path length and deposit their energy within the cells which accumulate the radiopharmaceutical, allowing a more selective and targeted anti-tumour therapy [13]. In this context, ^{99m}Tc may be relevant for therapeutic applications, since this radiometal is also an Auger electron-emitter. DNA damage caused by Auger electron-emitting radiopharmaceuticals is dependent on the proximity of the radionuclide to the DNA [13]. This proximity can be promoted using the so called *bifunctional multicomponent* approach, which means to put together a *bioactive peptide*, a DNA intercalator and a ^{99m}Tc complex, through suitable linkages. This approach is schematically shown in *scheme 1(b).*

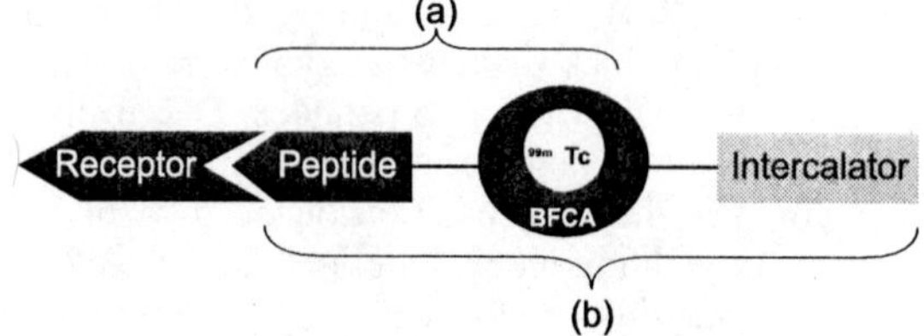

Scheme 1. Schematic drawing of a *bioactive complex* (a) and of a *multicomponent bioactive complex* (b)

Part of our ongoing projects involve design, characterization and *in vitro* and *in vivo* evaluation of *bioactive and multicomponent bioactive* ^{99m}Tc complexes. To achieve this goal we have been using pyrazolyl-containing ligands as bifunctional chelators and small bioactive peptides with recognized affinity for receptors overexpressed in tumour cells, namely prostate cancer and melanoma. To promote DNA intercalation we have used anthracenyl groups and anthrapyrazole derivatives. A summary of some of our results on this field will be discussed herein.

MATERIALS AND METHODS

The tridentate pyrazolyl ligands $\mathbf{L^1}$, $\mathbf{L^2}$, $\mathbf{L^3}$ and the starting material $(NEt_4)_2[Re(CO)_3Br_3]$ were synthesized as previously described [14-18]. ^{99m}Tc, in the form of $Na^{99m}TcO_4^-$, was eluted from a ^{99}Mo/^{99m}Tc generator, using 0.9% saline and the radioactive precursor *fac*-$[^{99m}Tc(OH_2)_3(CO)_3]^+$ (**1**) was prepared using a IsoLink® kit (Malinckrodt, Inc.). Solid phase peptide synthetic (SPPS) techniques, employing standard fmoc chemistry, were used to make all Pyrazolyl-α-MSH derivatives by methods previously described [16]. HPLC analysis of the Re and ^{99m}Tc complexes was performed on a Perkin-Elmer LC pump 200 coupled to a LC 290 tunable UV/Vis detector and to a Berthold LB-507A radiometric detector. Separations were achieved on a Nucleosil column (10μm, 250mm × 4mm), using a flow rate of 1mL/min; UV detection, 254 nm; eluents, A - aqueous 0.1% CF_3COOH solution, B-methanol; method, t = 0-3 min, 0% B; 3-3.1 min, 0-25% B; 3.1-9 min, 25% B; 9-9.1 min, 25-34% B; 9.1-20 min, 34-100% B; 20-22 min, 100% B; 22-22.1 min, 100-0% B; 22.1-30 min, 0% B.

Internalization assays were performed on B16F1 murine melanoma cells seeded at a density of 0.2 million/well in a 24-well tissue culture plates and allowed to attach overnight. The cells were incubated at 37°C for a period of 5 min to 4h with the HPLC purified radiolabelled compounds. The cellular internalized complexes were evaluated in the lysed cells (NaOH 1M, 10 min at 37°C) after washing the cells with acid buffer, to remove the membrane bound complex. The radiocomplexes internalized in the nucleus were determined in the nucleus fraction recovered by centrifugation (1300 g at 4°C, 1 min) from the lysed cells (Nonidet-P40, 15 min at 4°C). The *in vivo* studies were performed in normal or in melanoma-bearing C57BL/6 female mice, by intravenous injection of the radiolabelled complexes. The radioactivity uptake in the tumor and normal tissues of interest was expressed as a percentage of the injected radioactivity dose per gram of tissue (% ID/g).

RESULTS AND DISCUSSION

The pyrazolyl containing ligand L^1 has been synthesized, characterized, and its coordination capability towards the *fac*-$[M(CO)_3(H_2O)_3]^+$ (M = Re (**1**), ^{99m}Tc(**1a**)) precursors evaluated. L^1 reacts with **1** and **1a** yielding the complexes *fac*-$[M(CO)_3(k^3\text{-}L^1)]^+$ (M = Re (**2**), ^{99m}Tc (**2a**). The Re complex (**2**) has been characterized by the normal techniques in inorganic chemistry, namely X-ray diffraction analysis, ^{13}C and ^{1}H NMR spectroscopy and HPLC. The ^{99m}Tc complex (**2a**) was obtained in high radiochemical yield and with high radiochemical purity (> 95%) and its characterization was performed by HPLC comparison with the corresponding Re surogate (**2**) (*fig. 1*).

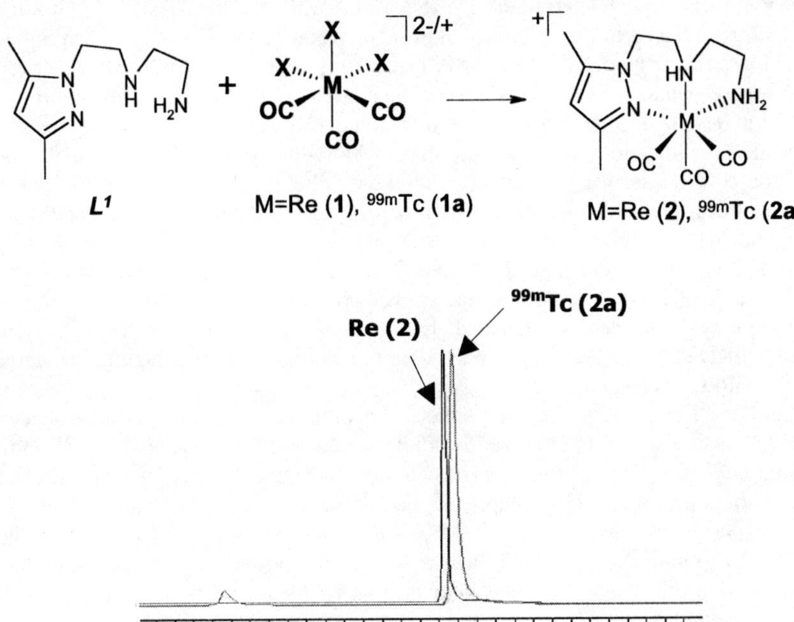

Fig. 1. Synthesis of complexes **2** and **2a** and characterization by HPLC

Complex **2a** is stable in the presence of histidine and cysteine (two biologically occurring chelating agents with recognized affinity for Tc(I)) (*fig. 2*), is hydrophilic (logP = - 0.24 ± 0.03), presents a fast clearance from blood and a fast overall excretion. Metabolic studies have also shown that **2a** is stable *in vivo*.

The high stability, biological profile and lipophilicity found for **2a** have shown that L^1 is an adequate ligand for the conjugation of a biologically active peptide and/or for the linkage of a DNA intercalator, being therefore a good candidate to pursue our studies.

Melanoma is one of the most aggressive tumours and has become a serious health problem with an increasing incidence and mortality rate. Moreover, metastatic melanoma deposits are difficult to detect and are resistant to conventional chemotherapy and external beam radiation therapy. So, there is a great need to develop new methodologies for early detection and therapy of melanoma

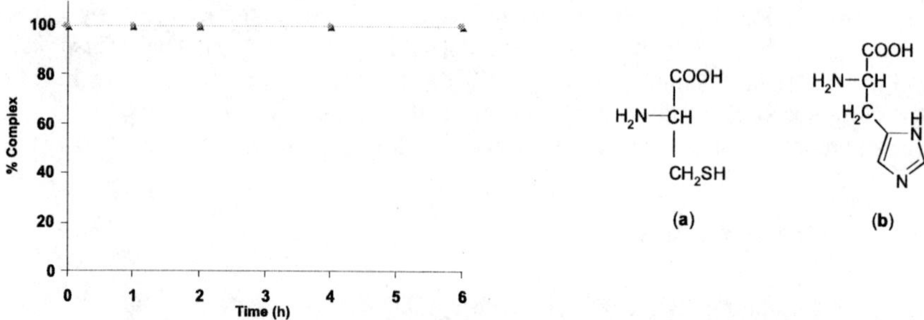

Fig. 2. Stability of **2a** in the presence of excess (1:100) of cysteine (a) and histidine (b)

and this justifies the interest on specific radiopharmaceuticals. Radiolabelled antibodies and antibody fragments have been investigated to target melanoma, but the success has been limited due to the slow clearance of antibodies and reduced tumor uptake [19]. One class of promising agents for melanoma imaging and therapy are peptides analogues of the endogenous α-melanocyte stimulating hormone (α-MSH). α-MSH is a tridecapeptide (Ac-Ser^1-Tyr^2-Ser^3-Met^4-Glu^5-His^6-Phe^7-Arg^8-Trp^9-Gly^{10}-Lys^{11}-Pro^{12}-Val^{13}-NH_2) which is involved in the control of skin pigmentation and its biological activity is mediated through interactions with melanocortin type 1 (MC1) receptors, being these MC1 receptors overexpressed in human and mouse melanoma cells [19]. Hence, analogues of α-MSH are promising biological targeting vectors for design and development of melanoma receptor specific imaging and therapeutic radiopharmaceuticals. Structure activity relationship (SAR) studies have shown that the biologically active part of the α-MSH are the four amino acids **His^6- Phe^7-Arg^8-Trp^9**. To pursue our studies we selected, among others, the analogues Ac-Nle-Asp-α-MSH_{6-11}-NH_2 and we have extended this peptide sequence with the pyrazolyl chelator **L^1**. This extension was made at the C-terminus of the peptide through an amide bond. The new conjugate Ac-Nle-Asp-α-MSH_{6-11}-NHCO-**L^1** (**L^2**) was synthesized by solid phase peptide synthesis, cleaved from the resin, and purified by RP-HPLC techniques. **L^2** was characterized by mass spectrometry (Calculated: 1348.8; Experimental: 1349.7 $[M-H]^+$). By reacting **L^2** with **1a**, the radiometallated peptide **3a** has been obtained in high yield and high radiochemical purity, as confirmed by HPLC analysis *(fig. 3).*

Complex **3a** has a high *in vitro* stability, either in fresh human serum or in the presence of a large excess of histidine and cysteine. Internalization studies of **3a** on B16F1 melanoma cells indicated that 60% of the total cell - associate activity (surface + internal bound activity) is taken and internalized by the cells at 4 hours post incubation. Externalization of **3a** from B16F1 melanoma cells is relatively slow, as efflux experiments have shown that 70% of the internalized activity remains inside the cells after 2 hours. In vivo pharmacokinetics of **3a** was studied in normal and in tumour-bearing mice. At 4 hours post injection, the results obtained indicate that 64-69% of the injected dose was excreted through the kidneys, and a significant amount was taken by the tumour (4.24±0.94 %ID/g of tissue). The retention of activity in stomach (1.06±0.96 %ID/g of tissue) was rather low, indicating a high stability of the radiometallated peptide towards *in vivo* oxidation. The kidney uptake was relatively low (4.5±2.4 %ID/g of tissue), a crucial issue if a compound is supposed to be used for therapy.

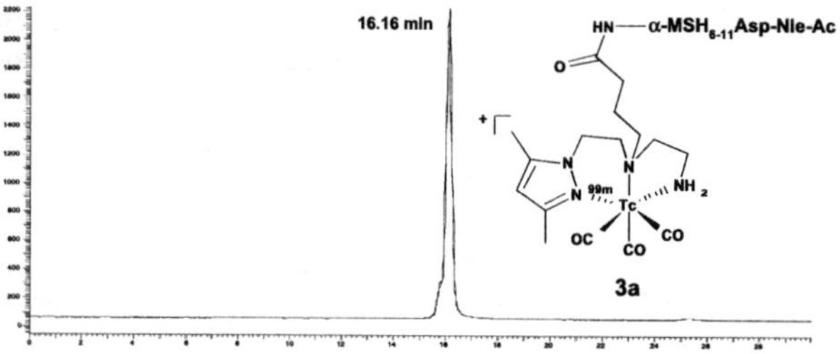

Fig. 3. HPLC chromatogram of the complex **3a**

Aiming to prove the radiotoxic potential of DNA targeting ^{99m}Tc complexes at the cellular level, we have prepared the novel pyrazolyl-containing ligand **L^3**, bearing an anthracenyl group in the C(4) of the azole, and we have evaluated its coordination capability towards the precursors **1** and **1a**. This study has shown that the introduction of the polycyclic moiety did not compromise the coordination capability of the ligand, being formed the complexes *fac*-[M(CO)$_3$(k^3-**L^3**)]$^+$ (M = Re (**4**), ^{99m}Tc (**4a**)) *(fig. 4)*.

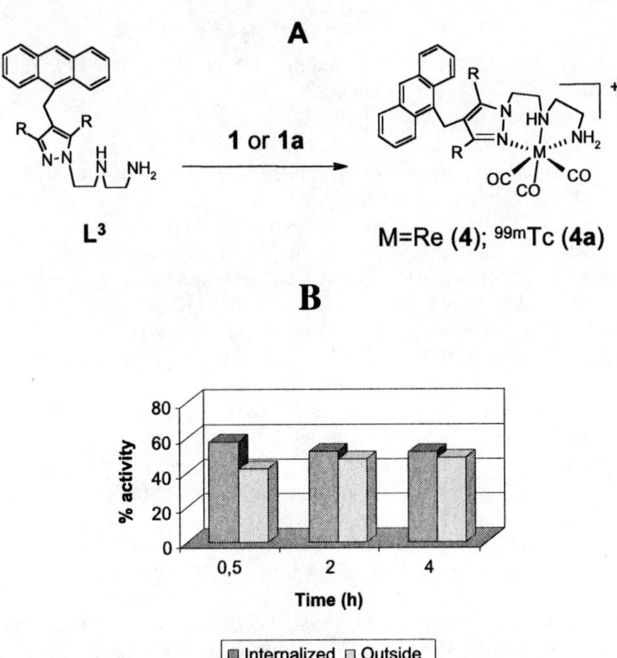

Fig. 4. Synthesis of complexes **4** and **4a** (**A**); Nuclear Internalization of **4a** in B16F1 cells (**B**)

The stability *in vitro* of **4a** was high and encouraged to pursue with the evaluation of the radiotoxicity and nuclear internalization for this complex. Complex **4a** has an enhanced capacity to kill B16F1 melanoma cells, when compared with the respective building block **2a** or with [^{99m}TcO$_4$]$^-$. This certainly reflects the fast and significant nuclear internalization found for **4a** (60% of the total cell-associate activity is taken by the nucleus, 30 minutes after incubation). Apparently, the presence of the intercalating moiety increased the internalization in the nucleus, as well as the cellular death.

CONCLUDING REMARKS

We have shown that **L^1** is an effective chelator for the stabilization of the *fac*-[M(CO)$_3$]$^+$ moieties (M = Re, ^{99m}Tc). Compound **L^1** is very versatile and can be easily linked to a biologically active peptide with affinity for MC1 receptors or to a DNA intercalator leading to **L^2** and **L^3**, respectively. With these two bifunctional ligands, the complexes *fac*-[^{99m}Tc(CO)$_3$(k^3-L)]$^+$ (**L** = **L^2** (**3a**), **L^3** (**4a**)) have been isolated and fully characterized. *In vitro* studies of these complexes have shown a high stability in serum and in the presence of cysteine and histidine. Complex **3a** presents a significant internalization in B16F1 melanoma cells, a favourable pharmacokinetics and a reasonable tumour uptake. Compound **4a** shows a high nuclear internalization and an enhanced radiotoxicity, if compared with the parent building block **2a**, suggesting that the presence of a DNA intercalator can improve the therapeutic potential of ^{99m}Tc as an Auger electron emitter. In order to go further towards a *multicomponent bioactive complex*, the coupling of $\mathbf{L}^3$ to a tumour-seeking peptide, such as the one used to prepare $\mathbf{L}^2$, is currently under study.

REFERENCES

1. P. Caravan, J. J. Ellison, T. J. McMurry, R. B. Laufer, *Chem. Rev.*, 1999, 99: 2293-2352.
2. S. Jurisson, J. D. Lydon, *Chem. Rev.*, 1999, 99: 2205-2218.
3. C. J. Anderson, M. J. Welch, *Chem. Rev.*, 1999, 99: 2219-2234.
4. S. Liu, D. S. Edwards, *Chem. Rev.*, 1999, 99: 2235-2268.
5. R. Alberto, In: *Contrast Agents III, Radiopharmaceuticals-From Diagnostic to Therapeutics*, W. Krause, ed., Springer-Verlag Berlin Heidelberg, 2005, 252: 1-44.
6. I. Santos, A. Paulo, J. D. G. Correia, In: *Contrast Agents III, Radiopharmaceuticals-From Diagnostic to Therapeutics*, W. Krause, ed., Springer-Verlag Berlin Heidelberg, 2005, 252: 45-84.
7. A. Boschi, A. Duatti, L. Ucceli, In: *Contrast Agents III, Radiopharmaceuticals-From Diagnostic to Therapeutics*, W. Krause, ed., Springer-Verlag Berlin Heidelberg, 2005, 252: 85-115.
8. S. Liu, In: *Contrast Agents III, Radiopharmaceuticals-From Diagnostic to Therapeutics*, W. Krause, ed., Springer-Verlag Berlin Heidelberg, 2005, 252: 117-153.
9. S. Liu, D. S. Edwards, *Bioconjugate Chem.*, 2001, 12: 7-34.
10. J. Fichna, A. Janeka, *Bioconjugate Chem.* 2003, 14: 1-14.
11. W. A. Volkert, T. J. Hoffman, *Chem. Rev.* 1999, 99: 2269-2292.
12. F. Rösch, E.Forsell-Aronsson, In: *Metal Ions in Biological Systems*, vol. 42: Metal Complexes in Tumour Diagnosis and as Anticancer Agents (A. Siegel and H. Siegel, eds) Marcel Decker, Inc., New York 2004, p. 77-108.
13. C. A. Boswell, M. W. Brechbiel, *J. Nucl. Med.*, 2005, 46: 1946-1947.
14. S. Alves, A. Paulo, J. D. G. Correia, Â. Domingos, I. Santos, *J. Chem. Soc., Dalton Transactions* 2002, 24: 4714-4719.
15. R. Vitor, S. Alves, J. D. G. Correia, A. Paulo, I. Santos, *J. Organomet. Chem.*, 2004, 25: 4764-4774.
16. S. Alves, A. Paulo, J. D. G. Correia, L. Gano, C. J. Smith, T. J. Hoffman, I. Santos, *Bioconjugate Chem.*, 2005, 16: 438-449.
17. R. Vitor, A. Paulo, I. Santos, I. Correia, J. C. Pessoa, *Fourth Annual Meeting of the Society for Molecular Imaging*, September 2005, Heidelberg, Germany.
18. R. Alberto, R. Schibl, A. Egli, A. P. Schubiger, U. Abram, T. A. Kaden, *J. Am. Chem. Soc.*, 1998, 120: 7987-7988.
19. S. Froidevaux, M. C-Christe, H. Tanner, A. N. Eberbe, *J. Nucl. Med.*, 2005, 46: 887-895.

ACKNOWLEDGMENTS

We thank Foundation for Science and Technology (FCT) (POCI/QUI/57632/2004) and Tyco-Mallinckrodt Med. Inc., Petten (The Netherlands) for finantial support. S. Alves and R. Vitor thanks FCT for PhD grants.

Metal Ions in Biology and Medicine: vol. 9. Eds Maria Carmen Alpoim, Paula Vasconcellos Morais, Maria Amélia Santos, Armando J. Cristóvão, José A. Centeno, Philippe Collery.
John Libbey Eurotext, Paris © 2006 pp. 9-1.

Synthesis and In Vitro Antitumor Activity of 2,3-Diaminoglucose-Based Platinum(II) Coordination Compounds

Berger Isabella, Nazarov Alexey A., Hartinger Christian G., Valiahdi Seied-M., Jakupec Michael A., Galanski Markus, Keppler Bernhard K.

Institute of Inorganic Chemistry, University of Vienna, Waehringer Str. 42, A-1090 Vienna, Austria

INTRODUCTION

Platinum complexes belong to the most widely used anticancer drugs in clinical practice. The first representative was cisplatin *(fig. 1)* which was developed by Rosenberg and co-workers in the 1960s [1]. It was included into the WHO list comprising the 17 essential anticancer drugs [2] necessary to treat the 10 most common cancers or category 1 or 2 cancers [3]. The development of new platinum-based drugs resulted in the approval of carboplatin [4] and oxaliplatin [5, 6], which are also in clinical use today *(fig. 1)*. Furthermore, nedaplatin, lobaplatin and heptaplatin have obtained regionally limited approval and several new platinum complexes are under clinical trials [7].

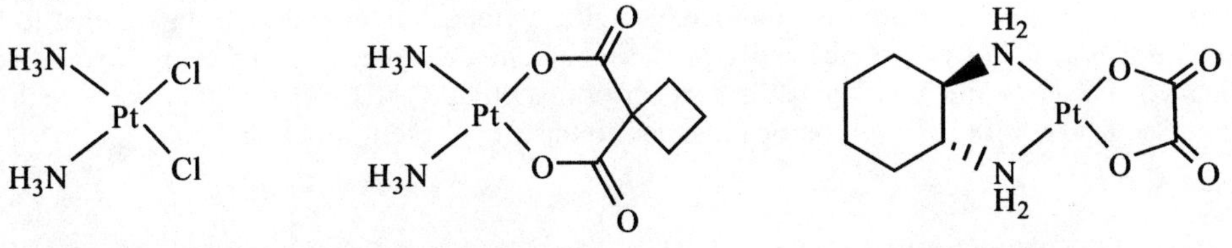

Fig. 1. Platinum complexes in worldwide clinical use: cisplatin (left), carboplatin (middle) and oxaliplatin (right)

Due to the inactivity of anticancer drugs against many tumor types, serious toxic side effects and acquired or intrinsic resistance phenomena, there is considerable interest in the development of new platinum-based drugs eliminating these disadvantages.

Oxaliplatin or (*SP*-4-2)-[(*1R,2R*)-cyclohexane-1,2-diamine-κ^2*N,N'*)(oxalato-κ^2*O,O'*)platinum(II) consists of the chelating oxalate ligand and the bulky cyclohexane-1,2-diamine (chxn) moiety. Schmidt *et al.* found for oxaliplatin a more efficient incorporation of intracellular platinum into DNA as compared to cisplatin. The cyclohexane-1,2-diamine ligand makes platinum-DNA adducts in average more cytotoxic [8] being in line with a stronger hindrance of replication [9, 10]. While cisplatin-induced DNA adducts are detected by mismatch repair proteins, those induced by oxaliplatin are not recognized [11-13].

The naturally occurring, inexpensive and enantiomerically pure carbohydrates with their well-known chemistry are structurally similar to the cyclohexane-1,2-diamine moiety of oxaliplatin. Sugars are of major importance to provide energy for cells. The increase of glycolytic activity in cancer cells is one of the fundamental metabolic alterations in malign tissues [14, 15]. In order to generate ATP, glucose is converted to lactate even in the presence of oxygen. The transport of glucose through the membrane occurs *via* transport proteins utilizing the diffusional gradient or by pumping glucose into cells against its concentration gradient [16]. In most primary and metastatic human cancers increased glucose uptake is accompanied by an upregulation of glucose transporters [17]. Exploiting the peculiar physiological properties of carbohydrates [18] might lead to enhanced assimilation of platinum complexes bearing carbohydrate ligands into the tumor cells.

Several platinum complexes of diamino-dideoxy sugars with anticancer activity were reported in literature [19-22]. In the present study, the carbohydrate 2,3-diamino-2,3-dideoxy-D-glucopyranose was chosen as ligand, in order to resemble the oxaliplatin-structure, and the respective platinum complexes with iodide **1**, oxalate **2** and malonate **3** as leaving groups were synthesized and characterized by NMR, MS, and elemental analysis. For comparison purposes (*SP*-4-3)-[(2,3-diamino-2,3-dideoxy-D-glucose-$\kappa^2 N,N'$)dichloroplatinum(II)] **4** was synthesized following the literature procedure [21, 22]. The four complexes were evaluated for their in vitro cytotoxicity by a colorimetric microculture assay (MTT assay) in the human cancer cell lines HeLa (cervix carcinoma), CH1 (ovarian carcinoma), SW480 (colon carcinoma), and U2-OS (osteosarcoma).

RESULTS AND DISCUSSION

2,3-Diamino-2,3-dideoxy-D-glucose dihydrochloride was obtained by a modified method of Meyer zu Reckendorf [23]. The commercially available 2-amino-2-deoxy-D-glucose hydrochloride was transformed by reaction with acetic anhydride to 2-acetamino-2-deoxy-D-glucose. Using a higher amount of benzyl alcohol for the preparation of benzyl-2-acetamido-2-deoxy-α-D-glucopyranoside increased the yield significantly (> 20%). Ultrasonification of the reaction mixture containing benzyl-2-acetamido-2-deoxy-α-D-glucopyranoside and $ZnCl_2$ in benzylaldehyde was utilized to obtain benzyl-2-acetamino-4,6-*O*-benzylidene-2-deoxy-α-D-glucopyranoside [24]. The latter compound was mesylated in pyridine, transformed into the corresponding allo-derivate and again mesylated. Displacement of the mesylgroup by azide, reduction to the diamine and cleavage of all protection groups resulted in the desired 2,3-diamino-2,3-dideoxy-D-glucopyranose hydrochloride. In contrast to literature reports, the stability of the benzyl group at the anomeric center was high in refluxing hydrochloric acid. Therefore, the hydrogenation was performed on Pd/C (10% Pd) at 5 bar in concentrated hydrochloric acid for 18 h. The modifications led to an overall yield of about 12%.

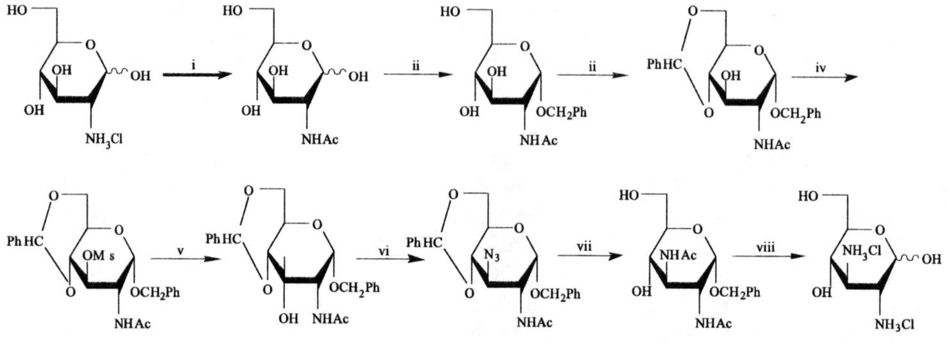

Fig. 1. The synthetic route to 2,3-diamino-2,3-dideoxy-D-glucopyranose dihydrochloride; (i) NaOMe, Ac_2O, rt, 18 h; (ii) $PhCH_2OH$, HCl, reflux, 30 min; (iii) PhCHO, $ZnCl_2$, 60 °C, 30 min, ultrasonification; (iv) MsCl, Py, 0 °C, 17 h; (v) CH_3CO_2Na, $CH_3OCH_2CH_2OH$, reflux, 48 h; (vi) MsCl, Py, 0 °C, 18 h; NaN_3, DMSO, 150 °C, 1 h; (vii) AcOH, 90 °C, 2 h; Pd/C, H_2, MeOH, rt, 4 h; Ac_2O, MeOH, rt, 3 h; (viii) Pd/C, H_2, HCl, rt, 18 h; HCl, 90 °C, 1 h.

In order to synthesize the coordination compounds with the diamine-ligand, $K_2[PtI_4]$ was formed *in situ* by mixing $K_2[PtCl_4]$ and potassium iodide. Though coordination experiments with $K_2[PtCl_4]$ were performed, following the method of Appleton and Hall [25] and yielding complex **4** at moderate yield (30%), tetraiodoplatinate(II) was chosen as starting material since the very good solubility of the dichloro-complex hampers the isolation of the product. The addition of an excess of 2,3-diamino-2,3-dideoxy-D-glucopyranose dihydrochloride in KOH solution to $K_2[PtI_4]$ led to complex **1**, which precipitated at 4 °C over night.

For syntheses of the other coordination compounds, **1** was activated by $AgNO_3$. The precipitated AgI was removed by centrifugation and the activated complex was reacted with sodium oxalate. After stirring for 12 h at room temperature (*SP*-4-3)-(2,3-diamino-2,3-dideoxy-D-glucose-(e*N,N'*)(oxalato-κ^2*O,O'*)platinum(II) **2** was precipitated by the addition of acetone. The analogous malonato complex **3** was synthesized in a similar way.

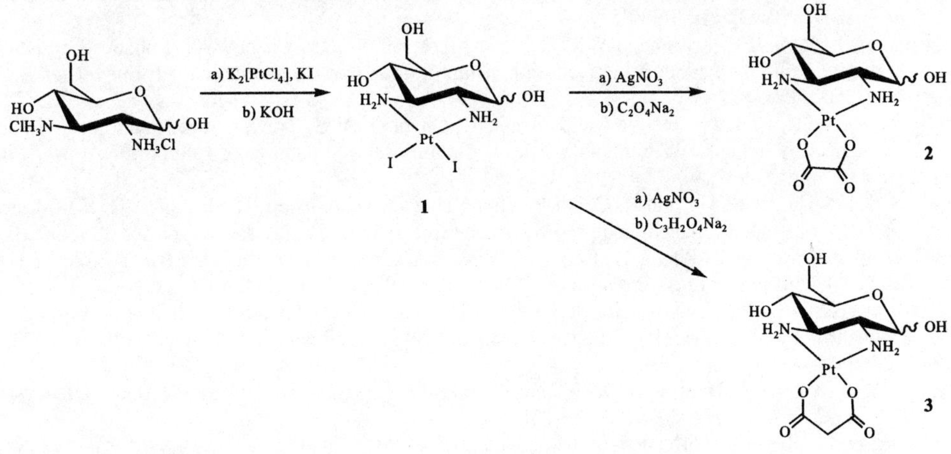

Fig. 2. Synthesis of platinum(II) carbohydrate complexes (*SP*-4-3)-diiodo(2,3-diamino-2,3-dideoxy-D-glucose-κ*N,N'*)platinum(II) **1**, (*SP*-4-3)-(2,3-diamino-2,3-dideoxy-D-glucose-κ^2*N,N'*)(oxalato-κ^2*O,O'*)platinum(II) **2**, and (*SP*-4-3)-(2,3-diamino-2,3-dideoxy-D-glucose-κ^2*N,N'*)(malonato-κ^2*O,O'*)platinum(II) **3**.

NMR spectra were obtained in D_2O and two sets of signals, assignable to the α- and β-anomers of the complexes, were found. The vicinal proton-proton coupling constants were within 9.5 and 12.5 Hz, which indicates that the corresponding protons of the pyranose ring are in *trans*-position to each other, the protons H2, H3, H4 and H5 were found to be in axial orientation. This clearly shows that the carbohydrate ligand is present in $^4C_1$ conformation.

The positive ion ESI mass spectra of compounds **1-4** showed the expected pseudo molecular ion peaks $[M+Na]^+$ at *m/z* 650, 484, 498, and 467, respectively. The observed isotopic patterns in the mass spectra were in good agreement with the calculated isotopic distribution.

Cytotoxicity of the platinum(II) complexes is strongly dependent on the cell line. For all compounds, sensitivity decreases in the following rank order: CH1 (ovary) > HeLa (cervix) > SW480 (colon) > U2-OS (osteosarcoma). Antiproliferative effects are moderate to pronounced, with IC_{50} values generally being in the micromolar range. Differences between the cytotoxic potencies of **1-4** are comparatively small, with compound **4** being the most potent in three of the four cell lines. Further structure-activity relationships cannot be generalized.

REFERENCES

1. Rosenberg B, VanCamp L, Trosko JE, Mansour VH. Platinum compounds: a new class of potent antitumour agents. *Nature* 1969; 222: 385-386.
2. Sikora K, Advani S, Koroltchouk V, Magrath I, Levy L, Pinedo H, Schwartsmann G, Tattersall M, Yan S. Essential drugs for cancer therapy: a World Health Organization consultation. *Ann Oncol* 1999; 10: 385-390.
3. WHO, National Cancer Control Programmes: Policies and Managerial Guidelines, 2002, pp. 203.

4. Wong E, Giandomenico CM. Current Status of Platinum-Based Antitumor Drugs. *Chem Rev* 1999; 99: 2451-2466.
5. Galanski M, Arion VB, Jakupec MA, Keppler BK. Recent developments in the field of tumor-inhibiting metal complexes. *Curr Pharm Des* 2003; 9: 2078-2089.
6. Jakupec MA, Galanski M, Keppler BK. Tumour-inhibiting platinum complexes-state of the art and future perspectives. *Rev Physiol Biochem Pharmacol* 2003; 146: 1-53.
7. Galanski M, Jakupec MA, Keppler BK. Update of the preclinical situation of anticancer platinum complexes: Novel design strategies and innovative analytical approaches. *Curr Med Chem* 2005; 12: 2075-2094.
8. Schmidt W, Chaney SG. Role of carrier ligand in platinum resistance of human carcinoma cell lines. *Cancer Research* 1993; 53: 799-805.
9. Mamenta EL, Poma EE, Kaufmann WK, Delmastro DA, Grady HL, Chaney SG. Enhanced replicative bypass of platinum-DNA adducts in cisplatin-resistant human ovarian carcinoma cell lines. *Cancer Res* 1994; 54: 3500-3505.
10. Woynarowski JM, Faivre S, Herzig MCS, Arnett B, Chapman WG, Trevino AV, Raymond E, Chaney SG, Vaisman A, Varchenko M, Juniewicz PE. Oxaliplatin-induced damage of cellular DNA. *Mol Pharmacol* 2000; 58: 920-927.
11. Aebi S, Kurdi-Haidar B, Gordon R, Cenni B, Zheng H, Fink D, Christen RD, Boland CR, Koi M, et al. Loss of DNA mismatch repair in acquired resistance to cisplatin. *Cancer Res* 1996; 56: 3087-3090.
12. Fink D, Nebel S, Aebi S, Zheng H, Cenni B, Nehme A, Christen RD, Howell SB. The role of DNA mismatch repair in platinum drug resistance. *Cancer Res* 1996; 56: 4881-4886.
13. Nehme A, Baskaran R, Nebel S, Fink D, Howell SB, Wang JYJ, Christen RD. Induction of JNK and c-Abl signalling by cisplatin and oxaliplatin in mismatch repair-proficient and -deficient cells. *Br J Cancer* 1999; 79: 1104-1110.
14. Kim J-W, Gardner LB, Dang CV. Oncogenic alterations of metabolism and the Warburg effect. *Drug Discovery Today: Dis Mech* 2005; 2: 233-238.
15. Warburg O. On the origin of cancer cells. *Science* 1956; 123: 309-314.
16. Wood IS, Trayhurn P. Glucose transporters (GLUT and SGLT): Expanded families of sugar transport proteins. *Br J Nutr* 2003; 89: 3-9.
17. Gatenby RA, Gillies RJ. Why do cancers have high aerobic glycolysis? *Nat Rev Cancer* 2004; 4: 891-899.
18. Dwek RA. Glycobiology: Toward Understanding the Function of Sugars. *Chem Rev* 1996; 96: 683-720.
19. Bitha P, Child RG, Hlavka JJ, Lin YI, EP186085, 1986.
20. Hlavka JJ, Child RG, Bitha P, Lin YI, US4587331, 1986.
21. Tsubomura T, Ogawa M, Yano S, Kobayashi K, Sakurai T, Yoshikawa S. Highly active antitumor platinum(II) complexes of amino sugars. *Inorg Chem* 1990; 29: 2622-2626.
22. Tsubomura T, Yano S, Kobayashi K, Sakurai T, Yoshikawa S. First synthesis and characterization of platinum(II) complexes of amino sugars having antitumor activity; crystal structure of dichloro(methyl 2,3-diamino-2,3-dideoxy-α-D-mannopyranoside)platinum monohydrate. *J Chem Soc, Chem Commun* 1986; 459-460.
23. Meyer zu Reckendorf W. Diamino sugars. V. Synthesis of 2,3-diamino-2,3-dideoxy-D-allose, 2,3-diamino-2,3-dideoxy-α-D-glucose, and 2,6-diamino-2,6-dideoxy-α-D-allose. *Ber* 1964; 97: 1275-1285.
24. Chittenden GJF. Acetalation studies. Part VI. Concerning the effects of ultrasound on the benzylidenation of some alkyl D-glycopyranosides. *Recl Trav Chim Pays-Bas* 1988; 107: 607-609.
25. Appleton TG, Hall JR. Complexes with six-membered chelate rings. I. Preparation of platinum(II) and palladium(II) complexes of trimethylenediamine and some methyl-substituted derivatives. *Inorg Chem* 1970; 9: 1800-1806.

ACKNOWLEDGEMENTS

This work was supported by the Austrian Council for Research and Technology Development, by Faustus Forschung Translational Drug Development AG and by COST D20.

Metal Ions in Biology and Medicine: vol. 9. Eds Maria Carmen Alpoim, Paula Vasconcellos Morais, Maria Amélia Santos, Armando J. Cristóvão, José A. Centeno, Philippe Collery.
John Libbey Eurotext, Paris © 2006 pp. 13-1.

Novel Mo(VI) complexes with potential biological relevance

Sílvia Chaves[1], Marco Gil[1], Ratomir Jelic[2], M. Amélia Santos[1]

[1]*Centro de Química Estrutural, Instituto Superior Técnico, Av. Rovisco Pais 1, 1049-001 Lisboa Portugal*
[2]*Faculty of Science, Chemistry Department, p.o. box 60, 34000 Kragujevac, Serbia and Montenegro*

ABSTRACT

Some oxomolybdenum complexes have been related to the lowering of plasma glucose levels and the amelioration of heart function defects associated with diabetes. With the purpose of developing new potential drugs with these therapeutic roles, the Mo(VI) complexation with two model compounds, a known iron-chelating pharmaceutical drug (Deferiprone, **DMHP**) and a novel thio analogue **(DMHTP)**, is studied to compare the *O,O*- versus *O,S*- metal binding properties. Solution equilibrium studies of these compounds are performed, namely the Mo(VI) complexation and electrochemical behaviour. The obtained results revealed that **DMHTP** presents higher affinity for the "soft-hard" metal ion Mo(VI) than the corresponding oxo analogue, avoiding the formation of polyoxomolybdates in acidic solution and retarding the emergence of MoO_4^{2-} at higher pH values. Moreover, as anticipated, the softer *O,S*-donor ligand significantly stabilizes the reduced complex species relative to the harder *O,O*-derivative.

INTRODUCTION

Molybdenum plays an important role in biological systems, being present in several redox enzymes that include the molybdopterin cofactor such as the xantine oxydase (XO). Siderophores proved to be involved in molybdenum uptake in nitrogen-fixing bacteria [1, 2], the amount of their release by the microbes being dependent on the concentration of molybdate in the growth medium. So, several studies on the interaction of molybdenum with cathecolate or hydroxamate type compounds have been performed [1-4]. Also, oxomolybdenum complexes have been bioassayed and some glucose-lowering activity [5, 6] as well as amelioration of heart function defects in diabetic rats has been reported [6]. Specifically, molybdenum complexes with naturally occurring hydroxypyrones or hydroxypyridinones have been recently tested for these therapeutical roles [6]. Moreover, the interest in molybdenum complexes with compounds containing sulfur donor atoms has been growing related to the study of the nature, composition and action mechanism of the active sites in molybdoenzymes.

As part of an ongoing project, the Mo(VI) complexation with two model hydroxypyridinone compounds, an orally active iron-chelating agent for the treatment of transfusion-induced iron overload in thalassemia (Deferiprone, **DMHP**) and its novel thio analogue **(DMHTP)**, is studied by using spectroscopic and cyclic voltammetric techniques. Our goal in this study is to analyze the Mo(VI) complexation in terms of the *O,O*- versus *O,S*- metal binding groups.

Investigations into the effects of these molybdenum compounds over heart dysfunctions of diabetic rats are under way and these studies should be most interesting, particularly if their therapeutical role could be related to redox properties and/or coordination modes.

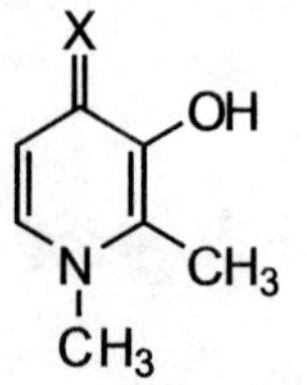

X = O Deferiprone (**DMHP**)
X = S **DMHTP**

Scheme

MATERIALS AND METHODS

The materials and methods used are according to the literature [7]. The synthesis of **DMHTP** was achieved following a similar procedure to the reported in the preparation of thiohydroxamic acids [8]. The protonation and stability constants were determined by fitting the spectroscopic data with the PSEQUAD [9] program. Cyclic voltammetry was performed using an AUTOLAB potentiostat, with a three-electrode cell consisting of hanging mercury drop work electrode, a graphite auxiliary and an Ag/AgCl reference electrodes (I = 0.1 M KNO_3, 15% CH_3OH aqueous solution). Complexes were generated in situ by using molybdic acid in 1:4 metal/ligand stoichiometry.

RESULTS AND DISCUSSION

The results of the equilibrium studies performed in 15% CH_3OH aqueous solution are presented in *table 1*. This solution medium was selected due to the lower solubility of the thio-derivative in water.

Table 1. Stepwise protonation constants (log K_i) of DMHP and DMHTP, as well as the global formation constants of their Mo(VI) complexes (I = 0.1 M KCl, 15% CH_3OH, T = 25.0 ± 0.1 °C)

Ligand	**DMHP**	**DMHTP**
log K_1	9.82(1) 9.75(4)[a]	9.70(1)
log K_2	3.74(2) 3.66(1)[a]	0.95(3)[b]
log $\beta_{MoO_2L_2}$	39.31(4) 40.22(4)[a]	41.48(6)
log β_{MoO_3L}	20.10(4) 20.0(1)[a]	21.82(5)

[a] ref. 10 (I=0.1 M KCl, in water); [b] determined by ^1H NMR titration

Spectrophotometry was chosen to study these Mo(VI)-systems because it is known that oxo-complexes containing dioxo-molybdenum core have intensive characteristic UV-band at λ_{max} ca 290 nm (2500 $M^{-1}cm^{-1}$), while polyoxo-molybdates and molybdate itself do not have any measurable band in this UV-region [11]. However, since the ligands have characteristic UV-bands in this energy region, the protonation behaviour was also studied by spectrophotometric titrations *(fig. 1a)*, except for the determination of the second protonation constant of **DMHTP** for which a ^1H NMR titration was performed due to the low value (< 2) of log K_2.

Both ligands were obtained as neutral species but they have two dissociable protons in the fully protonated form, namely in the hydroxyl and pyridine groups. The thio-derivative is more acidic than the corresponding oxo-derivative due to the higher stabilisation of the conjugate base, since sulfur is less electronegative and more polarizable than oxygen.

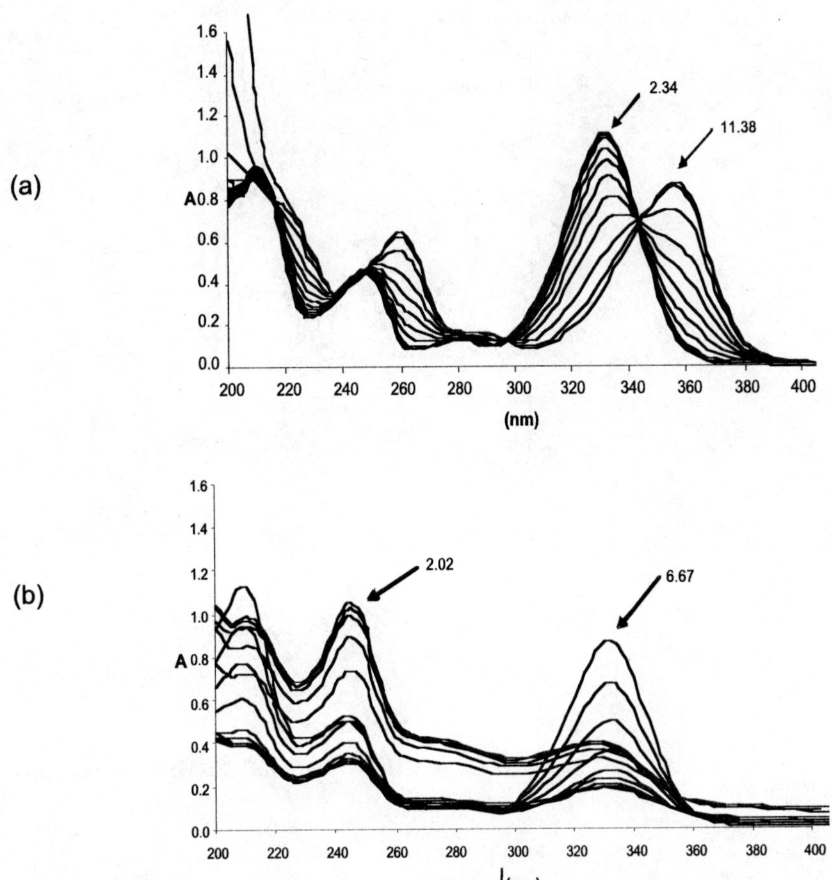

Fig. 1. UV/Vis spectra of **DMHTP** (a) and 1:2 Mo(VI)/**DMHTP** (b) systems at various pH values (C_L = 5.3 (10^{-5} M).

According to *table 1*, the softer *O,S*-donor ligand **(DMHTP)** evidences a better affinity for the "soft-hard" Mo(VI) and the results obtained for **DMHP** are analogous to the previously determined in water [10]. Moreover, the species distribution diagrams associated to the solution complex formation results *(fig. 2)* show that both ligands form two types of complexes, namely a bis-(MoO_2L_2) and a mono-chelated (MoO_3L) species, in acidic and neutral conditions, respectively. Nevertheless, while **DMHP** evidences some competition between the polyoxomolybdates and the complexes with the ligand till pH ca 5, the ligand **DMHTP** does not show that competition and retards the formation of MoO_4^{2-} to higher pH values.

Cyclic voltammetric studies were performed at pH 3.5-4.0 to make a brief evaluation of the electrochemical properties of the MoO_2L_2 complexes for both systems *(fig. 3)*.

DMHP presents three electrochemical processes with cathodic peaks (E_p^c) at -0.46, -0.83 and -1.19 V. The first two peaks show a quasi-reversible behaviour, while the third one seems to involve an irreversible process. **DMHTP** also evidences three reduction waves (E_p^c= -0.22, -0.49, -1.04 V), all of them without the anodic counterpart but the second one, which presents a quasi-reversible behaviour. A detailed analysis of the electrochemical mechanisms involved in these two systems is out of the aim of the present paper and, on the other hand, the thio-derivative seems to have some adsorption processes. Noteworthy is the fact that the reduction peaks of **DMHTP** are centred at less negative potential values than the oxo-derivative, which means that, under the

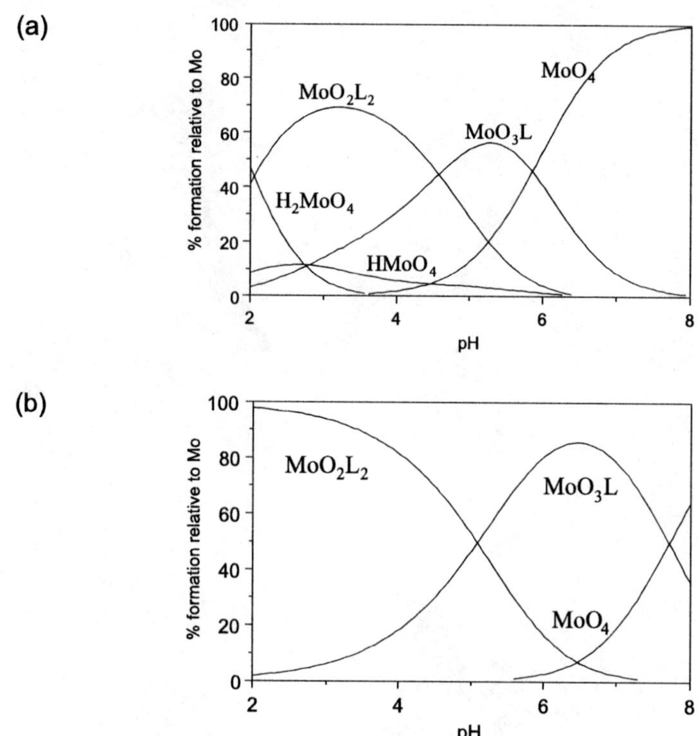

Fig. 2. Species distribution diagrams for the MoO_4^{2-}/**DMHP** (a) and MoO_4^{2-}/**DMHTP** (b) systems ($C_L = 5.3 \times 10^{-5}$ M, $C_L/C_M = 2$).

present experimental conditions, the ratio between the stability constants of the oxidized and reduced complex species is lower for the *O,S*-derivative than the *O,O*-analogue. This feature may be of relevance for the redox processes that are expected to be involved in the potential biological applications of these compounds.

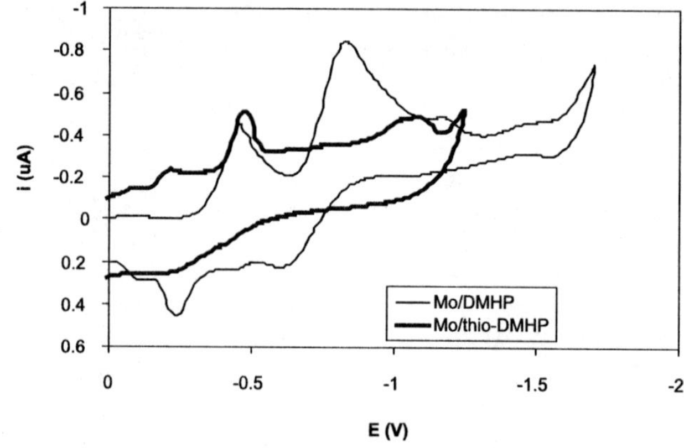

Fig. 3. Cyclic voltammograms of Mo(VI)/**DMHP** and Mo(VI)/**DMHTP** systems in 15% CH_3OH aqueous solution at a hanging mercury drop electrode (scan rate 300 mV s^{-1}, $I = 0.1$ M KNO_3).

REFERENCES

1. Duhme A-K, Dauter Z, Hider RC, Pohl S. Complexation of Molybdenum by Siderophores: Synthesis and Structure of the Double-Helical *cis*-Dioxomolybdenum(VI) Complex of a Bis(catecholamide) Siderophore Analogue. *Inorg Chem* 1996; 35: 3059-3061.
2. Duhme A-K. Synthesis, characterisation, and solution behaviour of two dioxomolybdenum(VI) complexes of a bis(catecholamide) siderophore analogue. *J Chem Soc Dalton Trans* 1997: 773-779.
3. Farkas E, Csóka H, Tóth I. New insights into the solution equilibrium of molybdenum(VI)-hydroxamate systems: ^{1}H and ^{17}O NMR spectroscopic study of Mo(VI)-desferrioxamine B and Mo(VI)-monohydroxamic acid systems. *Dalton Trans* 2003: 1645-1652.
4. Brown DA, Bogge H, Coogan R, Doocey D, Kemp TJ, Müller A, Neumann B. Oxygen Abstraction Reactions of N-Substituted Hydroxamic Acids with Molybdenum(V) and Vanadium(III) and -(IV) Compounds. *Inorg Chem* 1996; 35: 1674-1679.
5. Thompson KH, Chiles J, Yuen VG, Tse J, Mcneill JH, Orvig C. Comparison of anti-hyperglycemic effect amongst vanadium, molybdenum and other metal maltol complexes. *J Inorg Biochem* 2004; 98: 683-690.
6. Lord SJ, Epstein NA, Paddock RL, Vogels CM, Hennigar TL, Zaworotko MJ, Taylor NJ, Driedzic WR, Broderick TL, Westcott SA. Synthesis, characterization and biological relevance of hydroxypyrone and hydroxypyridinone complexes of molybdenum. *Can J Chem* 1999; 77: 1249-1261.
7. Santos MA, Gil M, Gano L, Chaves S. Bifunctional 3-hydroxy-4-pyridinone derivatives as potential pharmaceuticals: synthesis, complexation with Fe(III), Al(III) and Ga(III) and in vivo evaluation with ^{67}Ga. *J Biol Inorg Chem* 2005; 10: 564-580.
8. Prabhakar S, Lobo AM, Santos MA, Rzepa HS. A convenient method for the synthesis of N-hydroxythiobenzamides (C-arylthiohydroxamic acids). *Synthesis* 1984: 829-830.
9. Zékany L, Nagypál I. in *Computational Methods for the Determination of Stability constants*, New York, ed. D. Legget, Plenum, 1985, 291.
10. Santos MA, Gama S, Pessoa JC, Oliveira MC, Toth I, Farkas E. Complexation studies of molybdenum(VI)-hydroxypyridinone systems. *submitted.*
11. Farkas E, Csóka H, Micera G, Dessi A. Copper(II), nickel(II), zinc(II), and molybdenum(VI) complexes of desferrioxamine B in aqueous solution. *J Inorg Biochem* 1997; 65: 281-286.

Metal Ions in Biology and Medicine: vol. 9. Eds Maria Carmen Alpoim, Paula Vasconcellos Morais, Maria Amélia Santos, Armando J. Cristóvão, José A. Centeno, Philippe Collery.
John Libbey Eurotext, Paris © 2006 pp. 18-1.

Vanadium complexes - concerns about possible therapeutic apllications

Costa Pessoa[1], Cavaco I[1], Correia I[1], Gonçalves G[1], Tomaz I[1], Vale I[1], Ribeiro V[2], Castro MMCA[3], Geraldes CFGC[3], Delgado T[3], Jones JG[3], Meier B[4], Rehder D[5]

[1]*Instituto Superior Técnico, Centro Química Estrutural, Av. Rovisco Pais, 1049-001 Lisboa Portugal;*
[2]*Centro de Biomedicina Molecular e Estrutural, Universidade do Algarve, Portugal,*
[3]*Departmento de Bioquímica, Faculdade de Ciências e Tecnologia, Universidade de Coimbra, P.O. Box 3126, 3001-401 Coimbra, Portugal;*
[4]*85307 Entrischenbrunn 12, Germany,* [5]*Institute of Inorganic and Applied Chemistry, University of Hamburg, 21146 Hamburg, Germany*

INTRODUCTION

The presence of vanadium in biological systems and its insulin-enhancing action [1] and anti-cancer activity [2] has driven a considerable amount of research. Particular interest has been given to the study of the potential benefits of vanadium compounds (VCs) as oral insulin substitutes for the treatment of diabetes. Coordinated ligands are said to be able to improve the absorption and intracellular mobility of vanadium, reducing the dose necessary for producing equivalent effects. However, the molecular mechanisms by which the VCs exert their insulin enhancing effects *in vivo* and *in vitro* have not been clarified. In fact, in *in vitro* studies the nature of the vanadium species acting is often not known, and additionally in *in vivo* studies the role of serum proteins (eg. albumin, transferrin) and that of insulin, which may act synergistically, is also not understood.

Several vanadium complexes of the tetradentate Schiff base salen type ligands have been proposed for use as insulin enhancing agents, and for treatment of obesity and hypertension. The ability of $V^{IV}O$(salen) to reverse the hyperglycemic condition of alloxan-induced diabetic rats to near normal has been mentioned [3]. However, rats tended to become hypoglycemic, and withdrawal of treatment brought an immediate return to hyperglycemia.

In solution salen Schiff base (SB) compounds have the disadvantage of their hydrolysis. This instability can often be overcome by reduction of the SB to give an amine compound (hereafter designated by salan). This presents interesting possibilities, as salan ligands will be more flexible and not restrained to remain planar when coordinated. We have reported the preparation of several new salen- and salan-type compounds, and of their $V^{IV}O^{2+}$ complexes. Namely compounds derived from pyridoxal (pyr) and salicylaldehyde-5-sulphonate (SO_3-sal) with ethylenediamine were studied [1]. Most of the salen-type ligands and their VCs prepared so far are not water-soluble. Those prepared using pyr and especially SO_3-sal are soluble in water; therefore they may be particularly useful for therapeutic use.

(SO_3-sal)en ^-O_3S —OH HO— SO_3^- HOH$_2$C —NH HN— CH$_2$OH —OH HO— N CH$_3$ H$_3$C N pyran

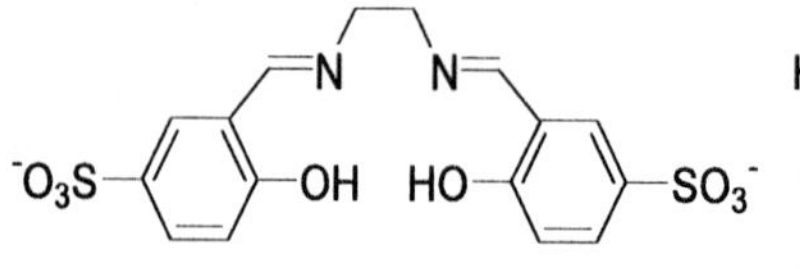

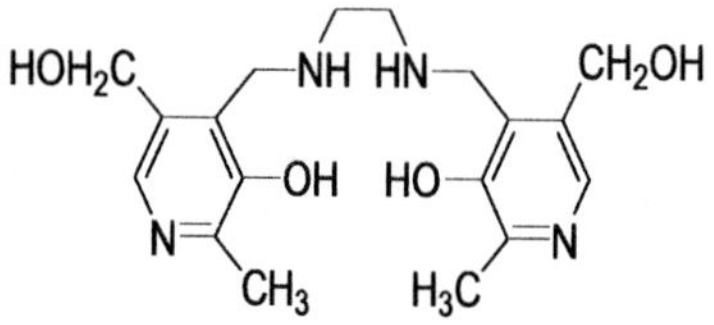

Both pyren and pyran proved to be efficient binders of vanadium(IV) and vanadium(V). We prepared several $V^{IV}O$- and V^VO_2-pyran complexes and studied their properties. Both ligands form

basically similar complexes coordinating through ($2{\times}O_{phenolate}$, $2{\times}N_{amine/imine}$). The solution speciation revealed that pyran formed much more stable complexes with both $V^{IV}O^{2+}$ and $V^{V}O_2^{+}$ than the corresponding SB.

Some of the vanadium(IV) complexes synthesized and characterized in the present and in previous reports [4] have been tested *in vitro* for their toxicity and insulin-mimetic behaviour [1]: $Cs_2[V^{IV}O(SO_3\text{-sal})en]$ **1**, $V^{IV}O$(salan) **2**, $V^{IV}O$(pyren) **3** and $V^{IV}O$(pyran) **4**. We now also present insulin-mimetic studies with: $V^{IV}O$(RsalDPA) **5** (RsalDPA = reduced SB of salicylaldehyde and diaminopropionic acid), $V^{IV}O$(sal-D-galacN) **6**, $V^{IV}O$(sal-*D*-glsmN) **7** (sal-*D*-glsmN and sal-*D*-galacN correspond to the SBs obtained from the condensation of salicylaldehyde with *D*-glucosamine and *D*-galactosamine, respectively), $V^{IV}O(dmpp)_2$ **8** (dmpp=3-hydroxy-1,2-dimethyl-4-pyridinonato) and $Na_6[(V^{IV}O)_2(Frutose)_5]\cdot 4H_2O$ **9**.

Studies of the effect of vanadium complexes on DNA have mainly concentrated on plasmid nicking caused by the VC itself or reactivity initiated by H_2O_2 or UV radiation. *In vivo* use of VCs therefore raises the issue of cellular toxicity due to DNA modification. Namely some (hydroxysal)en vanadium complexes have been shown to exhibit nuclease activity in the presence of an activating agent (mercaptopropionic acid or Oxone), whereas in the absence of an activating agent no cleavage of DNA was induced. The reaction occurs essentially at guanine residues [5].

In the present study we discuss some aspects related to the uptake and metabolic effects of two VCs in human erythrocytes, insulin mimetic studies of compounds **1-9**, some toxicity studies and nuclease activity of several salen and salan VCs.

RESULTS AND DISCUSSION

Toxicity tests

Some of the vanadium(IV) complexes synthesized and characterized in the present and in previous reports [1] have been tested *in vitro* for their toxicity and insulin-mimetic behaviour using transformed mice fibroblasts (cell line SV 3T3). Toxicity tests were carried out by incubating the fibroblasts with solutions of the VCs for 12, 24 and 36 h, followed by the addition of trypan blue. This dye penetrates the membrane of dead cells only, and these adopt a bluish colour. Most of these complexes are toxic at C(V)=1mM [except VO(pyran)], and negligibly toxic or non-toxic at C(V)=0.01mM and below.

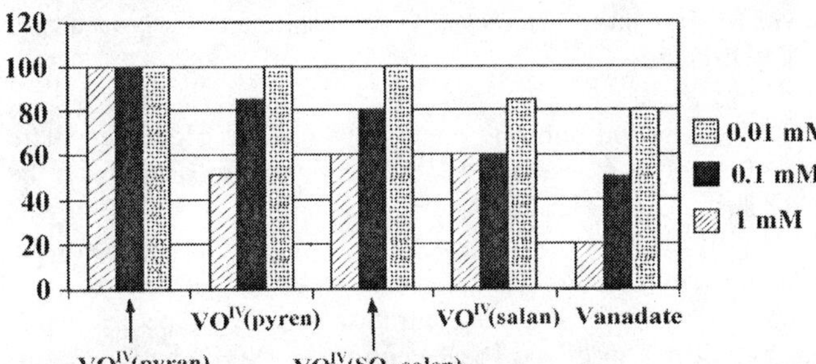

Fig. 1. Toxicity *in vitro* at 3 diferent VC concentrations, expressed as the number of cells (SV 3T3 mice Fibroblasts), which survived after 36 hours in contact with the compounds.

The oxidative stress induced by $VO(dmpp)_2$ and VO(pyran) in human erythrocytes was characterised measuring their effect on the pentose phosphate (PP) flux [6]. The oxidative stress induced by the VCs is not significant at 1 mM concentration, but became significant for both vanadate and oxidized $V^{IV}O(dmpp)_2$ at 5 mM.

Uptake of $VO(dmpp)_2$ and VO(pyran) by erythrocytes

In aerobic aqueous solution and at physiological pH $V^{IV}O$(pyran) **4** and $V^{IV}O(dmpp)_2$ **8** are oxidized to their V^V counterparts: V^VO_2(Hpyran), and V^VO_2 complexes of 1:1 and 1:2 stoichiometry with dmpp. The uptake of the oxidation products of **4** and **8** by human erythrocytes was studied by ^{51}V and ^{1}H NMR, and EPR spectroscopy.

When human erythrocyte suspensions were incubated with 1 mM oxidized $V^{IV}O(dmpp)_2$, the ^{51}V NMR spectra of the extracellular medium obtained as a function of time, at two different temperatures, 25°C *(fig. 2a)* and 37°C *(fig. 2b)*, showed a decrease in the intensity of the signals observed at -483 and -507 ppm, corresponding, respectively, to the 1:2 and 1:1 complexes, which is considerably faster at 37°C, and faster for the negatively charged 1:2 species at both temperatures and at all times. Similar ^{51}V NMR experiments carried out in the presence of DIDS, the anion channel blocker, showed no significant differences in the spectra relative to those obtained in its absence [6], thus indicating that none of the two negatively charged complexes $[V^{V}O_2L_2]^-$ and $[V^{V}O_2L(H_2O)(OH)]^-$ (L=dmpp), present as the major species in solution at physiological pH, enters the cells. The disappearance of both 1:1 and 1:2 complexes from the extracellular medium indicates that the neutral 1:1 complex $[V^{V}O_2L(H_2O)_2]$ is the only species taken up by the erythrocytes through passive diffusion, in a temperature dependent process. The entry of this neutral species into the cells and its subsequent intracellular reduction was corroborated through the EPR spectra of erythrocyte lysates obtained from cell suspensions incubated with $V^{IV}O(dmpp)_2$ oxidation products, at 37°C, which show initially a fast increasing signal intensity up to 60 min incubation time, followed by a constant value *(fig. 2c)*. However, the identity of the complex is not maintained inside the cells, where complexes involving a N_2O_2 or NO_3 binding modes form [6].

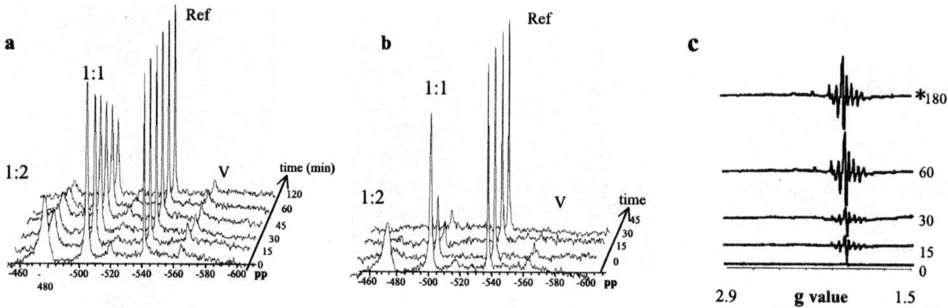

Fig. 2. ^{51}V NMR spectra of the extracellular medium of human erythrocyte suspensions (Hematocrit=50%) incubated with 1 mM oxidized $V^{IV}O(dmpp)_2$ as a function of time at (**a**) 25°C and (**b**) 37°C. $V^{V}O_2L_2$ is the 1:2 species, $V^{V}O_2L$ the 1:1 species (L=dmpp), V is free vanadate and Ref is the external reference. (**c**) EPR spectra (77 K) as a function of time (min.) of frozen human erythrocyte lysate samples previously incubated with 1 mM oxidized $V^{IV}O(dmpp)_2$ at t = 37°C [6].

Similar NMR and EPR experiments when carried out with complex **4** at 37°C. However, there were no significant changes with time in the intensity of the ^{51}V NMR signals measured for the extracellular medium of the erythrocyte suspensions, indicating that no significant uptake of this bulky complex is observed by ^{51}V NMR [6]. The EPR spectra of the lysates obtained from the erythrocyte suspensions showed low intensity signals that increase slowly with the incubation time, indicating the presence of a very low and slowly increasing concentration of a $V^{IV}O$-species inside the cells, resulting from very slow passive diffusion of the large neutral $[V^{V}O_2(HRpyr_2en)]$ complex. These EPR signals are very similar to those obtained in the erythrocyte lysates after incubation with either $V^{IV}O(dmpp)_2$ or vanadates.

Insulin mimetic tests

In one set of tests transformed mice fibroblasts (cell line SV 3T3) were used, as described in [1]. The glucose intake was determined by a vitality test based on MTT (addition of yellow MTT, the amount of MTT-formazan blue is measured spectrophotometrically, the absorbance being related to the amount of glucose incorporated by the cell [1]). Some data is presented graphically in *fig. 3*. Maximum activity is found in the range C(V) = 0.1 to 0.0001 mM. After 24h incubation in some cases some of the VCs appear to be more effective than insulin itself.

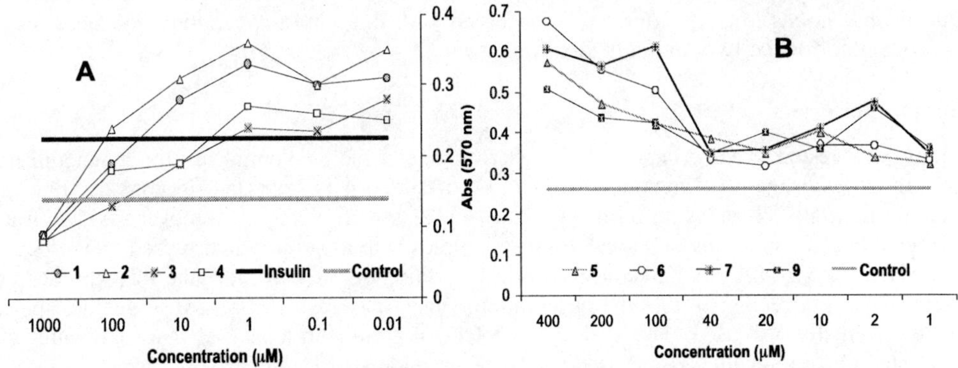

Fig. 3. Glucose intake by simian virus transformed 3T3 mice SV 3T3 fibroblasts in the presence of VCs after 24 h (**A**), after 4h (**B**). The ordinate is a measure for the reduction equivalents of glucose. The glucose intake from the extracellular medium containing complexes **4**, **8** or vanadates was also measured by the hexokinase method [6]. It was found that the glucose intake rates for the groups stimulated by vanadates and **4** did not significantly differ from the control. Only **8** had a significant effect on the glucose intake rate, this being probably related to the larger amount of vanadium taken up by the cells in the case of this complex.

DNA cleavage reactions

DNA cleavage was analysed by monitoring the conversion of supercoiled plasmid DNA (Sc) to nicked circular DNA (Nck) and linear DNA (Lin) - see *fig. 4*.

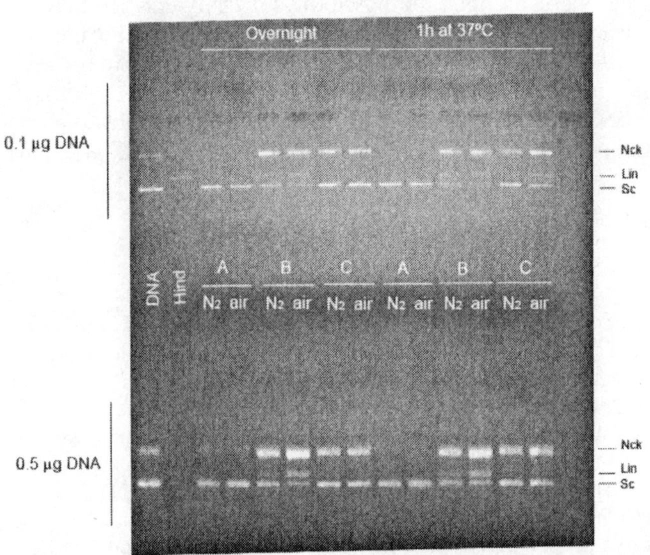

Fig. 4. Cleavage of supercoiled pA1 DNA (Sc) by complexes **1**, **4** and **5**. Nck and Lin refer to the nicked and linear DNA forms, respectively. The lanes marked DNA and Hind refer to the plasmid DNA and to the plasmid linearized by digestion with the restriction enzyme HindIII, respectively. Lanes marked A, B and C refer to the plasmid DNA incubated with **1**, **4** and **5**, respectively, in varying conditions of atmosphere, amount of DNA, incubation time and temperature.

Incubation of the plasmid with [VO(SO_3-sal)en] **1**, VO(pyran)] **4** and VO(RsalDPA) **5** show different results. Complex **1** caused no conversion of the Sc form to Nck form. Both **4** and **5** caused DNA cleavage, in all tested conditions and without the need of additional activating agents. Complex **5** converts Sc to Nck form. Complex **4** caused the most efficient cleavage, with conversion to Nck form and partial linearization of the plasmid DNA.

No significant difference can be observed between incubations done overnight at room temperature and for 1h at 37°C for **1**. With **5**, some DNA linearization is observed only after incubation for 1h at 37°C in aerobic conditions, but not at room temperature nor under N_2. The extent of DNA linearization observed after incubation with **4** is slightly higher if it is carried out in aerobic conditions, but no significant difference is observed with time and temperature. All these results are reproducible for the two amounts of DNA tested.

Final considerations

Many VCs tested *in vitro* here and elsewhere revealed their potential insulin-enhancing properties. If we envisage VCs for oral treatment of diabetes, it is important to consider that oral application normally provides an intimate contact of VCs with oxygen. Moreover, oxidation and the acidic stomach conditions will convert most complexes to a partially hydrolysed V(V) species. Most *in vivo* and *in vitro* studies concerning insulin mimetic VCs do not take this into account properly, or do not recognize that the observations made may result from a very distinct species from the originally VC used. The synergistic effect of serum proteins and that of insulin only recently started to be evaluated, but is far form being understood.

The speciation of the V(IV) and V(V) with pyran is well understood, and it is known that at pH=7 ~100% of vanadium is in the form of $V^{IV}O$-pyran or $V^{V}O_2$-pyran complexes. It was found to be non-toxic even at C(V)=1 mM. This may simply result from its low absorption from the cells, as found in human erythrocytes. However, while in the tests with mice fibroblasts *(fig. 3)* complex **4** was found to be an insulin-mimetic compound, in the tests measuring the glucose intake rates by the hexokinase method no significant stimulation was found. Moreover, *in vitro* enhanced insulino-mimetic activity was not found in rat adipocytes (by inhibition of free fatty acids release experiments made by K. Kawabe and H. Sakurai). The possibility of being an insulin-enhancing compound *in vivo* remains open.

As V-pyran complexes were found to cause DNA cleavage *(fig. 4)*, if they are significantly absorbed and keep their integrity inside the cells, then the possibility of DNA damage may be significant, and it would be toxic. At least with human erythrocytes it was found by EPR that the small amount of vanadium inside the cells is not in the form of $V^{IV}O$(pyran). This balance between the insulin mimetic effect of VCs and its possible DNA damage should be carefully evaluated before any compound could be considered for the treatment of diabetes. If the VC acts directly potentiating the tyrosine phosphorylation of the insulin receptor without entering the cell, problems of DNA damage could be ruled out.

REFERENCES

1. Rehder D, Costa Pessoa J, Geraldes CFGC, Castro MMCA, Kabanos T, Kiss T, Meier B, Micera G, Pettersson L, Rangel M, Salifoglou A, Turel I, Wang D. In vitro study of the insulin mimetic behaviour of vanadium(IV,V) coordination compounds. *J Biol Inorg Chem* 2002; 7: 384-396.
2. Evangelou AM. Vanadium in Cancer Treatment. *Crit Rev Oncol/Hemat* 2002; 42: 249-265.
3. Durai N, Saminathan G. Insulin-Like Effects of salen-oxovanadium(IV) Complex on Carbohydrate Metabolism. *J Clin Biochem Nutr* 1997; 22: 31-39.
4. Correia I, Costa Pessoa J, Duarte MT, Henriques RT, Piedade MF, Veiros LF, Jakusch T, Dörnyei A, Kiss T, Castro MMCA, Geraldes CFGC, Avecilla F. N,N'-ethylenebis(pyridoxylideneiminato) and N,N'-ethylenebis(pyridoxylaminato): synthesis, characterisation, potentiometric, spectroscopic and DFT study of their vanadium(IV) and vanadium(V) complexes. *Chem Eur J* 2004; 10: 2301-2317.
5. Verquin G, Fontaine G, Bria M, Zhilinskaya E, Abi-Aad E, Aboukais A, Baldeyrou B, Bailly C, Bernier JL. DNA modification by oxovanadium(IV) complexes of salen derivatives. *J. Biol Inorg Chem* 2004; 9: 345-353.
6. Delgado TC, Tomaz I, Correia I, Costa Pessoa J, Jones JG, Geraldes CFGC, Castro MMCA. Uptake and metabolic effects of insulin mimetic oxovanadium compounds in human erythrocytes. *J Inorg Biochem* 2005; 99: 2328-2339.

ACKNOWLEDGEMENTS

We thank the Fundo Europeu para o Desenvolvimento Regional, Fundação para a Ciência e Tecnologia, project POCI//QUI/56949/2004), and the COST D21 Action.

Metal Ions in Biology and Medicine: vol. 9. Eds Maria Carmen Alpoim, Paula Vasconcellos Morais, Maria Amélia Santos, Armando J. Cristóvão, José A. Centeno, Philippe Collery.
John Libbey Eurotext, Paris © 2006 pp. 24-1.

Impact of biological reductants on GMP binding of *trans*-[$Ru^{III}Cl_4(Hind)_2$]$^-$ and preparation of a model nucleobase adduct

Egger Alexander, Schluga Petra, Hartinger Christian G., Arion Vladimir B., Keppler Bernhard K.

Institute of Inorganic Chemistry, University of Vienna, Waehringer Str. 42, A-1090 Vienna, Austria

Platinum-based chemotherapeutics (cisplatin, carboplatin, oxaliplatin) have been used as anticancer drugs for over 30 years. Severe side effects and development of resistance during treatment motivate for investigation on other metal-based anticancer drugs for example based on ruthenium [1]. Two ruthenium complexes (H_2im)[*trans*-$RuCl_4$(DMSO)(Him)] (NAMI-A, Him = 1*H*-imidazole) and (H_2ind)[*trans*-$RuCl_4$(Hind)$_2$] (KP1019, Hind = 1*H*-indazole), have already finished clinical phase I trials and hence are potential new drugs for anticancer treatment *(fig. 1)*.

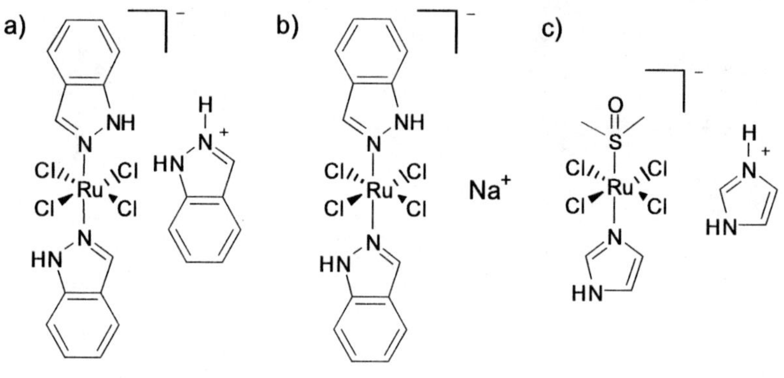

Fig. 1. Structural formulae of a) (H_2ind)[*trans*-$RuCl_4$(Hind)$_2$] (KP1019, FFC14A), b) Na[*trans*-$RuCl_4$(Hind)$_2$] (KP1339, FFC14), c) (H_2im)[*trans*-$RuCl_4$(DMSO)(Him)] (NAMI-A)

These Ru^{III} complexes share the physiologically accessible reduction potential Ru^{III}/Ru^{II}, which was recently reported for the analogous sodium salt of KP1019 (KP1339, *fig. 1*) to be in the range of 0.00 V to 0.03 V, independent of the pH (5.0 - 8.0) [2]. Ru^{III} complexes are considered as prodrugs which are activated by biological reductants as ascorbic acid or glutathione. Reduction leads to more reactive Ru^{II} species (activation by reduction hypothesis), which interact with biomolecules and subsequently cause cell death. In analogy to platinum-containing drugs, it is assumed that apoptosis is partly caused due to interactions with DNA, probably via N^7 of adenine and/or guanine [3]. Therefore, it is of paramount importance to investigate the influence of reducing agents on the oxidation state of KP1019 and the binding properties of KP1019 towards DNA-building molecules.

As tumour tissue is insufficiently vascularised, anaerobic metabolism is enhanced, leading to a lower pH compared to normal tissue. Therefore, the impact of pH on the reduction kinetics of

KP1019 in the presence of ascorbic acid (AA) or glutathione (GSH) and the influence of GSH on the binding of KP1019 towards guanosine 5'-monophosphate (GMP) was studied.

Finally, the synthesis and crystal structure of a Ru^{III} complex is presented, which was obtained by the reaction of the antitumour [*trans*-$RuCl_4(Hind)_2]^-$ complex anion with the nucleoside model 9-methyladenine, containing a methyl group as a substituent for the sugar moiety in adenosine.

REDUCTION OF KP1019 BY ASCORBIC ACID AND GLUTATHIONE

Experimental and methods

^{1}H NMR spectra were recorded with a Bruker Avance DPX 400 (Ultrashield™ Magnet) at 400.13 MHz and 25 °C in D_2O. KP1019 (0.5 mM) and GSH or AA were dissolved either in D_2O (pD approx. 3.5 due to the indazolium counter ion) or in 20 mM phosphate buffer (pD 6.0 and pD 7.4) prepared with D_2O at different molar ratios (1 : 1, 1 : 2 and 1 : 5 for GSH as well as 1 : 1 and 1 : 2 for AA). The reducing agent was added just before the start of the NMR experiment. Selected experiments were internally standardised for detection of possible release of indazole ligands during reduction.

Complete reduction was determined by the disappearance of the broad and strongly highfield-shifted indazole signals, coordinated to paramagnetic Ru^{III} and the simultaneously arising peaks of indazole coordinated to diamagnetic Ru^{II} at typical chemical shifts for indazole protons. Due to coordination, these peaks were slightly downfield shifted (0.1 ppm) compared to the free indazolium counter ion. These facts allowed to clearly distinguish between the amount of uncoordinated indazole, indazole bound to a Ru^{III} center and indazole coordinated to Ru^{II}.

Results and discussion

Table 1 summarises the duration until complete reduction of KP1019 ($E^{0'}$ = 0.00 - 0.03 V *vs.* NHE at pH 5.0-8.0 [2]) in the presence of GSH ($E^{0'}$ = -0.26 V *vs.* NHE at pH 7.0 [4]) or AA ($E^{0'}$ = 0.06 V *vs.* NHE at pH 7.0 [5]) at pH 3.5 or 6.0, obtained by a ^{1}H NMR study. AA was capable of reducing KP1019 much faster than GSH. While stoichiometric amounts of AA and KP1019 led to complete reduction within 4 h in unbuffered solutions, a fivefold excess of GSH was shown to be necessary for obtaining the same reduction kinetics. As expected, the change to a higher pD (6.0) accelerated reduction due to the increased reducing force of AA and GSH.

Table 1. Period until complete reduction of KP1019 in the presence of ascorbic acid (AA) or glutathione (GSH) at varying molar ratios and pH

	KP1019: AA		KP1019: GSH		
	1: 2	1: 1	1: 1	1: 2	1: 5
pD 3.5	~ 1 h	4 h	>22 h	16 h	5 h
pD 6.0	<5 min	n.d.	n.d.	3.5 h	45 min

When surveying the newly arising peaks in NMR spectra over time, indazole peak patterns of at least two different Ru^{II} complexes can be observed (*fig.* 2, top), whereupon the dark grey set of Ru^{II}-coordinated indazole peaks arises prior to the light grey one. However, we cannot definitely assign these peaks to the reduced species proposed by Ravera *et al.*, namely $[Ru^{II}Cl_4(Hind)_2]^{2-}$, $[Ru^{II}(H_2O)Cl_3(Hind)_2]^-$, and $[Ru^{II}(H_2O)_2Cl_2(Hind)_2]$ [6], as we can only discriminate between two Ru^{II}-coordinated indazole species. In accordance to Ravera's findings, kinetics and peak patterns were comparable and loss of coordinated indazole could not be detected.

Comparison of the integration of the first Ru^{II}-indazole signals with uncoordinated indazole closely reached the theoretical value of 2:1 only in case of a tenfold excess of AA, in which reduction was complete within seconds. Prolonged periods until complete reduction (achieved via lowering the amount of reducing agent) especially effected this ratio in GSH experiments, which was lowered to 1 : 1 for KP1019 : GSH = 1 : 5 in unbuffered solution at time of complete reduction (5 hours, see *fig. 2* bottom).

Precipitation, occurring especially in buffered settings over time, contributes to this effect as well as the above mentioned formation of a further Ru^{II}-coordinated indazole species.

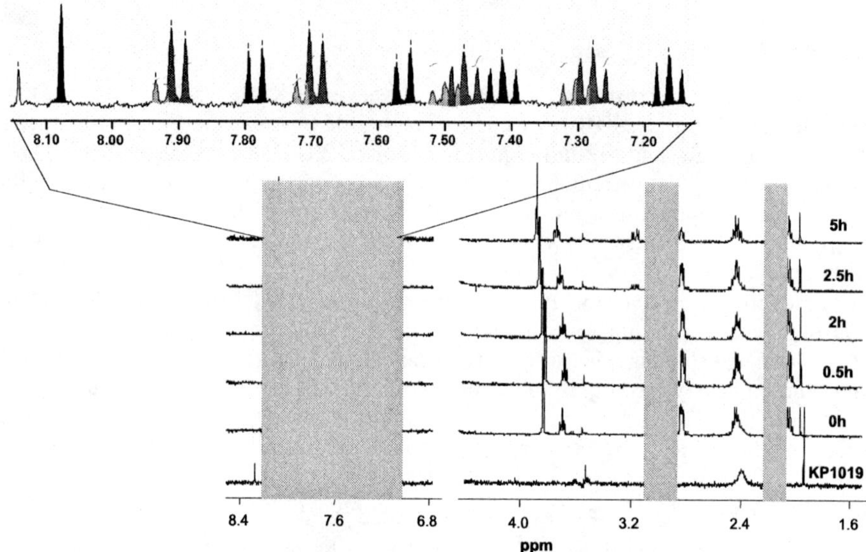

Fig. 2. Top: detailed view onto the ^{1}H NMR indazole signals after 5 h: black: uncoordinated indazole, dark grey: first arising Ru^{II}-indazole complex and light grey: second Ru^{II}-indazole complex
Bottom: Time dependent study by ^{1}H NMR spectroscopy of the reduction of KP1019 with GSH (KP1019 : GSH = 1 : 5) in D_2O at 25 °C, Ru^{III}-indazole signals at ca. 2.1 and 3.0 ppm as well as Ru^{II}-indazole and indazole signals between 7.0 and 8.0 ppm are marked in grey.

GMP BINDING OF KP1019 UNDER THE INFLUENCE OF GSH

Experimental and methods

All analyses were performed on a Hewlett-Packard ^{3D}Capillary Electrophoresis system equipped with a diode-array detector in fused-silica capillaries (50 µm ID, total length 50 cm, effective length 42 cm). A 50 mM NaH_2PO_4-Na_2HPO_4 buffer (pH 6.0 or 7.4) was used as background electrolyte (BGE). The temperature was kept constant at 37 °C and samples were dissolved in 20 mM NaH_2PO_4-Na_2HPO_4 buffer (pH 6.0 or 7.4). Voltage was maintained constant at 15 kV.

KP1019 (0.5 mM) was incubated in 20 mM NaH_2PO_4-Na_2HPO_4 buffer (pH 6.0 or 7.4) with GMP to obtain molar ratios of 1 : 2 (complex : GMP). GSH was added to the latter mixture, resulting in molar ratios of 1 : 2 : 2 and 1 : 2 : 10 (KP1019: GMP: GSH). The decrease of GMP was recorded at 200, 254 and 265 nm over 20 h. Each manipulation was repeated three times. The autooxidation of GSH was analysed under the same experimental conditions in the absence of KP1019 and GMP, and resulted in a decrease of GSH of approx. 26%.

Results and discussion

Table 2 summarises the decrease of unbound GMP under varying ratios of KP1019: GMP: GSH at pH 6.0 and 7.4 after 20 h of incubation determined by capillary electrophoresis.

Table 2. Decrease of free GMP upon reaction with KP1019 under the influence of pH and GSH. Incubation conditions: 20 mM phosphate buffer (pH 6.0 or 7.4) at 37 °C for 20 h

Molar ratio	pH 6.0	pH 7.4
KP1019: GMP (1: 2)	21.4±0.6%	11.1±2.3%
KP1019: GMP: GSH (1: 2: 2)	41.7±0.9%	18.2±1.5%
KP1019: GMP: GSH (1: 2: 10)	10.3±1.8%	n.d.

Upon addition of a twofold excess of GSH at pH 6.0, the decrease of GMP was much more pronounced than in the experiments without GSH (41.7 vs. 21.4%, respectively), whereas at pH 7.4 only a slight influence on GMP could be observed (18.2 vs. 11,1%). However, a tenfold excess of GSH did not further improve the binding of GMP to the ruthenium complex but even had an adverse effect. At pH 6.0 only a 10% reduction of the peak area of uncoordinated GMP was found, which is even lower than in the experiment without GSH (21.4%).

As discussed in the NMR-section, hydrolysis followed by precipitation can explain these findings: Küng *et al.* reported that the hydrolysis of $(H_2ind)[trans\text{-}RuCl_4(Hind)_2]$ shows a strong pH dependence, resulting in changes of the half-lives from 5.4 h at pH 6.0 to less than 0.5 h at pH 7.4 [7]. In addition, at pH 7.4 a blue precipitate was observed within one hour of incubation. In the present experiments, the addition of two equivalents of GSH accelerated the formation of precipitate up to half an hour at pH 7.4 and up to 5 h at pH 6.0.

Hence, reduction of KP1019 (in case of GSH addition), GMP binding to KP1019, and formation of insoluble, probably polynuclear ruthenium species are competing processes during the experiments. Therefore only a limited time frame for GMP binding is available. At pH 6.0, precipitation occurs much slower than at pH 7.4, and therefore, KP1019 can bind to GMP at a higher degree before insoluble species are formed. As uncoordinated GMP only decreased about 10% at a tenfold excess of GSH over KP1019 and no precipitation occurred under these settings, the formation of soluble KP1019-GSH adducts is suggested, which prevent GMP from coordination towards the ruthenium center. The analysis of this precipitate in acetone by ESI-MS and NMR could not enlighten its nature or chemical structure.

INSIGHT INTO DNA ADDUCTS: MODEL NUCLEOBASE 9-METHYLADENINE AS LIGAND IN $[Ru^{III}Cl_3(Hind)_2(9\text{-meade})]$

Synthesis and crystal structure of [*mer,trans*-trichlorobis(indazole)(9-methyladenine) ruthenium(III)], $[Ru^{III}Cl_3(Hind)_2(9\text{-meade})]$

0.11 g (0.2 mmol) of the tetramethylammonium salt of KP1019, $[NMe_4][trans\text{-}Ru^{III}Cl_4(Hind)_2]$, and 0.06 g (0.4 mmol) of 9-methyladenine were dissolved in 15 ml of ethanol. The solution turned deeply red while stirring under reflux for 1h. Subsequently, the solvent was removed by rotary evaporation under reduced pressure, the solid residue was extracted with $CHCl_3/MeOH$ (10:1) and the extract was further purified by column chromatography on silica by using a mixture of CH_2Cl_2/CH_3CN (5:2) as eluent. Yield: 0.04 g (15%). The complex was well soluble in chloroform and DMF and less soluble in methanol.

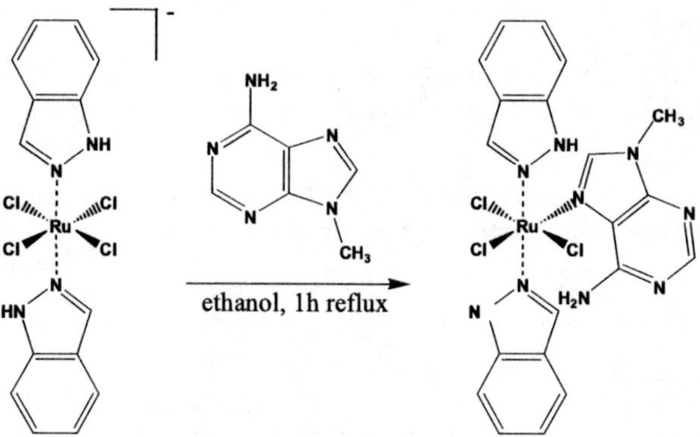

Fig. 3. Synthetic pathway for [*mer,trans*-$Ru^{III}Cl_3(Hind)_2$(9-meade)]. The methyl group at position 9 in adenine resembles the sugar moiety in adenosine and prevents from coordination to N^9 in analogy to deoxyadenosine.

The complex was characterised by elemental analysis, ESI-MS and IR. Crystals of X-ray diffraction quality were grown by slow diffusion of hexane into a dichloromethane solution of [$Ru^{III}Cl_3(Hind)_2$(9-meade)], containing a few drops of methanol. The structure was solved by direct methods and refined by full matrix least-squares techniques [8].

Results and discussion

In analogy to platinum-based drugs, which exhibit their toxic potential mainly due to coordination towards nucleobases via N^7 of adenine or guanine, it was suggested that ruthenium complexes cause apoptosis by binding to DNA. 9-methyladenine is an appropriate model nucleobase since the methyl group resembles the deoxyribose moiety in adenosine and therefore prevents coordination at N^9 in the same way as in DNA. The preparation and crystallisation of a KP1019-derived complex with a N^7 coordination of 9-methyladenine was successful. Interestingly, binding did not occur via the more basic ring nitrogen N^1. Instead, N^1 and the amino-group are involved in intermolecular hydrogen bondings, leading - like Watson-Crick interactions in DNA - to self-pairing of two complex molecules via their 9-methyladenine ligands *(fig. 4)*. These interactions probably determine the metal-binding site explaining the coordination via N^7.

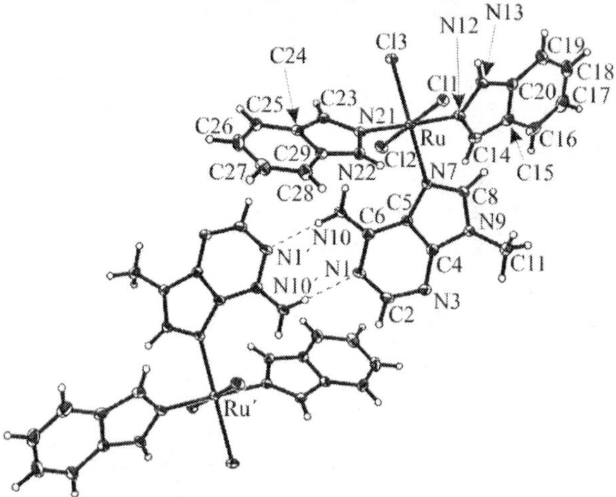

Fig. 4. Crystal structure of [$RuCl_3(Hind)_2$(9-meade)] shows that two complex molecules are paired via hydrogen bondings between N^1 and N^{10} of the 9-methyladenine ligand (dotted lines).
Ru: black, N: dark grey, C: grey, Cl: light grey, and H: white.

CONCLUSION

Based upon the activation of reduction hypothesis, physiological reducing agents (GSH and AA) were capable of reducing KP1019, whereas - at identical concentrations and ratios - AA, the extracellular reducing agent caused faster reduction than GSH, the main intracellular reducing agent. Binding of KP1019 towards GMP was enhanced when GSH was added to a mixture of GMP: KP1019 = 2: 1 at pH 6.0 and 7.4. Due to precipitation, especially at pH 7.4, reduction and binding of GMP are limited to a small time frame and complicate quantitative statements. Crystal structure of the KP1019 adduct with 9-methyladenine as ligand showed that two complex molecules are sticked together via hydrogen bondings between the amino-group and N^1 of 9-methyladenine in the same manner as Watson-Crick interactions in DNA. This finding may assert the preference for coordination towards N^7, although the basicity of N^1 is more pronounced and should therefore be the favoured target for coordination.

REFERENCES

1. Galanski M, Arion V B, Jakupec M A, Keppler B K. Recent Developments in the Field of Tumor-Inhibiting Metal Complexes. *Curr Pharm Design* 2003; 9: 2078-2089.
2. Schluga P, Hartinger C G, Egger A, Reisner E, Galanski M, Jakupec M A, Keppler B K. Redox behavior of tumor-inhibiting ruthenium(III) complexes and effects of physiological reductants on their binding to GMP. *Dalton Trans* 2006; in press.
3. Clarke M J. Ruthenium metallopharmaceuticals. *Coord Chem Rev* 2003; 236: 209-233.
4. Millis K K, Weaver K H, Rabenstein D L. *J Org Chem* 1993; 58: 4144.
5. Frasman G D. *CRC Handbook of Biochemistry and Molecular Biology*, Cleveland: CRC Press, 1976: 122.
6. Ravera M, Cassino C, Baracco S, Osella D. New Insights into the Redox Chemistry of Ruthenium Metallopharmaceuticals: The Electrochemical Behaviour of [LH][*trans*-$Ru^{III}Cl_4L_2$] (L=imidazole or indazole) Complexes. *Eur J Inorg Chem* 2006; 740-746.
7. Küng A, Pieper T, Wissiack R, Rosenberg E, Keppler B K. Hydrolysis of the tumor-inhibiting ruthenium(III) complexes *trans*-$[RuCl_4(im)_2]^-$ and *trans*-$[RuCl_4(ind)_2]^-$ investigated by means of HPCE and HPLC-MS. *J Biol Inorg Chem* 2001; 6: 292-299.
8. Egger A, Arion V B, Reisner E, Cebrian-Losantos B, Shova S, Trettenhahn G, Keppler B K. Reactions of Potent Antitumor Complex *trans*-$[Ru^{III}Cl_4(indazole)_2]^-$ with a DNA-Relevant Nucleobase and Thioethers: Insight into Biological Action. *Inorg Chem* 2005; 44: 122-132.

ACKNOWLEDGEMENT

This work was supported by the Austrian Science Fund (FWF), the Austrian Council for Research and Technology Development, Faustus Forschung Translational Drug Development AG and COST.

Markus Galanski is gratefully acknowledged for measuring ^1H NMR kinetics.

Metal Ions in Biology and Medicine: vol. 9. Eds Maria Carmen Alpoim, Paula Vasconcellos Morais, Maria Amélia Santos, Armando J. Cristóvão, José A. Centeno, Philippe Collery.
John Libbey Eurotext, Paris © 2006 pp. 30-1.

Divergent effects of complexation with gallium(III) or iron(III) on the antitumor potency of 2-acetylpyridine-^4N-dimethylthiosemicarbazone

Eichinger Renè, Kowol Christian R., Arion Vladimir B., Jakupec Michael A., Keppler Bernhard K.

Institute of Inorganic Chemistry, University of Vienna, Waehringer Strasse 42, 1090 Vienna, Austria

INTRODUCTION

α-*N*-Heterocyclic thiosemicarbazones have been explored for their applicability as antitumor agents for about half a century [1]. Their main target was identified as the enzyme ribonucleotide reductase [2]. They are known to be the strongest inhibitors of this enzyme that catalyzes the conversion of ribonucleotides to deoxyribonucleotides, making the enzyme crucial for rapidly proliferating cells like tumor cells, where it is highly expressed. Inhibition of this enzyme results in the depletion of cellular deoxyribonucleotide pools, disruption of DNA synthesis, cell cycle arrest in the S phase and, in the case of irreversible cell damage, induction of apoptosis. Ribonucleotide reductase is composed of two subunits (R1, R2) that are binding the substrates and allosteric effectors as well as iron stabilizing the active centre, which consists of a tyrosyl radical.

Originally the activity of α-*N*-heterocyclic thiosemicarbazones has been explained by their iron-chelating properties, either by coordination of iron from the active center of ribonucleotide reductase or by formation of an iron chelate which then inhibits the enzyme, implying that iron complexes might be the actually active species. The observation that the preformed iron(II) chelates are more potent inhibitors of ribonucleotide reductase in the absence of additional iron than the uncomplexed thiosemicarbazones supports the latter hypothesis [2, 3]. On the other hand, it was proposed that oxidation of the ferrous form of the iron chelate results in the destruction of the catalytically active tyrosyl radical of the enzyme by a one-electron reduction [4]. Furthermore it has been reported that 3-aminopyridine-2-carboxaldehyde-thiosemicarbazone (3-AP, triapine) induces iron-dependent free radical damage, behaving distinctly different from classic iron-chelating drugs [5]. The major problem encountered in the development of α-*N*-heterocyclic thiosemicarbazones is their high general toxicity and their low therapeutic index. Anyway, 3-aminopyridine-2-carboxaldehyde-thiosemicarbazone (3-AP, triapine) entered the clinical stage of development with the well-founded prospect of overcoming these problems [6].

Gallium(III) is able to inhibit the activity of ribonucleotide reductase and is endowed with clinically useful antiproliferative properties [7]. Due to its ability to compete with iron(III), gallium(III) can interact directly with ribonucleotide reductase, displacing iron from the R2 subunit of the enzyme [8]. The rationale for preparing gallium(III) complexes of α-*N*-heterocyclic thiosemicarbazones is based on the fact that it would be a possible way to produce highly potent ribonucleotide reductase inhibitors that benefit from a cooperative action of the two components. A prototypic gallium complex with 2-acetylpyridine-^4N-dimethylthiosemicarbazone has been shown to be highly cytotoxic to cancer cells, with IC_{50} values being in the low nanomolar range [9]. The concentration-effect curves of this complex closely parallel that of the uncomplexed thiosemicarbazone, indicating that the pharmacologic properties of the complex are largely governed by the ligand. However, the observed increase in cytotoxic potency gained by complexation with gallium seemed explainable by the metal-to-ligand stoichiometry of 1:2, raising the question whether gallium(III) makes a specific contribution to the biological activity or whether the same effect might be achieved by complexation to iron.

METHODS

The ligand 2-acetylpyridine ^4N-dimethyl thiosemicarbazone (HL) has been prepared as described in the literature [10].

Synthesis of $[GaL_2][PF_6]$

To a solution of 2-acetylpyridine-^4N-dimethyl thiosemicarbazone in dry ethanol a solution of gallium(III) nitrate in ethanol was added in 2:1 molar ratio at room temperature. After the addition of 2 equiv ammonium hexafluorophosphate yellow precipitate was formed. The precipitate was filtered off, washed with ethanol and dried *in vacuo*. Yield: 0.27 g (91%). Anal. (%) calcd for $C_{20}H_{26}N_8S_2GaPF_6$ (M_r = 657.29 g/mol): C, 36.55; H, 3.99; N, 17.05. Found,%: C, 36.28; H, 3.86; N, 16.80. ^1H NMR (400.13 MHz, dmso-d_6): d = 8.25-8.20 (m, 4H, py), 7.92 (d, 2H, py), 7.60-7.54 (m, 2H, py), 3.25 (br. s, 12H, $N(CH_3)_2$), 2.83 (s, 6H, CCH_3).

Synthesis of $[FeL_2][PF_6]$

To a solution of 2-acetylpyridine-^4N-dimethyl thiosemicarbazone in ethanol iron(III) nitrate nonahydrate was added in 2:1 molar ratio at room temperature. To the black solution 2 equiv ammonium hexafluorophosphate were added and the mixture stirred for 1.5 h at room temperature and subsequently refluxed for 1 h. After the reaction mixture cooled down to room temperature the black precipitate was filtered off, washed with ethanol and dried *in vacuo*. Yield: 0.32 g (72%). Anal. (%) calcd for $C_{20}H_{26}N_8S_2FePF_6$ (M_r = 657.29 g/mol): C, 37.33; H, 4.07; N, 17.42. Found,%: C, 37.03; H, 3.86; N, 17.20. ESI-MS in H_2O (positive), *m/z*: 498, $[FeL_2]^+$. Crystals suitable for X-ray data collection were obtained from chloroform saturated with *n*-hexane.

Cell Culture and MTT-Assay

Cytotoxicity was determined by means of a colorimetric microculture assay (MTT assay, MTT = 3-(4,5-dimethyl-2-thiazolyl)-2,5-diphenyl-2H-tetrazolium bromide). 41M (ovarian carcinoma) and SK-BR-3 (mammary carcinoma) cells were grown in Minimal Essential Medium (MEM) supplemented with 10% heat-inactivated fetal bovine serum, 1 mM sodium pyruvate, 2 mM *L*-glutamine and 1% non-essential amino acids (100×) (all purchased from Gibco/Invitrogen). Cultures were maintained at 37 °C in a humidified atmosphere containing 5% CO_2. They were harvested from culture flasks by trypsinization and seeded into 96-well microculture plates (Iwaki). A cell density of 4×10^3 cells/well was chosen in order to ensure exponential growth throughout drug exposure. After a 24 h pre-incubation, cells were exposed to solutions of the test compounds in 200 μL/well complete culture medium for 96 hours. For this purpose, the compounds were dissolved in DMSO and then serially diluted in complete culture medium such that the effective DMSO content did not exceed 0.05%. At the end of exposure, drug solutions were replaced by 100 μL/well RPMI1640 culture medium (supplemented with 10% heat-inactivated fetal bovine serum, 1 mM sodium pyruvate and 4 mM *L*-glutamine) plus 20 μL/well MTT solution in phosphate-buffered saline (5 mg/ml PBS). After incubation for 4 hours, the medium/MTT mixtures were removed, and the formazan crystals formed by the mitochondrial dehydrogenase activity of vital cells were dissolved in 150 μL DMSO per well. Optical densities at 550 nm were measured with a microplate reader (Tecan Spectra Classic). The quantity of vital cells was expressed in terms of T/C values by comparison to untreated control microcultures, and IC_{50} values were calculated from concentration-effect curves by interpolation. Evaluation is based on means from at least three independent experiments, each comprising six microcultures per concentration level.

RESULTS AND DISCUSSION

Crystal Structure

Perspective views of [bis-(2-acetylpyridine-^4N-dimethyl thiosemicarbazonato)-*N,N,S*-iron(III)] hexafluorophosphate ($[FeL_2][PF_6]$) with the labeling schemes are shown in *fig. 1*. The iron atom is coordinated by the two approximately planar tridentate ligands. The coordination polyhedron approaches an octahedron, where the two ligands are bound to Fe atom through a nitrogen atom of the pyridine ring, and a nitrogen and sulfur atom of the thiosemicarbazide group in a meridional arrangement. In comparison the deviation of the coordination polyhedron from the ideal octahedron of the corresponding gallium(III) complex with $[GaCl_4]^-$ as counter ion [9] is more evident, the angle <N2-Ga1-N6 is at 171.18(9)° compared to <N2-Fe1-N6 = 176.08(7)°.

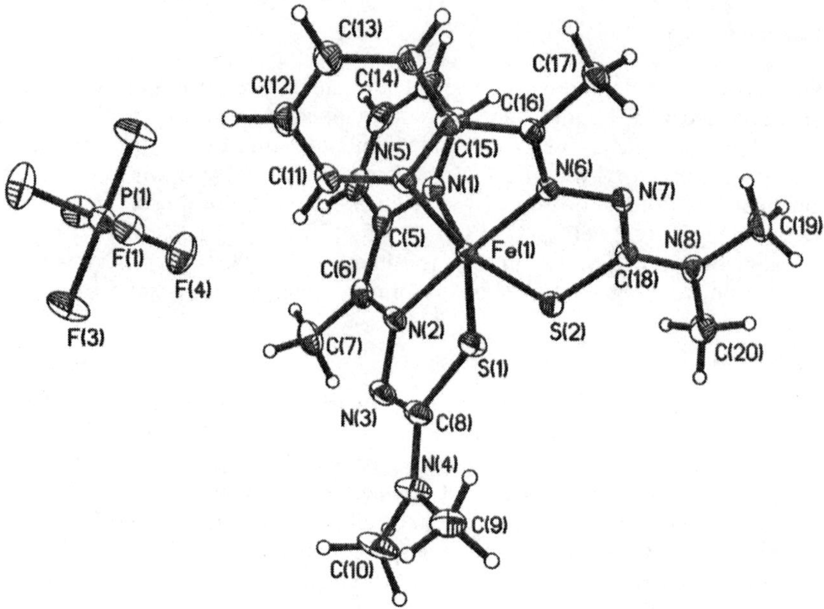

Fig. 1. ORTEP drawing of $[FeL_2][PF_6]$ (HL = 2-acetylpyridine ^4N-dimethyl thiosemicarbazone) with thermal ellipsoids depicted at 50% probability.

Cytotoxicity Testing

The cytotoxic potencies of the thiosemicarbazone (2-acetylpyridine ^4N-dimethylthiosemicarbazone (HL)) and the complexes $[GaL_2]PF_6$ and $[FeL_2]PF_6$ were investigated in the human tumor cell lines 41M (ovarian carcinoma) and SK-BR-3 (mammary carcinoma). Generally, 41M cells are more sensitive to the test compounds, giving 5-10 times smaller IC_{50} values than SK-BR-3 cells. Both the complexes and the ligand have very high cytotoxic potencies, with IC_{50} values ranging from picomolar to nanomolar concentrations *(table 1)*.

Table 1. IC_{50} values (nM; means ± standard) deviations after 96 h of incubation with the introduced compounds. Values were obtained from at least three independent experiments

	41M	SK-BR-3
$[GaL_2][PF_6]$	0.053±0.017	0.43±0.25
$[FeL_2][PF_6]$	126±32.3	452±36.3
HL	0.22±0.13	2.7±1.4

Concentration-effect curves of both the complexes and HL are rather flat, gently declining over a range of three orders of magnitude *(fig. 2)*, which contrasts with the steep concentration-effect curves usually observed with classic platinum drugs and many other tumor-inhibiting metal compounds. This suggests that the mode of action is mainly governed by the thiosemicarbazone ligands, which are highly cytotoxic themselves, while complexation to metal ions rather serves to modulate the cytotoxic potency. Nevertheless, the modulating effects of the central metal ion on the cytotoxic potency of HL are very pronounced. Complexation to iron(III) weakens the cytotoxic properties to a remarkable extent. IC_{50} values for the iron(III) complex are at 130 and 450 nM for the two cell lines 41M and SK-BR-3, respectively, indicating an about 170 to 500-fold lower cytotoxicity than that of the uncomplexed ligand. In contrast, complexation to gallium(III) increases the cytotoxicity 4-6 times, which is higher than could be explained by the stoichiometry (considering that the complex contains two ligand molecules).

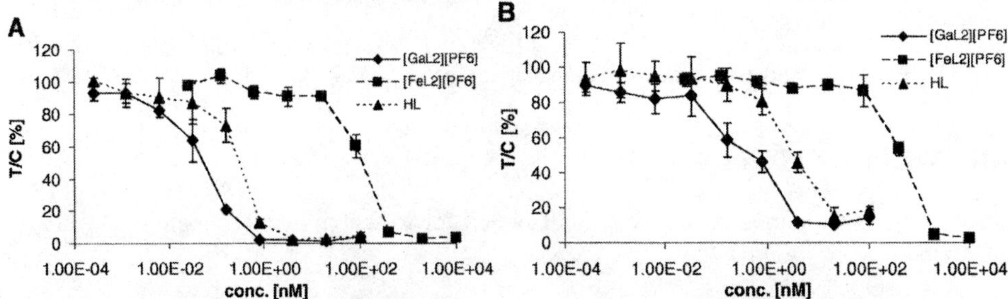

Fig. 2. Concentration-effect curves of 2-acetylpyridine-^4N-dimethylthiosemicarbazone and its gallium(III) and iron(III) complexes, obtained by the MTT assay in **(A)** 41M and **(B)** SK-BR-3. In both cell lines. HL (▲) is less toxic than its gallium complex (◆) but much more toxic than the iron complex (■).

While in the case of the gallium complex with 2-acetylpyridine-^4N-dimethylthiosemicarbazone with tetrachlorogallate(III) as the counterion [9], structural rearrangements in solution resulting in a mixture of species with 1:2 and 1:1 metal-to-ligand stoichiometry had been recognized, the complexes presented here are not susceptible to such rearrangements. The work presented here clearly indicates that gallium(III) is able to enhance the cytotoxicity of α-*N*-heterocyclic thiosemicarbazones to an extent largely exceeding that of mere stoichiometric effects, whereas complexation to iron(III) is not only disadvantageous in comparison to gallium(III), but even results in a marked attenuation of the activity by about two orders of magnitude. This is in sharp contrast to the enhancing effects of complexation with iron(III) on the cytotoxicity and the ribonucleotide reductase-inhibitory potency (in the absence of external iron) of 2-formylpyridine- and 1-formylisoquinoline-thiosemicarbazone [3][4]. The increase of cytotoxicity obtained with complexation with gallium(III) can be ascribed to gallium and seems not to be the result of complexation in general or the geometry of the complex.

Whether the conclusions drawn from our in vitro findings, in particular the favorable effects of complexation with gallium(III), can be transferred to the in vivo setting is subject to ongoing studies in animal tumor models.

REFERENCES

1. R.W. Brockman, J.R. Thomson, M.J. Bell, H.E. Skipper, Observations on the antileukemic activity of pyridine-2-carboxaldehyde thiosemicarbazone and thiocarbohydrazone. *Cancer Res* 1956; 16: 167-170.
2. Moore E.C., Sartorelli A.C., Inhibition of ribonucleotide reductase by alpha-(N)-heterocyclic carboxaldehyde thiosemicarbazones. *Pharm Ther* 1984; 24: 439-447.
3. Saryan L. A., Ankel E., Krishnamurti C., Petering D. H. Comparative cytotoxic and biochemical effects of ligands and metal complexes of α-*N*-heterocyclic carboxaldehyde thiosemicarbazones. *J Med Chem* 1979; 22: 1218-1221.
4. Thelander L., Gräslund A. Mechanism of inhibition of mammalian ribonucleotide reductase by the iron chelate of 1-formylisoquinoline thiosemicarbazone. Destruction of the tyrosine free radical of the enzyme in an oxygen-requiring reaction. *J Biol Chem* 1983; 258: 4063-4066.
5. Chaston T. B., Lovejoy D. B., Watts R. N., Richardson D. R. Examination of the antiproliferative activity of iron chelators: multiple cellular targets and different mechanism of action of triapine compared with desferrioxamine and the potent pyridoxal isonicotinoyl hydrazone analogue 311. *Clin Cancer Res* 2003; *9*: 402-414.
6. Wadler S., Makower D., Clairmont C., Lambert P., Fehn K., Sznol M. Phase I and Pharmacokinetic Study of the Ribonucleotide Reductase Inhibitor, 3-Aminopyridine-2-Carboxaldehyde Thiosemicarbazone, Administered by 96-Hour Intravenous Continuous Infusion. *J Clin Oncol* 2004; 22: 1553-1563.
7. Jakupec M. A., Keppler B. K. Gallium in cancer treatment. *Curr. Top. Med Chem* 2004; 4: 1575-1583.
8. Narasimhan J., Antholine W. E., Chitambar C. R. Effect of gallium on the tyrosyl radical of the iron-dependent M2 subunit of ribonucleotide reductase. *Biochem Pharmacol* 1992; 44: 2403-2408.
9. Arion V.B., Jakupec M.A., Galanski M., Unfried P., Keppler B.K. Synthesis, structure, spectroscopic and in vitro antitumour studies of a novel gallium(III) complex with 2-acetylpyridine (4)N-dimethylthiosemicarbazone. *J Inorg Biochem* 2002; 91: 298-305.
10. Klayman D. L., Scovill J. P., Bartosevich J. F., Mason C. J. 2-Acetylpyridine thiosemicarbazones. 2. N^4, N^4-disubstituted derivatives as potential Antimalarial Agents. *J Med Chem* 1979; 22: 1367-1373.

ACKNOWLEDGEMENT

This work was supported by the Austrian Council for Research and Technology Development and by COST.

Metal Ions in Biology and Medicine: vol. 9. Eds Maria Carmen Alpoim, Paula Vasconcellos Morais, Maria Amélia Santos, Armando J. Cristóvão, José A. Centeno, Philippe Collery.
John Libbey Eurotext, Paris © 2006 pp. 35-1.

New Hydroxypyrimidinones as Inhibitors of Matrix Metalloproteinases

M. Alexandra Esteves[1], Anabela Cachudo[1], Cláudia Ribeiro[1], Sílvia Chaves[2], Armando Rossello[3], M. Amélia Santos[2]

[1]*INETI, Estrada do Paço do Lumiar, 1649-038 Lisboa, Portugal*
[2]*IST, Centro de Química Estrutural, Av. Rovisco Pais, 1049-001 Lisboa, Portugal*
[3]*Dipartimento di Scienze Farmaceutiche, Università degli Studi di Pisa, Via Bonanno 6, 56126 Pisa, Italy*

ABSTRACT

Matrix metalloproteinases (MMPs) are a particular type of endopeptidases, which are known to catalyze the turnover of extra-cellular matrix components, and abnormal MMP activities are linked to the genesis and promotion of serious diseases such as cancer and arthritis.

This work describes a set of results on three new matrix metalloproteinase inhibitors (MMPis) of 1-hydroxy-2(1*H*)-pyrimidinone type with different modifications at the heterocyclic 4-position, including aminoalkylamino and sulfamoyl-alkyl-amino groups. This paper will focus on results of solution studies, namely the acid-base properties and chelating abilities of the compounds towards Zn(II), as well as of bioassays on their enzyme inhibitory activity against several MMPs. The solution equilibrium studies revealed that the hydroxypyrimidinone is the zinc-binding group, independently of the presence of the sulfonamide moiety; the results of preliminary bioassays showed that the inhibitory activity is of micromolar order and it improves with the introduction of the aryl sulfonamide as a side chain substituent of the hydroxypyrimidinone ring, namely for the MMP-2 and MMP-9 gelatinases.

INTRODUCTION

The hydroxypyrimidinones are chelators with high affinity for hard metal ions and recent research has been mostly focused on their potential application as hard metal decontaminants for environmental and pharmacological purposes [1]. Moreover, taking into account that the 1-hydroxy-2(1*H*)-pyrimidinones include an endocyclic hydroxamate functional group and that acyclic hydroxamic acid derivatives are known to be by far the strongest class of MMPis, the assessment of the potential role of hydroxypyrimidinones as MMPis sorted out as an interesting challenge. In fact, these zinc-containing enzymes are involved in several processes associated to matrix degradation, namely tumor cell invasion and joint destruction in arthritic diseases, and so they have been an important target for drug design aimed at the rational MMP inactivation in several disease situations [2]. The inhibition activity is quite determined by the binding strength of the inhibitor molecule to the zinc at the active site, thus explaining the fact that the hydroxamate group is the preferred metal-binding group for the inhibition. However, in order to be highly active and specific, the inhibitors should further include extra-functional groups to enhance their interaction with sub-sites at the neighborhood of the zinc active site and thus their accommodation within the enzyme active site. The incorporation of sulfonamide groups in the scaffold of hydroxamate inhibitors has shown to improve their activity against some MMPs [3].

We have developed a small series of 1-hydroxy-2(1*H*)-pyrimidinones substituted at the 4-position with aminoalkylamino groups, which further included an arylsulfonamide moiety *(fig. 1)*, aimed at achieving eventual enhancements on the enzymatic inhibitory activity of these compounds.

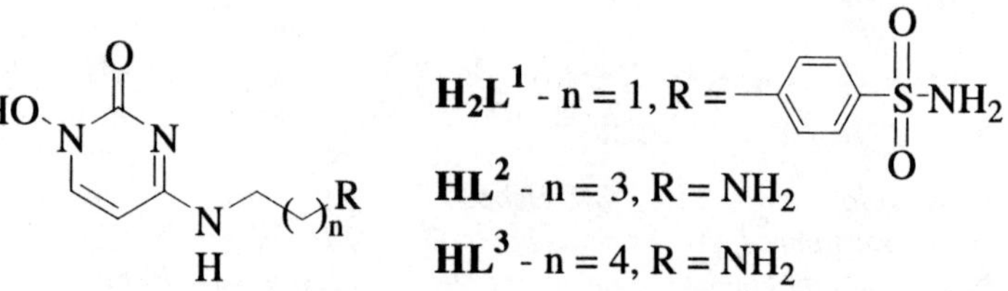

H_2L^1 - n = 1, R = $-C_6H_4-SO_2NH_2$

HL^2 - n = 3, R = NH_2

HL^3 - n = 4, R = NH_2

Fig. 1. Structural formulae for the set of 4-substituted 1-hydroxy-2(1*H*)-pyrimidinones

Herein, we present the results of solution studies of these compounds and their Zn(II) complexes, to evaluate the corresponding coordination modes, as well as the bioassay results on their inhibitory activity against a set of enzymes (MMP-2, -7, -9, -14), to assess their potential as MMP inhibitors and to establish some eventual structure-activity relationships.

MATERIALS AND METHODS

All reagents were of analytical grade and the methods used were according to previously [1, 4]. The general procedure for the preparation of the hydroxypyrimidinone compounds (**H_2L^1, HL^2** and **HL^3**) involved protecting group strategies, prior to the coupling between the heterocycle and the amine side chain, as well as activation of the heterocycle at the point of attachment (4-position) with a triazol group. The last step involved the removal of the protecting groups by standard catalytic hydrogenolysis.

The potentiometric measurements were carried out at $T = 25.0 \pm 0.1$ °C and ionic strength *(I)* of 0.1 M KNO_3 in 5% DMSO aqueous solution. Protonation and stability constants of the zinc(II) complexes were determined by fitting the potentiometric curves with HYPERQUAD 2000 program [5].

The MMP inhibition assays were performed according to the literature, namely in terms of activation of the pro-enzymes, type and concentration of the substrate and methods for controlling the substrate hydrolysis. Percent inhibitions were calculated from control reactions without the inhibitor [6].

RESULTS AND DISCUSSION

Acid-Base properties

All the ligands were obtained as neutral species but they have three dissociable protons in the fully protonated form. The calculated protonation constants (log K_i) for ligands **H_2L^1** and **HL^3** are reported in *table 1*. Based on our previous studies, the sequence of protonation of **H_2L^1** follows the order: terminal primary amine, hydroxyl and 4-imine groups [7]. Also there is a slight increase of the basicity of the proton-labile groups with the length of the alkyl side chain, which can be explained by the increase of electron-donation effects. The protonation constants calculated for **H_2L^1** are identical to those of **HL^3**, except for the first protonation, which is attributed to the sulfonamide group.

Table 1. Stepwise protonation constants (log K_i) of H_2L^1 and HL^3 and global formation constants of the corresponding Zn(II) complexes

Ligand	H_iL log K_i	$Zn_pH_qL_r$ (pqr) log $\beta_{Zn_pH_qL_r}$
$\mathbf{H_2L^1}$	10.16(1) 7.09(2) 2.90(2)	(101) 6.85(4) (111) 15.07(2) (122) 29.20(3) (201) 9.81(2)*
$\mathbf{HL^3}$	10.45(1) 7.11(3) 2.99(3)	(111) 15.30(1) (122) 29.59(2)

* Value obtained from the potentiometric titration curve with 2-fold zinc excess (C_L/C_{Zn} = 0.5)

Zinc complexation

Potentiometric titrations of Zn(II) with $\mathbf{H_2L^1}$ and $\mathbf{HL^3}$ were performed at 1:1, 1:2 and 2:1 metal-to-ligand molar ratios. The values calculated for the global formation constants of the complexes *(table 1)* reveal that this set of compounds is able to form very stable complexes with Zn(II). Moreover, the solution complexation studies of $\mathbf{H_2L^1}$ with Zn(II) indicates the formation of 1:1 ($ZnHL^1$ and ZnL^1) and 1:2 ($ZnH_2L^1_2$) species, involving only the hydroxamate moiety, according to what is observed for $\mathbf{HL^3}$. The interaction of Zn(II) with the sulfamoyl group is only detected in the presence of a two-fold metal ion excess (see *fig.* 2).

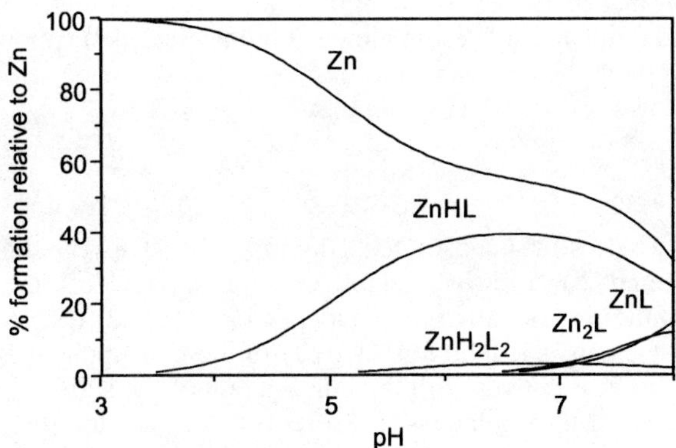

Fig. 2. Species distribution diagram for the Zn(II)/ $\mathbf{H_2L^1}$ system ($C_L = 7 \times 10^{-4}$ M, C_L/C_{Zn} = 0.5)

MMP inhibition

The bioassay results depicted in *table 2* show that the inhibitory activities of these hydropyrimidinone ligands against MMP-2, MMP-7, MMP-9 and MMP-14 are of micromolar order. The similarity presented by the inhibitory activity of these compounds as well as the results of solution studies indicate that the endocyclic hydroxamate groups should be responsible for the interaction with the Zn cofactor. The improvements observed for the sulfonamide derivative, namely against MMP-2 and MMP-9, may be due to a better accommodation of the inhibitor to the enzyme active site, as a result of extra interactions, through either H-bonding with the sulfonamide oxygen atoms or binding of the aryl group with the enzyme lipophilic sub-sites.

Table 2. Inhibitory activity (%) of H_2L^1, HL^2 and HL^3 towards a series of MMPs

Ligand	MMP-2		MMP-7		MMP-9		MMP-14	
H_2L^1	100 μM	86%	100 μM	38 %	100 μM	67%	100 μM	48%
	30 μM	19.6%			10 μM	9%		
	3 μM	7.4%			1 μM	6%		
HL^2	300 μM	88%	100 μM	29%	100 μM	26%	100 μM	28%
	3 μM	22%	3 μM	9%	3 μM	6%		
	30nM	16%			30nM	1%		
HL^3	100 μM	24%	100 μM	30%	100 μM	23%	100 μM	42%
	3 μM	9%	3 μM	1%	3 μM	3%	3 μM	7%

Noteworthy is the fact that, at our best knowledge, this is the first reported example of MMP inhibitors based on the hydroxypyrimidinone compounds. On the other hand, the MMP inhibitory activity of these compounds seems to be determined by a secondary hydroxamic acid as the zinc binding group (ZBG) but only primary hydroxamic acids are known to be strong MMP inhibitors [8]. Therefore, the important role of the N-H proton on the potent activity of primary hydroxamic acid inhibitors, through the establishment of a strong hydrogen bond with enzyme aminoacid residues at the active site, must be overcome, in the hydroxypyrimidinone derivatives, by some other type of binding modes. Furthermore, the fact that these compounds, as endocyclic secondary hydroxamic acids, are much more stable than the acyclic primary derivatives, and thus with higher potential bioavailability, makes the development of new hydroxypyrimidinones a major challenge for virtual screening and rational drug design aimed at biomedical applications. Further studies are presently on course.

CONCLUSIONS

Solution studies on a series of 4-substituted 1-hydroxy-2-(1*H*)-pyrimidinone derivatives have shown that these compounds can form very stable complexes with Zn^{2+}, the heterocyclic α keto-*N*-hydroxy moiety being the zinc-binding group, independently of the presence of sulfamoyl groups in the scaffold of the side chain. The inhibitory activity of these compounds against several MMPs is of micromolar order and it improves with the introduction of the sulfonamide group, namely in the cases of MMP-2 and MMP-9 gelatinases. Moreover, the fact that the hydroxypyrimidones present much higher bioavailability than the primary hydroxamic acids makes these compounds interesting targets for drug design.

REFERENCES

1. Esteves MA, Cachudo A, Chaves S, Santos MA. Synthesis and metal-complexing properties of a new hydroxypyrimidinone-functionalized sepharose. *Eur J Inorg Chem* 2005: 597-605.
2. Whittaker M, Floyd CD, Brown P, Gearing AJH. Design and therapeutic application of matrix metalloproteinase inhibitors. *Chem Rev* 1999; 99: 2735-2776.
3. Marques S, Chaves S, Scozzafava A, Supuran CT, Rossello A, Santos MA. Carbonic Anhydrase and Matrix Metalloproteinase Inhibitors. Sulfonamide Incorporating Iminodiacetic and Hydroxamate Moieties. *Eurobic-7*; Garmisch-Partenkirchen, Germany, 29, 2004.
4. Boyd SA, Fung KL, Baker WR, Mantei RA, Stein HH, Cohen J, Barlow JL, Klinghofer V, Wessale JL,

Verburg KM, Polakowski JS, Adler AL, Calzadilla SV, Kovar P, Yao Z, Hutchins CW, Denissen JF, Grabowski BA, Cepa S, Hoffman DJ, Garren KW, Kleinert HD. Nonpeptide renin inhibitors with good intraduodenal bioavailability and efficacy in dog. *J Med Chem* 1994; 37: 2991-3007.

5. Gans P, Sabatini A and Vacca A. Investigation of equilibria in solution. Determination of equilibrium constants with the HYPERQUAD suite program. *Talanta* 1996; 43: 1739-1753.
6. Rossello A, Nuti E, Orlandini E, Carelli P, Rapposelli S, Macchia M, Minutolo F, Carbonaro L, Albini A, Benelli R, Cercignani G, Murphy G and Balsamo A. New N-arylsulfonyl-N-alkoxyaminoacetohydroxamic acids as selective inhibitors of gelatinase A (MMP-2). *Bioorg & Med Chem* 2004; 12: 2441-2450.
7. Esteves MA, Cachudo A, Chaves S, Santos MA. Synthesis and complexing properties of new 4-aminoalkyl hydroxypyrimidinone ligands. *XIX Encontro Nacional da Sociedade Portuguesa de Química*, Coimbra, Portugal, 2004, QO6.
8. Santos MA, Marques S, Gil M, Tegoni M, Scozzafava A, Supuran CT. Protease inhibitors: synthesis of bacterial collagenase and matrix metalloproteinase inhibitors incorporating succinyl hydroxamate and iminodiacetic acid hydroxamate moieties. *J Enzyme Inhibit & Med Chem* 2003; 18: 233-242.

Metal Ions in Biology and Medicine: vol. 9. Eds Maria Carmen Alpoim, Paula Vasconcellos Morais, Maria Amélia Santos, Armando J. Cristóvão, José A. Centeno, Philippe Collery.
John Libbey Eurotext, Paris © 2006 pp. 40-1.

Ruthenium(II)-arene complex with heterocyclic ligands as prospective antitumor agent

John Roland O., Arion Vladimir B., Jakupec Michael A., Keppler Bernhard K.

Institute of Inorganic Chemistry, University of Vienna, Waehringer Strasse 42, 1090 Vienna, Austria

INTRODUCTION

Side-effects and resistances developed against platinum drugs during the cancer therapy forces scientists to search for new metal-based substances for the treatment of malignant tumor. The preclinical anticancer activity of ruthenium complexes has been well documented in the literature [1]. The lower general toxicity of ruthenium complexes as compared to that of cisplatin has been attributed to the ability of ruthenium compounds to accumulate in cancer tissue and to their likely activation by reduction under hypoxic conditions.

In recent years ruthenium(II)-arene complexes entered the field of anticancer research and have been investigated for their ability to inhibit cancer cell growth. Some ruthenium(II)-arene compounds with ethane-1,2-diamine (en) as a bidentate co-ligand have already been reported by Sadler and co-workers as efficient antiproliferative agents in a number of tumor cell lines [2]. Organoruthenium complexes with various arene ligands and 1,3,5-triaza-7-phosphaadamantane (PTA) have been prepared by Dyson's group [3].

Our aim was to synthesize a different type of ruthenium(II)-arene complex with heterocyclic ligands, such as pyrazole (Hpz) and 8-quinolinole (oxine),especially since antitumor activities have been documented for oxine complexes of gallium, tin and bismuth [4].

SYNTHESES AND CHARACTERIZATION

General

All manipulations were performed under an inert atmosphere of argon by using Schlenck techniques. All chemicals were standard reagent grade and used without further purification. The solvents were purified according to standard procedures [5]. The deuterated solvents were purchased from Aldrich and dried over 4 Å molecular sieves.

$[Ru(\eta^6\text{-}p\text{-cymene})Cl_2]_2$ [6], K[oxine] [7] and $Ru(\eta^6\text{-}p\text{-cymene})(oxine)(\kappa^1(O)\text{-}CF_3SO_3)$ **(2)** [8] have been prepared according to the literature. A simplified procedure for $Ru(\eta^6\text{-}p\text{-cymene})(oxine)Cl$ **(1)** and an improved synthesis of $[Ru(\eta^6\text{-}p\text{-cymene})(oxine)(\kappa^1\text{-Hpz})]CF_3SO_3$ **(3)** is reported.

$Ru(\eta^6\text{-}p\text{-cymene})(oxine)Cl$ (1)

To a suspension of K[oxine] (0.71 g, 32.7 mmol) in ice-cooled CH_2Cl_2 (8 mL), $[Ru(\eta^6\text{-}p\text{-cymene})Cl_2]_2$ (1.0 g, 16.3 mmol) was added stepwise, and the reaction mixture was stirred until the room temperature was reached. Precipitation of an orange product was completed by addition of Et_2O (15 mL). The suspension was transferred to a centrifugation tube and centrifuged at 4000 rpm for 2 min. Afterwards the residue was twice extracted with CH_2Cl_2 (10 mL) and centrifuged. The clear CH_2Cl_2 solution was evaporated to dryness and redissolved in CH_2Cl_2 (10 mL).

Upon addition of Et_2O again an orange precipitate formed, which was washed with Et_2O (4 × 2 mL) and dried in vacuo.

TLC: R_f ((v/v) CH_2Cl_2/Acetone 1:1) = 0.47.

Yield: 1.24 g (92%) orange tan powder.

$C_{19}H_{20}ClNORu$, MW: 414.89	Calc., %:	C, 55.00	H, 4.86	N, 3.38
	Found, %:	C, 54.81	H, 4.86	N, 3.47

NMR ($CDCl_3$, 20 °C): ^{1}H, d = δ 8.93 (bs, 1H, hc^2), 8.09 (d, $^3J_{HH}$ = 8.6 Hz, 1H, hc^4), 7.34 (vt, $^3J_{HH}$ = 7.8 Hz, 1H, hc^6), 7.33 (bs, 1H, hc^3), 7.05 (bd, $^3J_{HH}$ = 7.8 Hz, 1H, hc^5), 6.85 (d, $^3J_{HH}$ = 7.8 Hz, 1H, hc^7), 5.58 (m, 1H, cy), 5.48 (m, 1H, cy), 5.41 (m, 1H, cy), 5.30 (m, 1H, cy), 2.81 (m, 1H, C*H*(Me)$_2$), 2.32 (s, 3H, Me), 1.19 (d, $^3J_{HH}$ = 6.2 Hz, 3H, CH(*Me*)$_2$), 1.16 (d, $^3J_{HH}$ = 6.4 Hz, 3H, CH(*Me*)$_2$);

^{13}C{^{1}H}, δ = 169.0 (hc^8), 149.7 (hc^2), 144.8 (hc^{8a}), 138.1 (hc^4), 130.9 (hc^6), 130.7 (hc^{4a}), 122.5 (hc^3), 115.6 (hc^5), 111.1 (hc^7), 101.8 (cy^1), 99.3 (cy^4), 83.1, 82.5, 81.8, 81.3 (cy^{2,3,5,6}), 31.6 (*C*HMe$_2$), 23.1, 22.7 (CH*Me*$_2$), 19.3 (*Me*).

[Ru(η^6-*p*-cymene)(oxine)(κ^1-Hpz)]CF_3SO_3 (3)

To a solution of Ru(η^6-*p*-cymene)(oxine)Cl (0.10 g, 0.24 mmol) and $AgCF_3SO_3$ (0.065 g, 0.25 mmol) in THF (5 mL) stirred at room temperature for 2 h, pyrazole (0.017 g, 0.24 mmol) was added. After stirring the reaction mixture for 2 h, the solution was filtered and the solvent removed under reduced pressure. The solid residue was dissolved in CH_2Cl_2 (2 mL). Upon addition of Et_2O a yellow precipitate formed, which was collected on a glass frit, washed twice with Et_2O and dried in vacuo.

Yield: 96 mg (67%) bright yellow powder.

$C_{23}H_{24}F_3N_3O_4RuS$, MW: 596.16	Calc., %:	C, 46.31	H, 4.06	N, 7.04	S, 5.37
	Found, %:	C, 46.14	H, 4.04	N, 6.94	S, 5.21

NMR ($CDCl_3$, 20 °C): ^{1}H, δ = 13.00 (bs, 1H, pz^{NH}), 9.60 (d, 1H, $^3J_{HH}$ = 4.5 Hz, hc^2), 8.07 (d, 1H, $^3J_{HH}$ = 8.5 Hz, hc^4), 7.56 (d, 1H, $^3J_{HH}$ = 2.0 Hz, pz ^{3,5}), 7.48 (q, 1H, $^3J_{HH}$ = 4.5 Hz hc^3), 7.39 (d, 1H, $^3J_{HH}$ = 2.0 Hz, pz^{3,5}), 7.32 (t, 1H, $^3J_{HH}$ = 8.0 Hz, hc^6), 7.03 (d, 1H, $^3J_{HH}$ = 8.0 Hz, hc^5), 6.85 (d, 1H, $^3J_{HH}$ = 8.0 Hz, hc^7), 6.12 (m, 1H, pz^4), 6.04 (d, 1H, $^3J_{HH}$ = 6.0 Hz, cy), 5.83 (t, 2H, $^3J_{HH}$ = 7.0 Hz, cy), 5.79 (d, 1H, $^3J_{HH}$ = 6.0 Hz, cy), 2.39 (m, 1H, $^3J_{HH}$ = 6.9 Hz, *CH*(Me$_2$)), 1.87 ((s, 3H, *CH$_3$*), 1.11(d, 3H, J= 6.5 Hz, CH*(Me$_2$)*), and 0.89 (d, 3H, J= 7.0 Hz, CH*(Me$_2$)*);

^{13}C{^{1}H}, d = 167.6 (hc^8), 151.6 (hc^2), 143.3 (hc^{8a}), 140.1 (pz^3), 138.5 (hc^4), 133.4 (pz^5), 130.5 (hc^6), 130.4 (hc^{4a}), 123.1 (hc^3), 114.8 (hc^5), 112.3 (hc^7), 106.8 (pz^4), 103.7 (cy^1), 101.3 (cy^4), 85.1, 82.3, 82.2, 68.1 (cy^{2,3,5,6}), 31.2 (*C*HMe$_2$), 22.8, 21.7 (CH*Me*$_2$), 18.2 (*Me*).

Physical measurements

^{1}H and ^{13}C-{1H} NMR spectra were recorded on a Bruker DPX400 Ultrashield™ Magnet spectrometer at 400.13 and 100.62 MHz.

Elemental analyses were carried out on a Carlo Erba microanalyser at the Microanalytical Laboratory of the University of Vienna. Infrared spectra were obtained from CsI pellets with a Perkin-Elmer FT-IR 2000 instrument (4000-200 cm^{-1}). UV/Vis spectra were recorded on a Perkin-Elmer Lambda 20 UV/Vis-spectrophotometer using samples dissolved in methanol. Electrospray ionization mass spectrometry was carried out with a Bruker Esquire 3000 instrument (Bruker Daltonic, Bremen, Germany). Expected and experimental isotope distributions were compared.

Crystallographic Structure Determination

X-ray data for **3** were collected on a Siemens Smart CCD area detector diffractometer using graphite monochromated MoKa radiation and 0.3° ω scan frames. Corrections for Lorentz and polarization effects, for crystal decay, and for absorption were applied. All structures were solved by direct methods using the program SHELXS97. Structure refinement on F^2 was carried out with program SHELXL97. Non-hydrogen atoms were refined anisotropically. Hydrogen atoms were in most cases inserted in idealized positions and were refined riding with the atoms to which they were bonded.

Cytotocicity tests in cancer cell lines

Cytotoxicity was determined by means of a colorimetric microculture assay (MTT assay, MTT = 3-(4, 5-dimethyl-2-thiazolyl)-2,5-diphenyl-2H-tetrazolium bromide). Colon carcinoma (HT29, SW480) and ovarian carcinoma (A2780, CH1) cells were grown in Minimal Essential Medium (MEM) supplemented with 10% heat-inactivated fetal bovine serum, 1 mM sodium pyruvate, 2 mM L-glutamine and 1% non-essential amino acids (100×) (all purchased from Gibco/Invitrogen). Cultures were maintained at 37 °C in a humidified atmosphere containing 5% CO_2. Cells were harvested from culture flasks by trypsinization and seeded into 96-well microculture plates (Iwaki). The following cell densities were chosen in order to ensure exponential growth throughout drug exposure: 5×10^3 cells/well for A2780 and HT29, 2.5×10^3 cells/well for SW480 and 1.5×10^3 cells/well for CH1. After a 24 h pre-incubation, cells were exposed to solutions of the test compounds in 200 μL/well complete culture medium for 96 hours. For this purpose, freshly made stock solutions of the substance were used, because it is known that metal coordination complexes can undergo ligand substitution reactions with components of the media. At the end of exposure, drug solutions were replaced by 100 μL/well RPMI1640 culture medium (supplemented with 10% heat-inactivated fetal bovine serum) plus 20 μL/well MTT solution in phosphate-buffered saline (5 mg/ml). After incubation for 4 hours, the medium/MTT mixtures were removed, and the formazan crystals formed by the mitochondrial dehydrogenase activity of vital cells were dissolved in 150 μL DMSO per well. Optical densities at 550 nm were measured with a microplate reader (Tecan Spectra Classic). The quantity of vital cells was expressed in terms of T/C values by comparison to untreated control microcultures, and IC_{50} values were calculated from concentration-effect curves by interpolation. Evaluation is based on means from at least three independent experiments, each comprising six microcultures per concentration level.

RESULTS AND DISCUSSION

Under argon atmosphere and using Schlenck techniques, treatment of the precursor [Ru(η^6-*p*-cymene)Cl_2]$_2$ with two equivalents of K[oxine] in ice-cooled CH_2Cl_2 afforded the half sandwich complex Ru(η^6-*p*-cymene)(oxine)Cl (**1**) as an orange air-stable complex in 92% yield *(scheme 1)*.

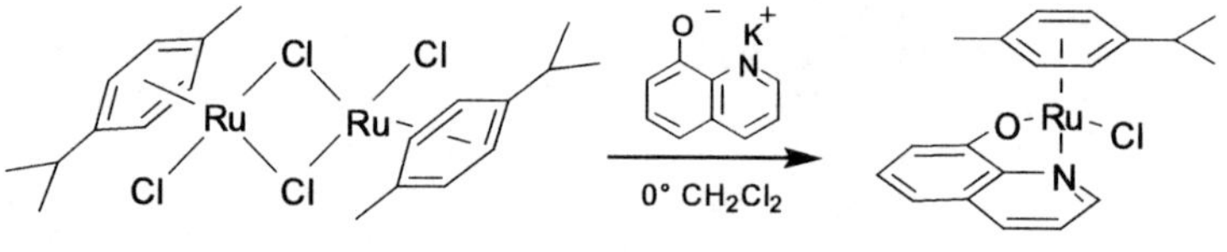

Scheme 1. Synthesis of complex Ru(η^6-*p*-cymene)(oxine)Cl (**1**)

Complex **1** has been characterized by elemental analysis as well as ^1H and $^{13}C\{^1H\}$ NMR spectroscopy. The ^1H NMR spectrum shows six distinct multiplets for the oxine ligand with the chemical shifts and multiplicities in the expected range for N, O-coordination.

The *p*-cymene ligand gives rise to four multiplets centered at 5.58, 5.48, 5.41, and 5.30 ppm, respectively, assignable to the aromatic hydrogen atoms of the *p*-cymene ligand. The methyl groups of the *i*-Pr moiety are diastereotopic, exhibiting two distinct doublets centered at 1.14 and 1.12 ppm. The $^{13}C\{^1H\}$ NMR spectrum is also in agreement with the structure proposed.

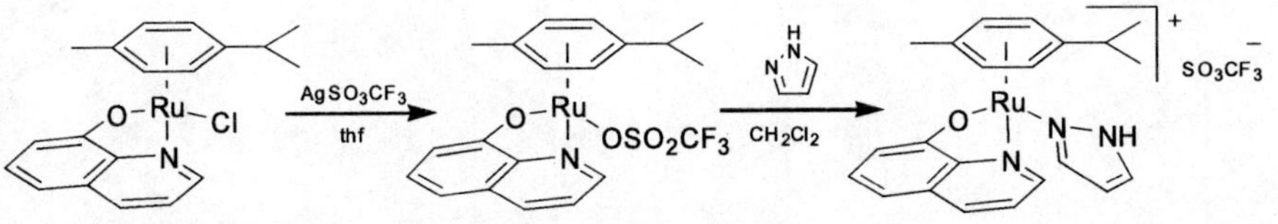

Scheme 2. Preparation of [Ru(η^6-*p*-cymene)(oxine)(κ^1-Hpz)]CF_3SO_3 **(3)**

Substitution of the Cl atom in **1** for the weakly nucleophilic $CF_3SO_3^-$ anion was investigated with the intention of generating a reactive complex bearing a weakly coordinating ligand occupying a latent coordination site. In fact, chloride abstraction from **1** with one equivalent of $AgCF_3SO_3$ affords, on workup, a complex with the formula Ru(η^6-*p*-cymene)(oxine)(CF_3SO_3) **(2)** *(scheme 2)*. This formulation agrees with the elemental analysis and the ^1H and $^{13}C\{^1H\}$ NMR spectra of the 18e complex **1**. However, in view of the ability of $CF_3SO_3^-$ to coordinate to Ru(II) as well as the orange color of the complex (all known 16e half-sandwich complexes of Ru(II) are dark blue to dark violet), we suppose that the formula should be Ru(η^6-*p*-cymene)(oxine)(κ^1(O)-CF_3SO_3). It should be noted that several ruthenium complexes with the κ^1(O)-CF_3SO_3 ligand are known and have even been characterized structurally. The lability of the $CF_3SO_3^-$ ligand in complex **2** was apparent by the reaction with pyrazole as ligand, giving a product of the formula [Ruη?^{6}-*p*-cymene)(oxine)(κ^1-Hpz)]CF_3SO_3 **(3)** (see also *scheme 2*).

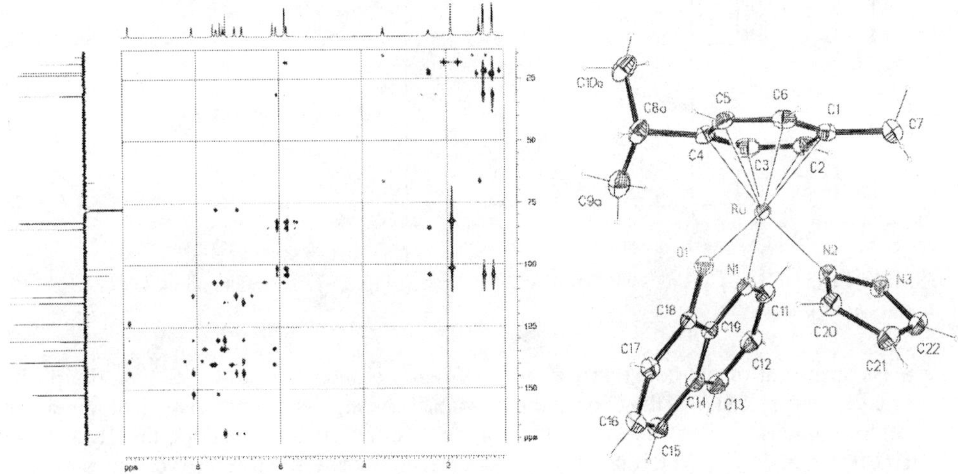

Fig. 1. 2D-NMR spectra of Complex **3**

Fig. 2. ORTEP Diagram of **3**

Compound **3** has been characterized by ESI-MS, UV/Vis-, IR- and NMR-spectroscopy as well as by X-ray crystallography *(fig. 1)*.

An ORTEP diagram is depicted in *fig. 2*. The [Ru(η^6-*p*-cymene)(oxine)(κ^1-Hpz)]CF_3SO_3 complex adopts a three-legged piano stool conformation. The Ru-N(Hpz), Ru-N, and Ru-O distances are 2.118(2), 2.091(2), and 2.063(2) Å, respectively, with N(Hpz)-Ru-N, N(Hpz)-Ru-O, and N-Ru-O angles of 85.1(1), 82.8(1), and 79.4(1)°. In the solid state the compound exhibits an orientation disordered isopropyl group (not shown in *fig. 2*).

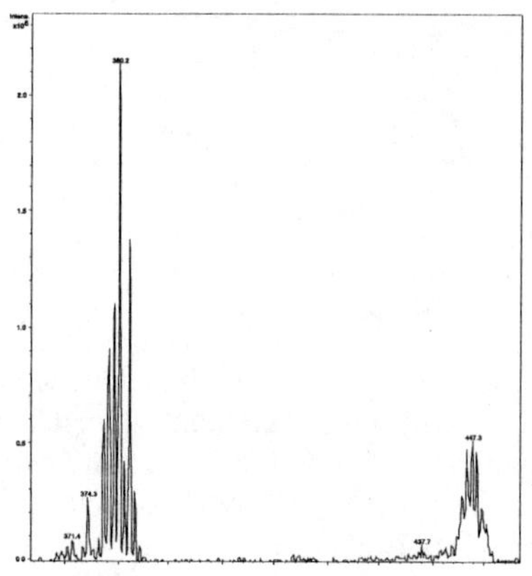

Fig. 3. ESI-MS spectra (positive and negative modes)

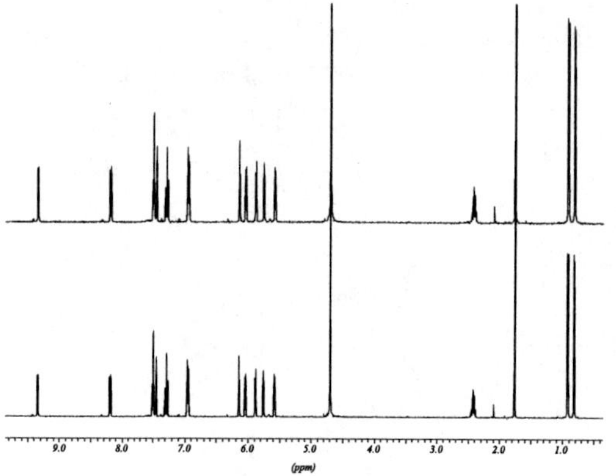

Fig. 4. NMR spectra of **3** in D_2O measured immediately, and 3 months after dissolution

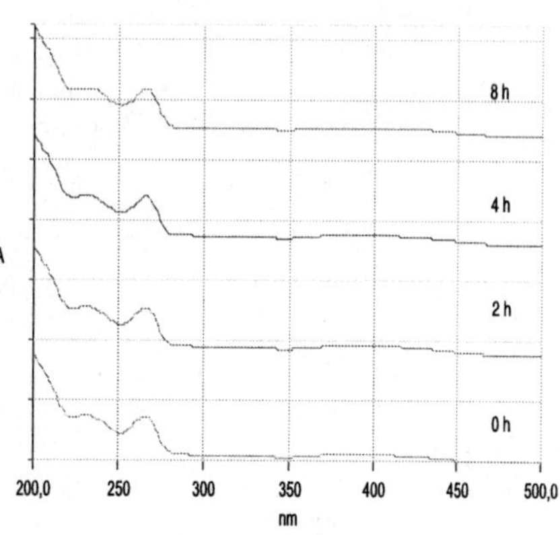

Fig. 5. Time-independent UV/Vis spectra

The mass spectrum of the complex [Ru(η^6-*p*-cymene)(oxine)(κ^1-Hpz)]CF_3SO_3 in the positive mode, displayed in *fig. 3*, shows the expected molecular peak and its characteristic isotopic pattern, but the highest intensity was found for the ion with *m/z* 380 attributed to the [Ru(η^6-*p*-cymene)(oxine)]$^+$ fragment, of which nearly no further decomposition was observed.

Under moderate conditions the complex **3** seemed to be stable, and no change of absorption spectra was found during 8 h in methanol solution *(fig. 5)*. A NMR study within three months showed no hydrolysis of the complex **3** either, in contrast to the behavior reported for ruthenium(II)-arene PTA complexes and Ru(η^6-*p*-cymene)Cl(en)]PF_6.

We were interested to check whether organoruthenium compounds showing no hydrolysis would have cytotoxic effects in tumor cells. So we tested [Ru(η^6-*p*-cymene)(oxine)(κ^1-Hpz)]CF_3SO_3 **(3)** on different colon (HT29, SW480) and ovarian (A2780, CH1) cancer cell lines.

Table 1. IC_{50} values and standard deviations after 96h of incubation

IC50 (µM)	SW480	HT29	CH1	A2780
complex **3**	7.57±1.94	31.69±1.71	5.54±1.22	7.22±1.39
KP1019	40.60±4.02	25.00±2.23	34.4±8.89	n.d.

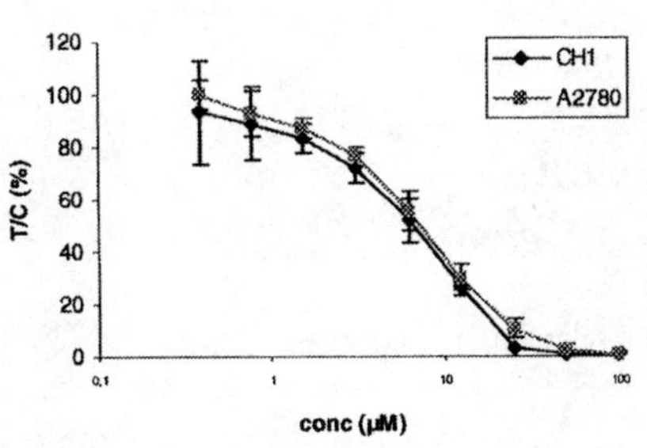

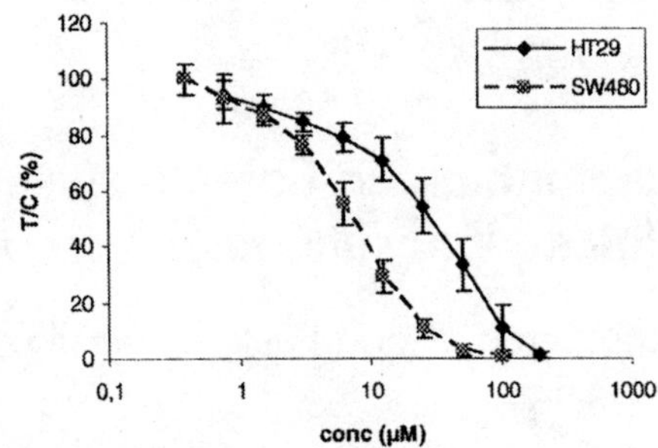

Fig. 6. Concentration-effect curves of [Ru(η^6-*p*-cymene)(oxine)(κ^1-Hpz)]CF_3SO_3 (**3**)

The investigated ovarian cancer cells (A2780, CH1) showed a higher sensitivity to the treatment with the new ruthenium(II)-arene complex **3** than the colon cancer cell lines (HT29, SW480). The IC_{50} values of complex **3** have been compared *(table 1)* to those of KP1019, a ruthenium coordination compound, which was developed in our group and has already successfully completed a clinical phase I trial [9]. Unexpectedly, **3** showed nearly the same (HT29) or up to six times higher cytotoxicity (SW480, CH1) than KP1019, therefore we are intriguingly looking forward for further investigations in preclinical tumor models.

REFERENCES

1. Clarke M J, Ruthenium metallopharmaceuticals, *Coord Chem Rev*, 2003; 236: 209-33.
2. Morris R E, Arid R E, Murdoch P del S, Chen H, Cummings J, Hughes N D, Parsons S, Parkin A, Boyd G, Jodrell D I, Sadler P J, Inhibition of Cancer Cell Growth by Ruthenium(II) Arene Complexes, *J Med Chem* 2001; 44: 3616-21.
3. Scolaro C,Bergamo A, Brescacin L, Delfino R, Cocchietto M, Laurenczy G, Geldbach T J, Sava G, Dyson P J, In Vitro and in Vivo Evaluation of Ruthenium(II)-Arene PTA Complexes, *J Med Chem* 2005; 48: 4161-71.
4. Huang, R, Wallquist A, Covell D G, Anticancer metal compounds in NCI's tumor-screening database: putative mode of action, *Biochemical Pharmacology* 2005; 69: 1009-39.
5. Armarego W L F, Chai C, *Purification of Laboratory Chemicals*, New York, Elsevier, 2003, 609.
6. Bennett M A, Smith A K, Arene ruthenium(II) complexes formed by dehydrogenation by cyclohexadienes with ruthenium(III) trichloride, *J Chem Soc, Dalton Trans* 1974; 2: 233-41.
7. Sue, P; Wetroff, G, Combinations of 8-hydroxyquinoline with alkali metals and zirconium, *Bull soc chim*, 1935; 5: 1002-07.
8. Gemel C, John R, Slugovc C, Mereiter K, Schmid R, Kirchner K, Synthesis and characterization of ruthenium quinolin-8-olate complexes. Unexpected formation of a κ 1-hydrotris(pyrazolyl)borate complex, *Dalton*, 2000; 15: 2607-12.
9. Dittrich C, Scheulen M E, Jaehde U, Kynast B, Gneist M, Richly H, Schaad S, Arion V B, Keppler B K, Phase I and pharmacokinetic study of sodium trans-[tetrachlorobis(1H-indazole)ruthenate(III)] / indazolehydrochloride (1:1.1)(FFC14A, KP1019) in patients with solid tumors - a study of the CESAR Central European Society for Anticancer Drug Research - EWIV, *Proc Am Assoc Cancer Res,* 2005; 46: 472.

ACKNOWLEDGMENT

This work was supported by the Austrian Council for Research and Technology Development and by COST.

Metal Ions in Biology and Medicine: vol. 9. Eds Maria Carmen Alpoim, Paula Vasconcellos Morais, Maria Amélia Santos, Armando J. Cristóvão, José A. Centeno, Philippe Collery.
John Libbey Eurotext, Paris © 2006 pp. 46-1.

Radiolanthanide Complexes with a Novel Bis(methylphosphonate) Tetraazamacrocycle

Sara Lacerda, Maria Paula Campello, Fernanda Marques, Lurdes Gano, Isabel Santos

Departamento de Química, Instituto Tecnológico e Nuclear, Estrada Nacional 10, 2686-953 Sacavém, Portugal

Lanthanide complexes have been considered useful tools for imaging and therapy in magnetic resonance and nuclear medicine. The main goal of this study was the synthesis of radiolanthanide complexes with the novel bis(methylphosphonate) tetraazamacrocycle ligand *trans*-H_6do2a2p (1,4,7,10-tetraazacyclododecane-4,10-bis(carboxymethyl)-1,7-bis(methylphos phonic acid)) and their *in vitro* and *in vivo* biological evaluation to assess the potential clinical interest of these complexes. The novel *trans*-H_6do2a2p was synthesized and characterized by multinuclear NMR spectroscopy (^{1}H, ^{13}C, ^{31}P). ^{153}Sm/^{166}Ho-*trans*-H_6do2a2p complexes were prepared in high yield and their stability and biological behaviour evaluated and compared with the results found for the corresponding complexes with dota and dotp. The negatively charged ^{153}Sm/^{166}Ho-*trans*-do2a2p complexes are hydrophilic, stable under physiological conditions, and present a moderate plasmatic protein binding. A relative high *in vitro* hydroxyapatite adsorption was found for ^{166}Ho-*trans*-do2a2p, while ^{153}Sm-*trans*-do2a2p binds in a lowest percentage. Biodistribution studies in mice indicated that all complexes are stable *in vivo* showing fast tissue clearance from most organs and a rapid total excretion from whole animal body. A moderate bone uptake was observed, which rapidly decreases with time. These results, when compared with the biological profile of ^{153}Sm/^{166}Ho-dota and ^{153}Sm/^{166}Ho-dotp, predict the interest of preparing radiolanthanide complexes with 12-membered tetraazamacrocycles and the possibility of modulating their medical application (internal radiotherapy or bone pain palliation) by changing the nature of the pendant arms.

INTRODUCTION

Tetraazamacrocyclic ligands, due to their cyclic and preorganized nature, form lanthanide complexes with high thermodynamic stability and kinetic inertness. Therefore, the chemistry of lanthanide complexes based on dota (1,4,7,10-tetraazacyclododecane-1,4,7,10-tetraacetic acid) and dotp (1,4,7,10-tetraazacyclododecane-1,4,7,10-tetra(methylenephosphonic acid)) has been largely studied and their potential for biomedical applications, such as magnetic resonance imaging (MRI) or therapy in nuclear medicine, evaluated [1-3]. For MRI, the majority of the approved contrast agents are based on Gd^{3+} complexes, due to the high effective magnetic moment and relatively long electron spin relaxation time of the Gd(III) ion [1]. A variety of agents based on dota or dotp, to treat tumours or as palliative of pain associated to bone metastasis, is under investigation [3].

The selection of a suitable radionuclide and a targeting biomolecule is essential for the design of an effective radiotherapeutic agent. Radionuclides that decay by beta emission have been extensively used for therapeutic applications, and among them radiolanthanides offer a wide range of beta energies and physical half-lifes that can be matched with the biological target and the medical application [3,4].

Macrocycles containing methylcarboxylate pendant arms (*e.g.*, dota) have been proposed as bifunctional agents for labelling biomolecules (peptides or monoclonal antibodies) for targeted radionuclide therapy [5-6]. The *in vitro* and *in vivo* studies of $^{153}Sm/^{166}Ho/^{177}Lu$-dota conjugated to biomolecules indicated that some of these complexes show very promising tumour uptake [7-8]. Macrocycles having methylphosphonate pendant arms are particularly adequate to develop radiopharmaceuticals for bone pain palliation/therapy. In fact, ^{153}Sm-dotp has efficacy in the treatment of painful osseous metastases and ^{166}Ho-dotp appears to be an effective agent for bone marrow ablation in multiple myeloma patients [9-10]. More recently, the ^{166}Ho-tritp complex (tritp = 1,4,7,10-tetraazacyclotridecane-1,4,7,10-tetra(methylenephosphonic acid)) has been reported as a promising candidate for bone targeting, due to its considerable bone uptake [11].

Herein, we report on the synthesis and characterization of the novel *trans*-H_6do2a2p ligand. Data on the *in vitro* and *in vivo* properties of $^{153}Sm/^{166}Ho$-*trans*-do2a2p complexes are also presented and compared with the biological behaviour, in the same animal model, of the well established $^{153}Sm/^{166}Ho$-dota and $^{153}Sm/^{166}Ho$-dotp.

MATERIALS AND METHODS

The bis(methylphosphonate) tetraazamacrocycle, *trans*-H_6do2a2p, was synthesized as previously described [12]. The ligands dota and dotp were obtained from Strem Chemicals. Enriched Sm_2O_3 (98.4% ^{152}Sm) and natural Ho_2O_3 (99.9%) were obtained from Campro Scientific and from Strem Chemicals, respectively. ^{153}Sm and ^{166}Ho were produced by thermal neutron bombardment of isotopically enriched $^{152}Sm(NO_3)_3$ or natural $Ho(NO_3)_3$ in the ITN Portuguese Research Reactor. The radionuclidic purity of the ^{153}Sm and ^{166}Ho solutions was assessed by γ-ray spectrometry, using a Ge (Li) detector coupled to an Accuspec B Canberra multichannel analyser. The radiolabelling efficiency and the stability of the radiocomplexes were assessed by ascending instant thin layer chromatography using silica gel strips (Polygram, Macherey-Nagel). Radioactive distribution on the ITLC strips was detected using a Berthold LB 505 γ detector coupled to a radiochromatogram scanner. The overall complex charge was determined by electrophoresis in 0.1 M Tris-HCl buffer (pH 7.4) for 1 h. Lipophilicity was assessed by determination of the partition coefficient *(P)* *n*-octanol/ saline and expressed as log *P*. Plasmatic protein binding was determined by gel filtration on Sephadex G-25 using saline as eluant, after 1 h incubation. The radioactivity of the samples was measured using a gamma counter (Berthold LB 2111). The biodistribution studies of the radiocomplexes were performed in female CD-1 mice (randomly bred Charles River, from CRIFFA, Spain) weighing approximately 20-22 g after intravenous (i.v.) injection through tail vein at 30 minutes, 2 h and 24 h post administration. Results were expressed as percentage of injected dose per gram of organ (% I.D./ g organ ± SD).

RESULTS AND DISCUSSION

Briefly, the novel *trans*-H_6do2a2p was synthesized by the Mannich reaction of 1,7-bis(acetic acid tert-butyl ester)-1,4,7,10-tetraazacyclododecane with triethylphosphite and dried paraformaldehyde in dry benzene. After work-up, the intermediate 1,7-bis(acetic acid tert-butyl ester)-4,10-bis(methanephosphonic acid diethyl ester)-1,4,7,10-tetraazacyclododecane (**1**) was obtained and its acidic hydrolysis provided 1,4,7,10-tetraazacyclododecane-1,7-bis(carboxymethyl)-4,10-bis(methylphosphonic acid) (*trans*-H_6do2a2p) as a white powder *(scheme 1)*. This compound was then characterized by ^1H, ^{13}C and ^{31}P NMR spectroscopy.

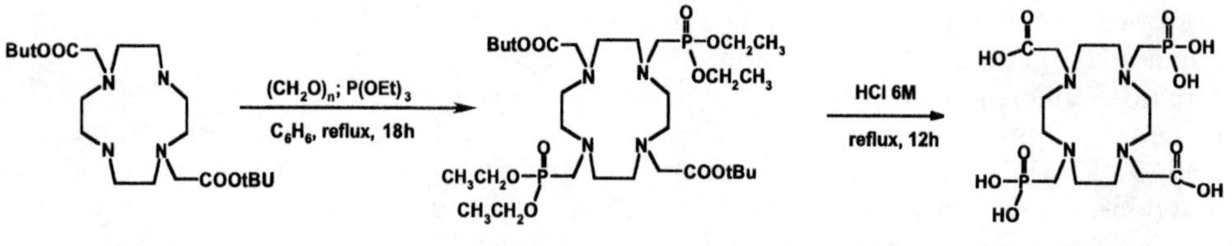

Scheme 1. Synthesis of the compound *trans*-H_6do2a2p

The $^{153}Sm/^{166}Ho$-*trans*-do2a2p complexes were synthesized by reacting $^{153}Sm/^{166}Ho(NO_3)_3$ with *trans*-H_6do2a2p in bidistilled water in a 1:2 metal to ligand molar ratio, at pH 8-9. The complexes were obtained quantitatively (η > 98%) after 2 hours at room temperature or after 30 min at 70°C.

Both complexes are stable up to five days at 37°C in several physiologic solutions, namely in saline and phosphate buffer (pH 7.4), and up to two days in human serum. Their lipo-hydrophilic character and plasmatic protein binding are presented in *table 1*. For comparison, the values determined for the analogues dota and dotp complexes are also shown. As can be seen, all the complexes are hydrophilic and present a low to moderate binding to plasmatic proteins.

Table 1. Human serum protein binding and lipo-hydrophilic character (log *P*) of $^{153}Sm/^{166}Ho$-tetraaza-macrocycles.

Ligand	**^{153}Sm complexes**		**^{166}Ho complexes**	
	% protein binding	log *P*	% protein binding	log *P*
dota	**7.0**	-2.02	1.4	-1.64
trans-do2a2p	**14.6**	-1.93	15	-1.32
dotp	-	-2.00	-	-1.90

The *in vitro* binding of $^{153}Sm/^{166}Ho$-*trans*-do2a2p onto hydroxyapatite (HA), the main mineral component of bone, was studied trying to anticipate the potential of the complexes to be taken *in vivo* by the bone tissue. *Table 2* shows the values found after incubation with 50 mg of HA in Tris-HCl buffer (pH 7.4, 0.1 M). ^{166}Ho-*trans*-do2a2p binds more to HA than ^{153}Sm-*trans*-do2a2p but both present lower and slower HA binding than the ^{153}Sm-dotp complex [9].

Table 2. Comparative study of binding to HA of tetraazamacrocycle phosphonate complexes with radiolanthanides.

Adsortion onto 50mg HA at 1-2 h incubation (%)		
^{153}Sm-dotp[9]	**^{153}Sm-*trans*-do2a2p**	**^{166}Ho-*trans*-do2a2p**
>95%, 2h	~ 13%, 1h	~ 34%, 1h

Although the adsorption values of the *trans*-do2a2p complexes were not very high, in comparison with those of dotp, the stability, log P and protein binding results were encouraging to pursue *in vivo* studies.

Biodistribution of $^{153}Sm/^{166}Ho$-*trans*-do2a2p complexes was evaluated in mice and, just for comparison, the analogues complexes with dota and dotp were also studied using the same animal model. Data for the most relevant organs are graphically presented in *fig. 2 and 3*.

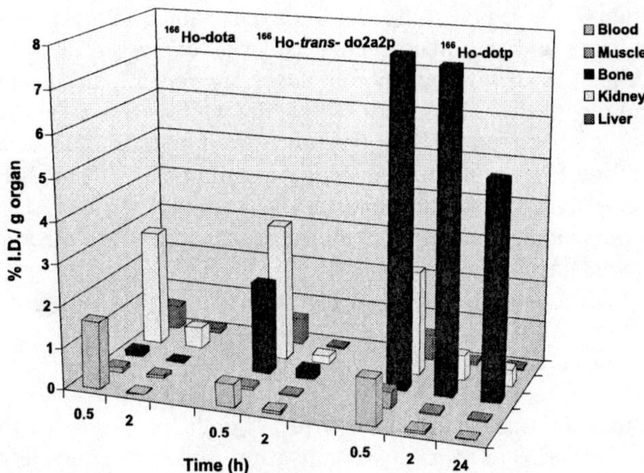

Fig. 2. Biodistribution data (% I.D./g organ) for ^{166}Ho-dota, ^{166}Ho-*trans*-do2a2p and ^{166}Ho-dotp, as a function of time after i.v. administration in CD-1 mice (*n*=4-5).

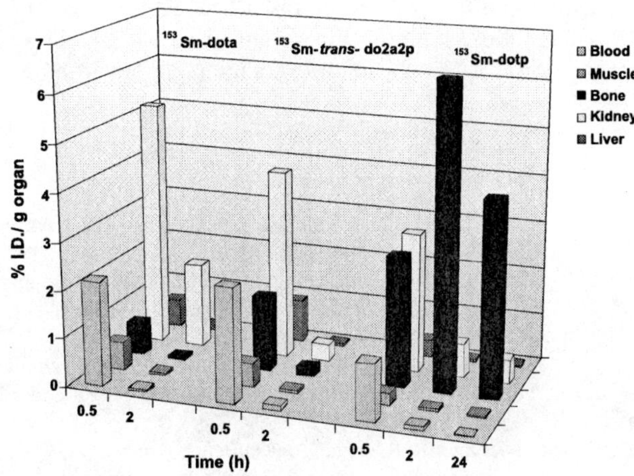

Fig. 3. Biodistribution data (% I.D./g organ) for ^{153}Sm-dota, ^{153}Sm-*trans*-do2a2p and ^{153}Sm-dotp, as a function of time after i.v. administration in CD-1 mice (*n*=4-5).

All complexes undergo a rapid blood and tissue clearance in accordance with their hydrophilic character and low plasmatic protein binding. In general, the *in vivo* behaviour of all the compounds is very similar to the one found for ^{153}Sm/^{166}Ho-dota in the same animal model. At 2 h after administration there is no significant radioactivity retention in any main organ, except in the organs involved in the excretion pathways. Metabolization of the complexes was assessed by urine ITLC analysis making evident their high *in vivo* stability, since they are excreted as intact complexes.The main difference in the biological profile of ^{153}Sm/^{166}Ho-*trans*-do2a2p and ^{153}Sm/^{166}Ho-dota is related with the degree of bone uptake. The moderate bone uptake found for ^{153}Sm/^{166}Ho-*trans*-do2a2p at 30 minutes is due to the presence of two methylphosphonate pendant arms in the molecular structure of the ligand. Nevertheless, the bone uptake is significantly lower than the value found for ^{153}Sm/^{166}Ho-dotp, and rapidly decreases over time, affecting the clinical application of these complexes on bone targeting. In fact, ^{153}Sm-dotp and ^{166}Ho-dotp have a bone uptake of 5.6% and 7.6% two hours after injection and these values increase over time.

Whole body excretion of the radioactivity was assumed as the difference between the measured radioactivity in the injected and sacrificed animal and was expressed as percentage of injected dose (% I.D.). The $^{153}Sm/^{166}Ho$-*trans*-do2a2p complexes are very rapidly excreted (> 93% at 2 h after injection) as found for $^{153}Sm/^{166}Ho$-dota (> 94% at 2h, while $^{153}Sm/^{166}Ho$-dotp present a slower whole body excretion: 79.8 ± 2.3 and 77.7 ± 0.3 for ^{153}Sm-dotp and ^{166}Ho-dota, respectively.

Taking into account the favourable biodistribution profile of the $^{153}Sm/^{166}Ho$-*trans*-do2a2p, in terms of blood clearance, overall excretion and in vivo stability, the chance to modify the type and/or number of phosphonate pendant arms in the basic structure of the macrocyclic ligand could be explored in order to enhance the bone uptake.

CONCLUDING REMARKS

The novel 12- membered tetraazamacrocycle, *trans*-H_6do2a2p, containing two acetate and two methylphosphonate pendant arms in *trans*-position, was prepared and characterized by ^{1}H, ^{13}C and ^{31}P NMR spectroscopy. $^{153}Sm/^{166}Ho$-*trans*-do2a2p have also been prepared quantitatively using a 1:2 metal to ligand molar ratio, at pH 8/9. The biodistribution profile of these complexes is very similar to that found for the analogue complexes with H_4dota in the same animal model, although with a significantly superior bone uptake that rapidly decreases over time. The *in vivo* behaviour of these novel complexes, i.e. rapid total excretion, fast washout from main organs, in addition to the high *in vivo* stability, make these building blocks attractive for labelling biomolecules or for bone pain palliation, if the nature of the phosphorus containing pendant arms is modified.

REFERENCES

1. P. Caravan, J. J. Ellison, T. J. McMurry, Gadolinium(III) Chelates as MRI Contrast Agents: Structure, Dynamics and Applications. *Chem. Rev.* 1999, 99: 2293-2352.
2. V. Jacques, J-F. Desreux: Synthesis of MRI Contrast Agents II. Macrocyclic Ligands. In: *The Chemistry of Contrast Agents in Medical Magnetic Resonance Imaging*, A.E. Merbach and Eva Toth eds, John Wiley & Sons, Ltd, New York 2001, 157-191.
3. F. Rösch, E. F. Aronsson, Radiolanthanides in Nuclear Medicine. In: *Metal Ions in Biological Systems*: Metal Complexes in Tumour Diagnosis and as Anticancer Agents, A. Siegel and H. Siegel, eds, Marcel Decker, Inc., New York.: 2004, 42: 77-108.
4. W. A.Volkert, T. J. Hoffman, Therapeutic Radiopharmaceuticals. *Chem. Rev.* 1999, 99: 2269-2292.
5. S. Liu, D. S. Edwards, Bifunctional Chelators for Therapeutic Lanthanide Radiopharmaceuticals. *Bioconjugate Chem.* 2001, 12: 7-34.
6. L. L. Chappell, D. E. Milenic, K..Garmestani, V. Venditto, M. P. Beitzel, M.. W. Brechbiel, Synthesis and Evaluation of Novel Bifunctional Chelating Agents Based on 1,4,7,10-Tetraazacyclododecane-*N,N',N'',N'''*-Tetraacetic Acid for Radiolabeling Proteins, *Nucl. Med. Biol.* 2003, 30: 581-595.
7. R. E. Weiner, M. L Thakur, Radiolabeled Peptides in the Diagnosis and Therapy of Oncological Diseases. *Appl. Radiat. Isot.* 2002, 57: 749-763.
8. N. Oriushi, T. Higuchi, H. Hanaoka, Y. Iida, K. Endo, Current Status of Cancer Therapy with Radiolabeled Monoclonal Antibody. *Ann. Nucl. Med.* 2005, 19: 355-365.
9. F. C. Alves, P. Donato, A. D. Sherry, A. Zaheer, S. Zhang, A. J. M. Lubag., M. E. Merritt, R. E. Lenkinski, J. V. Frangioni, M. Neves, M. I. M. Prata, A. C. Santos, J. J. P. de Lima, C. F. G. C Geraldes, Silencing of Phosphonate-Gadolinium Magnetic Resonance Imaging Contrast by Hydroxyapatite Binding. *Invest. Radiol.* 2003, 38: 750-760.
10. H. Breitz, R. Wendt, M. Stabin, L. Bouchet, B. Wessels, Dosimetry of High Dose Skeletal Targeted Radiotherapy (STR) with ^{166}Ho-DOTMP. *Cancer Biotherapy & Radiopharmaceuticals* 2003, 18: 225-230.
11. F. Marques, L. Gano, M. P. Campello, S. Lacerda, I. Santos, L. M. P. Lima, J. Costa, P. Antunes, R. Delgado, 13- and 14-Membered Macrocyclic Ligands Containing Methylcarboxylate or Methylphosphonate Pendant Arms: Chemical and Biological Evaluation of their ^{153}Sm and ^{166}Ho Complexes as Potential Agents for Therapy or Bone Pain Palliation. *J. Inorg. Biochem.* 2006, 100: 270-280.

12. M. P. Campello, F. Marques, L. Gano, S. Lacerda, I. Santos, Radiochemical and Biological Behaviour of ^{153}Sm and ^{166}Ho Complexes Anchored by a Novel Bis(methylphosphonate) Tetraazamacrocycle. Radiochimica Acta, submitted.

ACKNOWLEDGEMENTS

The authors acknowledge the financial support from FCT and POCTI, with co-participation of the European Community Fund FEDER **(POCTI/2000/CBO/35859)**. S. Lacerda thanks FCT for the PhD grant (SFRH/BD/19168/2004). COST ACTION D18 is also acknowledge.

Metal Ions in Biology and Medicine: vol. 9. Eds Maria Carmen Alpoim, Paula Vasconcellos Morais, Maria Amélia Santos, Armando J. Cristóvão, José A. Centeno, Philippe Collery.
John Libbey Eurotext, Paris © 2006 pp. 52-1.

Activation of anticancer platinum complexes by tumoral acidity

Meelich K.[1], Galanski M.[1], Arion V. B.[1], Jakupec M. A.[1], Schluga P.[1], Hartinger C.G.[1], Graf v. Keyserlingk N.[2], and Keppler B. K.[1]

[1] *Institute of Inorganic Chemistry, University of Vienna; Währinger Str. 42, A-1090 Vienna, Austria*
[2] *Faustus Forschungs Compagnie Translational Cancer Research GmbH, D-04109 Leipzig, Germany*

Since the successful introduction of cisplatin, the first metal based anticancer drug [1, 2], a wide spectrum of platinum compounds has been synthesized and tested [3]. Nevertheless, only a limited number made their way into clinical trials, just three of them have been approved for a worldwide clinical use *(fig. 1)*. Low selectivity of most anticancer agents is still a major problem; severe side effects or ineffective treatment are the results. The search for a more selective and tumor targeted therapy was the stimulus for the design of pH-sensitive platinum complexes *(fig. 2)*. It is known that most solid tumors display increased hypoxia, which results in a decrease of pH (5.5-7.4). The acidic environment, which is usually a problem for weak base organic drugs, could advantageously be used for the introduction of pH sensitive agents, such as aminoalcoholato platinum(II) complexes. These substances show a pH-driven reversible intramolecular ligand exchange reaction in aqueous solution *(fig. 3)*. At pH 7.4 ring-closed species are formed which display a relatively low reactivity. Also a low cytotoxicity of the mentioned ring-closed forms could be found. On the other hand, the ring-opened complexes, which are formed at lower pH, as found in tissues of solid tumors, are far more reactive. Respectively a much stronger cytotoxic effect was observed at pH 6. Three pH-sensitive aminoalcoholato complexes have been studied in detail: synthesis, characterization, chemical behavior, and cytotoxicity are described. In all three cases, the ring-closed species appear to be remarkably stable substances, also in an aqueous solution at pH 7.4 and at a chloride ion concentration of 100 mM (as present in blood).

These interesting results provide evidence that the concept of administration of rather unreactive drugs and activation under acidic pH conditions can be realized.

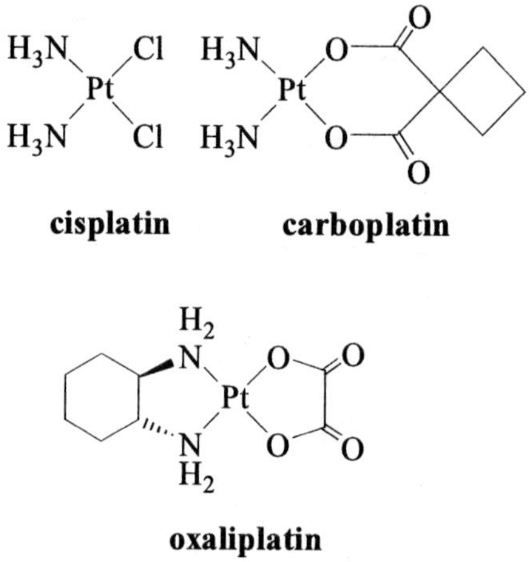

Fig. 1. Cisplatin, carboplatin, and oxaliplatin - the only platinum complexes approved for worldwide clinical use.

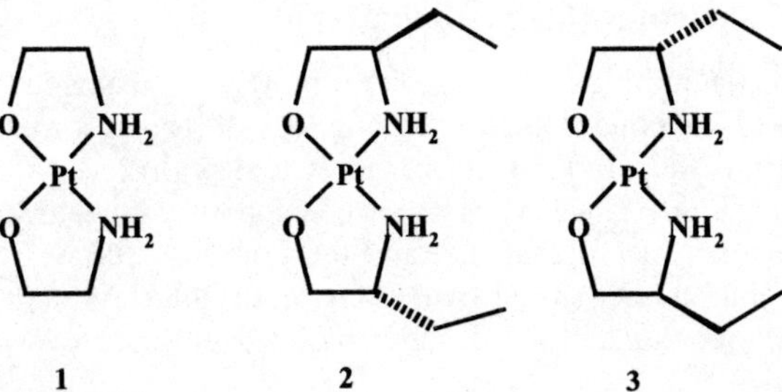

Fig. 2. Novel pH-sensitive platinum compounds - (*SP*-4-2)-bis(aminoethanolato-κ^2*N*,*O*)platinum(II) (**1**), (*SP*-4-2)-bis((S)-2-aminobutanolato-κ^2*N*,*O*) *platinum(II)* (**2**), (*SP*-4-2)-bis-((R)-2-aminobutanolato-κ^2*N*,*O*)platinum(II) (**3**).

Fig. 3. pH-dependent equilibrium of the dichloro, monochloro, and doubly ring-closed species.

EXPERIMENTAL

All chemicals were purchased from commercial suppliers; K_2PtCl_4 was obtained from Johnson Matthey. Deionised water (reverse osmosis) was doubly distilled before use. All reactions were carried out under protection from light, and for stirring a glass coated magnetic stirrer was used. The ^{1}H, ^{13}C, and ^{195}Pt NMR spectra were recorded with a Bruker DPX 400 (Ultrashield^{TM} Magnet) at 400.13, 100.62, and 85.99 MHz respectively. Elemental analysis was carried out with a Perkin Elmer 2400 CHN Elemental Analyser by the micro analytical laboratory of the Faculty of Chemistry, University of Vienna.

(SP-4-2)-Bis(aminoethanol-κN)diiodoplatinum(II)

K_2PtCl_4 (1500 mg; 3.61 mmol) was dissolved in 15 ml water, mixed with KI (3000 mg; 18.07 mmol), and stirred for 30 minutes at room temperature in the dark. The color turned from red to dark brown, and the solution showed a metallic luster. Ethanolamine (485 mg; 7.94 mmol; in 3 ml water) was added slowly. The mixture was stirred for three hours; a brownish yellow precipitate was formed, which was filtered off, washed with cold water three times, and dried in vacuum over P_4O_{10}. Yield: 1154 mg (56%). Elemental analysis calculated for $C_4H_{14}I_2N_2O_2Pt$ (571.05 g/mol): C: 8.41, H: 2.47, N: 4.91; found: C: 8.32, H: 2.63, N: 4.95.

(SP-4-2)-Bis(aminoethanol-κN)dichloroplatinum(II)

(*SP*-4-2)-Bis(aminoethanol-κ*N*)diiodoplatinum(II) (1120 mg; 1.96 mmol) was suspended in 25 ml water. This suspension was mixed with $AgNO_3$ (633 mg; 3.73 mmol) and the reaction mixture was stirred for 24 hours at room temperature in the dark. AgI was filtered off and the clear solution was mixed with 6 M HCl (2.5 ml; 15.00 mmol). The volume was reduced to ca. 10 ml; Crystallization of the green product took place at room temperature and was completed at 4 °C. The product was filtered off, washed with cold water three times, and dried in vacuum over P_4O_{10}. Yield: 441 mg (61%). Elemental analysis calculated for $C_4H_{14}Cl_2N_2O_2Pt$ (388.15 g/mol): C: 12.38, H: 3.63, N: 7.22; found: C: 12.45, H: 3.42, N: 7.15.

(SP-4-2)-Bis(2-aminoethanolato-κ²N,O)platinum(II) *(1)*

The dichloroplatinum(II) complex (350 mg, 0.9 mmol) was suspended in 10 ml of water and treated with 30 ml of rinsed and conditioned Amberlite IRA-400 basic ion exchanger *(fig. 4)* (conditioning: 30 ml of Amberlite IRA-400, Cl^- form, are stirred with 2 M NaOH for 30 minutes and washed three times with 20 ml of water). The suspension was stirred at room temperature for 24 hours. The ion exchanger was filtered off, and the colorless filtrate was concentrated under reduced pressure. The solution was stored over P_4O_{10} until colorless crystals of **1** were formed. The crystal mass was filtered off and dried under reduced pressure over P_4O_{10} to yield 136 mg (48%) of a white solid.

Elemental analysis calculated for $C_4H_{12}N_2O_2Pt$ (315.23 g/mol): C: 15.24, H: 3.84, N: 8.89; found: C: 15.08, H: 3.60, N: 8.61. ^{1}H-NMR (400 MHz, H_2O/D_2O 9:1, 298 K): $\delta = 2.25$ [t, (^3J(H, H) = 5.5 Hz), 2H, CH_2NH_2], 2.96 [t, (^3J(H,H) = 5.5 Hz) 2H, CH_2O]. ^{13}C-NMR (100.62 MHz, H_2O/D_2O, 9:1 298 K): $\delta = 50.93$ (CH_2NH_2), 69.31 (CH_2O).

(*SP*-4-2)-Bis((S)-2-aminobutanolato-κ²*N,O*)platinum(II) **(2)** and (*SP*-4-2)-bis((R)-2-aminobutanolato-κ²*N,O*)platinum(II) **(3)** were synthesized in a similar way.

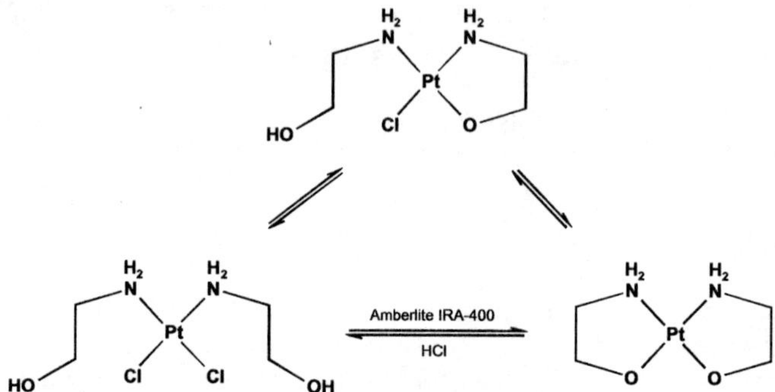

Fig. 4. pH-dependent behavior of (*SP*-4-2)-bis(2-aminoethanol-κ*N*)dichloloro platinum(II) and synthesis of (*SP*-4-2)-bis(2aminoethanolato-κ*N,O*)platinum(II) **(1)**.

Structure determinations by X-ray diffraction were performed on a Nonius Kappa CCD diffractometer. The data were processed using the Denzo-SMN software. The structure was solved by direct methods and refined by full-matrix least-squares techniques as a racemic twin.

In order to study the time-dependent binding to 5'-GMP at different pH values, the complexes (0.5 mM) were incubated with 5'-GMP (1 mM) at 37 °C corresponding to a molar ratio of 1:2 in phosphate buffer (20 mM, pH 7.4 and pH 6.0, respectively). For each pH value, the half life of 5'-GMP was determined by following the relative decrease of the peak area of 5'-GMP using capillary electrophoresis. The studies were recorded at 200 and 254 nm; the standard deviation was below 4%.

For determining the cytotoxicity at pH 7.0 and pH 6.0 the cisplatin sensitive human non-small cell lung cancer cell line A549 was used. Cells were grown as adherent monolayer cultures, expanded under appropriate culture conditions, and trypsinated. The cells were seeded in 100 µl of cell culture medium at the appropriate density of living cells into 96-well tissue culture plates and incubated at 37 °C and 5% CO_2 for 24 hours. The cell culture medium was either buffered at pH 7.0 with phosphate or at pH 6.0 with MES (2-(*N*-morpholino)ethanesulfonic acid). For a negative control 100 µl of cell culture medium was added to four wells (100% value). For a positive control all cells were deadened with phenol (0% value). The cells were incubated with the substances for further 48 hours at 37 °C and 5% CO_2. Cytotoxicity was determined by means of a microculture assay using resazurin which is metabolized by living cells. The amount of dye conversion in solution is measured fluorometrically. Fluorescence was monitored at a wavelength of

590 nm using a excitation wavelength of 560. Quantification was done by a fluorescence micro platereader (Genios, Tecan).

RESULTS AND DISCUSSION

With regard to structure-activity relationships of platinum anticancer drugs, bis(2-hydroxyalkyl)-substituted diaminedichloroplatinum(II) complexes and their ring-closed counter parts have been synthesized and characterized by elemental analysis, NMR spectroscopy, and crystal structure determination. Their pH-dependent behavior in aqueous solution has been studied in detail by ^{1}H and ^{195}Pt NMR experiments. Furthermore, their binding behavior to 5'-GMP, which is widely used as a model nucleobase to estimate the reactivity and toxicity of platinum-based antitumor agents towards DNA, has intensively been studied under various pH conditions and chloride ion concentrations [4]. Finally also cytotoxicity tests have been carried out at pH 6.0 and 7.0 [5].

Single crystals of the complexes **1**, **2**, and **3** could be isolated; here, the structures of **1** and **3** are shown *(fig. 5 and 6)* [6].

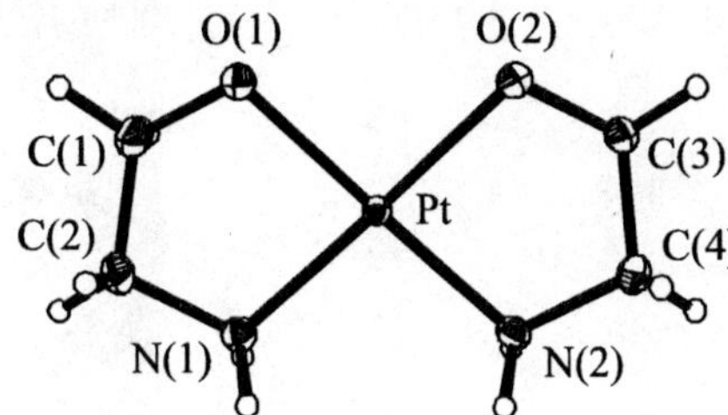

Fig. 5. Crystal structure of **1**.

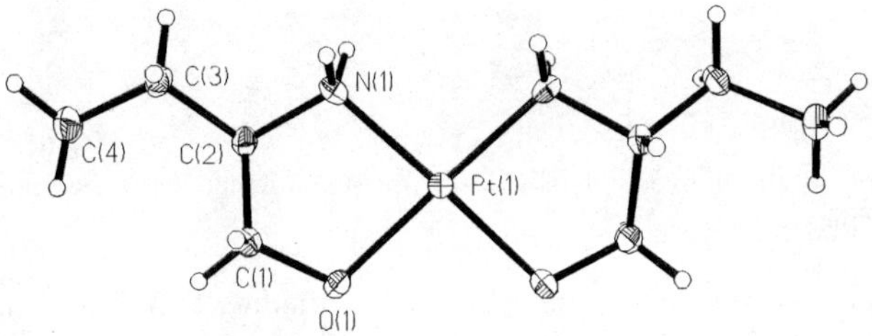

Fig. 6. Crystal structure of **3**.

In an aqueous solution of (*SP*-4-2)-bis(aminoethanol-κ*N*)dichloro platinum(II), a second and third set of methylene resonances could be observed in proton NMR spectra, which were increasing with time [7]. After addition of HCl these signals disappeared, and only two CH_2 resonances could be observed as expected for the corresponding diaminedichloro complex of **1** *(fig. 7)*. A further prove for the ring-closing reaction was achieved by ^{195}Pt NMR spectroscopy *(fig. 8)*. A solution of the diaminedichloro complex in D_2O treated with 0.5 equivalents of NaOD showed two significant resonances at -600 and -658 ppm **(a)**. These can be assigned to the monochloro and the dichloro complex, respectively. Further addition of 1.5 equivalents of NaOD **(b)** and further 0.5 equivalents after waiting over night **(c)**, lead to a decrease and finally vanishing of the dichloro complex. At the same time the signal of the monochloro complex had been decreased, and a new signal at -624 ppm had appeared. The latter derives from the doubly ring-closed species **1**. Full conversion into **1** could only be achieved by removal of the chloride ions by means of $AgNO_3$ **(d)**.

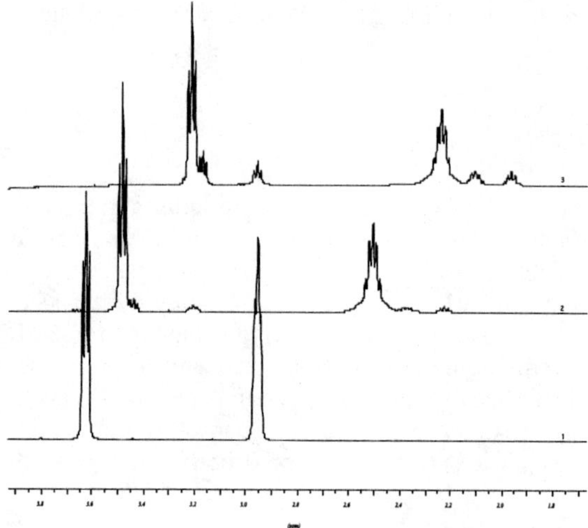

Fig. 7. ^1H NMR spectrum of (*SP*-4-2)-bis(aminoethanol-κ*N*)dicthloroplatinum(II) in D_2O/H_2O 9:1.

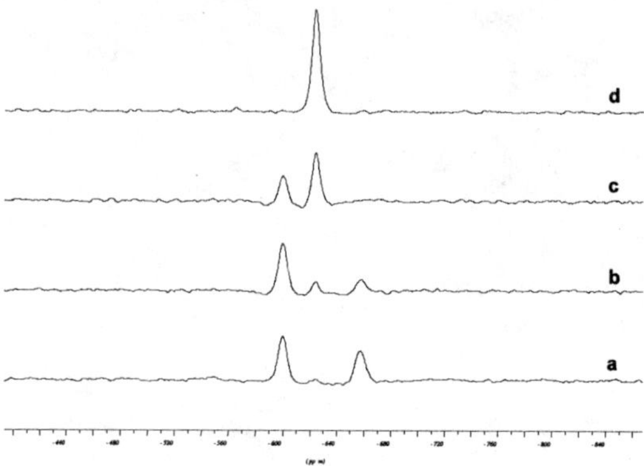

Fig.-8. ^{195}Pt NMR study of the conversion of (*SP*-4-2)-bis(aminoethanol-κ*N*)dichloroplatinum(II) into the doubly ring-closed complex **1** in D_2O.

Complexes **1**, **2**, and **3** displayed an unexpected slow binding to 5'-GMP under standard screening conditions at pH 7.4 in comparison to (*N,N*'-bis(2-hydroxyethyl)ethane-1,2-diamine)dichloroplatinum(II) and cisplatin. Therefore, the binding behavior of **1**, **2**, and **3**, as well as of their ring-opened dichloro counter parts was investigated under standard screening conditions (pH 7.4) as well as at pH 6.0, mimicking the pH of many solid tumors *(table 1, fig. 9)*. A significant difference in the half life of adduct formation could be observed both in presence and absence of chloride ions, which is of great interest with respect to the lower pH in solid tumors and also to decrease the general toxicity of anticancer platinum drugs in vivo.

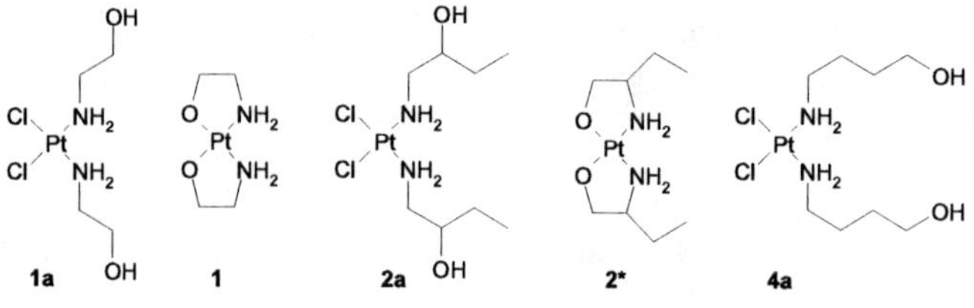

1a **1** **2a** **2*** **4a**

Fig. 9. Pt-complexes tested with 5'-GMP.

Table 1. Half time of 5'-GMP in binding studies with pH-sensitive Pt-complexes.

complex	half time [h] pH 7.4	half time [h] pH 6.0
1a	28.5	4.5
1	32.5	4.5
2a	66.3	6.1
2*	80.0	18.7
4a	10.6	6.0

Instead of complexes **2** and **3**, the results of the racemic complex **2*** and its dichloro counterpart **2a** are presented. Interestingly, in the case of **4a**, the difference in the half times between pH 7.4 and 6.0 is rather small, contrary to the other complexes. This result could be explained by a low tendency to form a seven-membered ring, which also supports our concept.

Cytotoxicity of **1a**, **1**, and **2** was investigated in the cisplatin sensitive human non-small cell lung cancer cell line A549 at pH 7.0 and pH 6.0 in comparison to cisplatin *(fig. 10)*. All substances showed a significant pH dependent cytotoxicity. At pH 7 the IC_{50} value was 110 μM for **1a** and 115 μM for **2**, whereas at pH 6.0 all complexes displayed a pronounced enhancement in their antiproliferative properties. In comparison, the IC_{50} values for cisplatin were found to be 2.69 μM at pH 7.0 and 1.50 μM at pH 6.0.

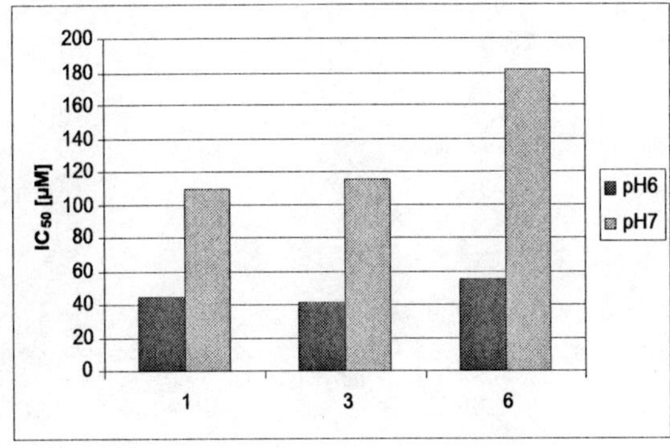

Figure 10: Cytotoxicity of 1a, 1, and 2*.

CONCLUSIONS

In conclusion, a new class of cytotoxic platinum(II) complexes is now available, showing a pH-dependent behavior. The compounds display a low reactivity at pH 7.4 and a significant activation under slightly acidic conditions, which could be highly interesting with respect to a lowered pH in many solid tumors. Moreover, general toxicity should positively be influenced. A variety of substituted ethanolamine compounds is accessible for fine tuning of important properties such as reactivity and lipophilicity, to set up structure-activity relationships and to learn more about the connection between chemistry and cytotoxic activity.

REFERENCES

1. Rosenberg B. Platinum complexes for the treatment of cancer *Interdiscip. Sci. Rev.* 1978; 3(2): 134-147.
2. Lippert B. (Ed.) Cisplatin: Chemistry and Biochemistry of a Leading Anticancer Drug. Zürich: Verlag Helvetica Chimica Acta, and Weinheim: WILEY-VCH, 1999, 564.
3. Galanski M, Jakupec MA, Keppler BK. Update of the Preclinical Situation of Anticancer Platinum Complexes: Novel Design Strategies and Innovative Analytical Approaches. *Curr. Med. Chem.* 2005; 12: 2075-2094.
4. Hartinger CG, Schluga P, Galanski M, Baumgartner C, Timerbaev AT, Keppler BK. *Electrophoresis* 2003; 24: 2038-2044.
5. Galanski M, Baumgartner C, Meelich K, Arion VB, Fremuth M, Jakupec MA, Schluga P, Hartinger CG, Graf v. Keyserlingk N, Keppler BK. Synthesis, crystal structure and pH dependent cytotoxicity of (*SP*-4-2)-bis(2-aminoethanolato-κ^2*N,O*)platinum(II) - a representative of novel pH sensitive anticancer platinum complexes. *Inorg. Chim. Acta* 2004; 357: 3237-3244.
6. Galanski M, Baumgartner C, Arion VB, Keppler BK. Bis(2-aminobutanol)dichloroplatinum(II) complexes and their singly and doubly ring-closed butanolato species - novel prodrugs for platinum-based antitumor chemotherapy? *Eur. J. Inorg. Chem.* 2003; 14: 2619-2625.
7. Galanski M, Zimmermann W, Baumgartner C, Keppler BK. The intramolecular ligand-exchange reaction of (*SP*-4-2)-dichlorobis(2-hydroxyethylamine)platinum(II) and (OC-6-22)-tetrachlorobis(2-hydroxyethylamine)-platinum(IV), a ^{1}H and ^{15}N,^{1}H-HMQC NMR study. *Eur. J. Inorg. Chem.* 2001; 5: 1145-1149.

ACKNOWLEDGMENTS

The support of COST and the Austrian Council for Research and Technology Development is gratefully acknowledged.

Metal Ions in Biology and Medicine: vol. 9. Eds Maria Carmen Alpoim, Paula Vasconcellos Morais, Maria Amélia Santos, Armando J. Cristóvão, José A. Centeno, Philippe Collery.
John Libbey Eurotext, Paris © 2006 pp. 59-1.

Copper complexes with heterocyclic sulfonamides, potential drugs for dermatological diseases

Torre M.H.[1], Chifflet S.[2], Foglia M.[2]

[1]Química Inorgánica, Facultad de Química, Gral Flores 2124, e-mail: mtorre@fq.edu.uy, and [2]Bioquímica, Facultad de Medicina; Gral. Flores 2125, e-mail: schiffle@mednet.org.uy, UDELAR, Montevideo, Uruguay

ABSTRACT

The SOD-like activity, the microbiological behavior and the penetration across the cell membrane in two different epithelial cell lines (MDCK, αTN4-1) were studied in copper(II)-sulfonamide complexes.

The results showed that the complexes with five-membered heterocyclic rings were more active than the free sulfonamides against *E. coli* and *S. aureus* and some of them presented SOD-like activity similar to those of pharmacological compounds.

The preliminary assays of the penetration tests showed that the studied complexes increased the copper content of cells.

INTRODUCTION

The skin is especially vulnerable to damage by reactive oxygen species such as superoxide anion (O_2^-) generated in physical and biological processes that can cause oxidative damage to cellular membrane lipids, proteins, and nucleic acids [1]. It is involved in various acute and chronic cutaneous changes such as erythema, connective-tissue degradation, photocarcinogenesis, among others. Cells located in the surface of the skin have strong antioxidant potential using specific enzymes that destroy the injuring species. Especially, superoxide dismutase is a copper-dependent oxidoreductase that catalyses the dismutation of superoxide, protecting against superoxide-mediated cytotoxicity [2]. When the copper level is low the activity of the enzyme decreases.

In spite of the fact that metal ions are usually unable to penetrate the unbroken skin, metal complexes with specific ligands can reach the circulation [3]. In particular it is known that some copper compounds have percutaneous absorption and cutaneous bioavailability of copper [4]. Besides, several copper complexes show an important superoxide dismutase (SOD)-like activity, and consequently they destroy the injurious superoxide radical [5, 6].

On the other hand sulfonamides are drugs extensively used in dermatology due to their antibacterial activity. Modified toxicological and pharmacological properties have been observed when some of these sulfonamides are administered in the form of their metal complexes [7-10]. For this reason and due to the versatility of coordination sites, this group of molecules was chosen as ligands with the aim of obtaining new interesting copper compounds useful for dermatological purpose. Especially we are looking for copper complexes with percutaneous absorption, and with SOD-like and antibacterial activities.

MATERIALS AND METHODS

The complexes [Cu(sulfadiazine)$_2$]·H_2O, [Cu(sulfamerazine)$_2$]·H_2O, [Cu(sulfapyridine)$_2$]·H_2O, [Cu(sulfachlorpyridazine)$_2$]·H_2O, [Cu(sulfamethoxypyridazine)$_2$]·H_2O, [Cu(sulfisoxazole)$_2$(H_2O)$_4$]·2H_2O, [Cu(sulfamethoxazol)$_2$(H_2O)$_4$]·3H_2O, [Cu(sulfamethoxazol)$_2$]·H_2O, [Cu(sulfamethoxazol)$_2$]·H_2O, reported in a previous work [11] and [Cu(sulfameter)$_2$]·H_2O, [Cu(sulfametazine)$_2$]·H_2O, and [Cu(sulfadimethoxine)$_2$]·H_2O, were synthesized according to the procedure described by Bult et al. [12], mixing each sulfonamide (SIGMA) in water with the addition of NaOH 1 M until total dissolution (pH=9-10). To the resulting solution, 50 mL of $CuSO_4$·5H_2O (FLUKA) 0.5 M were added. The precipitate formed was filtered, washed with water, dried at room temperature and protected from light.

The antimicrobial activity of each sulfonamide and the respective complex was tested using the agar dilution test. The minimal concentration of the antimicrobial agent required to inhibit or kill the microorganisms (MIC) was calculated. Every step was based on recommendations from the National Committee for Clinical Laboratory Standards [13]. A suspension in sterile water of the sulfonamides and the copper-sulfonamide complexes was incorporated in 20 mL of Mueller-Hinton agar. The pH of each batch of medium was in the range from 7.2 to 7.4. The dilution scheme for each antimicrobial agent covered a 128-0.25 µg of sulfonamide/mL range. The same process was carried out with a water dilution of $CuSO_4$·5H_2O. The standard strains used were *E. coli* ATCC 25922 and *S. aureus* ATCC 29213. All tests and inoculation on each dish were run in duplicate.

The SOD-like activity was evaluated by the method based on the inhibitory effect of SOD over the reduction of nitrobluetetrazolium by the superoxide anion generated by the xanthine/xanthine oxidase system.

The preliminary study of the penetration of the copper complexes across the membrane of cells was performed with [Cu(sulfadiazine)$_2$]·[H_2O and [Cu(sulfamethoxazole)$_2$(H_2O)$_4$]·3H_2O in cultured cells. Two different epithelial cell lines were used for this study, the immortal murine lens epithelial cell line αTN4-1 [14] and the kidney derived Madin Darby Canine Kidney (MDCK) cells. Both cell lines were cultured until confluence in 60 mm tissue culture dishes using standard procedures [14, 15]. The complexes were dissolved in DMSO in a concentration of 1mg/mL. Each cell plate was inoculated with 1 (L/mL of these solutions and left in the tissue culture incubator (37°C, 5% CO_2) for 24 hs. After removal of the culture medium the cells were washed thrice in 0.15 M NaCl and homogenized in 1 mL of distilled water. Copper content was determined by atomic absorption. Blanks were prepared with the same process above mentioned.

RESULTS

The MIC of free sulfonamides and their respective complexes are shown in *table 1*.

The new results are in accordance to our previous observation that showed that the complexes with five-membered heterocyclic rings were more active than the free sulfonamides against *E. coli* and *S. aureus* while the others had similar or less activity than the free ligands. In particular [Cu(sulfamethoxazol)$_2$(H_2O)$_4$]·3H_2O provided the highest antimicrobial potency [11].

Due to the insolubility of some complexes, the SOD-like activity was measured in DMSO/H_2O only for [Cu(sulfadiazine)$_2$]·H_2O (IC50=66 µM), [Cu(sulfameter)$_2$]·H_2O IC50 = 41µM, [Cu(sulfametazine)$_2$]·H_2O (IC50 = 98µM), [Cu(sulfamethoxipyridazine)$_2$]·H_2O (IC50 = 52µM) and [Cu(sulfamethoxazole)$_2$(H_2O)$_4$]·3H_2O (IC50 = 42 µM).

Although no relationship was found between the microbiological and the SOD-like activities, the Cu(sulfamethoxazole)$_2$(H_2O)$_4$]·3H_2O presented the best microbiological activity and one of the highest SOD-like activities, comparable with pharmacological active compounds.

The preliminary study of the penetration of copper complexes across the cell membrane is presented in *table 2*. The results were obtained by duplicate.

Table 1. MIC (μg/mL) of sulfonamides and their copper complexes

Heterocycle	Antimicrobial agent	S.aureus ATCC 29213	E.coli ATCC 25922
pyrimidine	Sulfameter $[Cu(sulfameter)_2]\cdot H_2O$	16 32	>128 > 128
	Sulfadiazine $[Cu(sulfadiazine)_2]\cdot H_2O$	32 >128	8 >128
	Sulfamerazine $[Cu(sulfamerazine)_2]\cdot H_2O$	32 >128	32 128
	Sulfametazine $[Cu(sulfametazine)_2]\cdot H_2O$	32 32	128 128
	Sulfadimethoxine $[Cu(sulfadimethoxine)_2]\cdot H_2O$	16 16	>128 >128
pyridine	Sulfapyridine $[Cu(sulfapyridine)_2]\cdot H_2O$	>128 >128	>128 >128
pyridazine	Sulfamethoxipyridazine $[Cu(sulfamethoxipyridazine)_2]\cdot H_2O$	8 8	32 32
isoxazole	Sulfisoxazole $[Cu(sulfisoxazole)_2(H_2O)_4]\cdot 2H_2O$	>128 128	>128 128
	Sulfamethoxazole $[Cu(sulfamethoxazole)_2(H_2O)_4]\cdot 3H_2O$ $[Cu(sulfamethoxazole)_2]\cdot H_2O$	16 4 16	128 32 16
diazomethizole	Sulfametizole $[Cu(sulfametizole)_2]\cdot H_2O$	64 32	64 32

Table 2. Copper concentration in the cell homogenates

Species	Cu concentration in αTN4-1 (ng/mL)	Cu concentration in MDCK (ng/mL)
$[Cu(sulfamethoxazole)_2(H_2O)_4]\cdot 3H_2O$	45	66
$[Cu(sulfadiazine)_2]\cdot H_2O$	69	77
Control	ND	ND

ND = (<20 ng/mL)

As shown in *table 2*, copper concentration in cell homogenates from treated cells is higher than those from the control ones. Further studies are necessary to determine whether drugs have reached the cell cytosol or have been retained at the level of the plasma membrane.

It is important to point out that neither cell morphology nor cell viability were altered after the treatment with either one of the drugs.

CONCLUSION

The results shown that the complexes with five-membered heterocyclic rings were more active than the free sulfonamides against *E. coli* and *S. aureus* while the others had similar or less activity than the free ligands. In particular [Cu(sulfamethoxazole)$_2$(H_2O)$_4$]·3H_2O, and [Cu(sulfameter)$_2$]·H_2O presented SOD-like activity similar to those of pharmacologically active compounds.

REFERENCES

1. H. Sasaki, H. Akamatsu and T. Horio, J. Invest. Dermatol., 114 (2000) 502.
2. N. P. Farrell, Uses of Inorganic Chemistry in Medicine, The Royal Society of Chemistry, Cambridge, 1999.
3. D. M. Taylor and D. R. Williams, Trace element medicine and chelation therapy, The Royal Society of Chemistry, Cambridge, 1995.
4. F. Pirot, J. Miller, Y. N. Kalia and P. Humbert, Skin Pharmacol. 9(4),(1996) 259.
5. N. Roberts and P. Robinson, Brit. J. Rheumatol., 24 (1985) 128.
6. G. Facchin, M. H. Torre, I. Viera, E. Kremer and E. J. Baran, Metal Ions in Biology and Medicine 7 (2002) 11.
7. J. E. F. Reynolds (Ed.), Martindale.The Extra Pharmacopoeia, London, 1996.
8. S. C. Chaturvedi, S. H. Mishra and K. L. Bhargava, Sci. Cult., 46 (1980) 401.
9. F. Blasco, L. Perelló, J. Latorre, J. Borrás and S. García-Granda, J. Inorg. Biochem., 61 (1996) 143.
10. G. Casanova, G. Alzuet, J. Borrás, J. Timoneda, S. García-Granda and I. Cándano-González, J. Inorg. Biochem, 56 (1994) 65.
11. E. Kremer, G. Facchin, E. Estévez, P. Alborés, E.J.Baran, J. Ellena and M. H. Torre, J. Inorg. Biochem., in press, 2006.
12. A. Bult, J. D. Uitterdijk and H. B. Klasen, Transition Met. Chem., 4 (1979) 285.
13. A. L. Barry, C. Thornsberry, E. H. Lennette, A. Balows, W. J. Hausler and H. J. Shadomy, Manual of Clinical Microbiology, Washington, 1985.
14. A. Spector, W. Ma, F. Sun, D. Li and N. J. Kleiman, Exp. Eye Res., 75 (2002) 573.
15. W. J. Nelson and R. W. Hammerton, J Cell Biol., 108 (1989) 893.

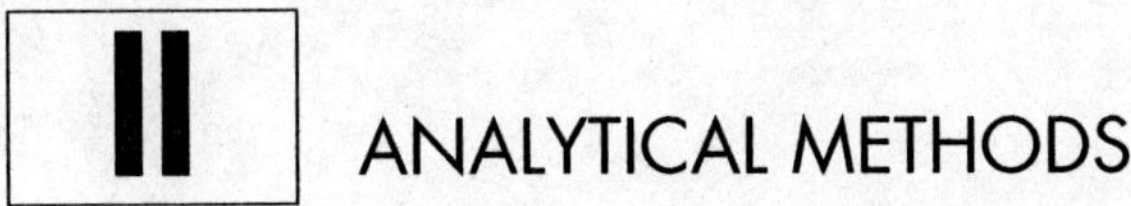

II ANALYTICAL METHODS

Metal Ions in Biology and Medicine: vol. 9. Eds Maria Carmen Alpoim, Paula Vasconcellos Morais, Maria Amélia Santos, Armando J. Cristóvão, José A. Centeno, Philippe Collery.
John Libbey Eurotext, Paris © 2006 pp. 65-1.

Simultaneous determination of potassium, calcium, sodium and magnesium ions in urine by capillary zone electrophoresis

Toshiko Fujii[1] and Kayo Sumida[2]

[1] *Department of Clinical Nutrition, Faculty of Medical Professions, Kawasaki University of Medical Welfare, 288 Matsushima, Kurashiki, 701-0193, JAPAN, e-mail: fujii@mw.kawasaki-m.ac.jp*
[2] *Master's Program in Clinical Nutrition, Graduate School of Health Science and Technology, Kawasaki University of Medical Welfare, 288 Matsushima, Kurashiki, 701-0193, JAPAN*

ABSTRACT

Capillary zone electrophoresis (CZE) was applied for the simultaneous determination of potassium (K^+), calcium (Ca^{2+}), sodium (Na^+) and magnesium (Mg^{2+}) ions in human urine samples.

Separations were carried out in a pH 4.2 carrier electrolyte containing 10 mM imidazol, 5 mM 2-hydroxy-iso-butyric acid, 2 mM 18-crown-6, and 0.2% acetic acid. Indirect UV detection was conducted at 215 nm. An aliquot (100 µl) of urine specimen with precipitate was diluted 1:100 with distilled water (9.9 ml), filtered through a 0.2 µm membrane filter, degassed using an ultrasonic generator, and then injected directly into the capillary. Twenty-four hours (24-h) urine samples were collected from 110 Japanese men and women aged 18-74 years.

The four cations were well separated in less than six minutes. The mean values of the cation concentrations in mg/l were K^+=1,372, Ca^{2+}=88, Na^+=3,072 and Mg^{2+}=62. The concentrations of K^+, Na^{2+} and Mg^{2+} were in agreement with those obtained in urine samples using an ion selective electrode meter for K^+ and Na^+ determination, and a colorimetric reaction method with xylidil blue for Mg^{2+} determination.

The proposed method is simple, rapid, and does not require any preliminary treatment of the urine samples except diluting.

INTRODUCTION

For adults in Japan, upper limits for the daily recommended dietary allowances of calcium and magnesium are 2,500 and 700 mg, respectively. Therefore, it is important to investigate the association between dietary intake and urinary excretion amount for the four main minerals: potassium, calcium, sodium and magnesium. The concentration of these metals in biological fluids, especially urine, could be an useful indicator of net dietary intake. The determination of the cations in urine has been approached in various ways [1, 2, 3]. The use of CZE for the analysis of ionic analytes has increased greatly, since it provides a number of advantages in analytical technique including rapid and efficient separations of charged components present in small sample volumes [4]. In a previous work utilizing CZE [5], a new electrolyte system based on imidazol was developed to separate the four cations in drinking water samples.

The aim of this study was to examine the possibility of simultaneously determining the four cations (potassium, calcium, sodium and magnesium) in human urine samples in a single analytical run.

MATERIALS AND METHODS

Chemicals and samples

Stock solutions (1,000 mg/l) of five cations (NH_4^+, K^+, Ca^{2+}, Na^+ and Mg^{2+}) and all other analytical-reagent grade chemicals were obtained from Wako Chemicals (Osaka, Japan). Working standard solutions were prepared daily by mixing and diluting appropriate amounts of stock solutions. All standard solutions were filtered through a 0.2 µm membrane filter and degassed for 10 minutes using an ultrasonic generator.

Twenty-four hours urine samples used for the simultaneous determination of the four cations were obtained from 110 healthy men and women. In order to detect any difference in urinary excretion of cations due to age, the subjects were divided into two groups, A and B. Group A consisted of 44 students (mean age=19 years, seven men and 37 women) and Group B consisted of 66 men and women (mean age=66 years, seven men and 59 women). Subjects of group B were from a rural area in Okayama prefecture. After collecting urine samples, the volume, concentration of creatinine and specific gravities were measured immediately. The samples were stored at -30°C until analyses were performed. An aliquot (1,000 µl) of urine sample with precipitate was diluted 1:100 with distilled water (100 ml) before CZE analysis.

Apparatus and operating conditions

A model CAPI-3300 capillary electrophoresis system (Otsuka Electronics, Osaka, Japan) equipped with a multi-wavelength photodiode-array detector and fused-silica capillaries (75 µm I.D., 72.5 cm L and 60 cm to detector) were used.

Separations were performed in a pH 4.2 carrier electrolyte containing 10 mM imidazol, 5 mM 2-hydroxy-iso-butyric acid, 2 mM 18-crown-6, and 0.2% acetic acid.

The samples were injected by raising the sample vial 25 mm above the level for 30 sec. The calculated injection volume was ca.10nl. The samples were run at 25 °C with an applied voltage of 25 kV. The indirect ultraviolet detection wavelength was set at 215 nm.

Each day before starting analysis, the capillary was rinsed sequentially with 0.05 mM oxalic acid, water, 0.1 M sodium hydroxide solution and water for 5-10 minutes each followed by carrier electrolyte for 10 minutes. Between each run, the capillary was rinsed for three minutes with carrier electrolyte.

RESULTS AND DISCUSSION

Capillary electropherograms

Fig. 1 shows representative capillary electropherograms of the standard mixtures of NH_4^+, K^+, Ca^{2+}, Na^+ and Mg^{2+} and a diluted urine sample (1:100). They show that all five compounds are completely separated in less than six minutes.

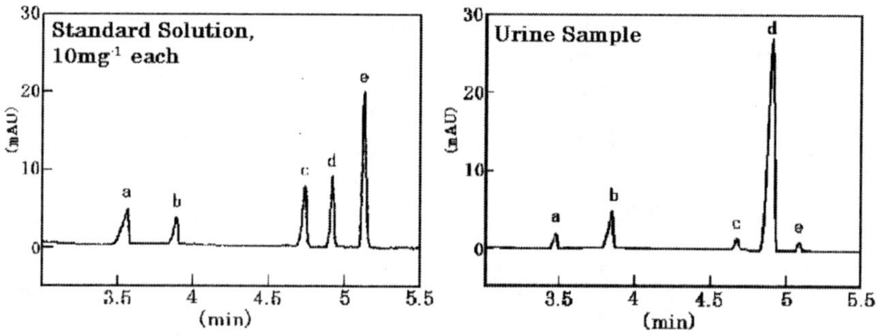

Fig. 1. Electropherograms of the standard cation solution and a diluted urine sample (1:100). Peak: a, NH_4^+; b, K^+; c, Ca^{2+}; d, Na^+; e, Mg^{2+}

The migration times in minutes at a concentration of 10 mg/l were 3.5 for NH_4^+, 3.8 for K^+, 4.7 for Ca^{2+}, 4.8 for Na^+ and 5.1 for Mg^{2+}, respectively.

Repeatability, intermediate precision and limits of detection

To determine repeatability for the CZE, the standard mixture was diluted to 10 mg/l from the stock cation solutions and injected sequentially nine times. Intermediate precision was determned by injecting the same standard mixture used above on six successive days of analyses. The LOD (limits of detection, mg/l) was calculated as the concentration of each metal ion that still gave a signal three times greater than the baseline noise.

Repeatability, intermediate precision and limits of detection are shown in *table 1.*

Table 1. Repeatability and intermediate precision of migration times and peak-ares using the CZE method at the concentration of 10 mg/l each, and LODs for the cations

Analyte	Repeatability (R.S.D.,%)		Intermediate precision (R.S.D.,%)		LOD (mg/l)
	Time	Peak-area	Time	Peak-area	
K^+	0.18	2.12	1.08	3.23	0.16
Ca^{2+}	0.26	3.18	1.14	3.96	0.07
Na^+	0.27	5.38	1.10	8.98	0.07
Mg^{2+}	2.54	2.50	1.17	3.58	0.03

R.S.D., Relative Standard Deviation (%); LOD, Limits of detection;
Repeatability in peak-area of the cations was validated on a given day and intermediate precision was validated over six succesive days.

Calibration and recovery

Linearity of peak areas for the CZE method was checked by measuring various concentrations: 12.5-100 mg/l range for K^+ and Na^+, 1.25-10.0 mg/l range for Ca^{2+}, and 0.625-5.0 mg/l range for Mg^{2+}. Calibration curves were obtained by plotting peak areas versus concentration. The analytical recovery was evaluated by assaying three urine samples spiked with 10 mg/l dilutions of the standard solutions for K^+ and Na^+ with 1 mg/l for Ca^{2+} and Mg^{2+}. The cation concentrations were calculated from peak areas. The average slopes and y-intercepts of the regression line, correlation coefficients and the analytical recovery are shown in *table 2.*

Table 2. Calibration graphs and analytical recovery for CZE.

Analyte	Calibration			Recovery (%)
	Regression line	r	Working range (mg/l)	(mean ± SD)
K^+	y=0.59x + 0.92	0.9985	12.5 - 100	100 ± 6.4
Ca^{2+}	y=2.11x + 0.13	0.9993	1.25 - 10	98 ± 6.7
Na^+	y=1.35x + 3.39	0.9988	12.5 - 100	99 ± 7.0
Mg^{2+}	y=3.37x - 0.39	0.9985	0.625 - 5	102 ± 5.6

x, Concentration (mg/l); *y*, Peak area; r, Correlation coefficient; SD, Standard deviation.

Correlation with concentrations determined using the proposed CZE method and other methods

Urinary concentrations of K^+, C^{2+}, Na^+ and Mg^{2+} were determined by the proposed CZE method. They were also determined using an ion selective electrode meter for urinary K^+ and Na^+, and the *o*-cresolphthalein complexone spectrophothometric method [6] and a colorimetric reaction with xylidil blue, respectively *(table 3)*.

Further study is necessary for determining Ca^{2+}, because the slope of the regression line is less than 0.6.

Table 3. Relation between cation concentrations using the CZE values for *y*-axis and values by other methods for *x*-axis

Analyte	Determination method		Relation	
	The *y*-axis mg/l	The *x*-axis mg/l	Regression line	r
K^+	CZE	Electrode metery[a]	$y=0.9984x + 28.95$	0.9210
Ca^{2+}	CZE	Spectrophothometery[b]	$y=0.5414x + 26.37$	0.8450
Na^+	CZE	Electrode metery[a]	$y=1.001x + 22.60$	0.9033
Mg^{2+}	CZE	Colorimetery[c]	$y=1.0472x - 2.70$	0.9146

r, Correlation coefficient (n=110);
a, Using an ion selective electrode meter:
b, An *o*-cresolphthalein complexone spectrophotmetric method;
c, A colorimetric reaction method with xylidil blue

Age differences in urine cation concentrations

The mean values of the cation concentrations in mg/l were K^+=1,372, Ca^{2+}=88, Na^+=3,072 and Mg^{2+}=62. In order to determine any differences of 24-h excretion rates of the four cations, subjects were divided into two age groups. Cations levels were expressed as the creatinine ratio.

Table 4 shows the concentrations of the four cations corrected by creatinine determined by the proposed CZE method.

Table 4. Cation concentrations in 24-h urine samples corrected by creatinine in two different age groups

Cation	Group A Concentration[a]	Group B Concentration[a]
	(mean ± SD)	(mean ± SD)
K^+	1,141 ± 419*	1,874 ± 862*
Ca^{2+}	89 ± 34	100 ± 47
Na^+	2,743 ± 1,123*	3,970 ± 1,661*
Mg^{2+}	67 ± 17	66 ± 39

a, Creatinine ratio (mg/mg creatinine); *, $p<0.05$ (group A vs. group B);
Group A, Mean age = 19 years (n = 44; seven men and 37 women)
Group B, Mean age = 66 years (n=66; seven men and 59 women)

The 24-hour of outputs of the four cations using the proposed CZE method are shown in *table 5*. K^+ and Na^+ values of group B were significantly higher than group A.

This data suggests that group B subjects may have consumed more foodstuffs that are rich in these cations, e.g., sodium chloride and vegetables.

Table 5. Daily amounts of cations excreted in urine by age groups

Cation	Group A mg/24-h urine	Group B mg/24-h urine
	(mean ± SD)	(mean ± SD)
K^+	1,185 ± 348*	2,002 ± 817*
Ca^{2+}	96 ± 36	108 ± 44
Na^+	2,888 ± 110*	4,230 ± 1,740*
Mg^{2+}	73 ± 19	70 ± 27

*, $p<0.05$ (group A vs. group B)
Group A, Mean age = 19 years (n=44; seven men and 37 women)
Group B, Mean age = 66 years (n=66; seven men and 59 women)

CONCLUSION

The proposed method is simple, rapid and does not require any preliminary treatment of urine samples except diluting. Further study is necessary with respect the determination of Ca^{2+}.

REFERENCES

1. Olšauskaite V, Paliuonyte V, Padarauskas A. Rapid analysis of cation constituents of urine by capillary electrophoresis. Clinica Chimica Acta 2000; 293:181-186.
2. Safarineejad MR. Urinary mineral excretion in healthy Iranian children. Pediatr Nephrol 2003;18:140-144.
3. Kimira M, Kudo Y, Takachi R, Haba R, Watanabe S. Associations between dietary intake and urinary excretion of sodium, potassium, magnesium, and calcium. Jpn J Hyg 2004; 59:23-30.
4. Li SMF. Different modes of capillary electrophoresis. In: Capillary electrophoresis. Amsterdam: ELSEVIER, 1992: 4-30.
5. Fujii T, Yanai R. Simultaneous determination of potassium, calcium, sodium and magnesium ions in drinking water samples by capillary electrophoresis. Metal ions in biology and medicine 2004; 8:23-30.
6. Lorentz K. Improved determination of serum calcium with 2-cresolphthalein Complexone. Clin Chem Acta 1982; 126:327-334.

ACKNOWLEDGEMENTS

Authors are thankful for the Interdepartmental Research Fund of Kawasaki University of Medical Welfare [2005] for financial assistance.

Metal Ions in Biology and Medicine: vol. 9. Eds Maria Carmen Alpoim, Paula Vasconcellos Morais, Maria Amélia Santos, Armando J. Cristóvão, José A. Centeno, Philippe Collery.
John Libbey Eurotext, Paris © 2006 pp. 70-1.

Characterization of Arsenic Species by Raman-microspectroscopy

Charity N. Mosley[1], Todor I. Todorov[2], Chin-Hsiao Tseng[3], Jose A. Centeno[2]*

[1]Jackson State University, College of Science, Engineering, and Technology, Department of Chemistry, Jackson, Mississippi, USA
[2]Armed Forces Institute of Pathology, Division of Biophysical Toxicology, Department of Environmental and Infectious Disease Sciences, Washington, DC, USA
[3]Division of Endocrinology and Metabolism, Department of Internal Medicine, National Taiwan University Hospital, No. 7 Chung-Shan South Road, Taipei, Taiwan

ABSTRACT

Background: Arsenic is a metalloid element found ubiquitously in nature. Human beings can be exposed to arsenic from either natural (i.e. contaminated drinking water, air) or anthropogenic sources (i.e., herbicides, animal feeds). Although a known system toxicant with a high degree of carcinogenicity in humans, the biochemical and molecular mechanisms by which arsenic exerts its toxic action remain to be elucidated. Because the toxicity of arsenic is strongly dependent upon its chemical species (inorganic forms are more toxic than organic forms), it is necessary to develop a methodology to speciate and characterize its molecular properties.

Aims: The aims of this investigation were to determine the structural characteristics of arsenicals with biological significance using Raman microspectroscopy and to create a library of these spectra.

Methods: The arsenic species being studied are inorganic arsenic (IAs^{3+}, IAs^{5+}), and those species known as "metabolites" (monomethylarsonic acid (MMA^{5+}) and dimethylarsinic acid (DMA^{5+}). Raman spectra was collected from the solid compounds using a 633 nm He-Ne laser.

Results: Raman spectra of inorganic arsenic compounds in the 200 - 1000cm^{-1} region, demonstrated vibrations attributed to the As–O stretch and deformation modes. The Raman spectra of the methylated arsenicals were recorded in the 200cm^{-1}-800cm^{-1} region corresponding to the presence of the As–C bend and stretch vibrations, along with the As–O stretch. Raman vibrations in the 2700 - 2900 cm-1 region were attributed to the anti-symmetric and symmetric vibrations of the methyl C – H bonds.

Conclusion: From the spectral library, molecular information will be available which may lead to a better understanding of the chemistry, structure-function relationship, and eventually activity and health effects of these arsenical compounds

Key words: Raman spectroscopy; arsenic; species

ACKNOWLEDGEMENTS

This research was supported by the National Science Foundation's Louis Stokes Mississippi Alliance for Minority Participation (LSMAMP) Bridge to the Doctorate Program (Grant # HRD-0115807) at Jackson State University and the Armed Forces Institute of Pathology.

* *Author for correspondence. Email: centeno@afip.osd.mil*

INTRODUCTION

Arsenic is a ubiquitous element found in the earth's crust. Arsenic and its compounds are found in the contents of manufactured glass, in medical drugs and in contaminated water. It is also found in herbicides and food products [1, 2]. Therefore, human contact with arsenic-containing products is inevitable. The effects of arsenic exposure vary from cancer to cardiovascular problems [1-8]. Worldwide millions of people are exposed to dangerously high levels of arsenic through contaminated drinking water. Once in the body, arsenic binds to hemoglobin, plasma proteins, and leukocytes and is redistributed to the liver, kidney, lung, spleen, and intestines. Arsenic produces cellular damage through various mechanisms. It binds to enzyme sulfhydryl groups, and deactivates the enzyme [9-11]. As a result of being deactivated arsenic binds to dihydrolipoic acid, a pyruvate dehydrogenase cofactor, blocking the conversion of pyruvate to acetyl coenzyme A, inhibiting gluconeogenesis [6]. Arsenic then competes with phosphates for adenosine triphosphate, forming adenosine diphosphate monoarsine, causing the loss of high-energy bonds. Phosphate and arsenate are analogues and share similar physiochemical behavior in soils, competing directly for the same sorption sites on soil particle surfaces [10]. Addition of phosphate to soil may enhance the downward movement of arsenic, leading to increased leaching from the topsoil or increase the availability of arsenic in the soil solution, resulting in higher uptake by plants [10]. Arsenic has the capability, once ingested, to exert a direct toxic effect on blood vessels and major organs [6]. Chronic exposure results in nerve damage, leading to lung, skin, or liver cancer [4-6]. Arsine gas is the most acutely toxic form, followed by inorganic (trivalent) As^{3+} compounds, inorganic (pentavalent) As^{5+} compounds and organic (pentavalent) As^{5+} compounds. Inorganic arsenic is found mostly embedded in geologic materials such as underground rocks and soils whereas the organic forms, arsenobetaine and arsenocholine are found in fish, shellfish, and some plants.

Arsenic is considered a metalloid because of its ability to form complexes with metals as well as the elements carbon, hydrogen, and oxygen [12]. Arsenosugars contain hydroxyl, phosphate, and or sulfate groups, and, they exist, as uncharged or anionic species at neutral pH [11]. In this study, we used Raman spectroscopy to investigate the structural properties of arsenic compounds. Raman spectroscopy probes the molecular composition and structure without being destructive to the sample [13]. It is a method of chemical analysis that enables real-time reaction monitoring and characterization of compounds in a non-contact manner. The sample is illuminated with a laser and the scattered light is collected. The wavelengths and intensities of the scattered light can be used to identify functional groups in a molecule [13]. Because of its small sample requirement, minimal sensitivity toward water interference, and spectral detail, Raman spectroscopy has proven to be a powerful tool for analysis and chemical monitoring [13].

The four main regions of interest within the Raman spectra represent the major bonds within the structures of the arsenic compounds. The bonds of interest are As–O, As–C, C–H, and O–H. The As–O stretch and bends are observed at 875 cm^{-1} and 100-250 cm^{-1}, respectively [12-15]. Previous studies on arsenic and its derivatives indicate the As–C vibration due to bending mode is observed at 224 cm^{-1}; however, its stretch has been observed at 595 cm^{-1} and 610 cm^{-1} [12-15]. For the methyl group stretching and bending modes result in Raman bands at 2926 cm^{-1} and 1409 cm^{-1}, respectively. The final bond of interest, the O–H bond exhibits a stretching vibration near 3200 cm^{-1} [12-15]. Deformational modes are observed within the 100-450 cm^{-1} region.

The aims of this investigation were to examine the chemical spectra and structural characteristics of inorganic arsenic (IAs^{3+}, IAs^{5+}), and the metabolites (monomethylarsonic acid (MMA^{5+}) and dimethylarsinic acid (DMA^{5+}), using Raman microspectroscopy, and to create a library of these Raman spectra. Moreover, the Raman spectrum of each arsenic species will be presented and structural features will be discussed.

MATERIALS AND METHODS

Trivalent inorganic arsenic in the form of sodium *m*-arsenite (**IAs^{3+}**, $NaAsO_2$), cacodylic acid (**DMA^{5+}**, $C_2H_6AsO_2Na$) and sodium arsenate, dibasic (**IAs^{5+}**, $Na_2HAsO_4 \cdot 7H_2O$) were purchased from Sigma (St. Louis, MO, USA); disodium methyl arsenate (**MMA^{5+}**, $CH_3AsO_2Na_2$) was purchased from Chem Services (West Chester, PA, USA).

The crystals were placed and oriented on an aluminum-coated glass slide on the stage of an Olympus BH50 microscope, which is equipped with 10 and 100X objectives. The microscope is part of a Jobin Yvon LabRam n° 6/178 IM (Edison, NJ, USA) Raman microscope system. Raman spectra were excited by an integrated 633 nm He/Ne excitation laser at a resolution of 2 cm^{-1} in the range between 50-4000 cm^{-1} region. Repeated acquisition using the highest magnification was accumulated to improve the signal to noise ratio in the spectra. Spectra were calibrated using the 520.5cm^{-1} laser line of a silicon wafer. Spectroscopic manipulation such as baseline adjustment and cosmic-ray filtering were performed using the Spectracalc software package GRAMS 32 (Galactic Industries Corporation, NH).

RESULTS AND DISCUSSION

The Raman spectra of the inorganic arsenic compounds, IAs^{3+} and IAs^{5+} in the 200-1000cm^{-1} region are presented in *figure 1*.

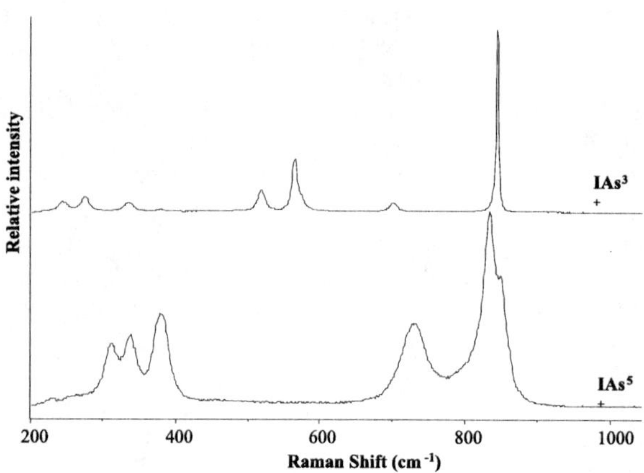

Fig. 1. Raman spectra of inorganic arsenic compounds: IAs^{3+}, IAs^{5+} in the 200-1000 cm^{-1} region

The spectrum of IAs^{3+} has As–O bends at 240, 279, and 332. The peaks at 522 cm^{-1} and 567 cm^{-1} in the IAs^{3+} spectrum denote the presence of an As–O bend. These peaks seem to only be Raman active in IAs^{3+} because they are not observed in IAs^{5+}. The presence of an As–O stretch is observed in both spectra near 703 cm^{-1} and 845 cm^{-1}. The spectrum of the IAs^{5+} has As–O deformation peaks present at 314 and 378, respectively. The peaks present due to the As–O stretching mode are observed at 735 and 833 cm^{-1}. This spectrum was used as a reference to compare the Raman shifts attained from other spectra.

The Raman spectra of the methylated arsenicals are presented in the 200-800 cm^{-1} in *figure 2* region. The As–C bend and stretch, along with the As–O stretch are observed in this region. In the MMA^{5+} spectrum, the peak associated with the As–C bend is observed at 268 cm^{-1}. The peaks at 370 and 395 cm^{-1}, respectively represent deformation modes due to the As–O bond. DMA^{5+} also has the As–C bend near 230 cm^{-1}. The As–C stretch and asymmetric stretch in DMA^{5+} produce vibrations at 604 and 637 cm^{-1}, respectively. MMA^{5+} exhibits only a symmetric stretch at 604 cm^{-1}. The vibration at 833 cm^{-1} for both MMA^{5+} and DMA^{5+} is attributed to the As–O stretching mode.

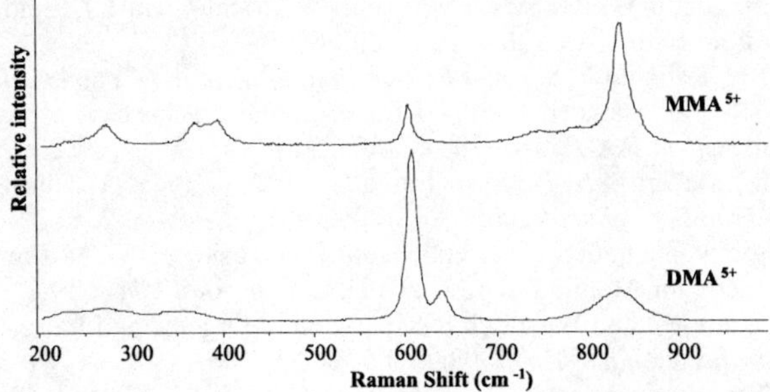

Fig. 2. Raman spectra of methylated arsenic compounds: MMA^{5+} and DMA^{5+} in 200-900 cm^{-1} region

The C – H stretching region is shown in *figure 3*. Both MMA^{5+} and DMA^{5+} show strong vibrations at 2931 cm^{-1} corresponding to the symmetric C – H stretch. The weaker broader band at 3007 cm^{-1} is due to the asymmetric C – H stretch. In the MMA^{5+} spectrum also a broad vibration is present at 3359 cm^{-1} caused by water molecules absorbed in the sample.

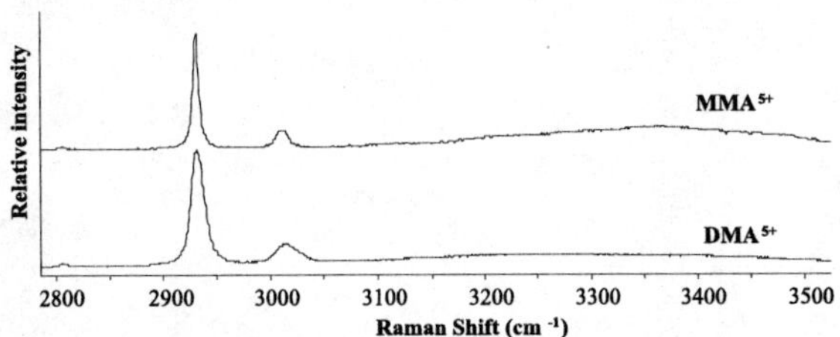

Fig. 3. Raman spectra of methylated arsenic compounds: MMA^{5+} and DMA^{5+} in 2800-3500 cm^{-1} region

CONCLUSION

Raman spectroscopy allows the molecular identification of compounds, providing insight into the molecular characteristics of arsenic compounds. The Raman spectra of inorganic arsenic compounds, methylated arsenicals, and organic arsenic species has been collected. From this library of spectra, the peak assignments of the As–C, As–O, and C–H, and their respective bending and stretching modes has been designated. With this information further studies to establish the structure-function relationship of arsenicals, their activity and toxicology can be investigated.

REFERENCES

1. Chen YC, Amarasiriwardena CJ, Chitra J, Hsueh YM, and Christiani DC, Stability of Arsenic Species and Insoluble Arsenic in Human Urine. *Cancer Epidemiol Biomarkers Prev* 2002, 11:1427-1433.
2. Tchounwou PB, Patolla AK, and Centeno JA, Carcinogenic and Systemic Health Effects Associated with Arsenic Exposure - A Critical Review. *Toxicol Pathol* 2003, 31:575-588.
3. Tchounwou PB, Centeno JA, and Patolla AK, Arsenic toxicity, mutagenesis, and carcinogenesis - a health risk assessment and management approach. *Mol Cell Biochem* 2004, 255 (1-2): 47-55.
4. Mandal BK, Ogra Y, and Suzuki KT Identification of Dimethylarsinous and Monomethylarsonous Acids in Human Urine of the Arsenic-Affected Areas in West Bengal, India. *Chem Res Toxicol* 2001, 14:372-378.

5. Gong Z, Lu X, Cullen WR, Lee XC (2001) Unstable trivalent arsenic metabolites, monomethylarsonous acid and dimethylarsinous acid. *J Anal At Spectrom* 2001, 16: 1409-1413.
6. Arsenic Toxicity: http://www.emedicine.com/med/topic168.htm. Pgs. 1-11.
7. Tseng CH, Tseng CP, Chiou HY, Hsueh YM, Chong CK, and Chen CJ, Epidemiologic evidence of diabetaogenic effect of arsenic. *Toxicol Lett* 2002, 133:69-76.
8. Suzuki KT, Mandal BK, Katagiri A, Sakuma Y, Kawakami A, Ogra Y, Yamaguchi K, Sei Y, Yamanaka K, Anzai K, Ohmichi M, Takayama H, Aimi N, Dimethylthioarsenicals as Arsenic Metabolites and Their Chemical Preparations. *Chem Res Toxicol* 2004, 17(7): 914-921.
9. Abedin J, Cresser MS, Meharg AA, Feldman J, and Cotter-Howells J, Arsenic Accumulation and Metabolism in Rice. *Environ Sci Technol* 2002, 36(5): 962-968.
10. Le XC, Ma M, Wong NA Separation of Arsenic Compounds using HPLC at Elevated Temperature and Selective Hydride Generation Atomic Fluorescence Detection. *Anal Chem* 1996, 68(24): 4501-4506.
11. Londesborough S, Mattusch J, and Wennrich R Separation of Organic and Inorganic Arsenic Species by HPLC-ICP-MS. *Fresenius J Anal Chem* 1999, 363:577-581.
12. Watari F Vibrational spectra and normal coordinate calculations for $(CH_3)_3AsO$ and $(CD_3)_3AsO$, Spectrochimica Acta 1975, 31A:1143-1150.
13. Colthup NB, Daly LH, and Wiberley SE *Introduction to Infrared and Raman Spectroscopy*. Academic Press, San Diego, 1990.
14. Vansant FK, Van der Veken BJ, and Desseyn HO Vibrational Analysis of Arsenic Acid and Its Anions. *J Mol Struct* 1972, 15:425-437.
15. Simon VA and Schumann HD Raman and IR spectroscopic investigation of arsenic acid. I. Vibrational spectra of some alkali metal alkanearsonates. *Z Anorg Allg Chem* 1972, 393:23-38.

Metal Ions in Biology and Medicine: vol. 9. Eds Maria Carmen Alpoim, Paula Vasconcellos Morais, Maria Amélia Santos, Armando J. Cristóvão, José A. Centeno, Philippe Collery.
John Libbey Eurotext, Paris © 2006 pp. 75-1.

Analysis of inorganic arsenic in foods by hydride generation-cold trap-atomic absorption spectrophotometry

Megumi Hamano Nagaoka, and Tamio Maitani

National Institute of Health Sciences, Kamiyoga 1-18-1, Setagaya, Tokyo 158-8501, Japan

SUMMARY

The JECFA (the Joint FAO/WHO Expert Committee on Food Additives) has set a PTWI (provisional tolerable weekly intake) value of arsenic at a quantity of more toxic inorganic arsenic, since the toxicity of arsenic in foods differs greatly between inorganic arsenic and organic arsenic. To determine the inorganic arsenic contents in food samples such as seaweed, rice and water samples, a speciation analysis method by hydride generation-cold trap-atomic absorption spectrometry was applied. To extract inorganic arsenic efficiently, arsenic in foods was extracted with mixed acids (nitric acid and perchloric acid). When some water samples containing germanium as organic germanium compound at the high concentrations were applied to this system, the peak of germane was obviously detected at an earlier retention time than that of arsine in spite of the use of lamp for arsenic detection. Thus, arsine could be detected separately from germane by hydride generation-cold trap-atomic absorption spectrometry, even if both arsenic and germanium were present.

INTRODUCTION

Since the toxicity of arsenic in foods differs greatly between inorganic arsenic and organic arsenic, the JECFA (the Joint FAO/WHO Expert Committee on Food Additives) has established a PTWI (provisional tolerable weekly intake) value of arsenic at a quantity consistent with more toxic inorganic arsenic. As a part of the project for estimating the intake of inorganic arsenic through foods and water, a speciation analysis method by hydride generation-cold trap (HG-CT) -atomic absorption spectrometry was applied to determine the inorganic arsenic contents selectively in several foods and water samples.

MATERIALS AND METHODS

Reagents

Standard mixed solution of methylarsonic acid, dimethylarsinic acid and trimethylarsine oxide was purchased from Wako Pure Chemical Industries, Ltd. Inc (Osaka, Japan). Nitric acid (68%) and perchloric acid (70%) of ultrapure analytical grade (TAMAPURE-AA-100) were purchased from Tama Chemical Industry (Kanagawa, Japan). Other chemicals were of reagent grade or of the highest grade available commercially.

Equipment

Shimadzu ASA-2sp (Kyoto, Japan) was used as arsenic speciation pretreatment system for HG-CT process. Measurement principle is based on that arsenic compounds are separated according to the boiling points of the respective arsenic hydrides. Thermo Elemental Solaar M5 (Kanagawa, Japan) was used as an atomic absorption spectrophotometer (AAS).

Food and water samples

Food samples including infant formulae and baby foods and water samples were obtained in the Tokyo Metropolitan area and by mail order in Japan.

Sample preparation

Foods were first heated with nitric acid, and then perchloric acid was added. Heating was continued until white fume of perchloric acid appeared to remove nitric acid. After heating, water was added to prepare the solution for analysis. Water samples were analysed without heating after filtration with 0.45-μm filter.

Measurements

The acidic solution was applied to the ASA-2sp. Arsenic species in the solution were reduced to the respective hydrides with sodium boronhydride solution, introduced by a carrier gas (helium) to the U-tube filled with quartz wool cooled with liquid nitrogen, and then collected. Next, the U-tube was pulled out of the liquid nitrogen. Arsine, monomethylarsine, dimethylarsine and trimethylarsine were vaporized in turn, depending on their boiling points, and were introduced to the AAS for monitoring.

The optimal conditions for obtaining high sensitivity were examined for the combined ASA-2sp (Shimadzu) and AAS (Thermo Elemental) system. Several types of foods and some water samples were analyzed under the optimized conditions.

RESULTS AND DISCUSSION

To apply this speciation method to a solid food, food containing arsenic must be converted to a solution. Moreover, to be detected, all arsenic compounds must be present as species that can be transformed into hydrides. Whether or not the organic arsenic compounds were degraded into inorganic arsenic on heating was examined using commercially available reagents, namely, methylarsonic acid, dimethylarsinic acid, trimethylarsine oxide and arsenobetaine. These organic arsenic compounds were not converted into inorganic species at the temperature below 110°C. Thus, the conditions under which organic arsenic compounds in foods did not change into inorganic species were determined.

Since the original conditions of the ASA-2sp pretreatment system were set to be optimal for the atomic absorption spectrophotometer of said corporation, the optimum conditions with the Solaar M5 spectrophotometer were studied. First, with the quartz cell of the Solaar M5 system heated electrothermally, helium gas flow rate was optimized. However, atomic absorbance was only one-third of that with the Shimadzu spectrophotometer. Moreover, the resolution of dimethylarsine and trimethylarsine was insufficient. Furthermore, the background level was not steady even when the flow rate of helium gas was changed. Since quartz cells supplied by the two companies differ in shape, the quartz cell from the Shimadzu Company could not be fitted to the Solaar M5 system.

Next, therefore, another heating method, in which a quartz cell is heated with a flame, was investigated. For this purpose, a new quartz cell suited to the Solaar M5 system was prepared. The optimum conditions for various factors were selected. Under the optimum conditions selected, the detection limit obtained with standard arsenite solution was 0.022 ppb. When this method was applied to a dry hijiki sample, the coefficient of variation for arsine was 2.6%, a satisfactory value. This method was also applied to pulverized rice, baby foods, infant formulae and water samples.

When some water samples containing germanium as organic germanium compound at the high concentrations were applied to this system, a tiny peak of germane was obviously detected at an earlier retention time than that of arsine, in spite of the use of lamp for arsenic detection. Germanium is known to have a spectral line at 193.7 nm, which is also the wavelength of dominant spectral line of arsenic. Therefore, this method, hydride generation-cold trap-atomic absorption spectrophotometry, may be considered to be a useful technique to detect arsine and germane separately from foods and water samples containing both inorganic arsenic and germanium.

REFERENCE

1. Nagaoka MH, Taneike Y, Akiyama H, Maitani T. Application of speciation analysis by hydride generation-cold trap-atomic absorption spectrometry to arsenic in foods. *Yakugaku Zasshi. J Pharm Soc Japan* 2005; 125 suppl.1: 69-71.

Metal Ions in Biology and Medicine: vol. 9. Eds Maria Carmen Alpoim, Paula Vasconcellos Morais, Maria Amélia Santos, Armando J. Cristóvão, José A. Centeno, Philippe Collery.
John Libbey Eurotext, Paris © 2006 pp. 78-1.

Hydrogeochemistry of thermal spring and caldera waters in São Miguel island (Azores, Portugal) and possible applications in Spa treatments

Terroso, D.[1]; Ferreira da Silva, E.[2]; Patinha, C.[2]; Rocha, F.[1]; Forjaz, V.[3] & Santos, A.[1]

[1]MIA, Dep. Geociências, Univ. Aveiro, 3810-193 Aveiro, Portugal, frocha@geo.ua.pt
[2]ELMAS, Dep. Geociências, Univ. Aveiro, 3810-193 Aveiro, Portugal, eafsilva@geo.ua.pt
[3]ELMAS/Centro Vulcanológico dos Açores, Univ. Açores, Ponta Delgada, Portugal

Portugal is rich in excellent minero-medicinal waters, some of them of marked thermal character. Their diversity is great, in terms of chemical and physical properties, and they are being the object of a fine characterisation programme by the authors of the present communication. The characterisation program has started with Vale das Furnas, São Miguel island, Azores archipelago *(fig. 1)*, where more than two dozens of springs of hyperthermal, mesothermal and hypothermal waters do occur.

The experimental data available so far allowed us to conclude that all the studied spring and caldera waters have good potentialities to be used for polytherapy applications: Its use combined with other natural therapies has good potential for the introduction of new methodologies.

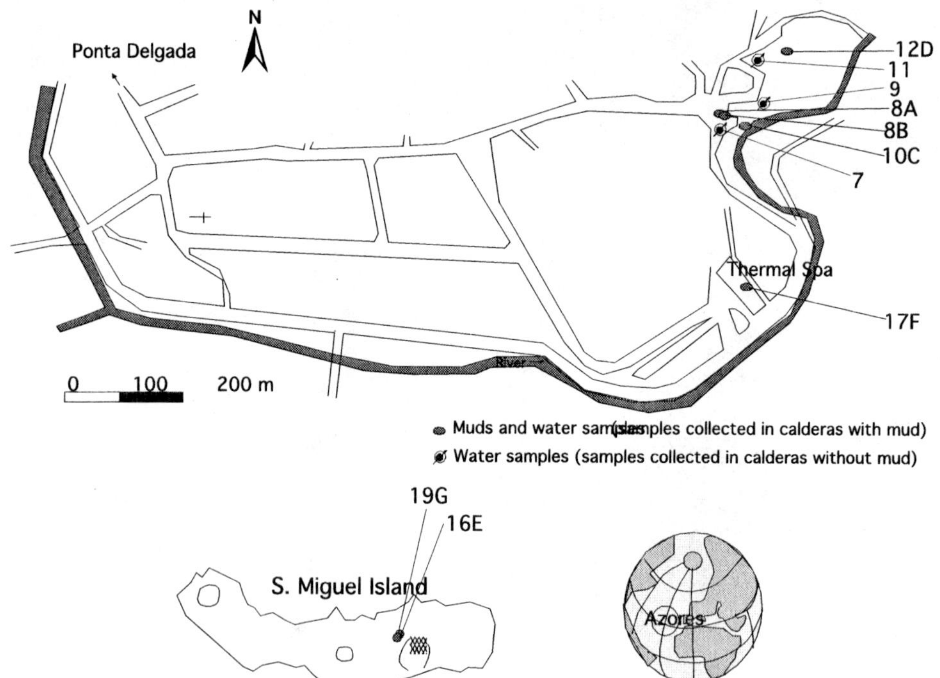

Fig. 1. Location of study area and sampling sites.

INTRODUCTION

The authors of the present study are involved in a research programme, whose main goal is the study of hydrochemical properties of the Portuguese thermal minero-medicinal waters starting with São Miguel island in Azores archipelago, particularly in what concerns their trace elements.

Numerous thermal and mineral springs are located in active volcanic regions all over the world, as a result of eruptive events, as well as obvious manifestations of long-lived hydrothermal systems. These springs are frequently developed as Spas, improving social and economic well-being (Cruz & França, 2005). Portugal Thermal Spas, most of them requiring revitalization through the renewal of infrastructures and the introduction of new methodologies and products in order to become real polytherapy centres (Gomes, 2002) can also benefit from the present characterisation program.

Amongst the various regions where thermal minero-medicinal springs and clays/muds do exist, S. Miguel island, Azores has been selected for the kick-off of the proposed project due to its great potential in thermal minero-medicinal springs as well as in muds/clays deposited by the thermal springs, associated to small calderas and fumaroles.

The characterisation program has started with Vale das Furnas, São Miguel island, Azores archipelago *(fig. 1)*, where more than two dozens of springs of hyperthermal, mesothermal and hypothermal waters do occur. Some of the hyperthermal springs deposit muds that are being used in the treatment of certain diseases.

MATERIALS AND METHODS

The Azores archipelago is composed of nine islands of volcanic origin and a few islets. It is located in the North Atlantic Ocean at about 1600 Km, West of Europe Continent, between latitudes 36°55'43''NS and 39°43'23''N and longitudes 24°46'15''W and 31°16'24''W (Cruz & França, 2005).

São Miguel island, in Azores archipelago, was formed around 4My ago starting with the formation of the basaltic shield volcano active till 1My before present. This volcanic event has been followed by three volcanic episodes yielding the three stratovolcanos, named Nordeste, Povoação and Furnas, all of them being of plinian and subplinian character. The volcanism character being initially basaltic did evolve to trachytic (Terroso, 2003).

Related with the Furnas stratovolcano two main calderas were formed, one of them occupied by a lake named Lagoa das Furnas. In both calderas there exist two fumarolic fields. From small ponds and rock cavities hot whitish smokes are emitted and profuse bubbling comes out from the hot mud that fills those ponds. Also, about two dozens of springs exist in Vale das Furnas, and the temperature of their waters goes up from the ambient temperature to 98°C. Muds are just deposited in the fumaroles yielding hyperthermal waters.

Nine hot springs (52°C ~ 98°C) were sampled *(fig. 1)* and analyzed to determine the physical and chemical characteristics of both muds and waters (samples 8A, 8B, 10C, 12D, 16E and 19G) or just for waters (7, 9 and 11). A sample (17F) representative of mud and water being used in the Vale das Furnas Thermal Spa was also collected.

Samples of water were collected from hot to warm springs which are located within the caldera. Samples were filtrated with 0.45 μm cellulose acetate membrane filter (Hunt & Wilson, 1986). Temperature, pH and conductivity were also measured in the place.

Chemical analyses were performed following the procedures described by EPA (1983) and ASTM (1984). Bicarbonates were measured by acid titration to pH 4.5 using a HCl (0.1N); major anions by Dionex Ion Chromatography (chloride, nitrate, sulphate); magnesium and calcium by atomic absorption spectrometry (AAS) and sodium, potassium by flame photometer at Geosciences Department of Aveiro University; trace metals by ICP-MS at a accredited Canadian laboratory (ACME Anal. ISO 9002 Accredited Lab-Canada).

Data Presentation

In order to characterize thermal and mineral water composition on the Azores archipelago a data table *(table 1)* was compose. Samples were divided in two main groups: Spring waters and Calderas waters. The second group comprises two different types of samples: samples collected in calderas yielding mud (WMUD) and water samples collected in calderas not yielding mud (WWMUD). Also note that samples 17 and 18 are spring waters that were collected in the Vale das Furnas Thermal Spa refered in *figure 1* on 17F location.

Geochemical data from all the analysed samples are plotted in *figures 2* and *3* on Piper trilinear diagram and in *figure 4* on a Cl- SO_4-HCO_3 ternary diagram.

RESULTS AND DISCUSSION

Spring waters show higher pH values (4.6-7.9) in comparison with Caldera waters (2.3-7.3) probably because of the higher content in sulfates in Caldera waters. Also conductivity (280-2020 μS/cm) and temperature (16-90 °C) values are generally lower for Spring waters samples. Spring waters show higher content in bicarbonates (85-824 ppm) and Caldera waters in sulphates (70-1022 ppm) and chlorates (8-301 ppm) and in some cases in bicarbonates (305-689 ppm).

In what concerns Calderas waters: the WMUD water type show high temperature (77 - 95 °C) and are characterized high concentrations of Al (6029 - 37356 ppb), Fe (17170 - 39835 ppb), Mn (879 - 3975 ppb), S (167 - 280 ppm) and Zn (98 - 366 ppb).

The WWMUD water type presents high concentrations of Cl (166 - 301 ppm), HCO_3 (305 - 689 ppm), Na (374 - 626 ppm), Li (247 - 402 ppb), As (619 - 1907 ppb), B (10253 - 16198 ppb) and Br (371 - 570 ppb).

Concentration of volcanic-gas derived species like Cl and SO_4 varies irregularly. SO_4 concentration increases in springs yielding mud (589 - 1022 mg/l) while in the springs not yielding mud SO_4 concentration varies in the rang 70 - 352 ppm. High Cl concentration was found in springs not yielding mud.

Some differences were observed in the Si concentration (WMUD with 79 to 199 ppm and WWMUD with 169 to 194 ppm).

The water samples data related to calderas yielding mud (WMUD) falls in the region of sodium sulphate type waters (with pH values ranging from 2.4 to 2.8) while the water samples chemical data collected in calderas not yielding mud (WWMUD) falls in the region of sodium-bicarbonate-chloride type waters (with pH ranging from 6.3 to 7.8).

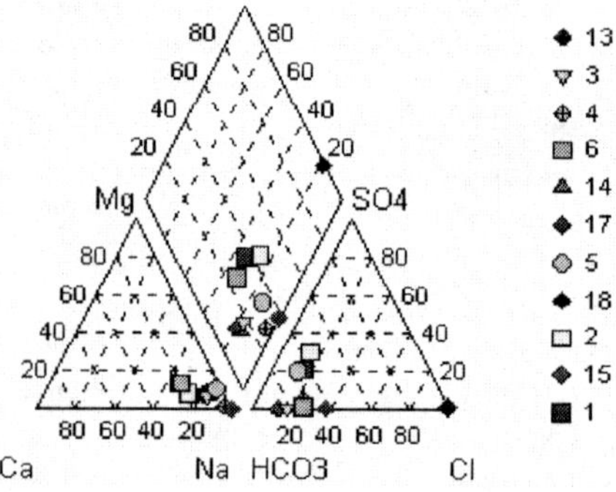

Fig. 2. Piper trilinear diagram showing the composition of the spring waters.

Table 1. Chemical data for the thermal spring and caldera waters in São Miguel island, Azores.

	No.	Location	pH	Cond (µS/cm)	Temp (ºC)	Ca (ppm)	Mg (ppm)	K (ppm)	Na (ppm)	Cl (ppm)	SO_4 (ppm)	HCO_3 (ppm)	Al (ppb)	As (ppb)	B (ppb)	Br (ppb)	Fe (ppb)	Li (ppb)	Mn (ppb)	Zn (ppb)
Spring Water	1	Azeda do Rebentão Spring	4,6	336	16	10	4	25	38	16	28	110	796	1	10	55	6020	8	704	15
	2	Prata Spring	4,8	337	37	11	3	24	50	19	51	122	1223	1	25	55	3157	14	998	9
	3	Caldeirão Spring	5,6	442	75	10	4	22	93	34	1	262	171	58	1289	87	1106	47	1021	5
	4	Santa Spring	6,9	895	90	7	1	16	224	82	22	427	73	322	4886	192	53	129	114	2
	5	Miguel Henriques Spring	4,9	400	20	2	4	32	64	21	42	183	699	3	10	56	6472	17	1022	17
	6	Dr Dinis Spring	4,6	280	17	10	4	25	39	17	1	85	943	3	10	61	7161	8	708	17
	13	Grutinha I/Ernesto Spring	5,8	1349	41	36	14	42	316	78	1	824	82	64	503	205	4358	267	717	0.25
	14	Grutinha II Spring	5,8	1304	45	31	13	37	305	75	1	793	104	62	519	195	6142	247	929	0.25
	15	Fria das Quenturas Spring	6,0	1261	58	35	14	49	281	65	1	732	4	22	902	179	1741	217	447	0.25
	17	Sulfurosas do Balneário Spring	7,9	2020	38	2	0	22	544	280	1	793	110	1786	18101	582	49	426	18	0.25
	18	Férricas do Balneário Spring	6,9	1305	n.d.	35	14	53	293	65	1	0	9	31	950	182	990	245	173	0.25

Table 1. Suite.

	No.	Location	pH	Cond (µS/cm)	Temp (ºC)	Ca (ppm)	Mg (ppm)	K (ppm)	Na (ppm)	Cl (ppm)	SO_4 (ppm)	HCO_3 (ppm)	Al (ppb)	As (ppb)	B (ppb)	Br (ppb)	Fe (ppb)	Li (ppb)	Mn (ppb)	Zn (ppb)
Caldera Water	7	Caldera Grande Water**	7,8	1958	83	2	0	27	548	301	70	689	130	1907	16198	579	39	336	24	2
	8	Caldera Barrenta Water*	2,4	1731	79	31	11	32	82	8	849	0	37356	120	10	19	39835	77	2649	366
	9	Caldera Asmodeu Water**	7,3	2320	82	2	0	29	626	273	353	628	335	1558	14741	542	150	402	28	1
	10	Rib. dos Tambores nearby Water*	2,8	2150	77	27	5	89	325	110	733	0	6029	268	7601	256	17452	113	3975	224
	11	Caldera do Esguicho Water**	6,3	1529	52	8	2	33	374	166	332	305	5138	619	10253	372	3307	247	540	20
	12	Santa Sprin nearby Water*	2,3	2400	80	66	10	45	86	11	786	0	6707	3	106	24	17170	64	2518	102
	16	Caldera da Lagoa Water*	2,4	1549	70	18	7	15	47	12	589	0	8273	4	104	39	15563	25	879	98
	19	Calderas da Ribeira Grande Water*	2,3	3060	n.d.	27	8	24	44	16	1022	0	34153	0.5	10	55	23080	23	971	144

* WMUD (Calderas with water yielding mud); ** WWMUD (Calderas not yielding mud).

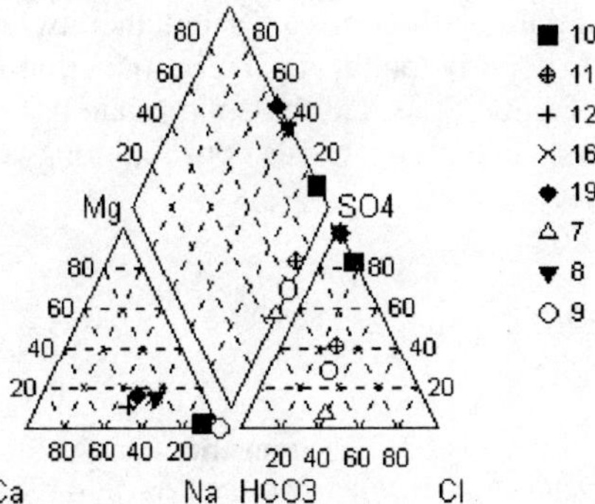

Fig. 3. Piper trilinear diagram showing the composition of the caldera waters.

The Piper diagram for spring waters illustrates that the general chemical character of the spring waters is mainly bicarbonated-sodium type, except for sample 18 (collected in Vale das Furnas Spa) that has chloride-sodium character. Caldera waters shows a chloride-sulphate-sodium facies, except for samples 19 that have a sulphate-sodium character and sample 7 that have sodium-bicarbonate character.

The chemical data for both studied groups of water are also represented in a $Cl-SO_4-HCO_3$ ternary diagram (Giggenbach, 1988) for thermal water composition *(fig. 4)*. This plot allows discrimination between water group giving insights: $Na-SO_4$ type waters are plotted in the steam-heated waters field, Na-Cl type waters plot in the field of mature waters, whereas other thermal discharges fall in the peripheral waters field (Cruz and França, 2005).

The chemical composition of the water samples in the ternary diagram *(fig. 4)* show also that most of the spring waters are represented in the peripheral waters field, except for sample 18 that is in the mature waters field. The caldera waters are represented in the steam heated waters field, excepted for samples 7 and 9 that are represented in the peripheral waters (these two samples correspond to WWMUD samples).

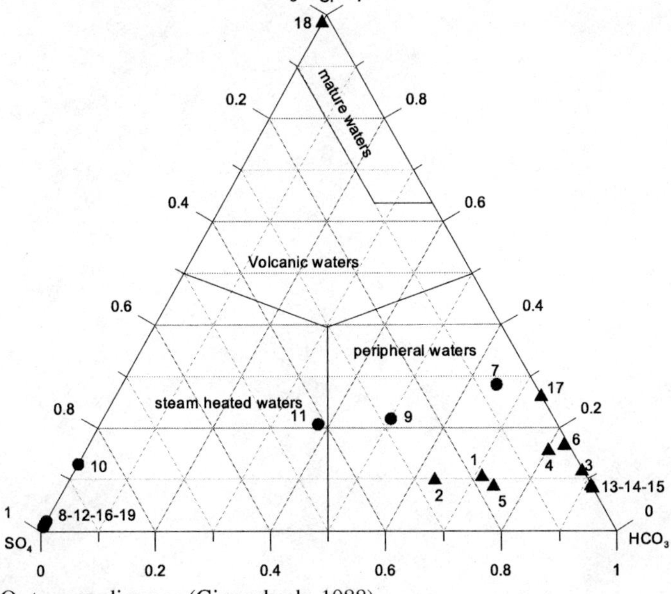

Fig. 4. $Cl-SO_4-HCO_3$ ternary diagram (Giggenbach, 1988).

The experimental data available so far allowed us to conclude that all the studied spring and caldera waters have good potentialities to be used for polytherapy applications: Its use combined with other natural therapies has good potential for the introduction of new methodologies.

The revitalization of some Termal Spas and the appropriate use of minerals and other mineral resources in geomedicine can reduce both pharmacs consumption and the number of working days people miss due to health problems.

REFERENCES

1. EPA, Environmental Protection Agency "Methods for Chemical Analysis of Water and Wastes. Inductively. Coupled Plasma - Atomic Emission Spectrometric: method for trace element analysis of water and wastes (method 200.7)". *United States Environmental Agency* 1983; 430 pp.
2. ASTM, American Society for Testing Materials, Annual Book of ASTM Standarts. *Water Environmental Technology*, 1984; Vol. 11.01.
3. Carretero, M. Isabel "Clay minerals and their beneficial effects upon human health. A review". *Applied Clay Science* 2002; 21: 155-163.
4. Gomes, Celso de Sousa Figueiredo "Argilas-Aplicações na Indústria" Aveiro, 2002. 338 p.
5. Gomes, C.; Silva, E; Rocha, F.; Patinha, C.; Forjaz, V.; Terroso, D. "Benefits of mud/clay and thermal spring water in the human health". *Environment 2010: Situation and Perspectives for the European Union, Porto, Portugal.* 2003 ; 269-270.
6. Terroso, D.; Gomes, C.; Rocha, F.; Forjaz, V.; Silva, E.; Patinha, C.; Gomes, V. "Muds deposited by fumaroles in Vale das Furnas, S. Miguel island, Azores archipelago: properties relevant for their use in mudtherapy". *Euroclay 2003 Abstracts Book*, Modena, Italy 2003: 269-270.
7. Gomes, C.; Sequeira, C.; Terroso, D.; Rocha, F.; Silva, E.; Patinha, C.; Forjaz, V.H.; Gomes, V. "Alunitic clay from Furnas do Enxofre fumarolic field, Terceira, Azores: Characterization for eventual applications in cosmetics and dermatological therapies". *XVIII Reunión Científica de la Sociedad Espanola de Arcillas*, Amagro 2003: 63-64.
8. Virgílio Cruz, J.; França, Zilda "Hydrogeochemistry of thermal and mineral water springs of the Azores archipelago (Portugal). *Journal of volcanology and geothermal research*, Article in press 2005.

Metal Ions in Biology and Medicine: vol. 9. Eds Maria Carmen Alpoim, Paula Vasconcellos Morais, Maria Amélia Santos, Armando J. Cristóvão, José A. Centeno, Philippe Collery.
John Libbey Eurotext, Paris © 2006 pp. 85-1.

Chemical and physical characterization of mud/clay from São Miguel and Terceira islands (Azores, Portugal) and possible application in Pelotherapy

Terroso, D.[1]; Rocha, F.[1]; Ferreira da Silva, E.[2]; Patinha, C.[2]; Forjaz, V.[3] & Santos, A.[1]

[1]MIA, Dep. Geociências, Univ. Aveiro, 3810-193 Aveiro, Portugal, frocha@geo.ua.pt
[2]ELMAS, Dep. Geociências, Univ. Aveiro, 3810-193 Aveiro, Portugal, eafsilva@geo.ua.pt
[3]ELMAS/Centro Vulcanológico dos Açores, Univ. Açores, Ponta Delgada, Portugal

S. Miguel island, in Azores archipelago, is a volcanic island formed around 4 My ago starting with the formation of the basaltic shield volcano active till 1My before present. In one of the three volcanic events, during the island formation, two main calderas were formed. In each one of the calderas there exist one fumarolic field where from small ponds and rock cavities hot whitish smokes are emitted and profuse bubbling comes out from the hot mud that fills those ponds. Muds are just deposited in the fumaroles yielding hyperthermal waters.

Also in Terceira island in Azores archipelago, can be found fumaroles where mud samples were collected. In this case the fumaroles do not yield hyperthermal waters.

The aim of this work is the geochemical and mineralogical study of samples of mud collected in selected fumaroles, some of them used in medical therapy, particularly in the Furnas spa (Centro Termal das Furnas).

INTRODUCTION

The appropriate use of minerals and other mineral resources in geomedicine can reduce both pharmacs consumption and the number of working days people miss due to health problems.

The use of minerals for medicinal purposes is almost as old as mankind itself (Carretero, 2002). Most of the materials used are muds/clays that have internal or external therapeutic applications in Mudtherapy or Pelotherapy (Gomes, 2003).

The main goal of the present communication is the study of some muds/clays being used in Portugal for health treatments, outdoors in the geological sites where they naturally occur or indoors in Thalassotherapy Centres or in Thermal Spas.

The Azores archipelago situated in the middle of the Atlantic Ocean comprises nine islands, all volcanic. These are classified accordingly to their geographic location into three groups: Western Group, Central Group and Eastern Group. São Miguel island belongs to the Eastern Group and Terceira island belongs to the Central Group.

Vale das Furnas, in S. Miguel island, Azores archipelago, is a particular case of a very restricted area where small ponds and rock cavities can be found with hot whitish smokes being emitted and profuse bubbling comes out from the hot mud that fills those ponds. Muds are just deposited in the fumaroles yielding hyperthermal waters.

Furnas de Enxofre is a fumarolic field located at 12 km, approximately, to the north of the town of Angra do Heroísmo, Terceira island, Azores.

MATERIALS AND METHODS

The Azores archipelago is composed of nine islands of volcanic origin and a few islets. It is located in the North Atlantic Ocean at about 1600 Km, West of Europe Continent, between latitudes 36°55'43''NS and 39°43'23''N and longitudes 24°46'15''W and 31°16'24''W.

In S. Miguel island, related with the Furnas stratovolcano two main calderas were formed, one of them occupied by a lake named Lagoa das Furnas. In both calderas there exist two fumarolic fields. From small ponds and rock cavities hot whitish smokes are emitted and profuse bubbling comes out from the hot mud that fills those ponds. Muds are just deposited in the fumaroles yielding hyperthermal waters *(fig. 1)*.

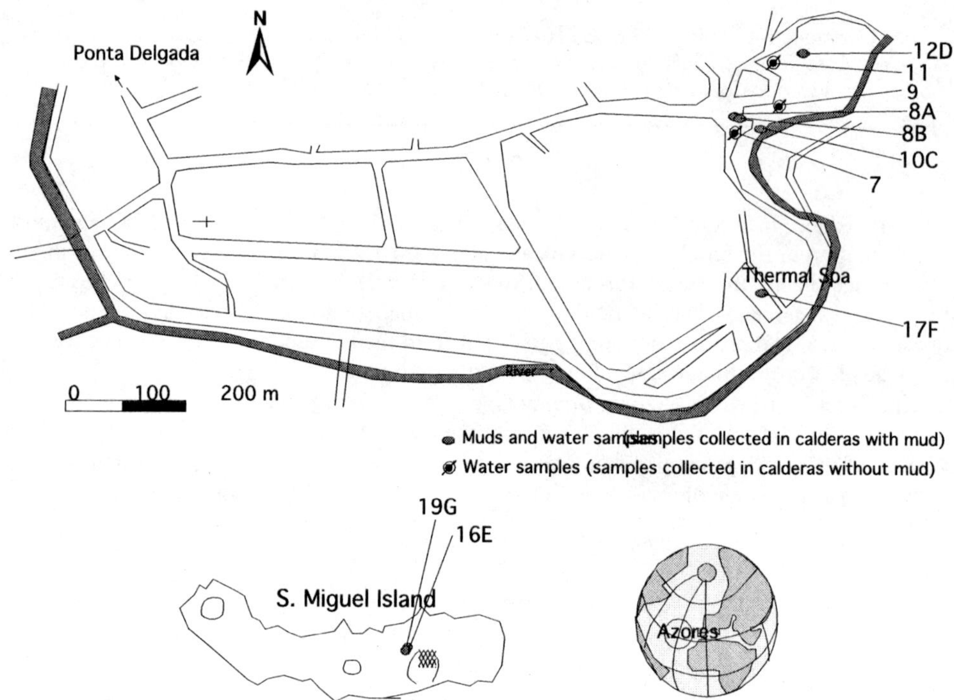

Fig. 1. Location of study area and sampling sites in São Miguel Island.

Furnas do Enxofre fumarolic field in Terceira island comprises two fumarolic subfields separated one from the other by a distance estimated at 200 meters, approximately, situated in the centre of the island *(fig. 2)*.

Efflorescences of sulphur, and sulphates such as mirabilite, $Na_2SO_4.10\ H_2O$, and alunite, $KAl_3(SO_4)_2(OH)_6$, are quite common, lying around the fumarole vent, more precisely. In fact this type of fumarole could be called solfatara. In the case of Furnas de Enxofre the solfataras do not expel liquid water. Local volcanic rock is a hyperalkaline trachyte containing more SiO_2, K_2O and Na_2O and less Al_2O_3 than the typical trachyte.

Around the solfatara vents trachyte is fully altered and as a result of that a whitish or reddish clay-like material, of deuteric origin, is produced. Four samples of the whitish and reddish clay-like material was studied and characterized (Gomes *et al.*, 2003).

Seven samples of mud/clays were collected in São Miguel island (8A, 8B, 10C, 12D, 16E, 17F and 19G) and four samples in Terceira island (I, J, L, M). Sample 17F is actually used in Vale das Furnas Spa for pelotherapy treatments.

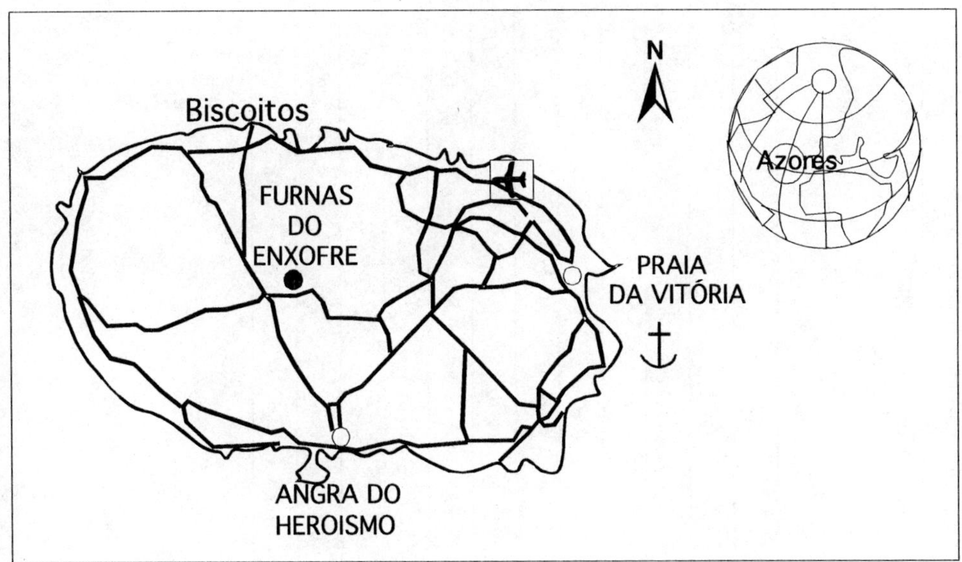

Fig. 2. Location of study area and sampling sites in Terceira Island.

Chemical and mineralogical composition, texture, pH, specific surface (SS), total ion exchange capacity, cooling rate, expandability (Exp), plasticity index (PI), abrasivity index (AI) and specific heat were studied.

As a matter of fact, the most relevant assets of peloids to be used in the form of warm patches or cataplasms are as follows: high specific surface area, high cation exchange capacity, high specific heat and low cooling rate.

All the properties referred to are dependent upon both granularity and mineral and chemical composition of clay or mud. Clay or mud particles can be smaller than bacteria and these whenever coated or encapsulated by clay particles lose activity and can be eliminated (Gomes *et al.*, 2003).

Data Presentation

In order to geochemicaly and physically characterize mud/clay on the Azores archipelago data tables *(tables 1, 2 and 3)* were composed. Samples were divided in two main groups: São Miguel and Terceira island. Another sample was added to all tables (VC) that was collected in Vale dos Cucos Spa in Portugal, this sample was also used in pelotherapy treatments and its data was compiled from previous studies (Gomes, 1988, 2002). Note that in this case not all properties were determined.

RESULTS AND DISCUSSION

All samples are finely grained muds that consist of two main mineral components: clay minerals and non clay minerals.

In what concerns the non clay minerals, the studied samples show (Terroso *et al.*, 2003) a mineralogical composition consisting mainly of alunite, feldspars, quartz, and amorphous alumi-nosilicates, accompanied by anhydrite and pyrite as accessory minerals.

Concerning clay minerals, small amounts of kaolinite, smectite and ilite-esmectite were found, the last only in some samples (Terroso *et al.*, 2003).

Table 1 shows the main physical and chemical characteristics of the studied samples.

Table 1. Main physical and chemical characteristics of mud/clay from São Miguel and Terceira islands, Azores.

Location		Fraction <0,063 mm (% of total sample)	Fraction <0,002 mm (% of <0,063 mm fraction)	pH	SS (m^2/g)	Ion exchange capacity (meq/100g)	Cooling rate (°C)	Exp (%)	PI (mm)	AI (g/m^2)	Specific heat (J/g °C)
S. Miguel	**8A**	95	25	2.1	5.0	8.20	19.5	9.73	1.3	71.8	0.57
	8B	99	58	1.7	23.2	22.60	20.0	6.40	8.5	27.5	1.38
	10C	98	30	3.3	32.4	18.60	19.0	21.13	10.8	36.4	1.25
	12D	86	13	2.4	12.4	13.20	19.5	16.86	2.9	60.3	0.88
	16E	98	21	2.6	12.1	7.60	19.0	22.66	5.7	68.2	0.49
	17F	76	71	3.8	25.1	18.40	19.5	26.46	37.7	17.4	1.19
	19G	99	35	2.0	17.4	5.20	19.0	11.70	5.9	52.5	0.39
Terceira	**I**	98	62	3.4	19.7	3.00	17.5	0.33	29.0	8.2	0.81
	J	59	73	4.0	20.1	3.80	15.5	10.80	n.d	26.2	0.89
	L	91	65	4.1	91.2	10.00	19.5	24.40	26.5	11.8	1.16
	M	79	10	6.1	87.6	29.20	28.5	13.90	n.d	23.6	3.87
VC*		-	-	-	18.0	11.00	19.8	12.00	8.0	-	3.45

* VC - Vale dos Cucos (Gomes, 2002).

Samples from Terceira show pH values similar to or slightly higher than reference sample, whereas samples from S. Miguel show lower ones.

In what concerns expandability, specific surface area and ion exchange capacity, only 3 samples (L and M from Terceira; 10C from S. Miguel) exhibit values similar to or slightly higher than those from the reference samples (17F and VC).

Similar considerations can be put forward concerning specific heat.

Table 2 shows the chemical data (Major Elements) of the studied mud/clay samples from São Miguel and Terceira islands, Azores.

In general terms, samples from S. Miguel show adequate values for calcium, potassium, magnesium, sodium and sulphur; on the other hand, Terceira samples show less adequate values for these particular chemical parameters, showing also higher contents in iron and aluminium.

All samples but J (from Terceira island) show high contents of fine (<0,063mm) fraction, ranging from 79 to 99%, always higher than reference sample 17F. In what concerns clay (<0,002 mm) fraction, only 4 samples (I, J and L from Terceira; 8B from S. Miguel) exhibit contents similar to the reference sample.

All samples but J show cooling rate values similar to or slightly higher than reference sample, behaviour quite similar to that one of the fine fraction contents, pointing out to some control of grain size over cooling rate.

In what concerns plasticity and abrasivity, only 6 samples (I, J, L and M from Terceira; 8B and 10C from S. Miguel) exhibit values similar to those from the reference samples (17F and VC), behaviour quite similar to that one of the clay fraction contents, once again pointing out to some control of grain size distribution.

Table 3 shows the chemical data (Minor and Trace Elements) of the studied mud/clay samples from São Miguel and Terceira islands, Azores.

In general terms, samples from S. Miguel show once again adequate values for the studied parameters (although sample 19G showing inadequate values for Pb), whereas Terceira samples show less adequate values for some particular chemical parameters, such as Zr, Zn, Ni, Co, Cr and V.

In regards to the studied physical and chemical parameters, almost all samples are in conformity in comparison with both reference samples (17F and VC) that are being used for pelotherapy treatments.

Actually, all samples are finely grained, have low pH, good specific surface, generally high Cationic Exchange Capacity, very good cooling rates and adequate chemical composition.

Nevertheless, it is possible to conclude that samples from Terceira show better physical results whereas samples from S. Miguel show better chemical ones.

Table 2. Chemical data (Major Elements) of the studied mud/clay samples from São Miguel and Terceira islands, Azores.

Location		Major Elements (%)											LOI (%)
		Fe_2O_3	MnO	TiO_2	CaO	K_2O	P_2O_5	SiO_2	Al_2O_3	MgO	Na_2O	SO_3	
S. Miguel	**8A**	1.63	0.05	0.70	0.27	2.55	0.13	53.61	13.65	0.06	1.42	7.82	17.72
	8B	2.17	0.05	0.85	0.19	2.86	0.24	40.38	20.49	0.13	1.27	9.97	20.56
	10C	8.63	0.12	0.74	0.65	3.17	0.33	53.07	15.84	0.39	2.01	5.20	9.00
	12D	1.79	0.06	1.00	0.40	3.98	0.19	50.08	15.97	0.13	3.07	8.32	14.77
	16E	3.39	0.06	1.28	0.46	3.94	0.26	45.11	17.06	0.20	3.36	9.91	15.00
	17F	1.76	0.03	1.24	0.17	2.45	0.19	52.16	19.79	0.27	1.20	4.84	15.34
	19G	1.01	0.01	1.45	0.12	2.70	0.25	43.37	15.06	0.05	1.52	11.22	22.63
Terceira	**I**	2.25	0.02	0.82	0.02	1.40	0.10	35.47	36.80	0.13	0.19	2.98	19.84
	J	3.98	0.02	10.66	0.04	0.27	0.63	74.85	2.89	0.40	0.10	0.96	5.73
	L	21.22	0.14	4.25	0.05	0.65	1.19	25.71	28.76	0.29	0.12	1.22	17.08
	M	22.94	0.32	5.34	0.19	0.62	2.77	18.32	25.68	0.46	0.79	0.08	21.90
VC*		5.15	0.08	0.75	17.21	2.57	0.13	38.49	17.21	2.61	0.91	0.58	5.04

* VC - Vale dos Cucos (Gomes, 2002); LOI - Lost on Ignition

Table 3. Chemical data (Minor and Trace Elements) of the studied mud/clay samples from São Miguel and Terceira islands, Azores.

Location		Minor and Trace Elements (ppm)															
		Ba	Sn	Nb	Zr	Y	Sr	Rb	Pb	As	Zn	W	Cu	Ni	Co	Cr	V
S. Miguel	**8A**	146	<5	273	1329	20	133	89	25	97	63	<5	24	9	<5	25	32
	8B	167	13	381	1772	20	220	75	30	152	64	<5	30	9	<5	33	45
	10C	93	5	193	908	26	89	113	15	279	92	14	5	10	<5	46	39
	12D	292	11	287	1345	22	243	107	28	<5	74	<5	83	11	<5	43	40
	16E	682	10	223	1042	22	480	98	16	<5	75	<5	14	10	<5	44	56
	17F	290	17	409	2021	30	304	66	28	39	78	<5	52	10	<5	23	55
	19G	290	19	391	1980	32	223	53	110	<5	8	<5	58	11	<5	28	52
Terceira	**I**	227	19	185	1457	14	10	<5	16	<5	25	<5	8	14	<5	9	39
	J	290	85	1295	9171	12	20	11	37	<5	<5	21	<5	13	7	27	253
	L	51	<5	61	473	25	47	53	17	<5	294	8	6	25	84	52	269
	M	407	18	181	1522	15	70	36	37	<5	207	6	<5	17	79	67	183
VC*		-	-	-	-	-	-	-	-	-	-	-	-	-	-	-	-

* VC - Vale dos Cucos (Gomes, 2002).

REFERENCES

1. Carretero, M. Isabel "Clay minerals and their beneficial effects upon human health. A review". *Applied Clay Science* 2002; 21: 155-163.
2. Gomes, Celso de Sousa Figueiredo *"Argilas-Aplicações na Indústria"* Aveiro, 2002. 338 p.
3. Gomes, C.; Silva, E; Rocha, F.; Patinha, C.; Forjaz, V.; Terroso, D. "Benefits of mud/clay and thermal spring water in the human health". *Environment 2010: Situation and Perspectives for the European Union, Porto, Portugal.* 2003 ; 269-270.
4. Terroso, D.; Gomes, C.; Rocha, F.; Forjaz, V.; Silva, E.; Patinha, C.; Gomes, V. "Muds deposited by fumaroles in Vale das Furnas, S. Miguel island, Azores archipelago: properties relevant for their use in mudtherapy". *Euroclay 2003 Abstracts Book*, Modena, Italy 2003: 269-270.
5. Gomes, C.; Sequeira, C.; Terroso, D.; Rocha, F.; Silva, E.; Patinha, C.; Forjaz, V.H.; Gomes, V. "Alunitic clay from Furnas do Enxofre fumarolic field, Terceira, Azores: Characterization for eventual applications in cosmetics and dermatological therapies". *XVIII Reunión Científica de la Sociedad Espanola de Arcillas*, Amagro 2003: 63-64.

Metal Ions in Biology and Medicine: vol. 9. Eds Maria Carmen Alpoim, Paula Vasconcellos Morais, Maria Amélia Santos, Armando J. Cristóvão, José A. Centeno, Philippe Collery.
John Libbey Eurotext, Paris © 2006 pp. 93-1.

Determination of trace metal speciation dynamics using Scanned Stripping Chronopotentiometry (SSCP)

Pinheiro, J.P.[1], Minor, M.[2], Van Leeuwen, H.P.[2]

[1] *Centro de Biomedicina Molecular e Estrutural, Dep. Química e Bioquímica/FCT Universidade do Algarve, Campus de Gambelas, 8005-139 Faro, PORTUGAL*
[2] *Laboratory of Physical Chemistry and Colloid Science Wageningen University, Dreijenplein 6, 6703 HB Wageningen, THE NETHERLANDS*

The interest in studying trace metal speciation is associated with health risks for living organisms due to the toxic nature of many trace metals. In most natural aquatic systems metal ions form stable complexes with a large variety of dissolved inorganic and organic ligands. Mostly, the metal ions are bound and/or adsorbed in natural macromolecules, colloids and particles while simultaneously are being taken up by micro organisms. Most of the interactions show both polyfunctional and polyelectrolytic characteristics and therefore cover a broad range of free energy of complex formation and a corresponding range of dynamic behaviour, thus controlling the bioavailability and mobility of the metal ions [1].

DYNAMIC TRACE METAL SPECIATION

It is increasingly recognized that a quantitative understanding of these relationships requires characterization of dynamic aspects, i.e. kinetic features of the interconversion of metal complex species. Many processes in natural aquatic systems involve consumption of a metal species at an interface, e.g. biouptake of a metal ion, which induces mass transport of metal species from the bulk to the consuming interface, followed by conversion to the surface active form. Thus understanding of dynamic bioavailability of metal species requires consideration of the overall flux towards the surface of the organism, as arising from the coupled diffusion and formation/dissociation involving the various metal species in the medium.

Let us consider the case of an electroactive metal ion, M, that forms an electroinactive complex, ML, with a ligand L,

$$\begin{array}{l} M + L \underset{k_a}{\overset{k_d}{\rightleftarrows}} ML \\ \downarrow\uparrow\ ne^- \\ M^0 \end{array} \qquad (1)$$

The rate constants of complex formation (k_a) are generally consistent with a mechanism in which formation of an outer-sphere complex between the metal and the ligand, with an electrostatically determined stability constant (K_{os}), is followed by a rate-limiting removal of water from the inner coordination sphere of the metal (k_{-w}), commonly known as the Eigen mechanism [2]. Complex systems are considered static if they are unable to restore equilibrium on the relevant time scale and dynamic if equilibrium is fully maintained in the bulk. The contribution of dynamic complexes to an overall metal flux depends on the relative magnitudes of the diffusive and kinetic fluxes and will range from fully labile (diffusion control) to non-labile (kinetic control) [3]. The system is dynamic or static if the rates for the volume reactions are fast or slow, respectively, on a time scale, t:

$$k_d t,\ k_a' t >> 1 \qquad \text{(dynamic)} \tag{2a}$$
$$k_d t,\ k_a' t << 1 \qquad \text{(static)} \tag{2b}$$

where k_a' is defined for conditions of excess of ligand:

$$k_a' = k_a c_{L,T} \text{ and } K' = k_a'/k_d = K c_{L,T} \tag{3}$$

where K is the stability constant of ML and $c_{L,T}$ is the total ligand concentration.

The concept of lability is used to define the contribution of metal species to an overall flux towards a consuming interface based on the relative magnitudes of their diffusive (mass transport) and kinetic (dissociation) fluxes. Dynamic theories for truly homogeneous solutions have been developed and successfully tested on a variety of model systems. However, the experimental assessment of the extent of lability of complexes is difficult, requiring variation of the effective timescale of the measuring technique over a sufficiently broad range. A helpful tool has been the establishment of lability criteria for various practical limiting cases. However questions have been raised about their applicability to colloidal and particulate ligand systems, namely, in a study of lead and copper binding in river water Botelho *et al.* [4, 5]. There it was found that "in particles covered with soluble organics, the surface complexes are inert whereas the desorbed soluble organic complexes are labile". Since the pertaining stabilities are similar, the conventional lability criteria for homogeneous solutions cannot explain the experimental observations. This raises the question as to whether the current dynamic theory for homogeneous solutions takes the colloidal nature of the systems into proper account. The key issue is that in colloidal systems the ligands are localized within the geometry of the particles whereas in true solutions the ligand distribution is taken as homogeneous over the solution volume.

Before we proceed in this discussion it is necessary to introduce SSCP and its ability to experimentally determine dynamic speciation parameters, which allowed us to further our studies in the dynamic speciation in colloidal systems.

SCANNING STRIPPING CHRONOPOTENTIOMETRY

Voltammetric stripping techniques have been widely employed to study metal speciation in natural waters [6] however their utility for measurements on environmentally relevant samples has been hampered by secondary effects such as adsorption of organic matter at the electrode surface. A further complicating factor is that the experimental assessment of the extent of lability of complexes is difficult, requiring the variation of the effective timescale of the technique over a sufficiently wide range.

The attractive features of depletive stripping chronopotentiometry [7], especially when operated in scanned deposition potential (SSCP) mode [8], include a detection limit comparable to that of pulsed stripping voltammetric modes, and an absence of adsorption interferences [9].

The deposition step in SSCP is the same as that in stripping voltammetry, but quantification (reoxidation) of the accumulated metal is effected by application of a constant oxidizing current. When the stripping current is sufficiently low, the accumulated metal is completely depleted from the electrode and simple application of Faraday's law yields a direct quantitative relationship between the analytical signal (the stripping or transition time, τ) and the pertinent species concentration in the sample.

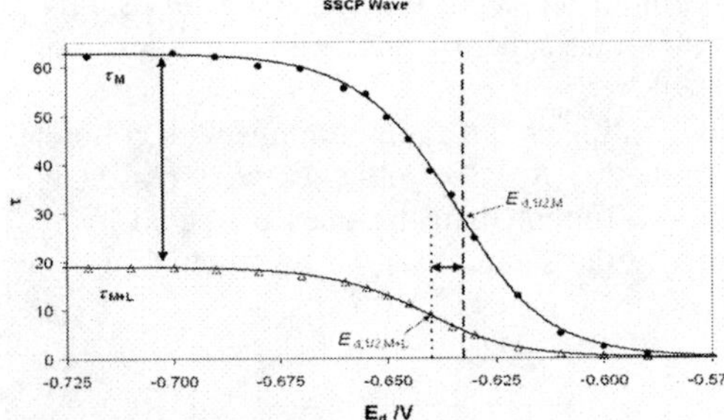

Fig. 1. A SSCP wave is constructed performing a series of deposition steps at different deposition potentials and representing the transition times vs. the deposition potential.

The relatively simple mathematical framework of SSCP, together with the far-reaching validity of the Koutecký-Koryta approximation (spatial division of the diffusion layer into a non-labile and a labile region, separated by the boundary of the reaction layer [10]) allowed a rigorous expression to be obtained for the full SSCP wave in the kinetic current regime [11].

Dynamic information obtained by SSCP

The ability of SSCP to obtain dynamic information derives from the fact that K, can be calculated from the shift in the half-wave deposition potential, $\Delta E_{d,1/2}$, (equivalent to DeFord-Hume expression) irrespective of the degree of lability [12]:

$$\ln(1 + K') = -(nF/RT)\Delta E_{d,1/2} - \ln(\tau^*_{M+L}/\tau^*_M) \tag{4}$$

while k_a' can be calculated from the limiting current value, for quasi-labile or non-labile complexes, using the thickness of the reaction layer, μ [13]:

$$\mu = (D_M/k_a')^{1/2} \tag{5}$$

This parameter can be obtained from the variation in the limiting transition time in presence (τ^*_{M+L}) and absence (τ^*_M) of complexing ligands:

$$\tau^*_{M+L}/\tau^*_M = \left[D_M (1 + K')/d_M ((\bar{d} - \mu)/\bar{D}(1 + K') + \mu/D_M)\right]^{-1} \tag{6}$$

where d_M and $\bar{d}$ are the thicknesses of the diffusion layer for a spherical electrode in absence and presence of complexing ligands respectively:

$$\bar{d} = (1/\delta + 1/r_0)^{-1} \tag{7}$$

and $\bar{D}$ is the average diffusion coefficient that describes the coupled diffusion of bound (c_{ML}) and free metal (c_M) in the labile region ($\mu < x < \delta$) of the diffusion layer,

$$\bar{D} = (D_M c_M + D_{ML} c_{ML})/(c_M + c_{ML}) \tag{8}$$

Detailed derivation of these SSCP equations can be found in references 8, 11 and 12.

Experimental dynamic parameters determined by SSCP

To evaluate the potential of SSCP for the determination of K in the kinetic current regime, we first studied the classical Cd-NTA system at pH 8 [12]. Using equation (4) and assuming an uncertainty of ± 0.002 V in the measured potential shift we obtained a log K of 9.81 ± 0.07 $dm^3.mol^{-1}$. This value agrees perfectly with the IUPAC recommended value of 9.8 (for I=0.1 $mol.dm^{-3}$, 20°C). From equation (6) we obtained a k_a value of $(3.2\pm1.2)\times10^9$ $dm^3mol^{-1}s^{-1}$. This is in good agreement with a k_a of 4.05×10^9 $dm^3mol^{-1}s^{-1}$ calculated on the basis of an Eigen type mechanism, using k_{-w} of 3×10^8 s^{-1} and a stability constant for the intermediate outer-sphere complex of $10^{1.13}$ dm^3 mol^{-1} (z_Mz_L=-4, I=0.1 $mol.dm^{-3}$) [2].

When we applied SSCP to the study of the interaction of lead and cadmium ions with colloidal dispersion of carboxyl modified latex particles *(fig. 2)* the log *K* values obtained were reasonable but the dynamic parameters were orders of magnitude different than the ones predicted by the Eigen mechanism *(table 1)*. This problem was essentially the same observed by Botelho *et al* in the particulate material in the river water [4, 5].

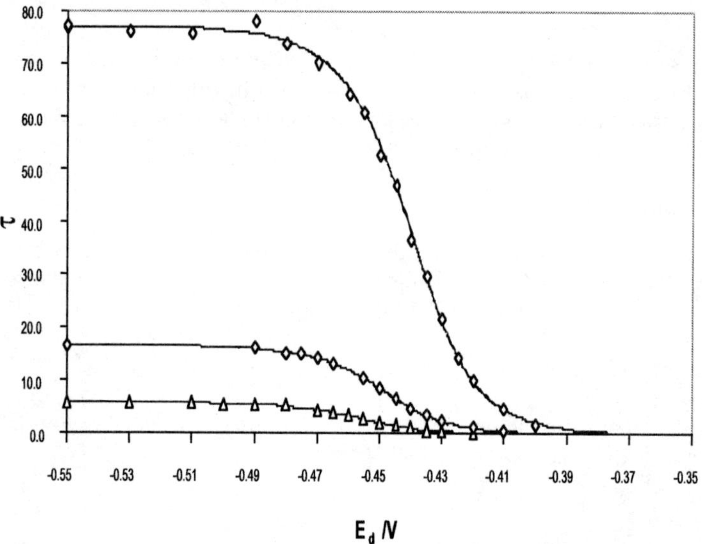

Fig. 2. Experimental and fitted SSCP waves for Pb/60.5 nm 0.1% latex dispersion at different pH. Experimental curves were measured for $3\times10^{-4}molm^{-3}$ Pb(II) in 0.1 $mol.m^{-3}$ KNO3, at 22 (•) and 58×10^{-3} $molm^{-3}$ COOH (Δ). The fitting parameters are presented in *table 1*, and additional parameters: $D=9.849\times10^{-10}ms^{-1}$, $A=4.0\times10^{-7}m^2$, $V=2.4\times10^{-11}m^3$, $\delta_M=2.8\times10^{-5}m$, t_d=90s and $I_s=1\times10^{-9}$ A.

DYNAMIC TRACE METAL SPECIATION IN COLLOIDAL DISPERSIONS

Until recently dynamic theories did not consider the nature of ligand distribution in macromolecular systems, seeing as it was taken as homogeneous over the solution volume, whereas in colloidal systems the concentrations of ligand and bound metal are constrained by the particle geometry.

Recently we demonstrated that the difference between colloidal ligand and the homogeneous systems appears due to an evolution from a chemically controlled reaction to a diffusion controlled one [14]. This was expressed in the modified rates of association and dissociation of the colloidal metal complexes, k_a^* and k_d^*, which now encompass kinetic and diffusive limits (detailed deduction of the new rates can be found in reference 14):

$$k_a^{*'} = k_a'/\left(1 + k_a'(4\pi aD_Mc_p)^{-1}\right) \quad (9a)$$

$$k_d^* = k_d/\left(1 + k_a'(4\pi aD_Mc_p)^{-1}\right) \quad (9b)$$

where a is the particle radius and c_p is the particle number density.

The term $k_a^{'}(4\pi a D_M c_p)^{-1}$ can be interpreted as the ratio of two characteristic times (τ_d/τ_a) which compares the residence time and the mean life time of a free metal ion in the shell layer.

The ratio of both times is the key parameter in the dynamic process. In the limiting situation where τ_d/τ_a is much smaller than unity, the chance of the metal reassociating with a ligand on the same colloidal particle is small. On the other hand if τ_d/τ_a is much larger than unity, the rate of reassociation of the metal is much larger than the diffusion rate, which then becomes the rate limiting step. It is now evident that the difference between k_d^* and k_d, and k_a^* and k_a is mainly due to evolution of a chemically controlled reaction compared to a diffusion controlled one, which derives from differences in spatial ligand distribution between a homogeneous solution and a colloidal ligand dispersion. In the latter systems the overall process is now affected, or even controlled, by diffusion.

Table 1 show the experimental association rate constants (k_a (experimental)), the corresponding value for the homogeneous solution based on k-w, which we denote as Eigen values (k_a (Eigen)), and the value ensuing from our colloidal ligand model calculated using equation (9a) (k_a^*). The most remarkable result is that, within error, the experimentally determined association rate constants agree with the values of k_a^* which differ significantly from their homogeneous counterparts, ka. For lead in the presence of 60.5 nm radius latex we observe a difference of three orders of magnitude when comparing the Eigen predicted value and the measured one, which suggests that the k_a^* value is totally controlled by diffusion to/from the particle.

Table 1. Experimental and calculated dynamic parameters for the lead and cadmium nanospheres systems of 60.5 nm radius at ionic strength 0.01 M.

Metal	$c_{L,t\,(COOH)}/10^{-3}$ mol.m^{-3}	K' ($\Delta E_{d,1/2}$) 10^2	$\mu/10^{-6}$ m	$k_a C_L$ (experimental) 10^3 s^{-1}	$k_a C_L$ (Eigen) 10^3 s^{-1}	$k_a^* C_L$ 10^3 s^{-1}
	21.7	0.48±0.04	0.72	0.9 [0.2 to 16]	555	0.76
Pb	58.8	0.78±0.03	0.77	1.6 [0.4 to 5.2]	1502	2.1
	65.0	2.58±0.20	0.78	1.6±0.7	1665	2.1
Cd	107	0.64±0.03	0.88	0.9 [0.16 to 38]	118	2.2
	118	1.13±0.04	0.86	0.95 [0.3 to 19]	130	1.6

One of the consequences is that a dynamic system for a homogeneously distributed ligand might become less dynamic, if the ligands are confined to local positions on dispersed particles. This is exactly what is reported by Botelho *et al.* [4, 5] for the binding of lead and copper in river waters. As stated above, it was found that Pb and Cu complexes with particles covered with soluble organics are inert, while the desorbed soluble organic complexes are labile; the formation constants were of the same order of magnitude. In this example, the soluble organics are very small, having a diffusion coefficient of the same order of magnitude of the metal, while the particles are the fraction retained in a 450 nm filter, so they are at least larger than 225 nm in radius. Evaluation of the kinetic features using the homogeneous approach shows that the system is dynamic with $k_a c_{L,t} t = 10^4 >> 1$ and $k_d.t = 10^2 >> 1$ (ligand concentration, 10^{-5} M, $k_a(Pb) = 10^{10}$ M.s^{-1}, experimental time scale of the technique used, 0.1s, $K \cong 10^7$). By comparison with *table 1* we can estimate a decrease of the rate constants by at least three orders of magnitude for the particulate system. Assuming the same ligand concentration, $k_a^* C_L t = 10$ and $k_d.t = 10^{-1}$ indicating that the surface complexes present in the particulate system are not dynamic.

CONCLUSIONS

We show that stripping chronopotentiometry at scanned deposition potential (SSCP) is a very good technique to determine the dynamic speciation features of metal complexes.

We propose the use of k_a^* and k_d^* instead of k_a and k_d in both the dynamic and the lability criteria to obtain a correct interpretation. The validity of the new approach is demonstrated for the speciation dynamics of lead and cadmium with carboxyl functionalized latex dispersions. Application of our theory to natural colloidal systems explains previous apparently puzzling observations on lead and copper behaviour in river water.

REFERENCES

1. J. Buffle, "Complexation reactions in aquatic systems. An analytical approach", Ellis Horwood, Chichester, 1988.
2. Morel, F.M.M.; Hering, J.G. Principles and applications of aquatic chemistry, John Wyley, New York, 1993.
3. H.P. van Leeuwen, *Electroanalysis*, 2001, 13, 826.
4. Botelho, C.M.S.; Boaventura, R.A.R.; Gonçalves, M.L.S.S. *Anal Chim Acta* 2002, 462, 73.
5. Botelho, C.M.S.; Boaventura, R.A.R.; Gonçalves, M.L.S.S., *Electroanalysis* 2002, 14, 1713.
6. A.M. Mota, M.M. Correia dos Santos, in A. Tessier, D. Turner, Metal speciation and bioavailability, John Wiley & Sons, New York, 1995, chapter 5.
7. R.M. Town, H.P. van Leeuwen, *J Electroanal Chem* 509 (2001) 58.
8. H.P. van Leeuwen, R.M. Town, *Environ Sci Technol* 37 (2003) 3945.
9. R.M. Town, H.P. van Leeuwen, *J Electroanal Chem* 523 (2002) 1.
10. H.P. van Leeuwen, J. Puy, J. Galceran, J. Cecília, *J Electroanal Chem* 526 (2002) 10.
11. H.P. van Leeuwen, R.M. Town, *J Electroanal Chem* 561 (2004) 67.
12. J.P. Pinheiro, H.P. van Leeuwen, *J Electroanal Chem* 570 (2004) 69.
13. J. Heyrovský, J. Kuta, Principles of Polarography, Publishing House of the Czechoslovak Academy of Sciences, Praha, and Academic Press, New York 1966.
14. J.P. Pinheiro, M. Minor, H.P. Van Leeuwen, *Langmuir* 21 (2005) 8635.

ACKNOWLEDGMENT

This work was performed within the framework of the projects BIOSPEC (funded by the European Commission RTD programme "Preserving the Ecosystem" (Key Action Sustainable Management and Quality of Water, contract EVK1-CT-2001-00086) and project FCT/POCI/QUI/56845/2004, Fundação para a Ciência e Tecnologia, Portugal.

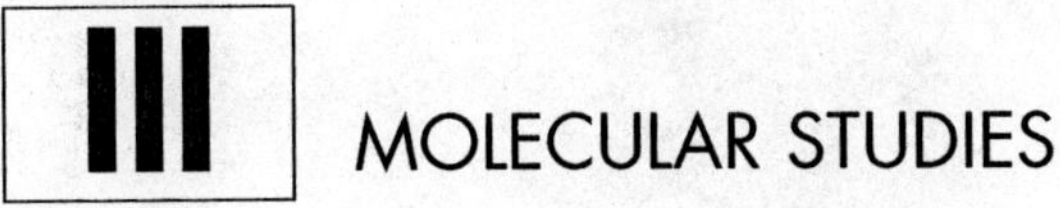

III MOLECULAR STUDIES

Metal Ions in Biology and Medicine: vol. 9. Eds Maria Carmen Alpoim, Paula Vasconcellos Morais, Maria Amélia Santos, Armando J. Cristóvão, José A. Centeno, Philippe Collery.
John Libbey Eurotext, Paris © 2006 pp. 101-1.

Hydroxamic acids as potential lead(II) sequestering agents: factors affecting lead(II) binding properties of hydroxamic acids

Etelka Farkas[1], Dávid Bátka[1], Péter Buglyó[1] and M. Amelia Santos[2]

[1]*Department of Inorganic and Analytical Chemistry, University of Debrecen, H-4010, Debrecen, POB 21. Hungary, fax:+36-52-489-667 e-mail:efarkas@delfin.klte.hu*
[2]*Centro de Química Estrutural, Complexo I, Instituto Superior Técnico, Av. Rovisco Pais, 1049-001 Lisbon, Portugal*

Hydroxamic acids (involving -CORNOH function) are naturally occurring metal chelating agents and hydroxamate-based siderophores play crucial role in the iron uptake of microbes [1, 2]. It is also known that siderophores might be involved not only in the iron but also in the molybdenum uptake in N_2-fixing bacteria [3, 4]. In addition to the two named metal ions, further metals (both essentials, e.g. zinc(II), nickel(II), copper(II), and toxic, e.g. aluminium(III), lead(II)) [5-7] can effectively be chelated by hydroxamic acids. Due to their metal binding ability, hydroxamic acids and aminohydroxamic acids (hydroxamic acid derivatives of amino acids) are often effective inhibitors of metalloenzymes (*e.g.* nickel(II)-containing urease, zinc(II)-containing MMP-s) [8-12]. Moreover, some metal complexes of aminohydroxamic acids are also planned to use as possible source of certain trace elements in animal nutrition [13].

Lead(II) is a highly toxic metal ion, which can be accumulated in the organs. Since there is no any really selective method for removal of lead(II), great effort is made to find it. The possible pathway can be via selective complexation by a sequestering agent. Since our earlier results show that hydroxamic acids may be good ligands for lead(II)ion [7, 14], our aim is to find hydroxamic acid derivatives that able to complexate the lead(II) with acceptable affinity and selectivity. To achieve this, evaluation of the main factors determining the lead(II) binding ability of hydroxamate based compound is an important task.

It is assumed that if the hydroxamic acid group is built in a natural molecule, the new compound obtained may have a lower toxicity and higher selectivity. That was our original motivation why a natural siderophore (desferrioxamine B, DFB) and hydroxamic acid derivatives of amino acids have been first of all investigated as possible lead(II) sequestering agents.

In a DFB molecule three hydroxamate chelating groups are involved, but due to the big space requirement of the $6s^2$ lone electron pair of this metal ion, maximum two hydroxamate chelates are able to co-ordinate to a lead(II) [7]. Taking this into account, dihydroxamic structural models of DFB were synthesized and their lead(II) binding ability was investigated.

Among the models, 2,5-DIHA ($x = 2$, $y = 5$) involves the same type of connecting chain as those in DFB. Compared to 2,5-DIHA, the position of the peptide group was changed in 3,4-DIHA and 3,3-DIHA. Change in the position of the peptide moiety compared to 2,5-DIHA resulted in the significant decrease of lead(II) binding ability. To evaluate the effect of the chain-length, the chain was systematically shortened in the order 2,5-DIHA > 2,4-DIHA > 2,3-DIHA > 2,2-DIHA and in the order 3,4-DIHA > 3,3-DIHA.

Table 1. The formulae of desferrioxamine B (DFB) and its structural model dihydroxamic acids

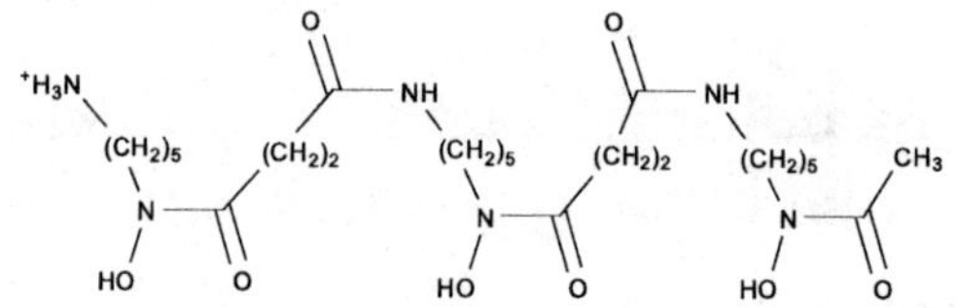

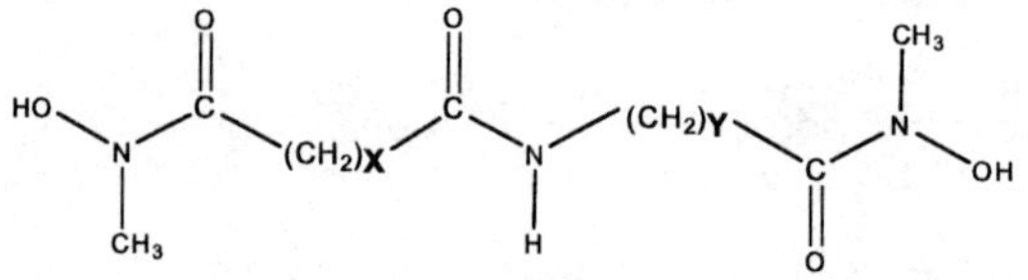

abbreviation of the molecules	X	Y
2,5-DIHA	2	5
2,4-DIHA	2	4
2,3-DIHA	2	3
2,2-DIHA	2	2
3,3-DIHA	3	3
3,4-DIHA	3	4

All the pH-potentiometric, ^1H NMR and ESI MS results show that the interaction between the lead(II) and DFB or its dihydroxamic models starts at pH ca. 3.5 with the formation of $[Pb(LH_3)]^{2+}$ or $[Pb(LH)]^+$, respectively. In these complexes, only one hydroxamate goup via its two oxygen atoms is coordinated to the metal ion, while the non-coordinated group(s) is(are) still protonated. By increasing the pH up to ca. 5.0-5.5, a second hydroxamate is able to coordinate to the metal ion. In addition to pH-potentiometry, ESI MS measurements were also performed to answer the question whether the two hydroxamates of a molecule is able to coordinate to the same metal ion, or, by sterical reasons, this is not favoured. Monomeric species is resulted in the former case and dimeric in the latter one. Based on the results, we could conclude that, in spite of the really large size of the Pb(II) ion, exclusively monomeric bis-chelated complex is formed even with the shortest ligand, 2,2-DIHA. It means that the stoichiometry of the bis-chelated complex with all the DIHA ligands is [PbL]. Surprisingly, the stability of the [PbL] formed with 2,2-DIHA is even higher than that with 2,5-DIHA (logβ values are 10.11 and 9.80, respectively [7]. Most probably, the rather packed arrangement of the four coordination sites of lead(II) *(scheme 1)* can explain why the effect of the connecting chain length on the stability trend is just the opposite with this metal compared to many other metals, including iron(III). As a final conclusion we could declare that lead(II) selectivity of 2,2-DIHA (having shorter connecting chain between the two chelating functions) is better than that of any other studied DFB models and also than that of the natural siderophore, DFB itself.

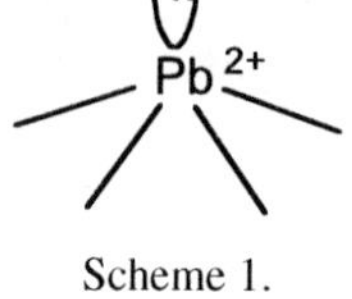

Pb^{2+}

Scheme 1.

In the amino acid derivatives, beside a hydroxamate function, at least one additional amino group is situated, what results in the possibility of new types of co-ordination modes. In our investigation, the role of the amino group in different positions (α-, β-,) in lead(II)-binding ability of the ligands have been studied.

Table 2. The formulae of the selected aminohydroxamic acids:

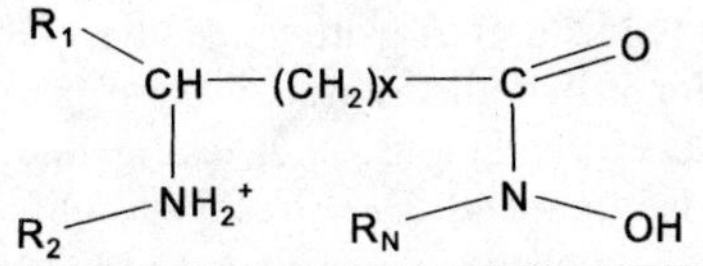

name of the molecule	R_1	R_2	X	R_N
α-alaninehydroxamic acid (α-Alaha)	$-CH_3$	-H	0	-H
N-methyl α-alaninehydroxamic acid (N-Me α-Alaha)	$-CH_3$	-H	0	$-CH_3$
β-alaninehydroxamic acid (β-Alaha)	-H	-H	1	-H
N-methyl β-alaninehydroxamic acid (N-Me β-Alaha)	-H	-H	1	$-CH_3$

When an amino group is situated at α- or β-position to the hydroxamic moiety and the substituent of the hydroxamate-N is hydrogen, chelates either via the two nitrogen donors or via the two oxygens, at least theoretically, can be realised (*scheme 2.* **I** and **II**). Moreover, mixed co-ordination mode is also possible **(III)** [14].

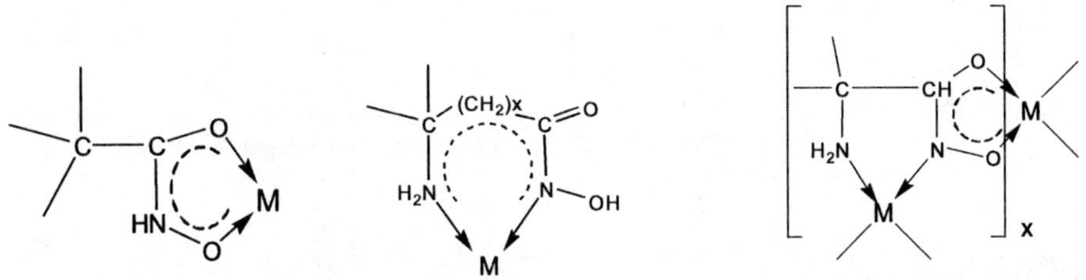

I. hydroxamate (O,O) chelate

II. ($N_{\alpha\text{-amino}}$-$N_{hydroxamate}$)type chelate

III. (N,N) (O,O) mixed coordination mode

Scheme 2.

Our results show that both the substituent of the hydroxamate-N and the position of the amino group have great effect on the stability and structure of complexes formed. Namely, if the substituent of the hydroxamate-N is a methyl group (secondary hydroxamic derivatives), only the hydroxamate oxygens are coordinated to the lead(II) ion Similarly to this behaviour, if the amino nitrogen atom is situated in β-position (β-Alaha), even if the substituent on the hydroxamate-N is hydrogen, the (N,N)-type coordination mode **(II)** does not occur and only hydroxamate type chelates are formed before the hydrolytic processes start. Moreover, the complexes formed in the above mentioned cases, have decreased stability compared to the simple hydroxamic acids due to the electron withdrawing effect of the amino groups. If however, the amino group is in α-position, the situation is much more complicated. Significant differences between the co-ordination modes of primary α- and β-derivatives (substituent of hydroxamate-N is hydrogen) appear above pH 6, where the amino-N starts to release its proton. With α-Alaha, the ^1H NMR results suggest the significant role of the hydroxamic-N in the co-ordination above pH 6. All the our results support that in this pH region, in addition to the hydroxamate-type (O,O)-chelate, the non-protonated amine-N together with the deprotonated hydroxamate-N form a five-membered (N,N)-type chelate (Structure **III**). The metal to ligand ratio in these stable, most probably polynuclear complexes is 1:1 and the pH-effect of their formation fits the formula $[PbLH_{-1}]_x$. In agreement with this suggestion, only polynuclear complexes (di-, tri- and tetranuclear) were found by ESI MS performed at pH 8.5 for the Pb(II)- α-Alaha system. Because this water soluble complex predominates by pH 9, under this condition a primary α-aminohydroxamic acid might be able to sequester Pb(II) effectively and with significant selectivity.

To try to evaluate that whether the natural trihydroxamate type DFB or the α-Alaha is better lead(II) chelator, speciation calculations for a hypothetic system were performed. Pb(II), DFB and α-Alaha were involved in a system in these calculations, and, taking into account the different number of chelating groups in the two ligands, the metal: DFB: α-Alaha ratio was chosen as 1:0.5:1. Out of the results, the total amount of lead(II) chelated by DFB or α-Alaha as a function of pH is shown in *figure 1*. The figure demonstrates some preference of α-Alaha over DFB at basic conditions.

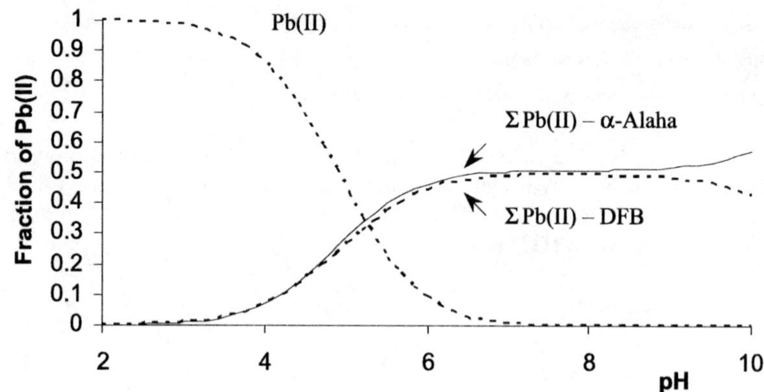

Fig. 1. Fraction of Pb(II) (dotted line), total amount of Pb(II) - α-Alaha complexes (continuous line) and Pb(II)-DFB complexes (dotted line) in hypothetical Pb(II) - DFB - α-Alaha system as a function of pH (c_{metal} = 5×10^{-3} mol dm^{-3}, Pb(II):DFB: α-Alaha ratio = 1:0.5:1)

REFERENCES

1. A-M. Albrecht-Gary and A. L. Crumbliss, in *Metal Ions in Biological Systems*, ed. A. Sigel and H. Sigel, Marcel Dekker, New York, 1998, vol. 35.
2. A. L. Crumbliss, in *Handbook of Microbial Iron Chelates*, ed. G. Winkelmann, CRC New York, 1991.
3. A-K. Duhme, Z. Dauter, R. C. Hider and S. Pohl, *Inorg. Chem.*, 1996, 35, 3059-3061.
4. A-K. Duhme, *J.Chem. Soc. Dalton Trans.*, 1997, 773-778.
5. A. Evers, R. D. Hancock, A. E. Martell and R. J. Motekaitis, *Inorg. Chem.*, 1989, 28, 2189-2195.
6. B. J. Hernlem, L. M. Vane and G. D. Sayles, *Inorg. Chim. Acta*, 1996, 244, 179-184.
7. E. Farkas, D. Bátka, Z. Pataki, P. Buglyó and M. A. Santos, *Dalton Trans.*, 2004, 1248-1253.
8. B. Kurzak. H. Kozlowski and E. Farkas, *Coord. Chem.Rev.*, 1992, 114, 169-200.
9. D. A. Brown, W. K. Glass, N. J. Fitzpatrick, T. J. Kemp, W. Errington, G. J. Clarkson, W. Haase, F. Karsten and A. H. Mahdy, *Inorg. Chim. Acta*, 2004, 357, 1411-1436.
10. C. M. Dooley, M. Devocelle, B. McLoughlin, K. B. Nolan, D. J. Fitzgerald and C. T. Sharkey, *Mol. Pharmacol.*, 2003, 63, 450-455.
11. M. Arnold, D. A. Brown, O. Deeg, W. Errington, W. Haase, K. Herlihy, T. J. Kemp, H. Nimir and R. Werner, *Inorg. Chem.*, 1998, 37, 2920-2925.
12. D. A. Brown, L. P. Cuffe, N. J. Fitzpatrick and Á. T. Ryan, *Inorg. Chem.*, 2004, 43, 297-302.
13. D. A. Brown, R. Geraty, J. D. Glennon and N. N. Choileain, *Inorg. Chem.*, 1986, 25, 3792-3796.
14. D. Bátka and E. Farkas, *J. Inorg. Biochem*, 2006, 100, 27-35.

ACKNOWLEDGEMENT

This work was supported by OTKA T049612 and TET P-7/03 (bilateral program between Portugal and Hungary).

Metal Ions in Biology and Medicine: vol. 9. Eds Maria Carmen Alpoim, Paula Vasconcellos Morais, Maria Amélia Santos, Armando J. Cristóvão, José A. Centeno, Philippe Collery.
John Libbey Eurotext, Paris © 2006 pp. 105-1.

Coadjuvation of a bis(3-hydroxy-4-pyridinone) with a deferiprone derivative: a new approach in chelation therapy

Sofia Gama[1], Marco Gil[1], Lurdes Gano[2], Etelka Farkas[3], M. Amélia Santos[1]

[1]*Centro de Química Estrutural, Instituto Superior Técnico, Lisboa, Portugal. e-mail: masantos@ist.utl.pt.*
[2]*Instituto Tecnológico Nuclear, Lisboa, Portugal.*
[3]*Department of Inorganic and Analytical Chemistry, University of Debrecen, Hungary.*

ABSTRACT

Iron overload is one of the causes of big helth problems namely associated to β-thalassemia and hematochromatosis. The better therapy for these ilnesses is based on iron chelation. The 3-hydroxy-4-pyridinones are known as highly effective and orally active iron chelators and thus, a big amont of recent research has being devoted to the development of new hydroxypyridinone derivatives with potential medical applications. A new arylpiperazine-containing bis-hydroxypyridinone was prepared (L^1) in order to explore its combination with the biomimetic mono-hydroxypyridinone ornithine-derivative (L^2) and to assess the potential benefits of a coadjuvation effect that could result from the administration of both compounds for the decorporation of hard metal ions. The iron(III) complexation behaviour of the ternary system was studied in solution and it showed improvements in terms of metal affinity. The first *in vivo* results indicated that the ^{67}Ga decorporation of overload mice proceeds through a more steady way than the bis-hydroxypyridinone derivative, mostly involving a hepatobiliar pathway.

INTRODUCTION

The 3-hydroxy-4-pyridinones (3,4-HP) are well known chelating agents with potential applications in medicinal chemistry. The importance of these compounds has been mostly associated to their high affinity towards hard trivalent metal ions (M = Fe, Al, Ga) and their potential use as metal decorporating agents in serious diseases resulting from Fe(III) and Al(III) accumulation [1].

Due to the potential clinical interest of those ligands, besides the polydenticity of 3,4-HP derivatives, their extra-functionalization was also explored aimed at improving the selectivity of the interaction with specific biological receptors. Therefore, a new arylpiperazine-containing bis-hydroxypyridone ligand was prepared (L^1) and its complexation behaviour was studied. The chelating properties of this ligand were further explored in combination with a biomimetic chelator, the mono-hydroxypyridinone ornithine-derivative (L^2), to assess potential improvement due to potential coadjuvating effects that could result from the administration of both compounds for the clearance of hard metal ions from specific body tissues.

This work reports a summary of solution and *in vivo* studies. Solution studies were performed to evaluate the iron chelating efficacy, as a simple binary and as a ternary system (L^1:L^2:Fe^{3+}), and also the lipo-hydrophilic character of the compounds. *In vivo* biodistribution studies were made to assess the ability of these chelating systems for the removal of a radiotracer (^{67}Ga) from overload mice.

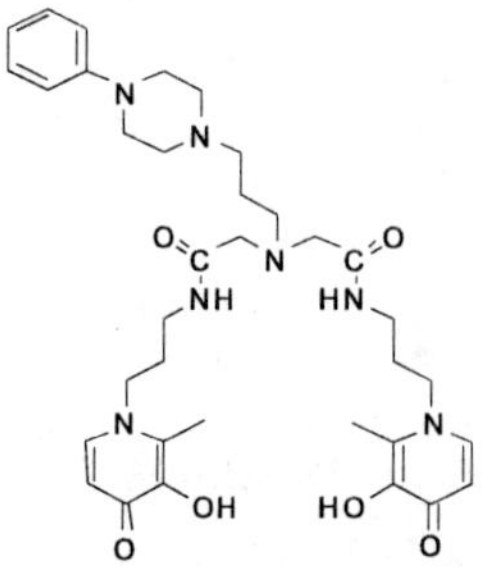

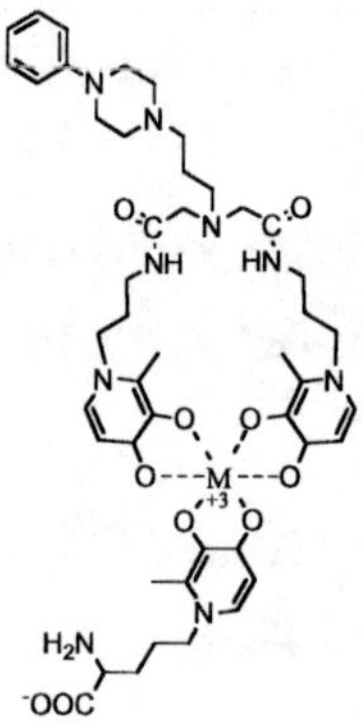

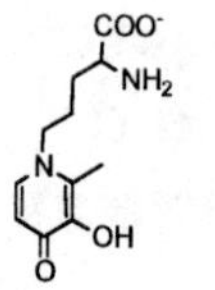

IDAPIPPr(3,4-HP)$_2$, L^1 ML^1L^2 Orn(3,4-HP), L^2

MATERIALS AND METHODS

The ligands were prepared using materials and methods described in the literature [2, 3]. Potentiometic and spectrophotometric methods were used to evaluate the acid-base properties and iron(III) complexation for each binary (L^1:M), (L^2:M) and the ternary (L^1:L^2:M) systems, according to published conditions [3, 4]. Distribution coefficients (log D) were determined from 1-octanol and a *Tris* buffered (pH 7.4) aqueous solution, based on previously reported methods [4]. The effect of the chelating agents on the *in vivo* biodistribution of ^{67}Ga-citrate overload mice was studied as described in the literature [4].

RESULTS AND DISCUSSION

The preparation of the bis(3-hydroxy-4-pyridinone) derivative, IDAPIPPr(3,4-HP), envolved firstly the coupling of the arylpiperazino-alkyl substituent to the amino group of the iminodiacetic acid (IDA) [5], followed by the condensation of the benzyloxy-hydroxypyridinone alkyl-amino side-chain to the carboxylic groups of the IDA skeleton. The last step was the catalytic hydrogenolysis of the benzylic protecting groups.

To evaluate the acid-base properties of the ligand L^1, potentiometric studies in aqueous solution were performed, allowing the determination of the corresponding six protonation constants. Its attribution was made according to chemical evidences, namely: the two highest values (10.03, 9.39) were ascribed to the hydroxypiridinone moieties [6]; the third protonation process (log K = 7.39) occurs on one of the pyperazine nitrogens; the two log K values around 3 (3.74 and 3.01) correspond to the protonation of the two pyridine nitrogen atoms; the lowest log K value (2.82) is attributed to the protonation of the IDA amine group.

Complexation studies of IDAPIPPr(3,4-HP)$_2$ with Fe^{3+} in aqueous solution were performed using spectrophotometric measurements because the very low water solubility of the complexes hindered the use of potentiometric measurements.

The studies of the Orn(3,4-HP) acid-base properties and the corresponding iron complexation were previously reported [3].

A comparison of iron affinity of ligands with diferent acid-base properties and denticities has to be based on the corresponding pFe values (pFe = - log [Fe], usually at the physiological pH (7.4) and diluted conditions, $C_L/C_M = 10$ with $C_M = 10^{-6}$ M), calculated from the complex stability constants. The pFe values, obtained for the present binary systems, as well as for a set of well known model ligands with clinical applications, are present in *table 1*.

Table 1. pFe* values and distribution coefficients (log D) of various ligands.

Ligand	pFe	Log D
IDAPIPPr(3,4-HP)$_2$ L^1	**25.7[a]**	**- 0.31**
Orn(3,4-HP)[b] L^2	**21.9**	**< -2**
Deferriprone (3, 4 - DMHP)[c,d]	**19.3**	**-1.03**
DTPA[e]	**24.6**	**< - 2**
DOTA[e]	**24.3**	**< - 2**
Desferrioxamine[f,g] (DFB)	**26.5**	**- 2**
Transferrin[h]	**20.3**	**-**

*pM = - log [M] with C_L/C_M = 10 and C_M = 10^{-6} mol/L at physiological pH 7.4; [a]This pFe was calculated from extrapolation of the system to pH 7.4, admitting there was no precipitation at that pH value; [b]Ref. [3]; [c]Ref. [6]; [d]Ref. [7]; [e]Ref. [8]; [f]Ref. [9]; [g]Ref. [10], [h]Ref. [11].

Analysis of *table 1* indicates that only Desferrioxamine (DFB) has higher affinity for Fe(III) than L^1, which is attributed to the DFB higher denticity. However, both ligands L^1 and L^2 are more speciffic for hard metal ions then other ligands used in clinical applications, such as DTPA and DOTA, and L^1 presents an even stronger iron affinity.

The octanol-water distribution coefficients indicate that L^2 present a much higher hydrophilic character than L^1, due to the considerable differences on the type of susbtituent groups, and the same correlation is expected for the corresponding iron complexes. This feature rendered in improvements on the water solubility of the ternary system (L^1:L^2:Fe), thus allowing the use of potentiometic techniques for the complexation studies. Three different stoichiometric ratios (L^1:L^2:M) were used (1:1:1, 2:1:1, 2:0.5:1). Under the potentiometric concentration conditions, some precipitation was observed at *ca.* pH 7, for the 1:1:1 molar ratio. The use of spectrophotometric measurements allowed a further qualitative analysis of the complex species in solution, giving support to the proposed model.

The model obtained for the ternary system is consistent with the formation of complex species with 1:1:1 stoichiometry at different protonation degrees, $FeH_xL^1L^2$ (x = 0, 1, 2, 3, depending on the protonation state of the non-coordinating sites.) The calculated global constants are as follows: log $\beta_{FeH_3L^1L^2}$ = 56.81, log $\beta_{FeH_2L^1L^2}$ = 54.30. Since hydrolysis started at pH around 7, values for the formation constants log $\beta_{FeHL^1L^2}$ and log $\beta_{FeL^1L^2}$ could not be determined. Anyway, if the value of the two stepwise protonation constants is subtracted from the last calculated global formation constant, log $\beta_{FeH_2L^1L^2}$, (most probably one of the pyperazine-*N* and the amino-*N* atoms are still protonated in this species), a rough evaluation of log $\beta_{FeL^1L^2}$ can be obtained (~ 54-10-7 = 37), which is in agreement with the expected value for a tris-chelated species [4]. *Fig. 1* presents the concentration distribution curves of the species calculated for the ternary system.

Although our model was only accurately determined above pH 6, because of the lake of data from L^1 due to precipitation, an extrapolation of ternary system equilibrium model was made up to pH 7.5, and pFe was calculated ($pFe_{7.4}$ = 29.9). The obtained result indicates a higher chelating efficacy of this ternary system when compared with the binary ones.

Fig. 2 presents the change of pFe with pH for the ligands L^1 and L^2, as well as for two clinically used compounds (DFB, 3,4-DMHP) and an important small size biological ligand (citrate).

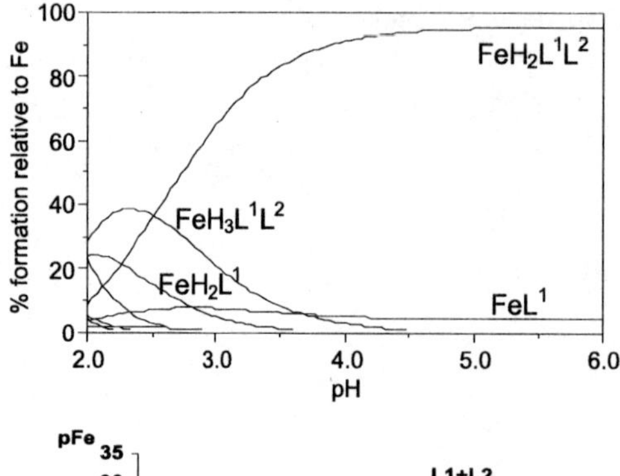

Fig. 1. Concentration distribution curves of the species formed in the system $L^1/L^2/Fe$ at (1:1:1) molar ratio, $C_{Fe} = 1.00 \times 10^{-3}$ M. $T = 25.0$ °C, $I = 0.2$ M KCl.

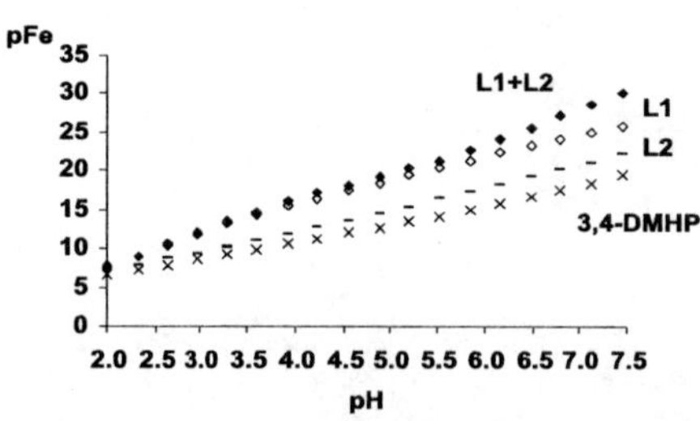

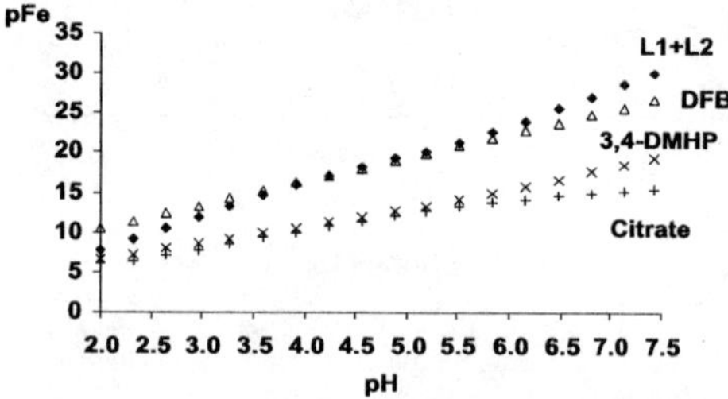

Fig. 2. pFe vs pH for the ternary system (Fe-L^1+L^2) and the binary systems: a) Fe(III)-L^1, Fe(III)-L^2, and Fe(III)-3,4-DMHP; b) Fe(III)-DFB, Fe(III)-3,4-DMHP and Fe(III)-citrate. pFe = -log[Fe] with $C_L/C_{Fe} = 10$ and $C_L = 1 \times 10^{-5}$ M.

Fig. 2a shows that the ternary system, involving the combination of the two ligands L^1 and L^2, presents higher iron affinity in the acid-neutral range (pH = 5 - 7.5) than any of the hydroxypiridinone binary systems. *Fig. 2b* further ilustrates that the combination of L^1 with L^2 seems to have higher affinity for iron than the chelating agents used in clinical applications (DFB and 3,4-DMHP).

The coadjuvation effect of the two 3,4-HP derivatives in the *in vivo* Ga(III) sequestration was evaluated in overload mice with ^{67}Ga-citrate. After administration of the radiotracer, a group of animals were injected with L^1 and another group with L^1 and L^2 at 1:1 molar ratio. Tissue distribution of the ^{67}Ga was assessed for the main organs, at 1 h, and this values are presented as percent of injected dose per total organ in *fig. 3*, which also includes the corresponding results previously reported for 3,4-DMHP and L^2 [3].

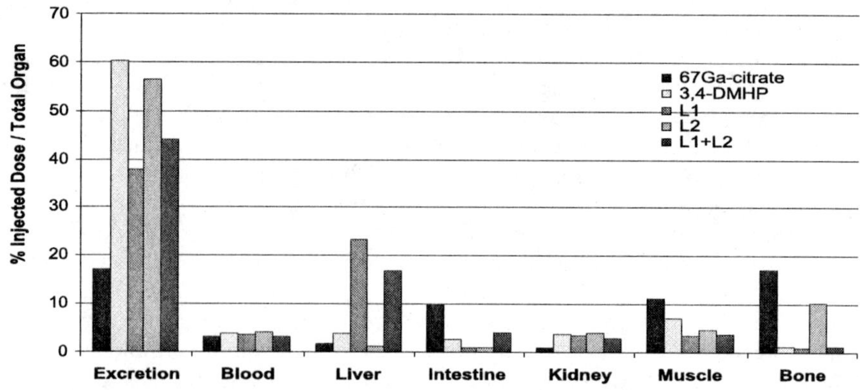

Fig. 3. Biodistribution data in percent of injected dose per total organ of ^{67}Ga-citrate and ^{67}Ga-citrate with simultaneous intraperitoneal injection of 3,4-DMHP, IDAPIPPr(3,4-HP)$_2$, Orn(3,4-HP), and a 1:1 mixture of IDAPIPPr(3,4-HP)$_2$/Orn (3,4-HP), 1 h after intravenous administration in mice.

These bioassays clearly demonstrate the ability of the chelating agents to complex *in vivo* and to eliminate the metal ion. In fact, the clearance of radioactivity from most organs and the rate of excretion from whole animal body are enhanced, as compared to those of ^{67}Ga-citrate.

Comparision of the biodistribution profiles associated to the use of chelating agent L^1, alone and combined with L^2, shows improvements for the combined system, namely on the excretion rate and the decrease of the liver retention. The excretion seems to involve mainly a hepatobiliar pathway, as suggested by the liver accumulation.

From these studies we can conclude that, for the stoichiometric conditions used in the combined system, there is some coadjuvating effect associated to the use of the mixture of two chelating agents with different physico-chemical properties (chelating affinity, molecular weight, distribution coefficient). However, further studies are in course aimed at optimizing that coadjuvation.

CONCLUSIONS

The potential coadjuvating effect associated to the use of a combination of chelating agents has been evaluated, regarding the iron complexation in aqueous solution and the *in vivo* sequestration of hard metal ions. The complexation studies with Fe(III) indicates improvements for the ternary system, namely some increasing on the complexation efficacy and a considerable increase on the solubility of the metal complexes, an important feature for the excretion process of the metal complex, upon the metal sequestration. The results of the *in vivo* studies with ^{67}Ga overload mice show differences on the biodistribution profiles of the radiotracer, upon the administration of each chelating agent, that are mainly ascribed to the differences of their extra-functional groups, namely their lipo-hydrophilic character. Administration of both chelating agents leads to a more steady metal mobilization, which may be attributed to an improved accessibility of the ligands to different cellular compartments. Further *in vivo* biodistribution studies with different L^1:L^2 molar ratios are in course to improve the coadjuvating effect on the metal decorporation.

REFERENCES

1. Santos MA, Hydroxypyridinone complexes with aluminium. In vitro/vivo studies and perspectives. *Coord Chem Rev* 2002; 228: 187-203.
2. Gama S, Gil M, Gano L, Farkas E, Santos MA, under publication.
3. Santos MA, Gil M, Gano L, Chaves S, Bifunctional 3-hydroxy-4-pyridinone derivatives as potential pharmaceuticals: synthesis, complexation with Fe(III), Al(III) and Ga(III) and in vivo evaluation with ^{67}Ga. *J Biol Inorg Chem* 2005; 10: 564-80.
4. Santos MA, Gama S, Gano L, Cantinho G, Farkas E, A new bis(3-hydroxy-4-pyridinone)-IDA derivative as a potential therapeutic chelating agent. Synthesis, metal-complexation and biological assays. *Dalton Trans* 2004; 3772-81.
5. Santos MA, Marques SM, Rossello A, Tuccinardi T, Carelli P, Panelli L, Design, synthesis and molecular modelling study of iminodiacetyl monohydroxamic acid derivatives as MMP inhibitors, in preparation.
6. Clarke ET, Martell AE, Stabilities of 1,2-dimethyl-3-hydroxy-4-pyridinone chelates of divalents and trivalent metal ions. *Inorg Chim Acta* 1992; 191: 57-63.
7. Yokel R, Datta AK, Jackson EG, Evaluation of potential aluminum chelators in vitro by aluminum solubilization ability, aluminum mobilization from transferrin and the octanol aqueous distribution of the chelators and their complexes with aluminum. *J. Pharmacol. Exp. Therapeutics* 1991; 257:100-6.
8. *Critically Selected Stability Constants of Metal Complexes Database*, ed. Martell AE, Smith RM, Motekaitis RJ, College Station TX, Version 4.0, 1997.
9. Farkas E, Enyedy EA, Csoka H, A comparison between the chelating properties of some dihydroxamic acids, desferrioxamine B and acetohydroxamic acid. *Polyhedron* 1999; 18: 2391-8.
10. Liu ZD, Hider RC, Design of iron chelators with therapeutic application. *Coord Chem Reviews* 2002; 232: 151-171.

11. Motekaitis RJ, Martell AE, Stabilities of the iron(III) chelates of 1,2-dimethyl-3-hydroxy-4-pyridinone and related ligands. *Inorg Chim Acta* 1991; 183: 71-80.

ACKNOWLEDGMENTS

The authors thank to the Portuguese FCT for the PhD grant SFRH/BD/8743/2002, the Hungarian-Portuguese Intergovern & the COST D21/001 programs for financial support. We also thank Dr. G. Cantinho, Instituto de Medicina Nuclear, Faculdade de Medicina de Lisboa, for her assistance and support.

Metal Ions in Biology and Medicine: vol. 9. Eds Maria Carmen Alpoim, Paula Vasconcellos Morais, Maria Amélia Santos, Armando J. Cristóvão, José A. Centeno, Philippe Collery.
John Libbey Eurotext, Paris © 2006 pp. 111-1.

The binding of ruthenium(III) anticancer complexes to serum proteins: an ESI-MS Study

Groessl Michael, Hartinger Christian G., Egger Alexander, Keppler Bernhard K.

Institute of Inorganic Chemistry, University of Vienna, Waehringer Str. 42, A-1090 Vienna, Austria

INTRODUCTION

In order to overcome severe side-effects and resistance in anticancer chemotherapy towards platinum-based drugs like cisplatin, a search for novel transition metal-based compounds has been initiated. Over the last few years, ruthenium(III) complexes such as indazolium [*trans*-(tetrachloro)bis(1*H*-indazole)ruthenate(III)] (KP1019, FCC14a) and imidazolium [*trans*-tetrachloro(1*H*-imidazole)(dimethylsulfoxide)ruthenate(III)] (NAMI-A) *(fig. 1)* have emerged as the most promising representatives of this substance class and have already successfully completed clinical phase I studies [1, 2].

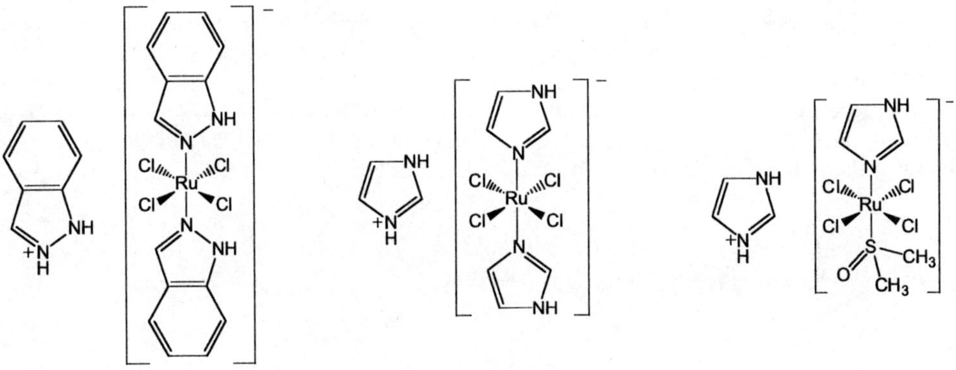

1 2 3

Fig. 1. Structural formulae of indazolium [*trans*-tetrachlorobis(1*H*-indazole)ruthenate(III)] (**1**, KP1019), imidazolium [*trans*-tetrachlorobis(1*H*-imidazole)ruthenate(III)] (**2**, KP418), and imidazolium [*trans*-tetrachloro(1*H*-imidazole)(dimethylsulfoxide)ruthenate(III)] (**3**, NAMI-A).

Antitumor ruthenium complexes exhibit, as compared to platinum-based chemotherapeutics, different properties such as octahedral geometry and the facility of the electron transfer for Ru^{II}/Ru^{III} couples without a change in both coordination number and of interatomic bond distances [3]. Therefore, the mode of action of ruthenium-based compounds might be characterized by distinct features: Ruthenium(III) complexes are reduced *in vivo* into their ruthenium(II) analogues, which is supported by the reductive environment inside the tumor. Consequently, the ruthenium(III) compounds are regarded as prodrugs and its reduction facilitates the interaction and coordination to biomolecules [4]. The altered cytotoxicity of KP1019 as compared to cisplatin might be explained by the formation of different DNA adducts [5], although DNA is not considered to be the ultimate target. The ruthenium complexes exhibit strong affinity to human serum proteins such as albumin (HSA) and transferrin (Tf) [6], and these transporter molecules are supposed to play a key role in the drugs' way to the cancer cells as well as in their metabolism. The iron transporting protein transferrin might serve as a "Trojan Horse", delivering "lethal" ruthenium instead of "required" iron which is highly demanded by the fast growing tumor cells [3]. This assumption is supported by the fact that transferrin is normally only to a degree of 30% saturated with Fe(III) [7] and that Ru(III) and Fe(III) exhibit comparable physical and chemical properties. Furthermore, human serum albumin, the most abundant plasma protein, acts as a carrier molecule for several drugs as shown in many investigations of the last decades [8], but also for physiological ligands in the human body such as vitamins, steroid hormones, non-esterified long-chain fatty acids, toxic metabolites and metal ions.

In order to improve the understanding of the mode of action of the ruthenium coordination compounds, their interactions with biomolecules are in the focus of interest. Timerbaev *et al.* studied the binding behavior of KP1019 towards HSA and transferrin utilizing capillary zone electrophoresis [6]. The determination of the rate and binding constants for the adduct formation elucidated that the binding to HSA is thermodynamically preferred, while the transferrin-drug conjugate is formed more rapidly. However, no structural characterization of the formed adducts can be extracted from that data.

Electrospray ionization (ESI) is the softest ionization method available in mass spectrometry and is therefore perfectly suited for studying the interactions of metal complexes and bio-macromolecules. This technique has already found application in characterization of interactions between anticancer agents and proteins [9-14]. For example, a number of research teams has examined the interactions of platinum- and ruthenium-based drugs with proteins resulting in the identification of the binding site of cisplatin in transferrin, namely threonine 457 [15]. However, there is still a controversial discussion about the preferred targets on proteins. There has also been extensive research on non-covalent complexes between polynucleotides and proteins with metal ions and small molecules utilizing ESI-MS [16].

In order to gain more information about the metabolism of KP1019 and its less active structural analogue imidazolium [*trans*-tetrachlorobis(1*H*-imidazole)ruthenate(III)] **2** (KP418; *figure 1*) and to elucidate the reason for the lower activity of KP418, a comparative ESI-MS study was performed.

MATERIALS AND METHODS

Chemicals

Indazolium [*trans*-tetrachlorobis(1*H*-indazole)ruthenate(III)] and imidazolium [*trans*-tetrachlorobis(1*H*-imidazole)ruthenate(III)] were synthesized as described elsewhere [17]. Human serum albumin, transferrin and ammonium bicarbonate were purchased from Sigma-Aldrich (Vienna, Austria) and were of analytical grade. Isopropanol and formic acid were obtained from Roth (Karlsruhe, Germany). High purity water used throughout this work was produced by a Millipore Synergy 185 UV Ultrapure Water system.

Mass Spectrometry

All MS-measurements were performed with an esquire 3000 ion trap mass spectrometer (Bruker Daltonics, Bremen, Germany) equipped with an orthogonal ESI source. For MS analysis of the complexes, the instrument was operated in negative ion mode, in case of the proteins and protein-metal complex adducts in positive ion mode. In order to assure best performance and lowest background and to simulate physiological conditions, sample solutions containing a varying drug-to-protein ratio from 1 : 1 to 10 : 1 were incubated at 37 °C in 20 mM hydrogencarbonate buffer at pH 7.4. The measurements were performed 15 min after start of the incubation and after a reaction time of 24 h. The sample solutions, isopropanol and formic acid (10%) were mixed in a

90 : 10 : 1 ratio just shortly before analysis for preventing interference with the binding process. The samples were introduced *via* flow injection at a rate of 4 µl/min using a Cole-Parmer 74900 single-syringe infusion pump. The ESI-MS instrument was controlled by means of the esquire-Control software (version 5.2), and all data were processed using DataAnalysis (version 3.2) (both Bruker Daltonics, Bremen, Germany).

RESULTS AND DISCUSSION

Mass spectrometry can deliver important information about the interactions of proteins with small molecules. Therefore, the mass spectrometric experiments were conducted with the aim of determining the stoichiometry of the binding of KP418 and KP1019, respectively, to the high abundant human serum proteins albumin and transferrin in dependence of their molar ratios and time of incubation.

Analyses of compounds **1** and **2** by ESI-MS in negative ion mode revealed in the mass spectra as most abundant peaks *m/z* 479.9 and 379.9 Da for KP1019 and KP418, respectively. Due to the very characteristic isotopic distribution pattern of ruthenium-chloride complexes, the respective peaks could be assigned unambiguously to the corresponding [*trans*-tetrachlorobis(1*H*-azole)ruthenate(III)] anions. The measured isotopic patterns were in very good accordance to the calculated peak distribution *(fig. 2)*.

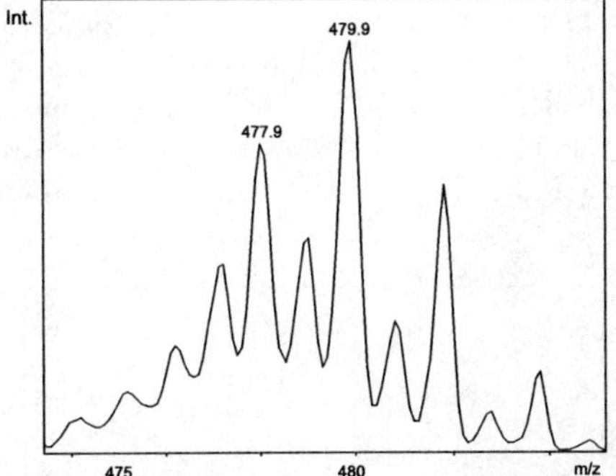

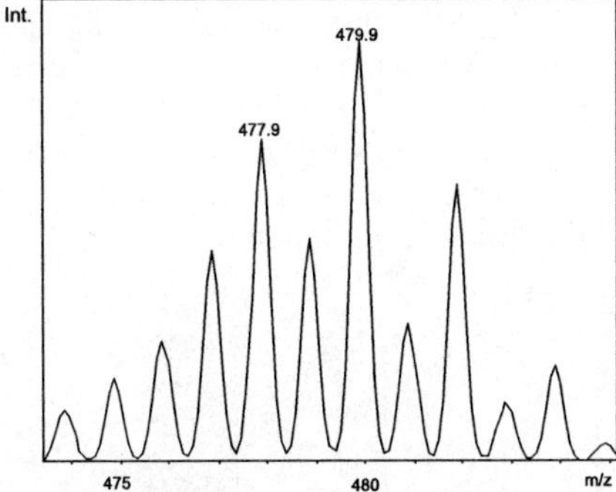

Fig. 2. Comparison of the measured (left) and the calculated (right) isotopic pattern for the complex anion of KP1019.

Prior to the analyses of the protein-metal complex adducts, solutions of HSA and Tf were used for optimizing the measurement parameters and determining the average molecular mass of the proteins: Charge deconvolution of the spectra yielded 66645±36 Da for HSA and 79635±37 Da for transferrin. Both values are slightly higher than the reported ones of 66478 Da for HSA and 79557 Da for transferrin. These minor deviations probably stem from alkali or ammonium adduct formation and/or different glycosylation of the protein product [18].

In an electrochemical study with NAMI-A and HSA, it was suggested that up to four complex anions can be bound unspecifically to HSA on the surface of the protein [19] while for KP1019 the specific binding of two ruthenium species into the iron binding pockets of transferrin were reported [20].

Incubation of KP418 with the two plasma proteins HSA and Tf for 15 min resulted in the attachment of at least one complex anion to both proteins.

At incubation ratios from 1 : 1 to 1 : 3 (HSA : drug), the most prominent HSA adducts were identified to be mono-adducts, indicated by a mass increase of only *ca.* 380 Da. However, in mass spectra of samples containing five- and ten-fold excess of the ruthenium compound, an additional peak corresponding to a mass increase of *ca.* 760 Da was assigned to a bisadduct. After allowing the samples to react for 24 h at 37 °C, a mass increase of even *ca.* 1150 Da was observed, indicating the binding of a third Ru-species.

In contrast, the binding to transferrin was found to take place at a similar rate but with a higher specificity than that to HSA [21]. Within the first 15 minutes of incubation, it can easily be distinguished between mono- and bisadducts, depending on the drug-to-protein ratio: At a 1 : 1 ratio, a mono-adduct was identified and at a two-fold excess of the drug, additionally a weak signal at 80400 Da assignable to the bisadduct appeared. Furthermore, raising the excess of the ruthenium species in the incubation mixture did not lead to the formation of higher adducts. Also, extending the reaction time to 24 h did not change the result. This finding might be explained by a loss of the metal-species during the ionization process.

In the same experiments with the drug candidate KP1019, the interpretation of the mass spectra was quite complicated. This is attributed to the rapid aquation of the complex under the incubation conditions, which probably results in poly-ruthenium species (gradual darkening of the solution). However, mass spectra confirming the interaction of KP1019 with HSA and transferrin were recorded.

For all HSA-ruthenium samples, the binding of at least one complex anion could be confirmed through a mass increase of approximately 480 Da. Additional peaks, especially at high drug-to-protein ratios but also after an incubation time of 24 h, are caused by the binding of either further complex anions or hydrolysis products/poly-ruthenium species.

The analyses of transferrin-containing solutions also showed clear indications of ruthenium-protein interaction. In accordance with the results obtained for KP418 and reported in literature for KP1019 [20], a mass increase of 480 Da and of 960 Da corresponding to the addition of one or two complex anions, respectively, can be observed. However, the resolution of the peaks for the protein and the metallocomplex adducts were much better than in ESI-MS studies reported recently [20]. Interestingly, the mass spectra of Tf-containing samples showed much narrower isotopic distribution patterns compared to those of HSA indicating specific binding of a limited number of ruthenium moieties.

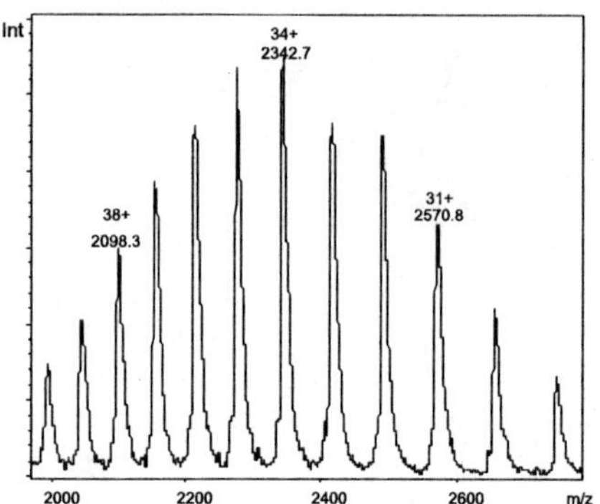

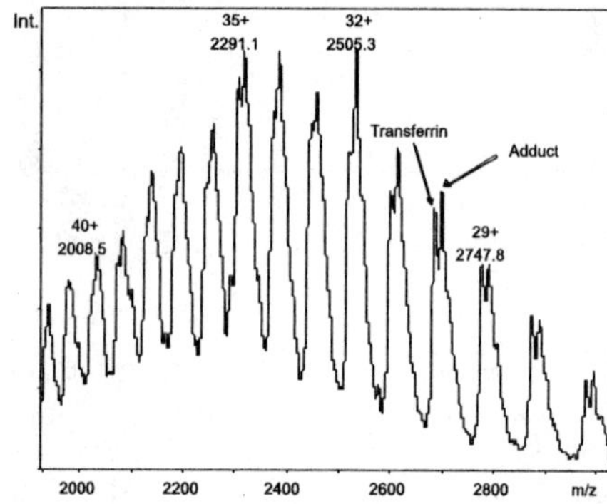

Fig. 3. Mass spectra of transferrin (left) and a transferrin-metal complex conjugate (right) at a drug-to-protein ratio of 1 : 1 after an incubation period of 15 min.

Nevertheless, the results for both studied compounds are not in line with previous reports in which up to 8-10 Ru-species were found to be bound to the protein [21]. Although ESI is considered as the softest ionization method, there is still potential that formed adducts can be destroyed during the spraying and ionization process. In general, due to the broad isotopic distribution pattern of ruthenium complexes, especially with chloro ligands, the adducts formed by these compounds with both proteins do not show sharp but rather broad and overlapping peaks which might also be caused by different adducts formed between the protein, hydrolysis products, and/or the complex anion. The low mass resolution of a mass spectrometer equipped with an ion trap analyzer did not allow distinguishing between all these species.

CONCLUSIONS

Electrospray ionization mass spectrometry was proven to be a suitable technique for the analyses of interactions between the high abundant serum proteins albumin and transferrin and the anticancer compounds KP418 and KP1019. It was possible to determine the stoichiometries of the binding under simulated physiological conditions at least at low metal complex-to-protein ratios. Especially for transferrin, the formation of preferably 1 : 1 and 2 : 1 drug-to-protein adducts (even at ten-fold excess) is a striking evidence for the probable specific binding of Ru-complex moieties into the iron binding pockets.

REFERENCES

1. Rademaker-Lakhai JM, van den Bongard D, Pluim D, Beijnen JH, Schellens JH. A Phase I and pharmacological study with imidazolium-trans-DMSO-imidazole-tetrachlororuthenate, a novel ruthenium anticancer agent. *Clin Cancer Res* 2004; 10: 3717-3727.
2. Dittrich C, Scheulen ME, Jaehde U, Kynast B, Gneist M, Richly H, Schaad S, Arion VB, Keppler BK. Phase I and pharmacokinetic study of sodium trans-[tetrachlorobis(1H-indazole)ruthenate(III)]/indazole hydrochloride (1:1.1) (FFC14A, KP1019) in patients with solid tumors - a study of the CESAR Central European Society for Anticancer Drug Research. 2005.
3. Reisner E, Arion VB, Hartinger CG, Jakupec MA, Pombeiro AJL, Keppler BK. From Synthesis to Antitumor Activity - NAMI-A and KP1019, Two Ruthenium Complexes in Clinical Trials. In: Trzeciak AM, ed. *Education in Advanced Chemistry, Perspectives of Coordination Chemistry*. 2005: 215-229.
4. Clarke MJ. Ruthenium metallopharmaceuticals. *Coord Chem Rev* 2003; 236: 209-233.
5. Malina J, Novakova O, Keppler BK, Alessio E, Brabec V. Biophysical analysis of natural, double-helical DNA modified by anticancer heterocyclic complexes of ruthenium(III) in cell-free media. *J Biol Inorg Chem* 2001; 6: 435-445.
6. Timerbaev AR, Rudnev AV, Semenova O, Hartinger CG, Keppler BK. Comparative binding of antitumor indazolium [trans-tetrachlorobis(1H-indazole)ruthenate(III)] to serum transport proteins assayed by capillary zone electrophoresis. *Anal Biochem* 2005; 341: 326-333.
7. Gomme PT, McCann KB, Bertolini J. Transferrin: structure, function and potential therapeutic actions. *Drug Discov Today* 2005; 10: 267-273.
8. Curry S. Beyond expansion: structural studies on the transport roles of human serum albumin. *Vox Sang* 2002; 83 Suppl 1: 315-319.
9. Mandal R, Kalke R, Li XF. Mass spectrometric studies of cisplatin-induced changes of hemoglobin. *Rapid Commun Mass Spectrom* 2003; 17: 2748-2754.
10. Peleg-Shulman T, Najajreh Y, Gibson D. Interactions of cisplatin and transplatin with proteins. Comparison of binding kinetics, binding sites and reactivity of the Pt-protein adducts of cisplatin and transplatin towards biological nucleophiles. *J Inorg Biochem* 2002; 91: 306-311.
11. Peleg-Shulman T, Gibson D. Cisplatin-protein adducts are efficiently removed by glutathione but not by 5'-guanosine monophosphate. *J Am Chem Soc* 2001; 123: 3171-3172.
12. Mandal R, Kalke R, Li XF. Interaction of oxaliplatin, cisplatin, and carboplatin with hemoglobin and the resulting release of a heme group. *Chem Res Toxicol* 2004; 17: 1391-1397.
13. Casini A, Gabbiani C, Mastrobuoni G, Messori L, Moneti G, Pieraccini G. Exploring Metallodrug/Protein Interactions by ESI Mass Spectrometry: the Reaction of Anticancer Platinum Drugs with Horse Heart Cytochrome c. *ChemMedChem* in press.
14. Zhao YY, Mandal R, Li XF. Intact human holo-transferrin interaction with oxaliplatin. *Rapid Commun Mass Spectrom* 2005; 19: 1956-1962.
15. Allardyce CS, Dyson PJ, Coffey J, Johnson N. Determination of drug binding sites to proteins by electrospray ionisation mass spectrometry: the interaction of cispaltin with transferrin. *Rapid Commun Mass Spectrom* 2002; 16: 933-935.
16. Loo JA. Studying noncovalent protein complexes by electrospray ionization mass spectrometry. *Mass Spectrom Rev* 1997; 16: 1-23.
17. Keppler BK, Henn M, Juhl UM, Berger MR, Niebl R, Wagner FE. New Ruthenium Complexes for the Treatment of Cancer. *Progr Clin Biochem Med* 1989; 10: 41-69.

18. Feng R, Konishi Y, Bell AW. High Accuracy Molecular Weight Determination and Variation Characterization of Proteins Up To 80 ku by Ionspray Mass Spectrometry. *J Am Soc Mass Spectrom* 1991; 2: 387-401.
19. Ravera M, Baracco S, Cassino C, Colangelo D, Bagni G, Sava G, Osella D. Electrochemical measurements confirm the preferential bonding of the antimetastatic complex [ImH][RuCl(4)(DMSO)(Im)] (NAMI-A) with proteins and the weak interaction with nucleobases. *J Inorg Biochem* 2004; 98: 984-990.
20. Pongratz M, Schluga P, Jakupec MA, Arion VB, Hartinger CG, Allmaier G, Keppler BK. Transferrin binding and transferrin-mediated cellular uptake of the ruthenium coordination compound KP1019, studied by means of AAS, ESI-MS and CD spectroscopy. *J Anal At Spectrom* 2004; 19: 46-51.
21. Szpunar J, Makarov A, Pieper T, Keppler BK, Lobinski R. Investigation of metallodrug±protein interactions by size-exclusionchromatography coupled with inductively coupled plasma mass spectrometry (ICP-MS). *Anal Chim Acta* 1999; 387: 135-144.

ACKNOWLEDGMENTS

The support of the FWF (Austrian Science Foundation), the Austrian Council for Research and Technology Development, Faustus Forschung Translational Drug Development AG and COST is gratefully acknowledged.

Metal Ions in Biology and Medicine: vol. 9. Eds Maria Carmen Alpoim, Paula Vasconcellos Morais, Maria Amélia Santos, Armando J. Cristóvão, José A. Centeno, Philippe Collery.
John Libbey Eurotext, Paris © 2006 pp. 117-1.

Iminodiacetyl-monohydroxamate derivatives as potent and selective MMP inhibitors

Sérgio M. Marques[1], Sílvia Chaves[1], Armando Rossello[2], Tiziano Tuccinardi[2] and M. Amélia Santos[1]

[1]*Centro de Química Estrutural, Instituto Superior Técnico, Av. Rovisco Pais 1, 1049-001 Lisboa Portugal;*
[2]*Dipartimento di Scienze Farmaceutiche, Università degli Studi di Pisa, Via Bonanno 6, 56126 Pisa, Italy.*

ABSTRACT

The matrix metalloproteinases (MMPs) are a family of zinc-dependent endopeptidases involved in the degradation of the major components of extracellular matrix [1]. Some of them, namely MMP-2 and -9, are associated to tumour invasion and angiogenesis in several neoplasias [2]. With the purpose of controlling the deregulated expression of these enzymes, several synthetic inhibitors have been developed in the last years.

Aimed at increasing the specific inhibitory activity for cancer-related MMPs, a set of *N*-derivatives of iminodiaceto-hydroxamic acids has been developed, bioassayed towards the MMP-2 and -7 inhibition, and studied in solution to evaluate the coordination modes to zinc(II) in equilibrium conditions.

The results of our studies on a series of iminodiaceto-hydroxamic acids containing *N*-arylsulfonyl or *N*-arylmethyl moieties indicated that, although the sulfamoyl group is not involved in the zinc-coordination, the sulphonamide-containing compounds are much more active than the amine analogues, due to favourable extra-functional interactions between the sulfonyl groups and amino-acid residues at the active site of the enzyme. Moreover, the inhibitory activity (nanomolar range) and the selectivity for MMP-2 can be achieved by inserting adequate aromatic substituents on the inhibitor scaffold.

INTRODUCTION

The human MMPs are a family of more than 20 zinc-containing enzymes, which are involved in the degradation of extra-cellular matrix. Although MMPs have important roles associated to the maintenance and repairing of tissues, unbalance of regulation processes can lead to their uncontrolled over-expression and promote a variety of diseases including arthritis, tumour metastasis, multiple sclerosis and periodontal degradation. Therefore, in the last decade, intensive research has been carried out in order to find new effective biomimetic inhibitors for these metalloenzymes. These inhibitors should be highly effective and selective for the targeted enzyme, a task that can be hard to achieve. When designing these inhibitors, another important point to take into account is to use lead molecules with feasible synthetic procedures and with expected good bioavailability to provide enhanced concentration at the target site. In the present case, the adopted design strategy is to make truncations in the structure of well known active inhibitors, namely on potent broad spectrum inhibitors such as the clinical stage drugs marimastat and batimastat, and create compounds containing some functional groups of recognized importance.

Aimed at developing selective inhibitors for some cancer-related enzymes, namely, MMP-2 and MMP-9, a series of compounds was developed *(scheme 1)*.

Herein, a set of the results is included, namely inhibition assays as well as docking simulations to aid the understanding of the biological results. Furthermore, solution equilibrium studies of the zinc(II) complexation with some inhibitors were performed to evaluate their binding modes and rationalize the inhibition results.

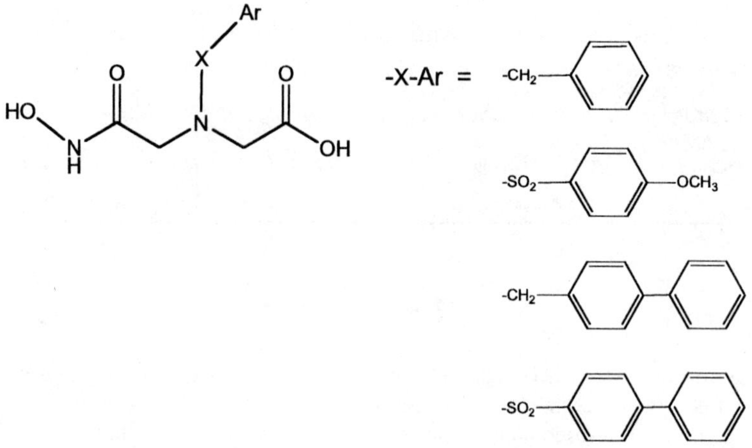

Scheme 1

MATERIALS AND METHODS

Compounds **1-4** were prepared by attaching the *N*-substituent groups to the iminodiacetic acid (IDA) through the respective chlorides, followed by nucleophilic substitution at one of the carboxylic moiety with hydroxylamine using standard methods [3]. The MMP inhibition assays were performed according to the literature, namely in terms of activation of the pro-enzymes, type and concentration of the substrate and methods for controlling the substrate hydrolysis [4]. The docking studies were performed using the AUTODOCK 3 program [5] while the molecular mechanics studies involved the AMBER 8 program using a modified AMBER forcefield [6]. The stability constants of the zinc(II) complexes were determined by fitting the potentiometric curves ($T = 25.0 \pm 0.1$ °C, $I = 0.1$ M KCl) with HYPERQUAD 2003 program [7].

RESULTS AND DESCUSSION

The inhibitory activity of the compounds towards MMP-2 and -7 are presented in *table 1*.

The sulphonamide-derivatives (**2** and **4**) showed, in general, higher activity than the corresponding amines (*ca* three orders of magnitude for MMP-2) laying in the sub-micromolar range (**2**) or nanomolar range (**4**). For MMP-7, that difference is not so large, but this is according to our aim of the enhancement of selectivity for MMP-2.

Table 1. Inhibitory activity (IC_{50}, μM) of compounds 1-4 towards MMP-2 and -7. In parentheses are the selectivities for MMP-2 in most relevant cases*.

	MMP-2	MMP-7
1	> 300	> 300
2	0.20 ± 0.02 (1.5)	0.30 ± 0.06
3	79 ± 7 (2.0)	161 ± 7
4	0.050 ± 0.002 (480)	24 ± 2

* Selectivity for MMP-2 over MMP-7 is expressed as the ratio of $IC_{50}^{(MMP-7)}$ / $IC_{50}^{(MMP-2)}$.

Compound **1** showed, unexpectedly, lower activity (IC_{50} > 300 μM) than in the previously reported studies [3], which can be rationalized in terms of the difference between the experimental conditions. Moreover, theoretical studies were performed to aid the understanding of the difference between the activities presented by compounds **1** and **2** (IC_{50} > 300 μM and ≈ 100 μM respectively).

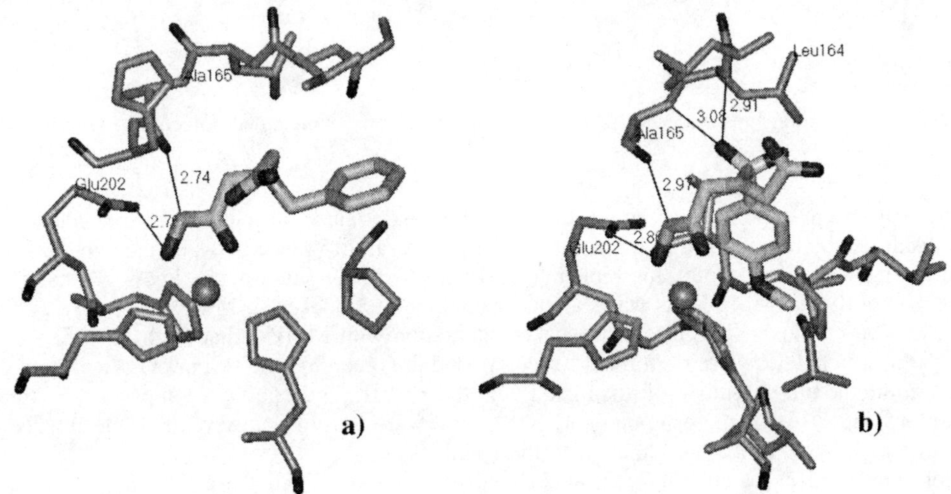

Fig. 1. Docking of compounds **1** (a) and **2** (b) to MMP-2 using *Ab initio* calculations.

These studies showed that ligand **1** *(fig. 1a)* is able to form only two hydrogen bonds, between the hydroxamate binding group with the amino-acid residues Glu202 and Ala165; the carboxylic group does not present any important interaction, while the phenyl substituent is out of the lipophilic S1' pocket and has only lower interaction. This result is in agreement with the biological results which present somehow low affinity for this enzyme. On the other hand, ligand **2** *(fig. 1b)* is able to form four hydrogen bonds, which reinforce the enzyme-inhibitor interaction: the same two H-bonds of the hydroxamate group with Glu202 and Ala165 and two new H-bonds of the sulfonamide oxygens with Leu164 and Ala165. Moreover, the presence of this new group gives to the phenyl substituent a specific spatial orientation so that it can be better inserted in the S1' binding pocket.

The difference between the inhibitory activity of **1** and **3** seems to be rationalized from the theoretical studies. It is shown that for ligand **3** a different orientation may render in a high stabilization within the enzyme site, because the biphenyl group can be well accommodated in the hydrophobic S2'-S3' valley *(fig. 2a)*, besides two extra hydrogen bonds which are possible to be formed through the NH-hydroxamate and the carboxylate group with Ala165 and His166, respectively *(fig. 2b)*.

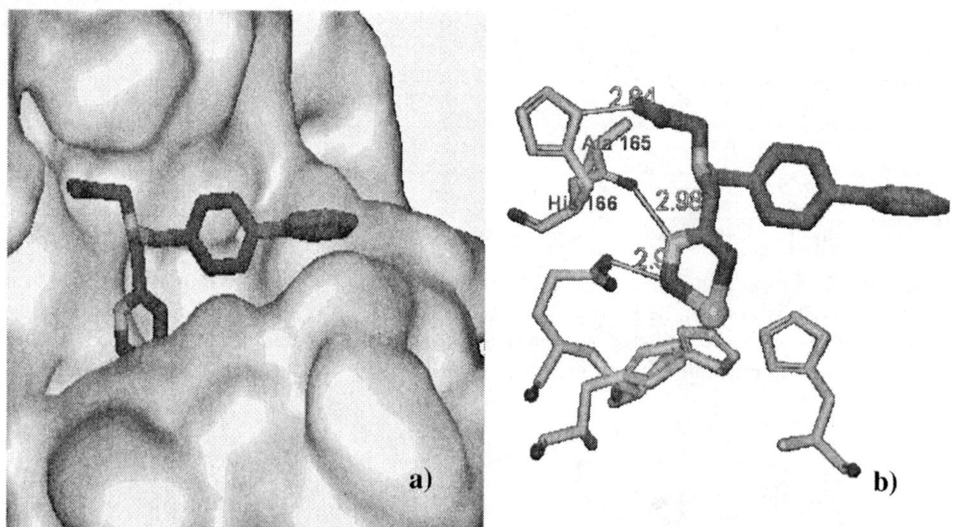

Fig. 2. Docking of compound **3** to MMP-2 using *Ab initio* calculations with Amber forcefield, in two different overviews of the enzyme active site.

It is interesting to notice that the most active compound, **4**, also presents the highest selectivity. This result can be rationalized in terms of a major structural difference between the two enzymes, since a longer aromatic group, the biphenyl, seems to be better fitted in the lipophylic cavity of MMP-2 than that of MMP-7 (as was shown for compound **3** docked to MMP-2 in *figure 2*). The sulfonyl group seems also to establish weaker interaction with MMP-7 than with MMP-2.

Equilibrium studies were performed for compound **2**, containing the sulfamoyl group, in order to determine the binding mode of this ligand with the zinc(II), and establish comparisons with the results previously reported for compound **1** [8], aimed at clarifying the eventual interference of the sulfamoyl group in the coordination to the metal ion.

For compound **2**, the stability constants found were $\log\beta_{ZNL} = 5.04(2)$ and $\log\beta_{ZNL_2} = 8.99(5)$. Comparison of these values with the corresponding values for GlyHA ($\log\beta_{ZNL} = 5.38$ and $\beta_{ZNL_2} = 10.07$ [9]) indicate that the complexation involves a pure hydroxamate type chelation. Consequently, the sulfamoyl should not be involved in the metal coordination and the potenciometric curves evidenced that the carboxylate group is also not coordinated to the zinc (II).

These results are not in accordance with those presented by **1** ($\log\beta_{ZNL} = 6.63$ and $\beta_{ZNL_2} = 11.06$), where the species ZnL evidenced the involvement of not only the hydroxamate, but also the amine-*N* atom and the carboxylate group [8].

The different behaviour presented by the two ligands regarding the coordination with the zinc(II) ion, does not seem to explain the difference found in the inhibitory activity, since the better inhibitor (**2**) forms complexes with lower stability constants. It is more probable, as shown by the theoretical calculations, that the structural differences between them, namely the ability to form other hydrogen bonds within the enzyme site are more determinant for the stability of the enzyme-inhibitor adduct than their ability to chelate the zinc ion.

On the other hand, the special type of coordination shown by **1** in the equilibrium studies may not be favoured when the inhibitor is accommodated within the enzyme active site, due to extra interactions with amino-acid residues, which can even force the coordination through the hydroxamate group.

CONCLUSIONS

Our studies on this set of compounds showed that the hydroxamate-sulfonamide inhibitors present, in general, a much higher activity against the set of metalloproteinases in study than the corresponding non-sulfonamide analogues, some of them with IC_{50} values for MMP-2 in the nanomolar range. These results can be rationalized in terms of extra-functional interactions between the sulfonyl groups and specific amino-acid residues, namely through hydrogen bonds and lipophilic interactions at the active site of the metalloenzyme. Furthermore, it was shown that the sulfamoyl group does not seem to be involved in the zinc-coordination.

REFERENCES

1. Becket RP, Davidson AH, Drummond AH, Huxley PH and Whittaker M. Recent advances in matrix metalloproteinase inhibitor research. *Drug Discovery Today* 1996; Vol 1 (1): 16-26.
2. Turpeenniemi-Hujanen T. Gelatinases (MMP-2 and -9) and their natural inhibitors as prognostic indicators in solid cancers. *Biochimie* 2005; 87: 287-297.
3. Santos MA, Marques S, Gil M, Tegoni M, Scozzafava A and Supuran CT. Protease inhibitors: synthesis of bacterial collagenase and matrix metalloproteinase inhibitors incorporating succinyl hydroxamate and iminodiacetic acid hydroxamate moieties. *J Enzyme Inhibit & Med Chem* 2003; 18: 233-242.
4. Rossello A, Nuti E, Orlandini E, Carelli P, Rapposelli S, Macchia M, Minutolo F, Carbonaro L, Albini A, Benelli R, Cercignani G, Murphy G and Balsamo A. New *N*-arylsulfonyl-*N*-alkoxyaminoacetohydroxamic acids as selective inhibitors of gelatinase A (MMP-2). *Bioorg & Med Chem* 2004; 12: 2441-2450.
5. Morris GM, Goodsell DS, Halliday RS, Huey R, Hart WE, Belew RK and Olson AJ. Automated docking using a Lamarckian genetic algorithm and an empirical binding free energy function. *J. Comp. Chem.* 1998; 19: 1639-1662.
6. Tuccinardi T, Martinelli A, Nuti E, Carelli P, Balzano F, Uccello-Barretta G, Murphy G and Rossello A. Amber force field implementation, molecular modelling study, synthesis and MMP-1/MMP-2 inhibition profile of *(R)*- and *(S)-N*-hydroxy-2-(*N*-isopropoxybiphenyl-4-ylsulfonamido)-3-methylbutanamides. *Bioorg & Med Chem*; in Press, Available online on 17 February 2006.
7. Gans P, Sabatini A and Vacca A. Investigation of equilibria in solution. Determination of equilibrium constants with the HYPERQUAD suite program. *Talanta* 1996; 43: 1739-1753.
8. Chaves S, Marques S and Santos MA. Iminodiacetyl-hydroxamate derivatives as metalloproteinase inhibitors: equilibrium complexation studies with Cu(II), Zn(II) and Ni(II). *J Inorg Biochem* 2003; 97: 345-353.
9. Paniago EB and Carvalho S. Formation constants and coordination in transition metal complexes of glycinehydroxamic acid. *Inorganica Chimica Acta* 1987; 136: 159-163.

ACKNOWLEDGMENTS

This work was supported by the Portuguese Foundation for Science and Technology (PhD grant SFRH/BD/10714/2002).

Metal Ions in Biology and Medicine: vol. 9. Eds Maria Carmen Alpoim, Paula Vasconcellos Morais, Maria Amélia Santos, Armando J. Cristóvão, José A. Centeno, Philippe Collery.
John Libbey Eurotext, Paris © 2006 pp. 122-1.

The Catalytically Competent Conformation of Prostaglandin G_2 at the Haem Site of Prostaglandin-Endoperoxide Synthase

Edelmiro Moman*, Anthony J. Chubb, and Kevin B. Nolan

Centre for Synthesis and Chemical Biology, Department of Pharmaceutical and Medicinal Chemistry, Royal College of Surgeons in Ireland, 123 St. Stephen's Green, Dublin 2, Ireland. emoman@rcsi.ie

Prostaglandin-endoperoxide synthase (PGHS) is a membrane enzyme that converts arachidonic acid into prostaglandin H_2 (PGH_2), the precursor of all prostaglandins and thromboxanes. The enzyme has two distinct catalytic sites: a cyclooxygenase site which catalyzes the conversion of arachidonic acid to prostaglandin G_2 (PGG_2); and a haem-containing peroxidase site which catalyses the reduction of the hydroperoxide bond of PGG_2 to the alcohol PGH_2. The peroxidase catalytic activity can continue independently of the cyclooxygenase site activity and is a source of free radicals which can contribute to tissue damage. We have combined molecular modeling and molecular biology to elucidate a plausible competent conformation of PGG_2 at the haem site of PGHS. In our binding model, the PGG_2 15-hydroperoxide group is in the proximity of the haem iron, whereas the carboxylate group forms salt bridges with Lys215 and Lys222. Site-directed mutagenesis showed that single mutation of Lys215 or Lys222 does not affect enzyme activity, whereas dual mutation of these residues significantly decreases turnover. This indicates that the conserved cationic pocket is involved in enzyme-substrate binding.

INTRODUCTION

Prostaglandin endoperoxide H synthase (PGHS) is a bi-functional membrane enzyme [1] that converts arachidonic acid into prostaglandin H_2 (PGH_2), the precursor of all prostaglandins, thromboxanes and prostacyclins [2]. These lipid mediators are intricately involved in normal physiology and numerous pathologies, including inflammation, and cardiovascular diseases. Two isoforms of PGHS with different expression patterns, PGHS-1 and PGHS-2, have been characterized over the past two decades [3]. The enzyme possesses two distinct catalytic sites. The cyclooxygenase site catalyzes the conversion of arachidonic acid to the lipid peroxide prostaglandin G_2 (PGG_2), and is the target for non-steroidal anti-inflammatory drugs (NSAIDs). The peroxidase site catalyses the two-electron reduction of the hydroperoxide bond of PGG_2 to yield the corresponding alcohol prostaglandin H_2 (PGH_2).

A simplified mechanistic scheme for the cyclooxygenase and peroxidase catalytic cycles [4] is shown in *figure 1*. The formation of a phenoxyl radical on Tyr385 couples the activities of the two sites [5]. The Tyr385$^{\bullet}$ radical is produced via oxidation by Compound I, an oxoferryl porphyrin π-cation radical, which is generated by reaction of the haemin resting state with PGG_2 or other hydroperoxides. The tyrosyl radical homolytically abstracts the 13*proS* hydrogen atom of arachidonic acid which initiates a radical cascade that ends with the stereoselective formation of PGG_2. PGG_2 then migrates from the cyclooxygenase (COX) site to the peroxidase (POX) site where it reacts with the haemin group to generate PGH_2 and Compound I. The heterolytic oxygen-oxygen bond cleavage is assisted by the conserved distal residues His207 and Gln203, mutation of which has been shown [6] to severely impair enzyme activity. Compound I, upon reaction with Tyr385$^{\bullet}$, gives Compound II which in turn is reduced to the haem resting state by one electron oxidation of reducing co-substrates, or undergoes reactions that result in enzyme self-inactivation.

The cyclooxygenase pocket is deeply buried within the protein [7] at the end of an essentially hydrophobic channel, the entrance of which is at the membrane binding domain and continues to Tyr385, adjacent to the haem group [8]. In contrast, the peroxidase pocket is a broad cavity on the surface of the protein. Peroxidase catalysis can continue independently of the cyclooxygenase site activity [9], and is a source of free radicals which contribute to tissue damage [10]. However, it is impossible to genetically eradicate both isoforms of PGHS in a living organism [11], and thus a chemical approach is necessary to elucidate the role of this peroxidase in pathophysiology. To facilitate the design of potent and selective inhibitors of this site, we decided to elucidate the catalytically active conformation of PGG_2 in PGHS-POX.

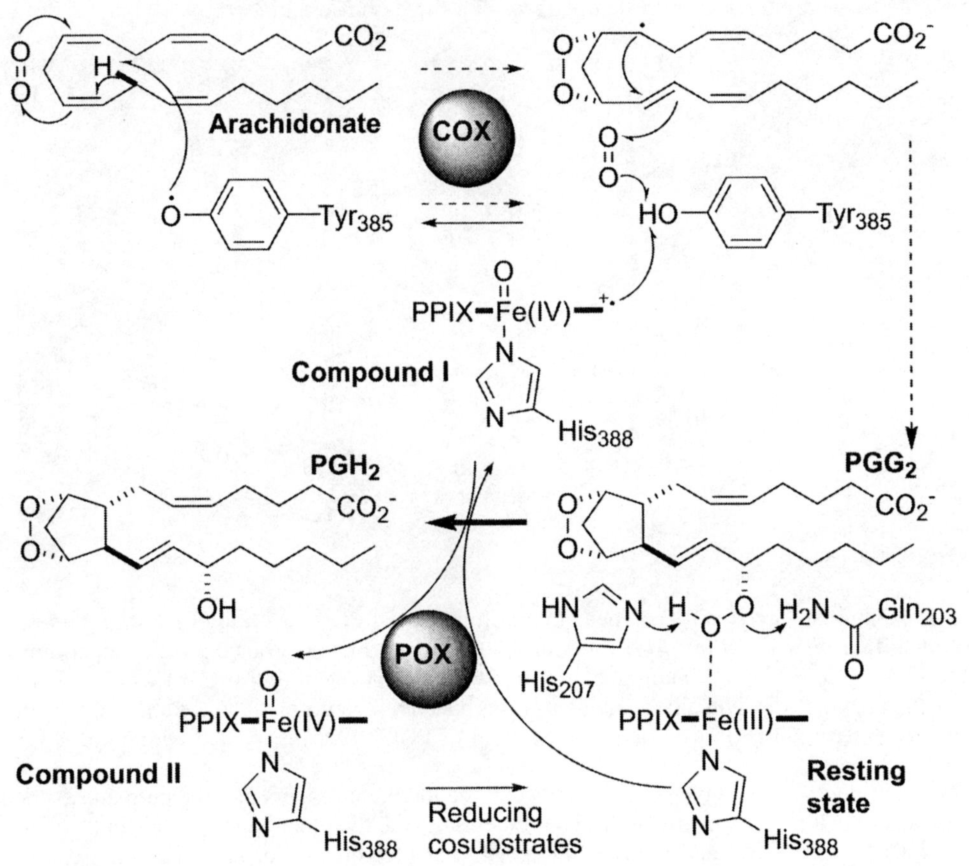

Fig. 1.

In order to gather relevant information on the structural features necessary for enzyme-substrate recognition and binding at the peroxidase site, we combined docking and molecular dynamics (MD) *in silico* studies with site-directed mutagenesis experiments. The recent publication of a theoretical MD study [12] using a non-natural PGG_2 analogue and a different docking methodology has prompted us to report our results with the natural substrate. Our computational and mutagenesis studies, correlated with previous knowledge in the field, provide a plausible binding model of PGG_2 within the peroxidase site of PGHS-1.

RESULTS AND DISCUSSION

Docking Studies. The first X-ray structure of ovine PGHS-1 (oPGHS-1) co-crystallized with a ligand, a serendipitous glycerol molecule, in the peroxidase site has recently been reported [13] (PDB code 1Q4G). This 2.0 Å resolution structure was used for the docking and MD experiments reported here. The structure of natural PGG_2 was docked into the peroxidase pocket of the protein using the Lamarckian genetic algorithm implemented in the automated docking program Autodock [14]. A conserved binding mode was identified *(fig. 2A)* for which the best docking energy was -15.7 kcal/mol.

A model of human PGHS-1 (hPGHS-1) was constructed using the Swiss-Model server and oPGHS-1 as a template, as there is 91% overall sequence identity between the ovine and the human enzymes and the POX site residues are entirely conserved. The docking results obtained with the human model were identical to those obtained with the ovine structure.

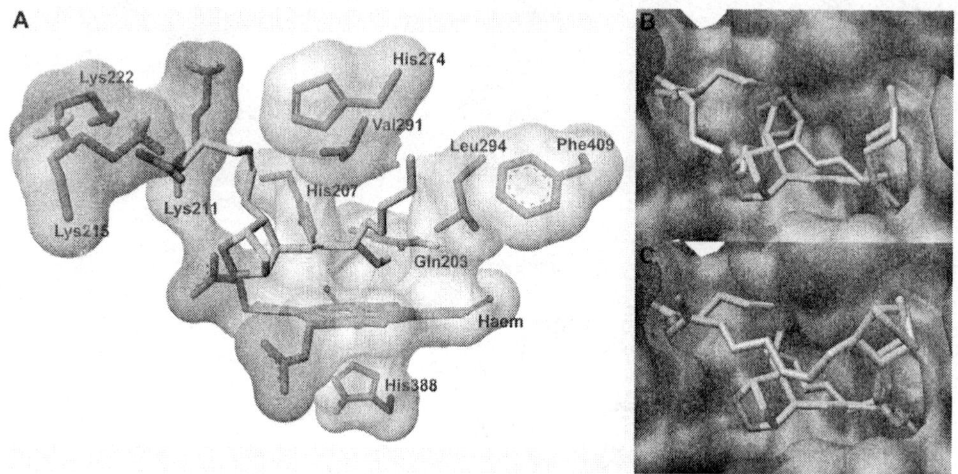

Fig. 2.

Two additional catalytically competent conformations of PGG_2, with higher docking energies, were identified. *figures 2B and 2C* represent the two conformers (carbons in grey) superimposed with the structure of the minimum docking energy conformer (carbons in blue) within the active site of the enzyme. Catalytically competent or "productive" conformations were defined as those in which the terminal hydroperoxide oxygen atom of PGG_2 (O26) is located within 4.0 Å of the iron.

The high degree of complementarity between the three conformers and the peroxidase pocket is noteworthy. All fulfill four structural requirements: (i) the hydroperoxide group is in the vicinity of the haem iron, His207 and Gln203, an established prerequisite for catalytic activity; (ii) the carboxylate group is near the cationic pocket comprising Lys215 and Lys222; (iii) a lipophilic moiety points towards the Val291, Leu294, His273 and Phe409 hydrophobic pocket; and (iv) another lipophilic moiety is inserted between Val291 and Lys211. Furthermore, the distance between the two polar anchor points, the iron on one side and the cationic pocket on the other, forces the substrate to adopt an extended conformation.

Molecular Dynamics. In order to account for protein flexibility and the possible participation of water molecules in substrate binding, the most favorable complex structure *(fig. 2A)* was hydrated with ~16,000 explicit water molecules, energy minimized, and a 500 ps molecular dynamics simulation performed at 300K using the Tripos force field, the NTV ensemble and periodic boundary conditions.

Slight conformational modifications that optimize substrate binding take place in the complex upon minimization. Namely, the Fe-O26 distance shortens, mainly due to the re-alignment of the haem iron into the protoporphyrin plane. This is likely to be a computational artifact due to the lack of adequate bending parameters for a pentacoordinated haem iron in the Tripos force field. However, we find this approximation to be acceptable for the purposes of this work.

Interestingly, the hydrogen bond network between PGG_2 15-hydroperoxide, His207 and Gln203 is modified upon minimization to incorporate a water molecule, almost equidistant between PGG_2-O26, His207 and Gln203. This hydrogen bond network incorporating the water molecule is maintained along the dynamics experiment *(figs. 3A and 3B)*. It has been hypothesized [15] that the ability to immobilize a water molecule coordinated to the haem iron might be an intrinsic structural feature of peroxidases, responsible in part for the different catalytic mechanisms of peroxidases (one electron oxidants) and catalases (two electron oxidants).

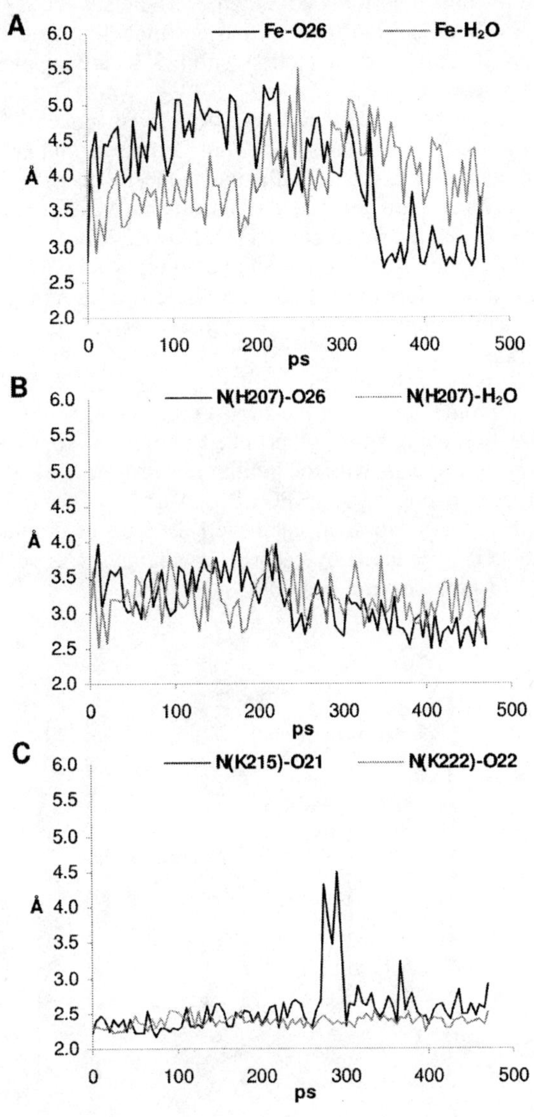

Fig. 3.

The overall folding of the protein is maintained along the dynamics experiment and the enzyme-substrate complex is stable. The evolution of various relevant enzyme-substrate distances along the 500 ps dynamics simulation is shown in *figure 3*. Interestingly, a water molecule and the terminal hydroperoxide oxygen (O26) alternately occupy a position close to the iron *(fig. 3A)*. Significantly, the salt bridges between Lys215 and Lys222 and PGG_2 carboxylate group are tightly conserved throughout the dynamics experiment *(fig. 3C)*, suggesting that this interaction plays a critical role in enzyme-substrate binding.

Site-Directed Mutagenesis. The presence of positively charged residues in the environment of the active site of a protein facilitates the binding of negatively charged substrates [16]. However, the roles of Lys215 and Lys222 at the PGHS peroxidase site in PGG_2 binding has not previously been demonstrated. In accordance with our model, the loss of the salt bridges between the PGG_2 carboxylate group and these two lysines, due to mutation, should result in a significant decrease of enzyme-substrate affinity and thus reduced enzyme efficiency. Lys211 is also located near Lys215 and Lys222 *(fig. 2A)* and, despite the fact that our modeling studies do not suggest participation of Lys211 in establishing a polar interaction with PGG_2 carboxylate, we decided to include Lys211 in our mutagenesis studies.

Site-directed mutagenesis of human PGHS-1 was performed sequentially, producing all combinations of single, double and triple mutations. Thus, fourteen mutants of the enzyme were constructed: three single mutants with a lysine to alanine replacement (K215A, K222A and K211A), three single mutants with a lysine to glutamic acid replacement (K215E, K222E and K211E), three double mutants with lysine to alanine replacements (K215A/K222A, K211A/K215A and K211A/K222A), three double mutants with lysine to glutamic acid replacements (K215E/K222E, K211E/K215E and K211E/K222E), one triple mutant with the three lysines replaced by alanine (K211A/K215A/K222E), and a triple mutant with the three lysines replaced by glutamic acid (K211E/K215E/K222E).

To test the enzymatic activity of the PGHS-1 mutants, transiently transfected COS-1 cells were allowed to react with arachidonic acid substrate for 15 min before the media were removed and assayed for PGE_2 accumulation using an enzyme-linked immunosorbant assay. Furthermore, preincubation of wild-type transfected cells with the inhibitor aspirin shows baseline activity, verifying that PGE_2 accumulation seen in this assay is PGHS dependent. The assays were performed in duplicate wells, with PGE_2 accumulation in each well assayed in duplicate, on three separate occasions. The amount of PGE_2 produced by each of the mutants was converted to a percentage of that produced by the wild type enzyme *(fig. 4)*.

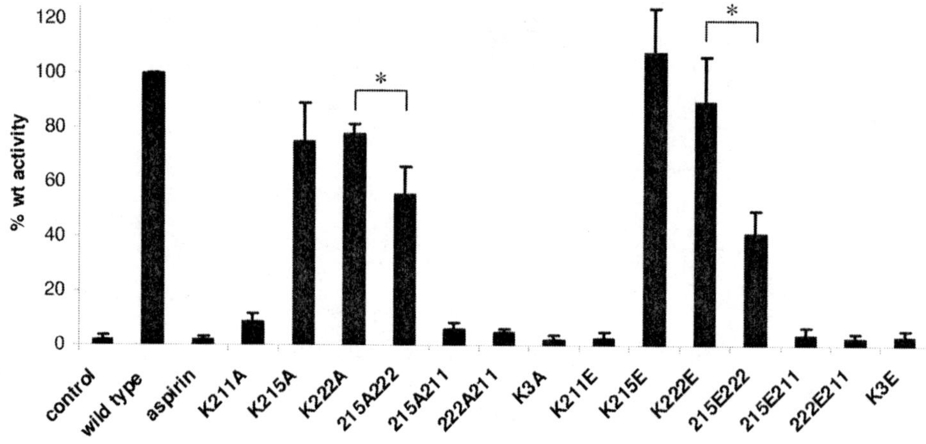

Fig. 4.

The most striking effect is the complete abolition of activity in all mutations involving Lys211. This effect is too dramatic to be attributed to a perturbation of ligand binding and is more consistent with a severe alteration of the structure of the enzyme. Indeed, this residue is totally conserved across both PGHS isoforms sequenced. Through formation of ionic linkages with the similarly conserved residues Asp236 and Glu290, Lys211 acts as a bridge between three poorly organized regions of the protein in the vicinity of the haem pocket [8] and is, therefore, likely to have a structural function.

Single mutations involving Lys215 and Lys222, to either alanine or glutamic acid, do not impair PGHS activity, with these mutants showing essentially wild-type conversion of PGG_2 to PGH_2. Importantly, when both of these residues are simultaneously mutated, a significant reduction of 27% and 58% was noted for alanine or glutamate respectively. This reduction is statistically relevant, with variance between the Lys222 and Lys215/Lys222 double mutants showing paired students t-test P values of 0.038 and 0.021 for the alanine and glutamate mutants, respectively. We propose that the presence of these two compensatory residues is a "safety mechanism" which highlights the importance of a positively charged region for substrate binding. Indeed, both residues are highly conserved in both isoforms of numerous species, and at least one of the two amino acids is always a lysine in mammals.

The proposed binding model is, thus, fully consistent with the commonly accepted mechanism of catalysis as well as with our, and other previously reported, site-directed mutagenesis studies. Based on the binding model presented here, which defines the minimal pharmacophore for specific enzyme-substrate recognition, we have designed a first generation of PGHS-peroxidase inhibitors which are expected to be highly selective and become valuable chemical tools for exploring the implication of this peroxidase in pathophysiology.

REFERENCES

1. Smith WL, DeWitt DL, Garavito RM. Cyclooxygenases: structural, cellular, and molecular biology. *Annu Rev Biochem*. 2000; 69: 145-82.
2. Simmons DL, Botting RM, Hla T. Cyclooxygenase isozymes: the biology of prostaglandin synthesis and inhibition. *Pharmacol Rev*. 2004, 56: 387-437.
3. Tanabe T, Tohnai N. Cyclooxygenase isozymes and their gene structures and expression. *Prostaglandins Other Lipid Mediat*. 2002, 68: 95-114.
4. Ullrich V, Ruf HH. Heme Proteins in Prostaglandin Biosynthesis. In: Sheldon RA, ed. *Metalloporphyrins in Catalytic Oxidations*. New York: Marcel Dekker, 1994: 157-92.
5. Tsai A, Hsi LC, Kulmacz RJ, Palmer G, Smith WL. Characterization of the tyrosyl radicals in ovine prostaglandin H synthase-1 by isotope replacement and site-directed mutagenesis. *J Biol Chem*. 1994, 269: 5085-91.
6. Landino LM, Crews BC, Gierse JK, Hauser SD, Marnett LJ. Mutational analysis of the role of the distal histidine and glutamine residues of prostaglandin-endoperoxide synthase-2 in peroxidase catalysis, hydroperoxide reduction, and cyclooxygenase activation. *J Biol Chem*. 1997, 272: 21565-74.
7. Kiefer JR, Pawlitz JL, Moreland KT, Stegeman RA, Hood WF, Gierse JK, Stevens AM, Goodwin DC, Rowlinson SW, Marnett LJ, Stallings, WC, Kurumbail RG. Structural insights into the stereochemistry of the cyclooxygenase reaction. *Nature*. 2000, 405: 97-101.
8. Picot D, Loll PJ, Garavito RM. The X-ray crystal structure of the membrane protein prostaglandin H2 synthase-1. *Nature*. 1994, 367: 243-9.
9. Song I, Ball TM, Smith WL. Different suicide inactivation processes for the peroxidase and cyclooxygenase activities of prostaglandin endoperoxide H synthase-1. *Biochem Biophys Res Commun*. 2001, 289: 869-75.
10. Wells PG, Bhuller Y, Chen CS, Jeng W, Kasapinovic S, Kennedy JC, Kim PM, Laposa RR, McCallum GP, Nicol CJ, Parman T, Wiley MJ, Wong AW. Molecular and biochemical mechanisms in teratogenesis involving reactive oxygen species. *Toxicol Appl Pharmacol*. 2005, 207: 354-66.
11. Reese J, Paria BC, Brown N, Zhao X, Morrow JD, Dey SK. Coordinated regulation of fetal and maternal

prostaglandins directs successful birth and postnatal adaptation in the mouse. *Proc Natl Acad Sci USA*. 2000, 97: 9759-64.
12. Seibold SA, Smith WL, Cukier CI. The peroxidase site of prostaglandin endoperoxide H synthase-1 docking and molecular dynamic studies with a prostaglandin endoperoxide analog. *J Phys Chem B*. 2004, 108: 9297-305.
13. Gupta K, Selinsky BS, Kaub CJ, Katz AK, Loll PJ. The 2.0 Å resolution crystal structure of prostaglandin H2 synthase-1: structural insights into an unusual peroxidase. *J Mol Biol*. 2004, 335: 503-18.
14. Morris GM, Goodsell DS, Halliday RS, Huey R, Hart WE, Belew RK, Olson AJ. Automated docking using a Lamarckian genetic algorithm and empirical binding free energy function. *J Comp Chem*. 1998, 19: 1639-62.
15. Jones P. Roles of water in heme peroxidase and catalase mechanisms. *J Biol Chem*. 2001, 276: 13791-6.
16. Riordan JF, McElvany KD, Borders CL. Arginyl residues: anion recognition sites in enzymes. *Science*. 1977, 195: 884-6.

Metal Ions in Biology and Medicine: vol. 9. Eds Maria Carmen Alpoim, Paula Vasconcellos Morais, Maria Amélia Santos, Armando J. Cristóvão, José A. Centeno, Philippe Collery.
John Libbey Eurotext, Paris © 2006 pp. 129-1.

Involvement of histones in nickel carcinogenesis: a study of Ni(II) interactions with the 30-aa N-terminal tail of histone H4

Maria Antonietta Zoroddu*[1], Massimiliano Peana[2], Serenella Medici[1]

[1]*Dipartimento di Chimica, University ofi Sassari, Via Vienna 2, 07100 Sassari, Italy. Email: Zoroddu@uniss.it*
[2]*CERM, Magnetic Resonance Center, University of Florence, Via L. Sacconi 6, 50019 Sesto Fiorentino, Florence, Italy*

Nickel compounds are established human carcinogens. Their carcinogenic activity is consistently related to the ability of Ni(II) to access chromatin and cause multiple types of cellular nuclear damage via direct or indirect mechanisms. The mechanistic concepts proposed for nickel carcinogenesis include promutagenic DNA damage [1, 2], epigenetic effects in chromatin [3-5], and impairment of DNA repair [6].

The core histone octamer (formed by two copies of histones H3, H4, H2A and H2B) together with the linker histone H1, package eukaryotic DNA into repeating nucleosomal units that are folded into higher order chromatin fibres. Due to its abundance inside the cell nucleus this histone octamer is a good target for nickel binding.

We focused our interest on histone H4, first of all because it has been reported that nickel(II) is a potent suppressor of histone H4 acetylation, in both yeast and mammalian cells [7], and this may lead to transcription errors and subsequent DNA modifications [8]. Secondly, an anchoring binding site for nickel ion on the terminal part of this protein, specifically histidine H_{18}, is close to sites for post-translational modifications involved in nickel toxicity.

All this evidence points to the H4 tail as a candidate for Ni(II) binding on the histone octamer, and the study of its N-terminal tail as a model for metal coordination can supply useful information in the effort of unveiling the mechanisms of nickel carcinogenesis.

We previously reported, by potentiometric and spectroscopic (NMR, Uv-Vis, CD) studies, about the interaction of Ni(II) with minimal models of the H4 tail: the two peptides with 6 amino acids Ac-AKRHRK-Am and with 22 amino acids Ac-SGRGKGGKGLGKGGAKRHRK VL-Am, respectively [9-11].

Here we present our recent results on the coordination ability of Ni(II) to the N-terminal tail of histone H4, the 30-amino acid peptide Ac-SGRGKGGKGLGKGGAKRH$_{18}$RKVLRDNIQGIT-Am, a more relevant model of the tail of the protein, achieved by the use of multidimensional NMR spectroscopy.

EXPERIMENTAL SECTION

Peptide synthesis

The peptide was chemically synthesized using solid phase Fmoc chemistry, purified and isolated by RP-HPLC. Fractions were collected and analyzed by MALDI-TOF MS. Fractions containing the peptide of the expected molecular weight were pooled and lyophilized.

NMR spectroscopy

NMR experiments were performed on Bruker Avance 600 or 700 MHz spectrometers equipped with a 5 mm TXI 1H-13C probe (Magnetic Resonance Center CERM, Florence). Samples used for NMR experiments were 5 mM in concentration and dissolved in 90/10 v/v H_2O/D_2O solutions. All acquisitions were performed at 298 K. The pH of the sample was adjusted to ranges of 2.7-10.0 by addition of 1 N NaOH or 1 N HCl. The titration experiments on Ni(II)-containing samples with peptide-to-metal molar ratio of 1:1 were performed at pH 8.7. Nuclear Overhauser Enhancement Spectroscopy (NOESY) with mixing times of 500 ms and Total Correlation Spectroscopy (TOCSY) with a mixing time of 50 ms were also performed. A combination of TOCSY and NOESY experiments was used to assign the spectra of both free and Ni(II)-bound peptide. Solvent suppression for 1D, TOCSY and NOESY experiments was achieved using WATERGATE pulse sequence or using excitation sculpting with gradients. All NMR data were processed using XWINNMR (Bruker Instruments) software on a Silicon Graphics Indigo workstation and analyzed using the Sparky 3.1 program.

UV-visible measurements

Absorption spectra of the peptide-Ni(II) system at 1:1 molar ratio were recorded on a Varian Cary 50 Scan spectrophotometer in the 600-300 nm range with changing the pH from 3.0 to 10.0. Solutions for UV-visible measurements had a 1.5 mM concentration.

RESULTS AND DISCUSSION

During the past years we reported our results for potentiometric and spectroscopic studies on the interactions of minimal models (6, 7, 11 and 22-amino acid fragments, respectively) of histone H4 with Ni(II) ions [9-11]. From the data we collected, it was evident that at pH values above 7 the N-terminal tail of H4 coordinates nickel in a stepwise fashion, starting from the imidazole nitrogen of His, that acts like an anchoring site for the metal, and following with the three amide nitrogens of His, Arg and Lys residues, respectively. The formation of stable five-membered chelate rings by consecutive nitrogens is the driving force of this process *(fig. 1)*.

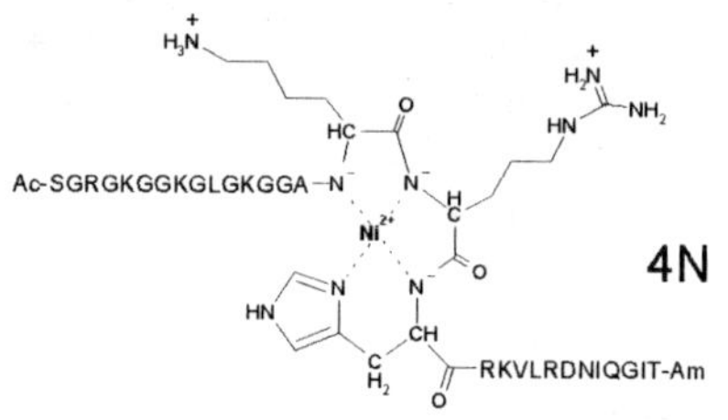

Ac-SGRGKGGKGLGKGGA–N⁻ ... Ni²⁺ ... RKVLRDNIQGIT-Am

4N

Fig. 1.

Ultraviolet-visible (UV-Vis) spectroscopy of Ac-SGRGKGGKGLGKGGAKRH$_{18}$RKVLRDNIQ-GIT-Am N-terminal tail of histone H4 confirmed the results we collected in our previous works. Spectra were recorded for a 1:1 mixture of Ni(II) ion with the 30-amino acid peptide by gradually changing the pH up to 10.0. The results are in good agreement with those collected from potentiometric and spectroscopic measurements performed on the comparable 22-amino acid fragment as we already reported [11]. From pH 9.0 to pH 10.0 the λ_{max} value at 437 nm (ε **??** = 110 and 156 dm^3 mol^{-1}cm^{-1} for pH = 9.0 and pH = 10.0, respectively) with a shoulder at 487 nm is characteristic of a planar coordination of Ni(II) ions in a 4N chromophore.

A detailed multidimensional NMR study was associated to UV-Vis spectroscopy in order to obtain more information about nickel binding to the peptide and evidences of structural modifications upon complexation. To verify the coordination mode of Ni(II) to our peptide to 1D, 2D ^{1}H homonuclear TOCSY and NOESY NMR spectra of H4 30-amino acid free peptide and of peptide-Ni(II) species at pH = 8.7 were recorded and compared. This pH was chosen since for the peptide-Ni(II) system it approaches maximum formation of the major planar diamagnetic species, as evidenced by potentiometric and spectroscopic measurements previously reported [11].

The resonances belonging to the 30-residues free peptide were assigned on the basis of 1D NMR spectra and 2D ^{1}H homonuclear TOCSY and NOESY experiments. The alkaline pH required for nickel binding has an evident effect on the protonation of the free peptide and causes exchange of the amidic protons with bulk water. Therefore their resonances were lost. Only the aromatic signals of the histidine residue (Hε_1 and Hδ_2 at 7.595 and 6.862 ppm, respectively) were present in the region between 6.6 and 8.5 ppm at this pH.

The binding mode of Ni(II) to the H4 tail was studied at pH = 8.7 with increasing nickel concentrations up to peptide/Ni molar ratio of 1:1. Clear information on the binding mode of the metal can be obtained from a series of 1D ^{1}H, 2D TOCSY and NOESY complex spectra recorded up to molar ratio of 1:0.8.

Figure 2 shows the aliphatic region of ^{1}H-^{1}H NMR TOCSY spectra for the Ni^{2+} bound peptide. It is evident that metal coordination causes deep changes to the peptide structure, as evidenced by the strong chemical shift differences recorded for the residues involved in metal binding.

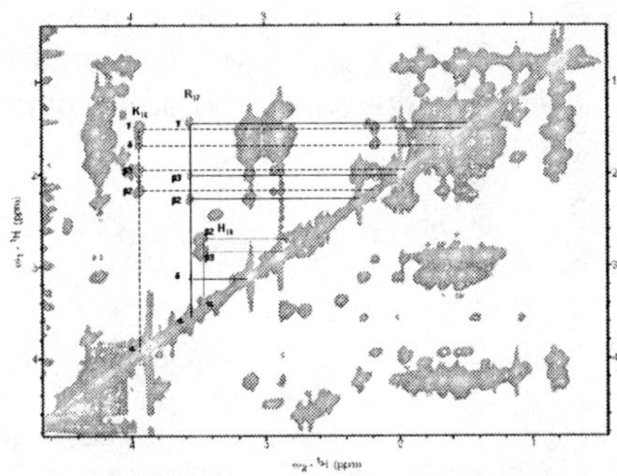

Fig. 2. Aliphatic region of ^{1}H-^{1}H NMR TOCSY spectra for the Ni^{2+} bound Ac-SGRGKGGKGLGKGGAKRH$_{18}$ RKVLRDNIQGIT-Am peptide at 1:0.8 molar ratio peptide-to-nickel. The new cross-peaks due to Ni-binding have been labelled.

When we compare the resonances of the free peptide with those recorded after addition of Ni(II) ions, we notice that only the signals relative to Lys$_{16}$, Arg$_{17}$, His$_{18}$ and Arg$_{19}$ appear shifted with respect to their original position, an evidence that only this part of the peptide is involved in the coordination process. Some of the largest changes in chemical shift are observed as strong upfield shifts attributable to the Hα protons of Lys$_{16}$, Arg$_{17}$, His$_{18}$ and to the Hε_1 proton of His$_{18}$, indicating, as expected, deprotonation and coordination of the amidic protons of these three residues, whilst the fourth donor is identified as the Nδ of the imidazole ring of His$_{18}$.

Smaller changes in chemical shifts were observed also for Arg$_{19}$, indicating that, although not directly involved in nickel complexation, this residue too is affected by its formation.

One of the most evident effect of Ni(II) coordination to the peptide is the dramatic upfield shift experienced by all the protons in the histidine residue, starting with the Hα signal (δ = -1.032 ppm). Both Hβ protons (δ = -0.165 ppm for Hβ_2; δ = -0.202 ppm for Hβ_3) and Hε_1 proton (δ = -0.123 ppm) show the same trend while the shielding effect is less pronounced for Hδ_2 (δ = -0.025 ppm).

Arg$_{17}$ Hβ protons are strongly shifted downfield (δ = 0.361 ppm for Hβ_2; δ = 0.554 ppm for Hβ_3, rispectively), while Qγ and Qδ protons show less pronounced differences in chemical shift with respect to the free peptide signals. Arg$_{19}$ chemical shifts are almost unaffected by nickel complexation except for Hβ_2 (δ = 0.161 ppm), indicating that this residue is not directly involved in the coordination mode of the complex, although coordination of the metal undoubtedly modifies its chemical environment.

Nevertheless, the most interesting feature of the Ni(II)-peptide complex is represented by Lys_{16} residue. Apart from its α proton, which is strongly shielded, as expected, after deprotonation and nickel binding, all the remaining protons show a clear downfield shift, their δ decreasing according to the order $\beta > \gamma > \delta > \varepsilon$. This behaviour can be explained if we consider the 2D NOESY spectra recorded for the Ni(II)-peptide complex. These bidimensional spectra show a set of NOE cross-peaks for histidine $H\varepsilon_1$ proton arising after nickel binding. Analysis of these cross-peaks pointed out the presence of interactions between His_{18} $H\varepsilon_1$ and all the aliphatic protons along the lysine chain. It seems thus evident that Lys_{16} points directly towards the histidine residue passing over the coordination plane, and that both the effect of the metal and of the ring current of the imidazolic moiety may play a role in determining the chemical shift changes observed for the lysyl protons.

CONCLUSIONS

The conformation of Lys_{16} side chain can be crucial in the enzyme recognition processes, i.e. in the acetylation mechanism promoted by the acetyltransferase enzyme HAT on lysine itself, which is located in the region close to histidine H_{18} of Histone H4, which represents the focus of nickel coordination. Any conformational change of Lys_{16} upon nickel binding may thus impair the activity of HAT leading to transcription errors and subsequent DNA modifications.

We believe that the results achieved in this study may add another piece to the puzzle of the mechanism of nickel carcinogenesis.

REFERENCES

1. Kasprzak, K.S. Possible role of oxidative damage in metal-induced carcinogenesis. *Cancer Invest.* 1995; 13:411-30.
2. Kasprzak, K.S. in: N. Hadjiliadis (Ed.), Cytotoxic, Mutagenic and Carcinogenic Potential of Heavy Metals Related to Human Environment, Vol. 26, Kluwer, Dordrecht, The Netherlands: NATO ASI Series 2, 1997, pp 73-92.
3. Costa, M. Molecular mechanisms of nickel carcinogenesis. *Annu. Rev. Pharmacol. Toxicol.* 1991; 31:321-37.
4. Salnikow, K., Cosentino, S., Klein, C., Costa, M. Loss of thrombospondin transcriptional activity in nickel-transformed cells. *Mol. Cell. Biol.* 1994; 14:851-58.
5. Lee, Y.-W., Klein, C.B., Kargacin, B., Salnikow, K., Kitahara, J., Dowjat, K., Zhitkovich, A., Costa, M. Carcinogenic nickel silences gene expression by chromatin condensation and DNA methylation: a new model for epigenetic carcinogens. *Mol. Cell. Biol.* 1995; 15:2547-57.
6. Hartwig, A. Current aspects in metal genotoxicity. *Bio-Metals* 1995; 8:3-11.
7. Broday, L., Peng, W., Kuo, M.H., Salnikow, K., Zoroddu, M.A., Costa, M. Nickel compounds are novel inhibitors of histone H4 acetylation. *Cancer Res.* 2000; 60:238-41.
8. Grunstein, M. Histone acetylation in chromatin structure and transcription. *Nature* 1997; 389:349-52.
9. Zoroddu, M.A., Schinocca, L., Kowalik-Jankowska, T., Kozlowski, H., Salnikow, K., Costa, M. Molecular mechanisms in nickel carcinogenesis: modeling Ni(II) binding site in histone H4. *Environ Health Perspect.* 2002; 110(5):719-23.
10. Zoroddu, M.A., Kowalik-Jankowska, T., Kozlowski, H., Molinari, H., Salnikow, K., Broday, L., Costa, M. Interaction of Ni(II) and Cu(II) with a metal binding sequence of histone H4: AKRHRK, a model of the H4 tail. *Biochim. Biophys. Acta* 2000; 1475:163-68.
11. Zoroddu, M.A., Peana, M., Kowalik-Jankowska, T., Kozlowski, H., Costa, M. The binding of Ni(II) and Cu(II) with the N-terminal tail of the histone H4. *J. Chem. Soc., Dalton Trans.* 2002; 3:458-65.

Metal Ions in Biology and Medicine: vol. 9. Eds Maria Carmen Alpoim, Paula Vasconcellos Morais, Maria Amélia Santos, Armando J. Cristóvão, José A. Centeno, Philippe Collery.
John Libbey Eurotext, Paris © 2006 pp. 133-1.

Cap43 protein interactions with Ni(II) ions: evidences of a possible detoxification role

Maria Antonietta Zoroddu*[1], Massimiliano Peana[2], Serenella Medici[1]

[1]*Dipartimento di Chimica, University of Sassari, Via Vienna 2, 07100 Sassari, Italy. Email : Zoroddu@uniss.it*
[2]*CERM, Magnetic Resonance Center, University of Florence, Via L. Sacconi 6, 50019 Sesto Fiorentino, Florence, Italy*

The Cap43 gene is induced by a rise in free intracellular Ca^{2+} following nickel exposure [1, 6]. No other metal compound significantly induced expression of this gene, indicating that it is expressed with marked specificity to Ni(II) exposure [5].

This finding makes the Cap43 protein an interesting candidate for studies of molecular mechanisms implicated in toxicity and carcinogenicity of nickel compounds, because a promising way to unveil these molecular events is to study the characteristics of the proteins expressed by genes specifically induced by these carcinogens.

For this reason we focused our attention on the ability of nickel(II) to interact with Cap43 protein.

Cap43 has no cysteine or histidine-rich motifs for metal binding, but it possesses a mono-histidine fragment composed by 10 amino acids (Thr-Arg-Ser-Arg-Ser-His-Thr-Ser-Glu-Gly) whose sequence is repeated consecutively three times, suggesting a nickel binding motif at the C-terminus. It should be mentioned that such mono-histidine fragments, e.g. octapeptide repeated regions in prion proteins, play a critical role in metal metabolism using sets of His imidazoles as the binding sites for metal ions [7].

We previously reported about our studies on Ni(II) binding to the 20-amino acid C-terminal sequence of the Cap43 protein -*TRSRSHTSEG-TRSRSHTSEG*-, and 30-amino acid sequence, *TRSRSHTSEG-TRSRSHTSEG-TRSRSHTSEG*, by combined pH-metric and spectroscopic (UV-VIS, CD, NMR) techniques [8, 9]. Here we discuss the results obtained from 2D multinuclear NMR experiments carried out to get a better insight into Ni(II) interaction with the C-terminal 30-amino acids sequence of Cap43 protein.

EXPERIMENTAL SECTION

Peptide synthesis

The peptide was chemically synthesized using solid phase Fmoc chemistry, purified and isolated by RP-HPLC. Fractions were collected and analyzed by MALDI-TOF MS. Fractions containing the peptide of the expected molecular weight were pooled and lyophilized.

NMR spectroscopy

NMR experiments were performed on a Bruker Avance 600 or 700 MHz spectrometer equipped with 5 mm TXI 1H-13 probe. Samples used for NMR experiments were 5 mM in concentration and dissolved in 90/10 v/v H_2O/D_2O solutions. All acquisitions were performed at the temperature of 298 K. A series of 1D spectra of the free peptide was recorded at various pH values between

2.7 and 10.0 by step of 1.0. The titration experiments of Ni(II)-containing samples with metal-to-ligand molar ratios of 1:1 and 2:1 were performed at pH 9.0 and for samples with 3:1 molar ratio were performed at pH 10.0. The pH of the sample was adjusted to reach the final pH by addition of 1 N NaOH or 1 N HCl. Nuclear Overhauser Enhancement Spectroscopy (NOESY) with mixing times of 500 ms, Rotating Frame Overhauser Enhancement Spectroscopy (ROESY) with mixing times of 250 ms and Total Correlation Spectroscopy (TOCSY) with a mixing time of 50 ms were also performed. The combination of TOCSY, NOESY and ROESY experiments was used to assign the spectra of both free and Ni(II)-bound peptides at various pH. Solvent suppression for 1D, TOCSY, NOESY and ROESY experiments was achieved using WATERGATE pulse sequence or using excitation sculpting with gradients. All NMR data were processed using XWINNMR (Bruker Instruments) software on a Silicon Graphics Indigo workstation and analyzed using the Sparky 3.11 program.

RESULTS AND DISCUSSION

The results of our previous studies on the interaction of Ni(II) ions with the fragments of Cap43 protein containing respectively two and three repeated -TRSRSHTSEG- amino acid sequences showed that each 10-amino acid fragment coordinates one metal ion. The coordination of the metal ion starts from the imidazole nitrogen atom of the histidine residue, and with increasing the pH, Ni(II) ions are able to deprotonate successive peptide nitrogen atoms, forming Ni(II)-N^- bonds, until a $NiH_{-3}L$ and $Ni_2H_{-6}L$ species for the 20- and $NiH_{-3}L$, $Ni_2H_{-6}L$ and $Ni_3H_{-9}L$ complexes for the 30-amino acid fragments, are formed (above pH 8). The formation of stable five-membered chelate rings by consecutive nitrogens is the driving force of the coordination process [8, 9].

At physiological pH (7.4) and mM concentrations of nickel(II), dependently on the metal-to-ligand molar ratio, the 20-amino acid fragment forms the Ni_2L complex (2:1 molar ratio), while the 30-amino acid fragment forms the NiL (1:1), Ni_2L (2:1), and Ni_3L (3:1) complexes, where each metal ion is coordinated by the imidazole nitrogen atom of the histidine residue of each 10-amino acid sequence *(fig. 1)*.

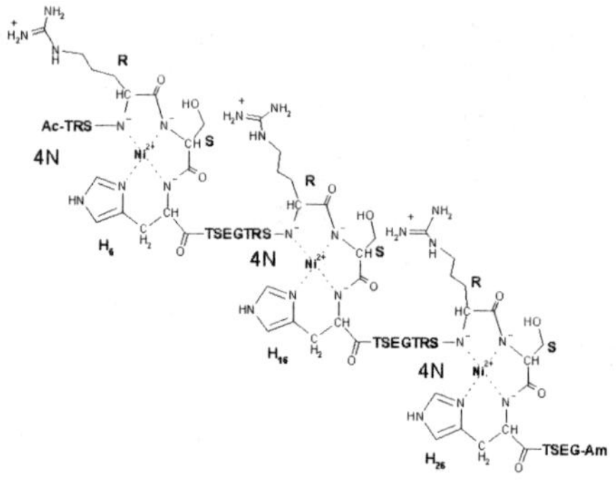

Fig. 1. Schematic representation of Ni(II) binding to the Ac-TRSRSHTSEG-TRSRSHTSEG-TRSRSHTSEG-Am 30-amino acid fragment of Cap43 protein

The Ni_2L and Ni_3L complexes of these peptides are more stable by about 0.7-1.5 orders of magnitude compared to the stability constants evaluated for these systems considering an independent coordination of each metal ion to a single *TRSRSHTSEG* amino acid sequence [8]. The coordination of two or three metal ions with the 4N $\{N_{Im}, 3N^-\}$ system on the whole fragment ($Ni_2H_{-6}L$, $Ni_3H_{-9}L$ complexes respectively) is not cooperative.

Based on this evidence, we performed a series of 1D and 2D multidimensional NMR experiments at different pH values in order to fully characterize both the free peptide and its Ni(II) complexes at different ligand/metal molar ratios.

For the 30-aa free peptide 1D, 2D ^{1}H homonuclear TOCSY and NOESY spectra were performed at various pH.

At pH 9.0 the resonances belonging to the 30 residues of the free peptide were assigned on the basis of 1D NMR spectra and 2D ^{1}H homonuclear TOCSY and NOESY experiments. In the region between 6.6 and 8.5 ppm, only the aromatic resonances of three histidine residues H_6, H_{16} and H_{26} were present, the three of them overlapping at the same chemical shifts (Hε_1 and Hδ_2, 7.607 ppm and 6.888 ppm respectively). All the amide resonances were in fast exchange with water at this pH and their resonances were lost. In the aliphatic region, the histidine Hα appeared at 4.600 ppm, under the water signal. Its assignment was based on the analysis of the TOCSY spectrum, where a correlation between histidinic Hα and Qβ was clearly visible (Qβ at 3.029 ppm). The TOCSY and NOESY spectra also allowed the assignment of the entire spin system of each amino acid.

For the peptide-Ni(II) species, in order to test the coordination properties of individual mono-histidinic motifs, the NMR study was performed at different Ni(II)-to-ligand molar ratios (1:1, 2:1 and 3:1, respectively). The pH was chosen to approach maximum formation of the major planar diamagnetic species, as previously evidenced by potentiometric and spectroscopic measurements (pH = 9 for 1:1 and 2:1, pH = 10.0 for 3:1) [9].

The binding mode of Ni(II) to the three TRSRSHTSEG mono-histidinic motifs of Cap43 peptide, monitored by collecting a series of 1D ^{1}H, 2D TOCSY and ROESY spectra at the different molar ratios (1:1, 1:2 and 1:3) for the peptide-metal system, is the same for the three cases. Analysis of the effects of nickel coordination on the chemical shift of the residue undergoing the strongest modifications allowed us to establish that the coordination mode of Ni(II) to our peptide involved H_{6+i} residues through imidazole and the amidic nitrogens, and R_{4+i} and S_{5+i} residues through their amidic nitrogens, respectively (where i = 0, 10, 20).

Figure 2 shows the aliphatic region of 1H-1H NMR TOCSY spectra for the Ni^{2+} bound to the 30-aa peptide at 1:3 molar ratio peptide-to-nickel.

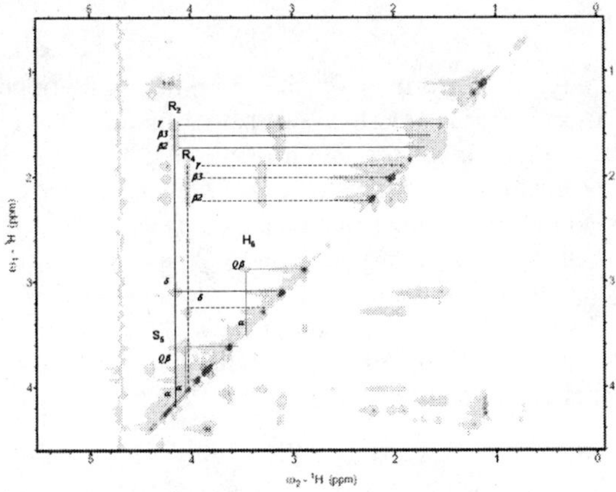

Fig. 2. Aliphatic region of 1H-1H NMR TOCSY spectra for the Ni^{2+} bound to Ac-TRSRSHTSEG-TRSRSHTSEG-TRSRSHTSEG-Am peptide at 1:3 molar ratio peptide-to-nickel. For simplicity the new cross-peaks seen in the Ni^{2+} bound peptide have been labelled only for the first 10-aa fragment.
The shifts found involve the resonances of Arg_{2+i}, Arg_{4+i}, Ser_{5+n} and His_{6+i} (where i = 0, 10 and 20). Conditions used were: [L] = 5.0 mM, 90/10 v/v H_2O/D_2O buffer, pH 9.0, T 298 K and 700 MHz proton frequency.

As expected, addition of increasing amounts of Ni(II), at pH 9, caused the incremental loss in intensity of a number of resonances, together with the simultaneous appearance of a new set of peaks. These new resonances increased in intensity with increasing additions of Ni(II), suggesting the progressive involvement in the metal binding of thearomatic protons $H\varepsilon_1$ and $H\delta_2$ for all the three histidines residues in the peptide sequence.

From the initial molar ratio 1:1 to the final 1:3, the two sets of the aromatic protons on the three histidines H_6, H_{16} and H_{26} showed exactly the same upfield shift with a $\delta = -0.176$ ppm for $H\varepsilon_1$ and $\delta = -0.019$ ppm for $H\delta_2$, respectively. The strong shift experienced by the $H\varepsilon_1$ protons respect to the $H\delta_2$ is due to their higher proximity to the metal ion. Strong shifts affected also the histidine $H\alpha$ and $Q\beta$ protons ($\delta = -1.156$ ppm for $H\alpha$; $\delta = -0.148$ ppm for $Q\beta$ respectively), as expected after deprotonation and coordination of the amidic nitrogen.

In the free peptide, the aliphatic protons of arginine R_2, R_4, R_{12}, R_{14}, R_{22} and R_{24}, experienced equivalent chemical environments resulting in an overlap of their resonances. On the contrary, the addition of Ni(II) ions caused a strong differentiation of their signals. In particular, we were able to assign a first set of resonances for R_4, R_{14}, R_{24} residues ($H\alpha = 4.024$ ppm; $H\beta_2 = 2.209$ ppm; $H\beta_3 = 2.032$ ppm; $Q\gamma = 1.914$ ppm; $Q\delta = 3.282$ ppm) and a second set of resonances for R_2, R_{12}, R_{22} ($H\alpha = 4.129$ ppm; $H\beta_2 = 1.726$ ppm; $H\beta_3 = 1.619$ ppm; $Q\gamma = 1.511$ ppm; $Q\delta = 3.094$ ppm).

This differentiation is due to the fact that the R_4, R_{14} and R_{24} residues are directly involved in the complex formation through their amidic nitrogen donors, and the metal binding causes stronger shifts on their proton resonances than for the R_2, R_{12}, R_{22} residues, which are not directly involved in the coordination process and remain, therefore, less perturbed. Consequently, the two different chemical environments for the arginine residues resulted in two new distinct spin systems that appeared in the TOCSY and ROESY spectra.

Threonine residues are located in position 1 and 7 in each repeated 10-amino acid fragment. From 1D and 2D spectra, small perturbations in the proton resonances after addition of nickel were clearly visible. Threonines in position 7 are closer to the coordination centre respect to those in position 1. For this reason they are more sensitive to the chemical environment changes caused by metal binding. This fact allowed us to fix the correct assignments. Notably, spin systems that are unaffected by Ni(II) addition include glutammate E_{9+i} and glycine G_{10+i} for every fragment.

CONCLUSIONS

The accurate NMR study we performed on the 30-amino acid fragment of Cap43 protein showed that its C-terminal sequence is able to coordinate 3 metal ions in a very effective way at various pH values. At pH = 9 maximum formation of the major planar diamagnetic species was observed, and the complex thus formed adopts a square-planar geometry. This complex shows a 4N $\{N_{Im}, 3N^-\}$ coordination mode involving a histidine residue through its imidazole and the amidic nitrogens, and two amidic nitrogens from arginine and serine residues, respectively.

The capability of this peptide to bind such a remarkable number nickel ions is an evidence of the possible role of Cap43 in metal detossification processes. The results we collected encourage us to expand the scope of our research to better understand the mechanisms behind the intriguing behaviour of Cap43 towards nickel ions.

REFERENCES

1. Zhou. D., Salnikow, K., Costa, M. Cap43, a novel gene specifically induced by Ni2+ compounds. *Cancer Res.* 1998;58(10):2182-9.
2. Salnikow, K., Blagosklonny, M.V., Ryan, H., Johnson, R., Costa, M. Carcinogenic nickel induces genes involved with hypoxic stress. *Cancer Res.* 2000; 60(1):38-41.
3. Piquemal, D., Joulia, D., Balaguer, P., Basset, A., Marti, J., Commes, T. Differential expression of the RTP/Drg1/Ndr1 gene product in proliferating and growth arrested cells. *Biochim. Biophys. Acta* 1999; 1450:364-73.

4. Kokame, K., Kato, H., Miyata, T. Homocysteine-respondent genes in vascular endothelial cells identified by differential display analysis. GRP78/BiP and novel genes. *J Biol Chem.* 1996; 271:29659-65.
5. Salnikow, K., Kluz, T., Costa, M. Role of Ca2+ in the regulation of nickel-inducible Cap43 gene expression. *Toxicol. Appl. Pharmacol.* 1999; 160:127-32.
6. Salnikow, K., Zhou, D., Kluz, T., Wang, C., M. Costa, in: A. Sarkar (Ed.), *Metal and Genetics*, Kluwer Academic, Plenum Publishers, New York, 1999; 131-44.
7. Viles, J.H., Cohen, F.E., Prusiner, S.B., Goodin, D.B., Wright, P.E., Dyson, H.J. Copper Binding to the Prion Protein: Structural Implications of Four Identical Cooperative Binding Sites. *Proc. Natl. Acad. Sci.* USA, 1999; 96, 2042-47.
8. Zoroddu, M.A., Kowalik-Jankowska, T., Kozlowski, H., Salnikow, K., Costa, M. Ni(II) and Cu(II) Binding with a 14-Amino Acid Sequence of Cap43 Protein, TRSRSHTSEGTRSR. *J. Inorg. Biochem.* 2001; 84, 47-54.
9. Zoroddu, M.A., Peana, M., Kowalik-Jankowska, T., Kozlowski, H., Costa, M. Nickel(II) binding to Cap43 protein fragments. *J. Inorg Biochem.* 2004; 98(6):931-9.

IV SOILS AND PLANTS

Metal Ions in Biology and Medicine: vol. 9. Eds Maria Carmen Alpoim, Paula Vasconcellos Morais, Maria Amélia Santos, Armando J. Cristóvão, José A. Centeno, Philippe Collery.
John Libbey Eurotext, Paris © 2006 pp. 141-1.

Chelate-enhanced solubility of metal increases phytoextraction of lead-contaminated soils by wheat *(triticum aestivum L.)*

Begonia G.B., Begonia M.T., Ntoni J., Miller G.S.

Department of Biology, Jackson State University, Jackson, MS 39217 USA

ABSTRACT

Phytoextraction is gaining acceptance as a cost-effective and environmentally friendly phytoremediation strategy for reducing toxic metal levels from contaminated soils. We hypothesized that the addition of synthetic chelates can increase the amount of bioavailable metal for root uptake, thereby improving the efficacy of phytoextraction. This study was therefore conducted to determine whether the addition of synthetic chelates can further enhance the root uptake and subsequent translocation of lead [Pb] to the shoots. Wheat [*Triticum aestivum* L.] seeds were planted in plastic tubes containing top soil and peat [2:1; v:v] spiked with various levels [0, 1000, 2000 mg Pb/kg dry soil] of lead nitrate. At six weeks after emergence, aqueous solutions [0, 1000 mg/kg dry soil] of ethylenediaminetetraacetic acid [EDTA] alone or in combination with acetic acid [HAc] were applied to the root zone. Plants were harvested at 7 days after chelate addition for biomass and metal content determinations. Results revealed that wheat was relatively tolerant to moderate levels of Pb as shown by non-significant differences in root and shoot biomass among treatments. An exception to this was a slight reduction in root biomass at the highest Pb treatment in combination with both chelates. Root Pb concentrations increased with increasing levels of soil-applied Pb. Further increases in root Pb were attributed to chelate amendments. Translocation index, a measure of the partitioning of the metal to the shoots, was significantly enhanced with chelate addition especially when both EDTA and HAc were used. Maximum translocation index occurred at 7 days after chelate addition. This observation coincided with the time when maximum amounts of Pb were bioavailable in the soil solution as shown in a corollary chelate-induced metal solubility study. Overall, this study demonstrated that the efficacy of phytoextraction can be further improved through the addition of synthetic chelates especially at a growth stage when the plants had attained maximum biomass.

INTRODUCTION

There has been an increasing interest in phytoextraction as a plant-based alternative for cost-effective and environmentally sound clean up of heavy metal-contaminated soils [1, 2, 3]. In phytoextraction, an efficient plant species must be able to absorb a substantial amount of the toxic metal into its roots and preferentially translocate the metal into the harvestable above-ground biomass for easier harvesting [4]. Through a cropping scheme, suitable species can be planted in succession ultimately leading to the reduction of soil metal concentrations to environmentally acceptable levels. In addition to a plant's high biomass yield and tolerance to toxic metal levels, the success of phytoextraction is also dependent upon the availability of the toxic metal in the soil for plant uptake. For instance, Pb, one of the most important environmental contaminants, has limited solubility in soils and its availability for plant uptake is minimal due to complexation with organic matter, sorption on oxides and clays, and precipitation as carbonates, hydroxides and phosphates [5]. Another requisite to Pb phytoextraction is to increase and maintain Pb concentrations in the soil solution. Chelates have been used to increase the solubility of metal cations in soils [6] and nutrient solutions and are reported to have significant effects on metal accumulation in plants [7, 8, 9]. Previous studies [10, 11] also demonstrated that addition of synthetic chelates to Pb-contaminated soils rapidly and dramatically increased Pb concentration in soil solution which consequently triggered a surge of Pb accumulation in shoots of corn, peas and Indian mustard. Using a modified hydroponics system [8] and Pb-amended sand [12], wheat [*T. aestivum L.* cv. TAM-109] was identified as a suitable phytoextraction species because of its high biomass yield under elevated Pb levels, and its ability to accumulate high amounts of Pb into its shoots. Also, wheat can be grown during the colder months of a year-round cropping scheme, thus ensuring ground cover of an otherwise barren, contaminated soil. The main objective of this study was to further evaluate the effectiveness of *T. aestivum* as a phytoextraction species. Specifically, this experiment was conducted to determine whether amendments of EDTA alone or in combination with HAc can further enhance the shoot uptake of Pb by wheat when grown on a Pb-contaminated soil.

MATERIALS AND METHODS

Solubility Study. Twelve mL of deionized, distilled water or chelate solution [1000 mg/L] were added to each 15 mL centrifuge tube containing 2 g of Pb-contaminated soil [i.e., 1000 mg Pb/kg dry soil; equilibrated for 7 weeks prior to metal extraction]. Soil suspensions were agitated in a platform shaker at room temperature for various extraction times. At the end of each designated extraction period, the soil suspensions were centrifuged at 5000 rpm for 30 min. The supernatant was filtered through a Whatman 0.45 μm filter paper. Pb contents of each filtrate were quantified using inductively coupled plasma-mass spectrometry [ICP-MS; Perkin Elmer Optima 3300 DV].

Plant Culture and Experimental Design. Seven weeks before planting, three concentrations [0, 1000, 2000 mg Pb/kg dry soil] of lead nitrate were mixed and equilibrated with the soil [2:1; v:v mixture of silty clay loam soil (pH 8.2, 1.5% organic matter) and peat]. Unless otherwise specified, five wheat [*T. aestivum* L. cv. TAM-109] seeds were sown in each 656 mL D40 Deepot tube containing the appropriate soil mixture. Emerged seedlings were thinned out to a desired population density [2 plants per tube] at 5 days after planting. Plants were irrigated every 2-3 days depending on the evaporative demand, with full strength nutrient solution. The volume of applied nutrient solution ensured that soil moisture content was maintained at field capacity. EDTA [0 or 1000 mg/kg dry soi]) was applied as a 100 mL aqueous solution one week before harvest. Moreover, 100 mL aqueous solutions of HAc were also added to some treatments one week before harvest. Also, a 10-cm diameter plastic saucer was placed beneath each tube to prevent cross contamination among treatments. Any symptoms of metal toxicity exhibited by plants were visually noted during the experimental period. Plants were maintained at the JSU greenhouse equipped with high intensity superhalide lamps that provided 12 hours of supplemental light. The photosynthetically active radiation [PAR; 400-700 nm] measured at the canopy level was no less than 1400 μmol photons m^{-2} s^{-1} as measured with a LI-COR 6200 portable photosynthesis system. All plants were harvested at seven weeks after emergence. During harvest, shoots and roots were separated, and roots were washed with distilled water to remove any adhering debris, then oven-dried at 70°C for 48 hours. Dried samples were weighed and ground in a Wiley mill equipped with a 425 μm [40-mesh] screen. Pb contents of each 200 mg dry, ground plant tissue were extracted using nitric acid-hydrogen peroxide [12]. Pb concentrations were quantified using ICP-MS as described above. Translocation index (%) was calculated as the ratio of shoot Pb concentration and total plant [shoot plus root] Pb concentrations. Treatments were arranged in a completely randomized design [CRD] with 4 replications. Data were analyzed using Statistical Analysis System [SAS]. Treatment separations were done using Fisher's Protected Least Significant Difference [LSD] test.

RESULTS AND DISCUSSION

Among the chelates tested, EDTA was the most effective in solubilizing soil bound Pb *(fig. 1)*. Pb concentration in soil solution increased with extraction time and remained relatively constant 6 to 7 days after chelate amendment. This indicated that soil Pb could be solubilized by EDTA in a short time and maintained at a high level afterward. The effectivity of EDTA in solubilizing Pb from the soil may be related to the high binding capacity of EDTA for Pb as shown in previous studies [10, 11]. The concentration of EGTA-extractable Pb in soil decreased with increasing extraction time from 5 days to 7 days. Also, HAc-extractable Pb began to decline 3 days after chelate amendment. These results indicated that these chelates are more rapidly degraded than EDTA.

Since total metal removal is a function of the metal concentration in the harvestable biomass [e.g., shoots], the first requisite in phytoextraction is the production of high plant biomass yield at the contaminated site. Generally, *T. aestivum* not only produced high biomass but was able to tolerate elevated levels of Pb / EDTA from the soil (table 1). There were no discernible toxic effects of Pb and chelates on wheat. However, there was a slightly significant reduction in root biomass at 2000 mg Pb / kg in combination with EDTA and HAc amendments. These observations confirm our previous findings regarding the relative tolerance of this wheat variety to various levels of Pb and EDTA [12].

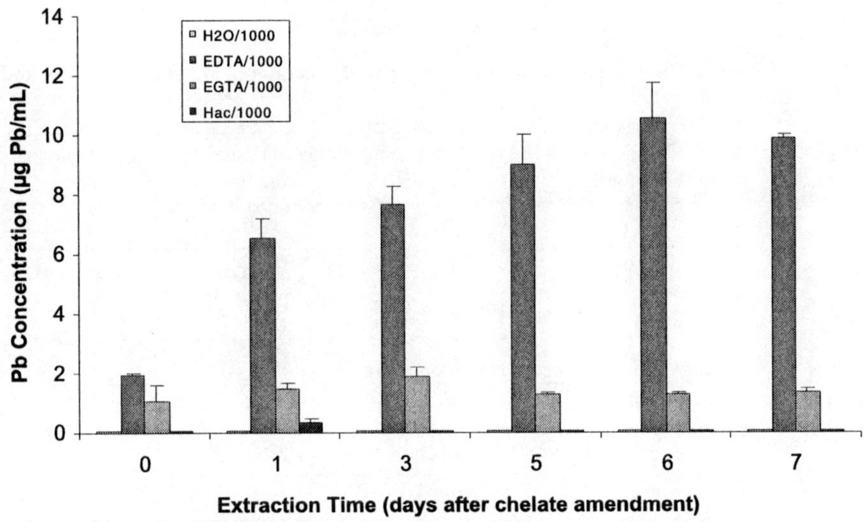

Fig. 1. Lead solubilization from a Pb-contaminated soil after application of chelates.

Root Pb concentrations increased with increasing levels of soil Pb treatments *(table 2)*. The addition of EDTA a week before harvest did not improve Pb uptake by the roots. This observation was in direct contrast to a previous study [11] which showed increased Pb accumulation in xylem sap of Pb-treated corn transplants 24 hours following EDTA application. However, when both EDTA and acetic acid were applied a week before harvest, there was a significant increase in root Pb uptake especially at the highest soil Pb treatment. Majority of the absorbed Pb remained in the roots when no chelate was applied. This could be due to Pb binding to ion exchangable sites in

Table 1. Effects of various concentrations of Pb and chelates on root and shoot dry biomass of wheat.

Treatment Lead [mg Pb/kg]	EDTA [mg/kg]	Dry Biomass [mg/plant] Root±SE	 Shoot±SE
0	0	12.8ab ± 1.1	37.5bc ± 1.3
0	1000	12.7ab ± 1.6	35.0c ± 3.5
1000	0	11.7ab ± 2.1	44.4ab ± 3.2
1000	1000	13.9 a ± 0.5	47.6a ± 1.8
1000	1000*	9.6b ± 0.7	39.0bc ± 1.7
2000	0	11.3ab ± 1.9	41.3abc ± 3.6
2000	1000	12.8ab ± 1.7	46.9a ± 1.7
2000	1000*	5.9c ± 0.8	35.0c ± 2.3

Means in a column with a common letter do not differ significantly according to Fisher's Protected LSD test ($P \leq 0.05$). * indicates that an aqueous solution of HAc [1000 mg/kg dry soil] was added following the application of the EDTA aqueous solution; SE=standard error of the mean [n = 4].

the cell wall and extracellular deposition mainly in the form of Pb carbonates deposited in the cell wall as previously demonstrated [13]. Another requisite to the success of phytoextraction is the enhancement of Pb accumulation in the harvestable biomass [e.g., shoots]. Vassil et al. [9] demonstrated that coordination of Pb transport by EDTA enhances the mobility within the plants of this otherwise insoluble metal ion, allowing plants to accumulate high concentrations of Pb in shoots.

Table 2. Effects of various Pb and chelate treatments on root and shoot Pb concen-trations and translocation indices of wheat.

Treatment Lead [mg Pb/kg]	EDTA [mg/kg]	Pb Conc. [µg Pb/g dry tissue] Root ± SE	 Shoot ± SE	Translocation Index (%) ± SE
0	0	0 f	0 d	0 f
0	1000	0 f	0 d	0 f
1000	0	1,970cd ± 193	436c ± 4	18.5e ± 1.4
1000	1000	1,199e ± 48	654c ± 62	35.1c ± 1.6
1000	1000*	2,095c ± 35	2,384b ± 133	53.1b ± 1
2000	0	3,260b ± 28	592c ± 14	15.7e ± 1.3
2000	1000	1,589de ± 13	690c ± 22	30.6d ± 1.8
2000	1000*	4,282a ± 303	9,150a ± 500	68.1a ± 1.8

See *table 1* for symbols and explanations.

In this study, Pb concentration in the shoot increased with increasing levels of soil-applied Pb *(table 2)*. EDTA amendment significantly increased shoot Pb uptake [e.g., 61% translocation index] especially in plants treated with the two highest soil Pb treatments. This was evidenced by an average increase in translocation index from 17% for non-EDTA exposed plants to 33% for EDTA-treated plants. Strikingly remarkable was the tremendous enhancement of shoot Pb concentration when both EDTA and HAc were applied one week before harvest, especially in wheat grown at

2000 mg Pb/kg soil. This additive effect of HAc on EDTA-mediated shoot Pb uptake by wheat is currently being undertaken in our laboratory, looking at the correlations between the amount of available soil Pb and Pb shoot uptake at different periods after chelate addition. We believe that EDTA especially in combination with acetic acid enhanced Pb desorbtion from soil to soil solution, facilitated transport into the xylem, decreased binding of Pb by the root tissue, and increased Pb translocation from the roots to the shoots as previously demonstrated in EDTA-mediated phytoextraction studies using corn (*Zea mays* L. cv. Fiesta), pea (*Pisum sativum* L. cv. Sparkle) and Indian mustard [*Brassica juncea* (L.) Czern.] [10, 11].

REFERENCES

1. Raskin I, Kumar PBAN, Dushenkov S, Salt DE. Bioconcentration of heavy metals by plants. *Curr Opin Biotechnol* 1994; 5: 285-290.
2. Salt DE, Smith RD, Raskin I. Phytoremediation. *Annu Rev Plant Physiol Plant Mol Biol* 1998; 49: 643-668.
3. Lasat M. Phytoextraction of toxic metals: A review of biological mechanisms, *J Environ Qual* 2002; 31: 109-120.
4. Kumar PBAN, Dushenkov V, Motto H, Raskin I. Phytoextraction: The use of plants to remove heavy metals from soils. *Environ Sci Technol* 1995; 29: 1232-1238.
5. McBride MB. *Environmental chemistry of soils*. Oxford University Press, 1994.
6. Means JL, Crerar DA. Migration of radioactive wastes: radionuclide mobilization by complexing agents. *Science* 1978; 200: 1477-1481.
7. Jorgensen SE. Removal of heavy metals from compost and soil by ecotechnological methods. *Ecol Eng* 1993; 2: 89-100.
8. Ghosh S, Rhyne C. A search for lead hyperaccumulating plants in the laboratory. *J Mississippi Acad Sci* 1998; 43: 11-12.
9. Vassil AD, Kapulnik YU, Raskin I, Salt DE. The role of EDTA in lead transport and accumulation by Indian mustard. *Plant Physiol* 1998; 117: 447-453.
10. Blaylock MJ, Salt DE, Dushenkov S, Zacharova O, Gussman C, Kapulnik Y, Ensley B, Raskin I. Enhanced accumulation of Pb in Indian mustard by soil-applied chelating agents. *Environ Sci Technol* 1997; 31: 860-865.
11. Huang, JW, Chen J, Berti WR, Cunningham SD. Phytoremediation of lead contaminated soils: Role of synthetic chelates in lead phytoextraction. *Environ Sci Technol* 1997; 31: 800-805.
12. Begonia GB, Begonia MFT, Miller GS, Kambhampati MS. Phytoextraction of lead-contaminated soils: Jackson State University research initiatives *In*: Centeno JA, Collery P, Vernet G, Finkelman RB, Gibb H, Etienne JC (eds). *Metal Ions Biol Med* 2000; 6: 672-675.
13. Dushenkov V, Kumar PBAN, Motto H, Raskin I. Rhizofiltration- the use of plants to remove heavy metals from aqueous streams. *Environ Sci Technol* 1995; 29: 1239-1245.

ACKNOWLEDGEMENTS

This research was made possible through support provided by NASA to Jackson State University through The University of Mississippi under the term of Grant No. NGT5-40098. Partial graduate support to NJ and MGS were provided by the U.S. Department of Education [Title III Program - Grant No. P031B440000-98].

Metal Ions in Biology and Medicine: vol. 9. Eds Maria Carmen Alpoim, Paulo Vasconcellos Morais, Maria Amélia Santos, Armando J. Cristóvão, José A. Centeno, Philippe Collery.
John Libbey Eurotext, Paris © 2006 pp. 146-1.

Influence of chelates on metal solubility: implications in the phytoextraction of lead-contaminated soils by tall fescue (*Festuca arundinacea* Schreb.)

Begonia M.T., Begonia G.B, Miller G.S., Ntoni J.

Department of Biology, Jackson State University, Jackson, Mississippi 39217 USA

ABSTRACT

Phytoextraction has emerged as a cost-effective and environmentally benign phytoremediation alternative for reducing toxic metal levels from contaminated soils. We hypothesized that the efficacy of phytoextraction can be further increased through chelate amendments. This study was therefore conducted to further evaluate the suitability of *Festuca arundinacea* as one of the potential crop rotation species for phytoextraction. Specifically, the objective of this experiment was to determine whether the addition of ethylenediaminetetraacetic acid [EDTA] alone or in combination with acetic acid [HAc] can further enhance the phytoextraction of lead [Pb]. Seeds were planted in plastic tubes containing top soil and peat [2:1, v:v] spiked with various levels [0, 1000, 2000 mg Pb/kg dry soil] of lead nitrate. At seven weeks after emergence, aqueous solutions [0, 1000 mg/kg dry soil] of EDTA and HAc were applied to the root zone. Plants were harvested 7 days after chelate addition. Results showed that tall fescue was relatively tolerant to moderate levels of Pb and chelates as shown by very slight reductions in root and shoot biomass. Root Pb concentrations increased with increasing levels of soil-applied Pb. Further increases in root Pb concentrations were attributed to chelate amendments. Translocation index, an indicator of the partitioning of the metal to the shoots, was significantly enhanced with chelate addition especially when both EDTA and HAc were used. Maximum translocation index occurred at 7 days after chelate addition. This observation coincided with the time when maximum amounts of Pb were bioavailable in the soil solution as shown in a preliminary chelate-induced metal solubility study. Overall, this study demonstrated that chelates can be added when plants have attained maximum biomass then harvested a week later in order to improve phytoextraction efficacy.

INTRODUCTION

Heavy metal phytoextraction has recently emerged as a promising, cost-effective alternative to the conventional engineering-based remediation [1]. The objective of phytoextraction is to reduce heavy metal levels below regulatory limits within a reasonable time frame. To achieve this objective, plants must accumulate high levels of heavy metals and produce high amounts of biomass. Early phytoextraction research dealt with hyperaccumulating plants, which have the ability to concentrate high amounts of heavy metals in their tissues [2]. However, hyperaccumulators often accumulate only a specific element and are slow-growing, low-biomass-producing plants with little known agronomic or horticultural attributes. Previous hydroponic studies revealed that uptake and translocation of heavy metals in plants are enhanced by increasing heavy metal concentration in the nutrient solution [3]. The bioavailability of heavy metals in the soil is therefore, of paramount importance for successful phytoextraction. Pb has limited solubility in soils, and its availability for plant uptake is minimal due to complexation with organic and inorganic soil colloids, sorption on oxides and clays, and precipitation as carbonates, hydroxides, and phosphates [4]. Therefore, successful phytoextraction must include mobilization of heavy metals into the soil solution that is in direct contact with the roots. In most soils capable of supporting plant growth, the readily available levels of heavy metals especially Pb, are low and do not allow substantial plant uptake if chelates are not applied. Chelates have been shown to desorb heavy metals from the soil matrix into soil solution, facilitate metal transport into the xylem, and increase metal translocation from roots to shoots of several fast-growing, high-biomass-producing plants [5, 6]. Using a Pb-amended sand [7], tall fesuce [*F. arundinacea* Schreb. cv. Spirit] was identified as a potential phytoextraction species because of its high biomass yield under elevated Pb levels and its ability to translocate high amounts of Pb into its shoots. The main objective of this study was to further evaluate the effectiveness of tall fescue as a phytoextraction species. We envisioned that this species can be used in a crop rotation scheme during the colder months, and also serves as a cover crop for an otherwise barren metal-contaminated soil. Specifically, this study was conducted to determine whether pre-harvest amendments of EDTA alone or in combination with HAc can further enhance the shoot accumulation [i.e., translocation index] of Pb by tall fescue grown on a Pb-contaminated soil.

MATERIALS AND METHODS

Solubility Study. Twelve mL of deionized, distilled water or chelate solution [1000 mg/L] were added to each 15 mL centrifuge tube containing 2 g of Pb-contaminated soil [i.e., 1000 mg Pb/kg dry soil; equilibrated for 7 weeks prior to metal extraction]. Soil suspensions were agitated in a platform shaker at room temperature for various extraction times. At the end of each designated extraction period, the soil suspensions were centrifuged at 5000 rpm for 30 min. The supernatant was filtered through a Whatman 0.45 μm filter paper. Pb contents of each filtrate were quantified using inductively coupled plasma-mass spectrometry [ICP-MS; Perkin Elmer Optima 3300 DV].

Plant Culture and Experimental Design. Seven weeks before planting, three concentrations [0, 1000, 2000 mg Pb/kg dry soil] of lead nitrate were mixed and equilibrated with the soil [2:1; v:v mixture of silty clay loam soil (pH 8.2, 1.5% organic matter) and peat]. Unless otherwise specified, 10 tall fescue [*F. arundinacea* cv. Spirit] seeds were sown in each 656 mL D40 Deepot tube containing the appropriate soil mixture. Emerged seedlings were thinned out to a desired population density [5 plants per tube] at 5 days after emergence. Plants were irrigated every 2-3 days depending on the evaporative demand, with full strength nutrient solution. The volume of applied nutrient solution ensured that soil moisture content was maintained at field capacity. EDTA [0 or 1000 mg/kg dry soi] was applied as a 100 mL aqueous solution one week before harvest. Moreover, 100 mL aqueous solutions of HAc were also added to some treatments one week before harvest. Also, a 10-cm diameter plastic saucer was placed beneath each tube to prevent cross contamination among treatments. Any symptoms of metal toxicity exhibited by plants were visually noted during the experimental period. Plants were maintained at the JSU greenhouse equipped with high intensity superhalide lamps that provided 12 hours of supplemental light. The photosynthetically active radiation [PAR; 400-700 nm] measured at the canopy level was no less than 1400 μmol photons m^{-2} s^{-1} as measured with a LI-COR 6200 portable photosynthesis system. All plants were harvested at 8 weeks after emergence. During harvest, shoots and roots were separated, and roots were washed with distilled water to remove any adhering debris, then oven-dried at 70°C for 48 hours. Dried samples were weighed and ground in a Wiley mill equipped with a 425μm [40-mesh] screen. Pb contents of each 200 mg dry, ground plant tissue were extracted using nitric acid-hydrogen peroxide [7]. Pb concentrations were quantified using ICP-MS as described above. Translocation index (%) was calculated as the ratio of shoot Pb concentration and total plant [shoot plus root] Pb concentrations. Treatments were arranged in a completely randomized design [CRD] with 4 replications. Data were analyzed using Statistical Analysis System [SAS]. Treatment separations were done using Fisher's Protected Least Significant Difference [LSD] test.

RESULTS AND DISCUSSION

Among the chelates tested, EDTA was the most effective in solubilizing soil bound Pb *(fig. 1)*. Pb concentration in soil solution increased with extraction time and remained relatively constant 6 to 7 days after EDTA amendment. This indicated that soil Pb could be solubilized by EDTA in a short time and maintained at a high level afterward. The effectivity of EDTA in solubilizing Pb from the soil may be related to the high binding capacity of EDTA for Pb as shown in previous studies [5, 6]. The concentration of EGTA-extractable Pb in soil decreased with increasing extraction time from 5 days to 7 days. Also, HAc-extractable Pb began to decline 3 days after chelate amendment. These results indicated that these chelates are more rapidly degraded than EDTA.

The Pb treatments alone did not significantly affect root biomass of tall fescue plants *(table 1)*. However, root biomass of plants grown at 1000 and 2000 mg Pb/kg were reduced by 24% and 28%, respectively with the addition of EDTA alone, and in combination with HAc. Both Pb and chelate amendments did not substantially affect shoot biomass *(table 1)*. No discernible phytotoxic symptoms were exhibited by the shoots. Specific high-affinity ligands have been shown to be activated at a certain EDTA threshold, and confer metal resistance in some plants by making the metal less toxic to the plant [8]. We are not certain whether this resistance mechanism also exists in tall fescue hence, further study is warranted. Vassil et al. [9] also demonstrated that free protonated EDTA (H-EDTA) was more phytotoxic to *Brassica juncea* than a Pb-EDTA complex. From earlier studies [10], we also observed the relative tolerance of wheat to Pb-EDTA complex. These previous findings support our present observation that a Pb-chelate complex was relatively non-phytotoxic to *F. arundinacea*, a monocotyledonous plant like wheat.

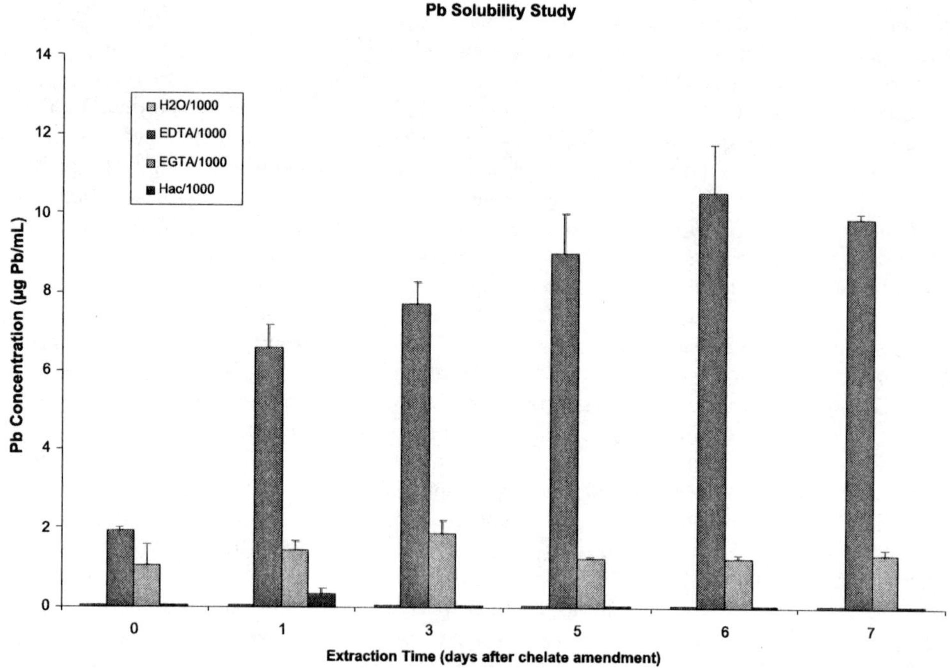

Fig. 1. Lead solubilization from a Pb-amended soil after application of chelates.

Table 1. Effects of various concentrations o Pb and chelates on root and shoot dry biomass of tall fescue.

Treatment		Biomass [mg/plant]	
Lead [mg Pb/kg]	EDTA [mg/kg]	Root ± SE	Shoot ± SE
0	0	130.3 ab ± 4.8	269.8 a ± 15.7
0	1000	132.8 a ± 8.4	248.8 ab ± 13.3
1000	0	121.8 a ± 2.5	249.8 ab ± 18.2
1000	1000	105.0 c ± 12.2	236.8 ab ± 8.4
1000	1000*	100.5 c ± 8.5	243.8 ab ± 12.2
2000	0	116.0 abc ± 6.4	228.8b ± 13.3
2000	1000	109.3 bc ± 9.6	219.8b ± 14.7
2000	1000*	107.3 c ± 4.8	225.5b ± 6.7

Means in a column with a similar letter do not differ significantly using Fisher's Protected LSD test ($P \leq 0.05$). * indicates that an aqueous solution of HAc [1000 mg/kg dry soil] was also added following EDTA amendment; SE = standard error of the mean of 4 replications.

Table 2. Root and shoot Pb concentrations and translocation indices of tall fescue grown at various levels of Pb and chelates.

Treatment		Pb Conc. [mg Pb/ kg dry tissue]		Translocation
Pb [mg Pb/ kg]	EDTA [mg/kg]	Root ± SE	Shoot ± SE	Index [%] ± SE
0	0	0 e	0 d	0.0 e ± 0.0
0	1000	0 e	0 d	0.0 e ± 0.0
1000	0	831 d + 27	29 d ± 5	3.3 e ± 0.4
1000	1000	1,041 d ± 34	2,471 c ± 269	69.8 b ± 3.0
1000	1000*	1,504 c ± 221	4,670 b ± 442	75.6 a ± 3.0
2000	0	1,592 bc ± 187	194 d ± 14	11.4 d ± 2.0
2000	1000	1,931 b ± 153	3,024 c ± 120	61.1 c ± 1.5
2000	1000*	2,408 a ± 188	5,618 a ± 395	70.9ab±1.7

See *table 1* for symbols and explanations.

Root Pb concentrations increased with increasing levels of soil Pb treatments *(table 2)*. The addition of EDTA improved Pb accumulation by the roots. However, when both chelates were applied, there was a significant increase in root Pb concentrations especially at the highest soil Pb treatment. Majority of the absorbed Pb remained in the roots when no chelate was applied. This could be due to Pb binding to ion exchangeable sites on the cell wall and extracellular deposition mainly in the form of Pb carbonates deposited on the cell wall as previously demonstrated [11]. When no chelates were applied, shoot Pb concentrations slightly increased with increasing levels of soil-applied Pb *(table 2)*. Dramatic increases in shoot Pb were observed with the addition of EDTA alone. However, when both chelates were amended, increases in shoot Pb were even more remarkable. In the absence of chelate(s), translocation indices of tall fescue plants grown at 1000 and 2000 mg Pb/kg were minimal, accounting for only 3.3% and 11.4%, respectively *(table 2)*. However, translocation indices dramatically increased to 66% and 73%, respectively when EDTA alone or both chelates were added simultaneously. For phytoextraction to be successful, there must be an enhanced metal accumulation in the harvestable biomass [e.g., shoots]. Vassil et al. [9] demonstrated that coordination of Pb transport by EDTA enhances the mobility within the plants of this otherwise insoluble metal ion, allowing plants to accumulate high concentrations of Pb in shoots. Pb forms a strong covalent bond not only with the soil, but with plant tissues as well [6]. It is believed that since the xylem cell walls have a high cation exchange capacity, the upward movement of metal cations are severely retarded [1]. Bringing the Pb into solution with a chelating agent, not only makes more Pb bioavailable for root uptake [5, 6] but also moves the Pb that is sequestered in the xylem cell wall upwards and into the shoots. We believe that EDTA enhanced Pb desorption from soil to soil solution and facilitated transport from roots to shoots as previously demonstrated in EDTA-mediated phytoextracton studies using high-biomass plants [5, 6, 9]. The results of this study indicated that tall fescue can be an efficient Pb-accumulating plant if chelates are amended to the Pb-contaminated soil to enhance metal bioavailability. Also, limiting the resident time of the chelate in the soil by applying it a few days before harvest lessens the mobility of bioavailable metals that can potentially migrate and serve as sources of secondary pollution to the ground water.

REFERENCES

1. Salt DE, Smith RD, Raskin I. Phytoremediation. *Annu Rev Plant Physiol Plant Mol Biol* 1998; 49: 643-668.
2. Chaney RL, Malik M, Li YM, Brown SL, Brewer EP, Angle JS, Baker AJM. Phytoremediation of soil metals. *Curr Opin Biotechnol* 1997; 8: 279-284.
3. Ghosh S, Rhyne C. Influence of EDTA on Pb uptake in two weed species, *Sesbania* and *Ipomoea* in hydroponic culture. *J Mississippi Acad Sci* 1999; 44: 11.
4. McBride MB. *Environmental chemistry of soils*. Oxford University Press, 1994.
5. Blaylock MJ, Salt DE, Dushenkov S, Zakharova O, Gussman C, Kapulnik Y, Ensley BD, Raskin I. Enhanced accumulation of Pb in Indian mustard by soil-applied chelating agents. *Environ Sci Technol* 1997; 31: 860-865.
6. Huang JW, Chen J, Berti WR, Cunningham SD. Phytoremediation of lead contaminated soils: Role of synthetic chelates in lead phytoextraction. *Environ Sci Technol* 1997; 31: 800-805.
7. Begonia MFT, Begonia GB, Ighoavodha M, Okuyiga-Ezem O, Crudup B. Chelate-induced phytoextraction of lead from contaminated soils using tall fescue *(Festuca arundinacea). J Mississippi Acad Sci* 2001; 46(1): 15.
8. Cunningham SD, Ow WD. Promises and prospects of phytoremediation. *Plant Physiol* 1996; 110: 715-719.
9. Vassil AD, Kapulnik Y, Raskin I, Salt DE. The role of EDTA in lead transport and accumulation by Indian mustard. *Plant Physiol* 1998; 117: 447-453.
10. Begonia MFT, Begonia GB, Butler A, Burrell M, Ighoavodha O, Crudup B. Chelate-assisted phytoextraction of lead from a contaminated soil using wheat *(Triticum aestivum L.). Bull Environ Contam Toxicol* 2002; 68: 705-711.
11. Dushenkov V, Kumar PBAN, Motto H, Raskin I. Rhizofiltration: The use of plants to remove heavy metals from aqueous streams. *Environ Sci Technol* 1995: 29: 1239-1245.

ACKNOWLEDGMENTS

This research was made possible through support provided by NASA to Jackson State University through The University of Mississippi under the terms of Grant No. NGT5-40098. Partial graduate support to NJ and MGS were provided by the U.S. Department of Education [Title III Program - Grant No. P031B440000-98].

Metal Ions in Biology and Medicine: vol. 9. Eds Maria Carmen Alpoim, Paula Vasconcellos Morais, Maria Amélia Santos, Armando J. Cristóvão, José A. Centeno, Philippe Collery.
John Libbey Eurotext, Paris © 2006 pp. 151-1.

Toxicity and accumulation of zinc in *Myriophyllum spicatum* L.

Canhoto C.[1], Martins R.[1], Pratas J.[2] & Canhoto J.M.[3]

[1]*IMAR, Department of Zoology, University of Coimbra, 3004-517 COIMBRA, Portugal.*
E-mail: ccanhoto@ci.uc.pt;
[2]*Earth Sciences Department, University of Coimbra, 3000-272 COIMBRA, Portugal.*
E-mail: jpratas@ci.uc.pt;
[3]*IAV, Department of Botany, University of Coimbra, 3001-405 COIMBRA, Portugal.*
E-mail: jorgecan@ci.uc.pt

Human activities have raised the level of trace elements and organic pollutants to values able to affect soil and water quality, biological structure, and human health. Phytoremediation, the capacity of plants to remove and detoxify polluted environments, has emerged in the last 10-15 years, as a potentially well-suited method to cleanup contaminated areas. Eurasian water-milfoil *(Myriophyllum spicatum)* is a freshwater rooted macrophyte, common in small streams of the Iberian Peninsula, frequently implicated in the removal and/or recovery of heavy metals (*e.g.* cadmium, lead, copper) from water. Herein we evaluate the toxicity and accumulation of Zinc in *M. spicatum*. This trace metal of environmental significance is a ubiquitous contaminant of industrial waste waters effluents. Increasing concentrations of zinc (0 to 4.5 mg/l) in the form of sulphate ($ZnSO_4.7H_2O$), were added to a growing media (Andrews modified medium) where axenic cultures of *M. spicatum* were previously obtained. After 15 days of exposure (70 r.p.m.; 25°C; 14h photoperiod) the apical shoots were measured for fresh weight, number of nodes, root and stem length. Plant metal uptake was also evaluated by atomic absorption spectophotometry. Results indicate that root length is the most sensitive parameter to Zn^{2+} (EC50%: number of nodes>>stem length>fresh weight>root length). All parameters were significantly ($p<0.05$) affected by zinc contents $\geq$ 0.9 mg/l. Maximum bioconcentration of Zinc, 4500 mg/Kg (DW), was observed in the more concentrated medium. A logarithmic pattern was found between zinc bioaccumulation and increasing zinc contents in the media. *M. spicatum* was capable to tolerate and efficiently remove high levels of zinc from the aqueous medium under laboratory conditions. Our findings tend to support the idea that this species can be successfully used as indicator of water contaminants (zinc included) and a reliable tool for the restoration of aquatic ecosystems.

INTRODUCTION

Rooted macrophytes *(e.g. Ceratophyllum, Elodea, Hippuris, Vallisneria)* are important components of aquatic ecosystems contributing to primary production, sediment stabilization, oxygen production and cycling of nutrients [1, 2]. *Myriophyllum spicatum* L. (eurasian water-milfoil), a submerged aquatic plant, is also one of these macrophytes. It belongs to the family *Haloragaceae* and is spread all over the Iberian Peninsula, usually in lakes, ponds and slow-moving waters but has a world wide distribution [3]. Due to its reproduction by vegetative stem fragmentation and runners, the number of individuals can rise very quickly and the plant can adversely impact aquatic ecosystems by forming dense canopies on the water surface. In the USA, especially in the northern tier of states, the eurasian water-milfoil is a troublesome plant, where it forms large masses that fill recreation and fishing lakes, degrading water quality and interfering with wildlife [4].

Since the industrial revolution, agricultural, industrial and other human activities have increased the level of trace elements and organic pollutants in soils and aquatic environments to values that seriously can affect biological structure, water quality and human health being an important cause of several ecosystems disturbances [5, 6]. Phytoremediation, the capacity of plants to remove and detoxify polluted environments, has emerged in the last 10-15 years, as a potentially well-suited method to cleanup contaminated areas [7]. Although phytoremediation has a few drawbacks, such as the small size of most hyperaccumulating species and their limited habitat range; its potential is mainly based on the relatively low cost of this process when compared with other techniques currently used [8].

Several studies have reported the ability of *M. spicatum* to remove heavy metals as cadmium, copper and lead from polluted waters [9, 10]. The potential use of this species in native areas, as an indicator of metal contamination and a phytoremediation vehicle, is though worth being explored. Zinc is a very important trace element for plant survival [11] since it is a component of several key enzymes such as superoxide dismutase [12] and RNA polymerase [13]. This element seems also to be required for auxin and chlorophyll synthesis and protein metabolism [14]. Nonetheless, it is also a trace metal of environmental significance as it is a ubiquitous contaminant of industrial waste waters [15]. The purpose of this study was to evaluate the potential of *M. spicatum* to grow, in axenic cultures, when exposed to non-physiological concentrations of zinc, and to determine the potential of this plant to accumulate this metal.

MATERIALS AND METHODS

Field growing plants of *M. spicatum* were collected in the Carreiras river, a tributary of the Guadiana river (South of Portugal). Plants were maintained in outdoor tanks at University of Coimbra. Apical and nodal segments were used to establish axenic cultures according with the procedures determined by the American Society for Testing and Materials for *Myriophyllum sibiricum* [16]. Stem segments (5-10 cm length) were excised and rinsed with sterilized water containing a few drops of a detergent (Tween 20). Plant material was then sterilized in a 7.5% hypochlorite calcium solution, for 20 minutes, in three consecutive days. Cultures were established in 50 or 100 ml glass vessels containing an Andrews modified medium [17] and 3% sucrose. Sucrose was added to rapidly verify which cultures were contaminated with fungi or bacteria and to faster plant growth. The cultures were kept in the dark, under agitation (60 r.p.m.). *In vitro* cultures were multiplied to obtain a great number of axenic cultures for further experiments. This was achieved through the culture of apical or nodal segments in an Andrews modified medium containing 0.2 mg/l benziladenine, a cytokinin.

To evaluate the effect of zinc on *M. spicatum* growth and development, apical segments (3 cm length) of *in vitro* growing plants were obtained, washed in sterilized water, weighed and the number of initial nodes counted. These apical segments were then transferred to 100 ml glass flasks containing 50 ml of Andrews modified medium and 3% sucrose. The pH of all media was adjusted to 5.8±0.1 prior autoclaving, at 121°C, for 20 min. The cultures were incubated in a greenhouse under a 14h photoperiod (96 µmol $m^{-2}s^{-1}$ by fluorescent tubes) and submitted to constant agitation (70 r.p.m.). The following concentrations of zinc (in the form of zinc sulphate - $ZnSO_4.7H_2O$) were tested: 0.9, 1.8, 2.7, 3.6 and 4.5 mg/l. Four replicates were used per treatment. The control corresponds to the concentration of Zn in the Andrews medium formulation (*i.e* 0.03 mg/l). In preliminary experiments, media without Zn or with extreme Zn concentrations (2µg/l $\leq$ Zn $\geq$ 9 mg/l) were also tested.

After 2 weeks of culture, four plant parameters were analyzed: fresh weight, number of nodes, root length and stem length. In all cases, growth indices (GI) were determined according with the formula:

$$IG = \frac{\text{final parameter at the concentration X - initial parameter at the concentration X}}{\text{final parameter in the control - initial parameter in the control}}$$

The EC50 values were obtained using a Probit analysis [18] and the "no observable effect concentration" (NOEC) was calculated for each concentration (ANOVA, log (x+1) transformed data, followed by a Fisher LSD).

To determine zinc concentration in plant material and in the culture media the plant material was dried at 60°C, for 24h, and then pulverized and homogenized. The material was then weighted (about 200 mg) and incinerated, for 24h, at 450°C. The resulting ashes were subsequently dissolved in nitric acid (2M) and directly measured by flame atomic absorption spectrophotometry in a Thermo Unicam SolaaR M6.

RESULTS

Segments of *M. spicatum*, cultured on Andrews modified medium (control conditions), reached an average shoot length of 8.8 cm (±0.29 SE) and a root length of 3.7 cm (±1.5 SE), after 14 days of culture. That corresponds to an increase of 4.1 mm/day and 2.6 mm/day, respectively. During the same period, fresh weight increased 5.9 mg/day while only three new nodes were produced. This value indicates a plastochron of about 5 days. Plantlets, maintained under control conditions, were phenotipically normal and appeared to be wealthy *(fig. 1A)*.

In a first set of experiments, extreme concentrations of Zn (≤ 2µg/l and ≥ 9 mg/l) were used to test *M. spicatum* development. The results of these initial experiments showed that Zn concentrations, higher than 9 mg/l, were completely inhibitory of plantlet growth; the explants rapidly became necrotic and died after a few days of culture *(fig. 1B)*. On the other hand, results obtained with low concentrations of the trace metal (2µg/l) were not statistically different from controls in all cases. When no Zn was added to the culture medium, explants did not grow, but remained green during the all culture period *(fig. 1C)*.

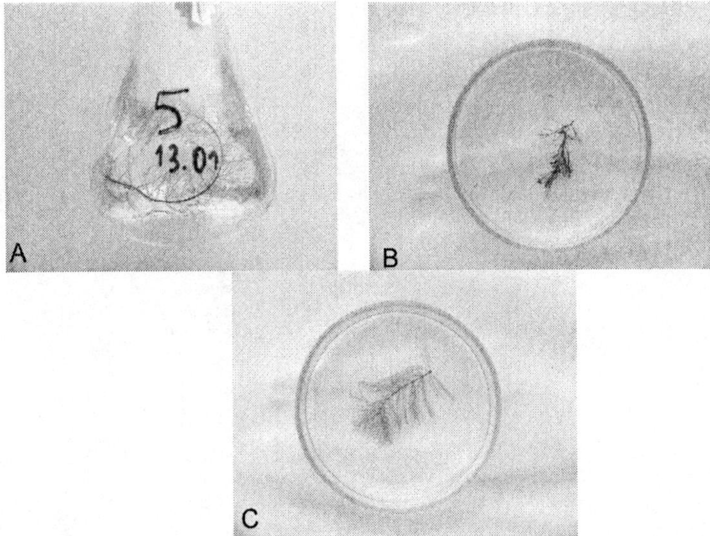

Fig. 1. *M. spicatum* plantlets tested on different culture conditions. A. Control. B. Medium with 9 mg/l Zn. C. Medium without Zn.

Based on these preliminary experiments, it was decided to test Zn concentrations between 0.9 mg/l and 4.5 mg/l. Root growth was strongly inhibited ($p<0.001$) by increasing Zn concentrations. A significant decrease in root length was observed in concentrations ≥ 1.8 mg/l. The effects of low Zn concentrations in root development, although not significant ($p>0.05$), were biologically relevant: a 50%

reduction in root growth was observed in plants maintained in media with 0.9 mg/l Zn *(fig. 2)*; IG_{root} values decreased exponentially and were almost zero (0.05) at the highest Zn concentration tested.

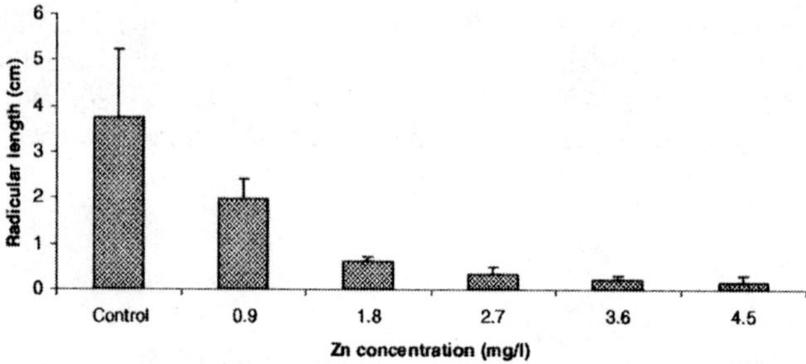

Fig. 2. Effect of Zn on root growth. Values are means ± SE. No significant differences (p>0.05) among means within the same line.

A Zn concentration of 0.9 mg/l was also enough to induce a significant reduction ($p<0.001$) on the fresh weight of the plantlets *(fig. 3)*. The lowest value was obtained when 4.5 mg/l Zn was used. At this concentration, the $IG_{freshweight}$ value was 0.12. A similar pattern was observed when shoot length was considered *(fig. 4)*. In this case, the highest Zn concentration determined an $IC_{shootlength}$ value of 0.28.

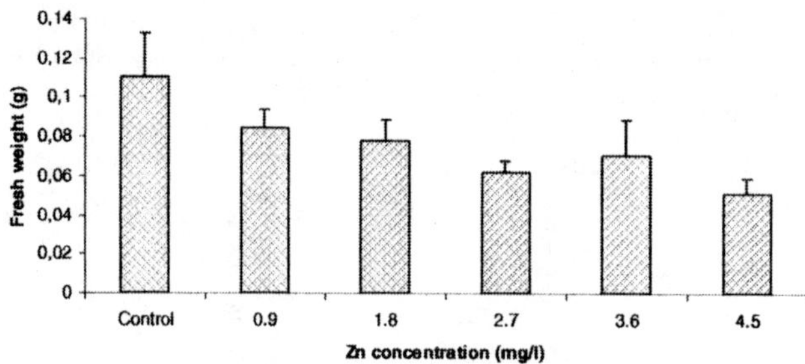

Fig. 3. Effect of Zn on *M. spicatum* fresh weight. Values are means ± SE. No significant differences (p>0.05) among means within the same line.

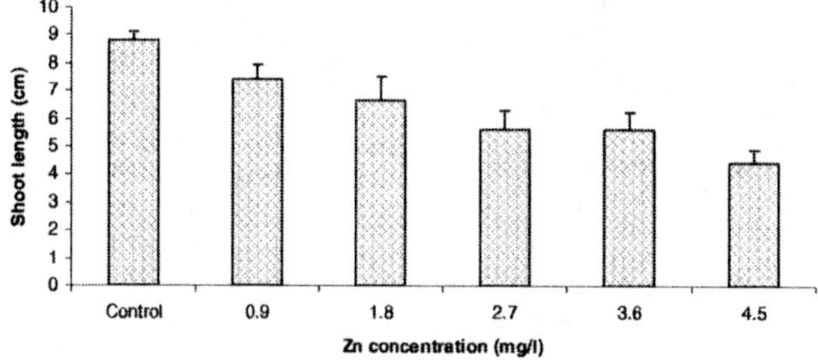

Fig. 4. Effect of Zn on *M. spicatum* shoot length. Values are means ± SE. No significant differences (p>0.05) among means within the same line.

The number of shoot nodes was the parameter less affected by the increase of Zn concentrations in the media. In fact, higher concentrations (3.6 mg/l) were needed to induce a significant decrease ($p<0.05$) in the formation of new nodes *(fig. 5)*. At the highest Zn concentration, IG_{nodes} value (0.4) was still 40% of the values observed in controls.

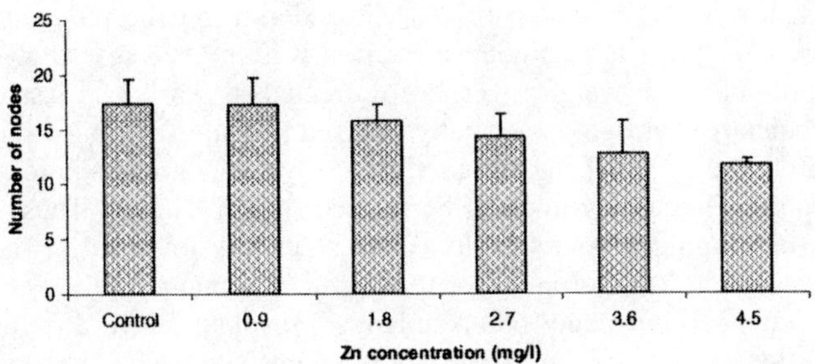

Fig. 5. Effect of Zn on *M. spicatum* number of nodes. Values are means ± SE. No significant differences (p>0.05) among means within the same line.

Results indicate a NOEC value of 0.9 mg/l of Zn for all the parameters except in the case of "node numbers" which was 3.6 mg/l. However, EC50 values suggest that root growth was the most sensitive factor to the trace metal (EC50 = 0.9 mg/l Zn; *table 1*).

Table 1. NOEC and EC50 values (mg/l) for the different parameters analyzed.

Parameters	NOEC (mg/l)	EC50 (95% CL)
Root length	0.9	1.45 (1.11-2.42)
Fresh Weight	0.9	1.35 (0.99-2.73)
Shoot length	0.9	0.9 (0.71-1.06)
Number of nodes	3.6	1.67 (1.67-2.31)

Results indicated that maximum bioaccumulation of Zn was 4500 ppm for a Zn concentration in the culture medium of 4.5 mg/l. At this concentration, the plants were able to remove about 80% of the initial Zn content. Bioaccumulation increased logarithmically (2514.8 ln(x) + 50.79; R^2=0.99) with increasing Zn concentration in the culture media *(fig. 6)*. A significant correlation could be detected between Zn accumulation and the remaining in the culture media (p<0.001).

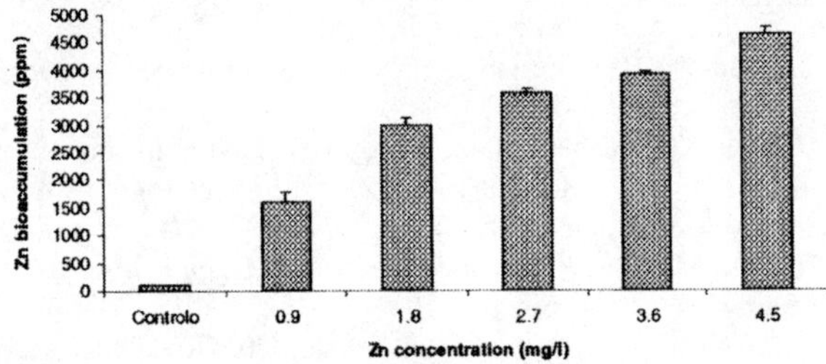

Fig. 6. Spectophotometry analysis of Zn in plants. Values are means ± SE. No significant differences (p>0.05) among means within the same line.

DISCUSSION

Previous studies have shown that *M. spicatum* is a good bioaccumulator of heavy metals [10]. and sensitive to several toxicants as creosote [19], glyphosate [17], and dichloroacetic acid [20].

In this work, we have made a first generic evaluation of the potential of *M. spicatum* to tolerate and accumulate high levels of the metal ion Zn. Considering all the parameters analyzed, root growth was the most sensitive whereas node formation was the less affected. The other two parameters (shoot length and fresh weight) were also affected by Zn but in less extent. These data were not surprising since root growth is normally referred as one of the most sensitive in response to abiotic stresses [21]. On the other hand the reduced effect of Zn in node formation reflects the long time that is required for a new node to be formed (about 5 days). Thus, in further studies, this parameter must be eliminated and substituted by other physiological or biochemical characteristic easy to analyze, such as chlorophyll or total protein content.

According to Baker [22] and many other authors [23], plants have different mechanisms to respond to increasing levels of metal ions in the environment. Thus, whereas some plants can avoid uptake, others possess detoxification mechanisms that allow the plants to accumulate high concentrations of metal ions in their tissues. Our data seem to indicate that *M. spicatum* behaves like an indicator plant since the spectophotometry analysis of Zn in the plant showed that the levels of Zn in tissues are strongly correlated with Zn concentrations in the culture medium. Similar results were obtained by Keskinkan *et al.* [10]. It seems though that *M. spicatum* can be used as an indicator plant for Zn concentrations between 0.03 mg/l (0.03 ppm) and 4.5 mg/l (4.5 ppm).

Considering a normal value of 10 μg/l (0.01 ppm) for Zn, in fresh waters (23), the results obtained in our study indicate that *M. spicatum* can withstand Zn concentrations of 1.8 mg/l (1.8 ppm) without a considerable reduction in growth rates. Such capacity to tolerate this and other metals ions (e.g. Cd, Cu, Pb) and toxicants, associated with its ability to propagate vegetatively may explain the competitive advantage of *M. spicatum* in some environments and its potential to become an invasive species. Further studies will be focused on the mechanisms of Zn toleration and in the potential of *M. spicatum* to remediate waters contaminated with excessive amounts of other pollutants such as nitrate and phosphate.

REFERENCES

1. Lewis MA. Use of freshwater plants for phytotoxicity testing: a review. *Environ. Pollution* 1995; 87: 319-336.
2. Cushing CE, Allan JD. Streams - their ecology and life. San Diego: Academic Press, 2001, pp. 366.
3. Cirujano S. *Myriophyllum* L. In: Castroviejo S et. al., eds. Flora Ibérica Vol. 8. Madrid: Real Jardín Botânico, 1997:3-7.
4. http://www.wapns.org/plants/milfoil.html. (Western Aquatic Plant Management Society USA).
5. Pilon-Smiths E. Phytoremediation. *Ann Rev Plant Biol* 2005; 56: 15-39.
6. Dean JG, Bosqui FL, Lanouette VH. Removing heavy metals from waste water. *Env. Sci Technol* 1972; 6: 518-522.
7. Salt DE, Blaylock M, Kumar NP, Dushenkov V, Ensley BD. Phytoremediation: a novel strategy for the removal of toxic metals from the environment using plants. *Biotechnology* 1995; 13: 468-474.
8. Tsao DT. Overview of phytotechnologies. *Adv Biochem Eng Biotechnol* 2003; 78: 1-50.
9. Sivaci ER, Sivaci A, Sökmen M. Biosorption of cadmium by *Myriophyllum spicatum* and *Myriophyllum triphyllum* orchard. *Chemosphere* 2004; 56: 1043-1048.
10. Keskinkan O, Goksu MZL, Yuceer A, Basibuyuk M, Forster CF. Heavy metal adsorption characteristics of a submerged aquatic plant *(Myriophyllum spicatum). Process Biochemistry* 2003; 39: 179-183.
11. Reugel Z. Heavy metals as essential nutrients. In: Prasad MNV, Hagemeyer J, eds. Heavy metal stress in plants - from molecules to ecosystems. Berlin: Springer, 1999: 231-251.
12. Chaknak I, Marschner H. Enhanced superoxide radical production in roots of zinc-deficient plants. *J Exp Bot* 1988; 39: 1449-1460.
13. Falchuk KH, Mazus B, Ulpino L, Vallee BL. *Euglena gracilis* DNA dependent RNA polymerase II: a zinc metalloenzyme. *Biochemistry* 1976; 15: 4468-4475.
14. Taiz CE, Zeiger E. Plant physiology 3rd ed. Sunderland: Sinauer Associated, Inc., Publishers, 2002, pp. 690.

15. Brooks RR, Robinson BH. Aquatic phytoremediation accumulator plants. In: Brooks RR, ed. Plants that hyperaccumulate heavy metals. Wallingford: CAB International, 1998: 203-226.
16. Anonymous. Standart guide for conducting static, axenic, 14 day phytotoxicity tests in test tubes with the submersed aquatic macrophyte *Myriophyllum sibiricum* Komarov. *American Soc. for Testing and Materials*; 2000: E 1913-97.
17. Carpio DS. Avaliação do potencial de *Myriophyllum spicatum* em ensaios de toxicidade in vitro. Coimbra: Universidade de Coimbra, 2004, pp. 63.
18. Finney DJ. Probit analysis. Cambridge: University Press, 1971, pp. 333.
19. McCann JH, Greenberg BM, Ulpino L, Solomon KR. The effect of creosote on the growth of an axenic culture of *Myriophyllum spicatum* L. *Aquatic Toxicology* 2000; 50: 265-274.
20. Hanson ML, Sibley PK, Mabury SA, Muir DC, Solomon KR. Field level evaluations and risk assessment of the toxicity of dichloroacetic acid to the aquatic macrophytes Lemna gibba, Myriophyllum spicatum and Myriophyllum sibiricum. *Ecot Environ Safety* 2003; 55: 46-63.
21. Baker AJM, Walker PL. The effect of Physiological responses of plants to heavy metals and the quantification of tolerance and toxicity. *Chem Speciation Bioavail* 1989; 1: 7-17.
22. Baker AJM. Accumulators and excluders - strategies in the response of plants to heavy metals. *J Plant Nut* 1981; 3: 643-654.
23. Greger M. Metal availability and bioconcentration in plants. In: Prasad MNV, Hagemeyer J, eds. Heavy metal stress in plants - from molecules to ecosystems. Berlin: Springer, 1999: 1-27.

Metal Ions in Biology and Medicine: vol. 9. Eds Maria Carmen Alpoim, Paula Vasconcellos Morais, Maria Amélia Santos, Armando J. Cristóvão, José A. Centeno, Philippe Collery.
John Libbey Eurotext, Paris © 2006 pp. 158-1.

Investigation of arsenate phytotoxicity in cucumber plants

Viktória Czech[1], Victor G. Mihucz[2,3,4], Pálma Czövek[1], Edit Cseh[1], Gyula Záray[2,3,4]

[1]Plant Physiology Department, L. Eötvös University, H-1518 Budapest, P.O. Box 120, Budapest, Hungary
[2]Joint Research Group of Environmental Chemistry of L. Eötvös University and Hungarian Academy of Sciences, H-1518 Budapest, P.O. Box 32, Budapest, Hungary
[3]Satellite Centre of Trace Elements Institute for UNESCO, H-1518 Budapest, P.O. Box 32, Budapest, Hungary
[4]Inorganic and Analytical Chemistry Department, L. Eötvös University, H-1518 Budapest, P.O. Box 32, Budapest, Hungary

Plant physiological experiments carried out with cucumber plants (*Cucumis sativus* cv. Joker F1) and arsenate in concentration of 2 and 10 μmol · dm^{-3} proved that the As(V) treatment inhibited considerably the growth of plants and caused turgor loss depending on the development stage of the plants. These phytotoxic symptoms were the most pronounced seven and nine days after the As(V) treatment had begun in the case of plants having two cotyledons. Turgor loss was supported by the K decrease of the roots of plants treated with 10 μmol · dm^{-3} As(V) and 10 μmol · dm^{-3} phosphate to about half compared with the values obtained for control plants. Severe perturbation in the Fe transport of the plants was also observed. Arsenic speciation in xylem saps by HPLC-ICP-MS demonstrated the reduction of As(V) to As(III), the latter being the predominant arsenic form in the saps. Moreover, As(V) reduction to As(III) was not observed in the case of arsenic speciation of the nutrient solutions, which were replaced every 48 hours. Turgor loss was the result of the membrane permeability caused by lipid peroxidation due to the possible formation of free radicals during the reduction of As(V) to As(III). Increase in the concentration of the stress marker, malonedialdehyde (MDA), as product of lipid peroxidation, has also been observed. If Fe(III)chloride of the nutrient solutions was replaced by Fe(III)ascorbate, MDA concentrations were similar to those of the control plants. Thus, Fe(III)ascorbate seems to be able to protect hypocotyls from As phytoxicity.

INTRODUCTION

Considering the relatively high As concentration (0.10-0.25 mg · dm^{-3}) of ground water in the south-eastern part of Hungary [1], the study of uptake and translocation processes of As in edible plants cultivated in this area is essential. As the predominant form of arsenic in groundwater is As(V), cucumber plants, chosen as models, were grown in modified Hoagland nutrient solutions containing arsenic as As(V) in concentration of 0.25-0.75 mg · dm^{-3} (2.0-10.0 μmol · dm^{-3}) and iron as Fe(III)chloride. Reduction of As(V) to As(III) can occur rapidly in the roots. The reduction process is accompanied by formation of reactive oxygen compounds, which can damage the cell walls [2]. Oxidative stress causes lipid peroxidation and MDA is one of the products of this reaction. Thus, the oxidative stress can be monitored determining the MDA formed during the arsenic treatment, like it was established in the case of heavy metal contaminated living organisms. The reduction capacity of cucumber roots is well known, thus in the case of an As(V) treatment its reduction was expected. Due to the similar chemical structure of phosphate and arsenate ions, there is an interaction between the transport of these two ions. Arsenate acts as a phosphate analogue and it is transported across the plasma membrane via phosphate co-transport systems [3]. However, the reduction mechanism of As(V) is not too much understood. Nevertheless, HPLC-ICP-MS hyphenation is an effective tool for the investigation of chemical speciation of As.

Cucumber plants grown in hydroponic cultures contaminated with different As(V) and phosphate concentrations were studied. The chemical form of As in the sap and the hydroponics were determined by an HPLC-ICP-MS method. Oxidative stress produced by the As treatment was monitored by MDA determination in order to extend the knowledge of As(V) toxicity.

MATERIALS AND METHODS

Plant growth

Cucumber seeds (*Cucumis sativus* cv. Joker F1) were germinated in in the dark. The seedlings were grown in modified Hoagland solution The composition of this solution was as it follows: 1.25 mmol/dm^3 KNO_3; 1.25 mmol · dm^{-3} $Ca(NO_3)_2$; 0.5 mmol · dm^{-3} $MgSO_4$; 0.25 mmol · dm^{-3} KH_2PO_4; 11.6 µmol · dm^{-3} H_3BO_3; 10.0 µmol · dm^{-3} $FeCl_3$; 4.5 µmol · dm^{-3} $MnCl_2 \cdot 4H_2O$; 0.19 µmol · dm^{-3} $ZnSO_4 \cdot 7H_2O$; 0.12 µmol · dm^{-3} $Na_2MoO_4 \cdot 2H_2O$; 0.08 µmol · dm^{-3} $CuSO_4 \cdot 5H_2O$. When the cotyledons of the plants were developed, twenty-five plants were exposed to light and divided into five groups. Five plants were kept as control plants. Other five received As(V) treatment right after they were taken out from the dark, the other three groups of plants were transferred into nutrient solutions containing As(V) in concentration of 10 µmol · dm^{-3} and phosphate in concentration 10 µmol · dm^{-3} 5, 7 and 9 days after they developed the cotyledons.

Xylem sap could be collected for one hour 14 days after the beginning of arsenic treatment with 2 µmol · dm^{-3} As(V) and 2 µmol · dm^{-3} phosphate, by cutting the root neck of the plants.

For the lipid peroxidase activity measurements, five plants were grown for seven days in the modified Hoagland nutrient solution containing Fe(III)cloride or Fe(III)ascorbate in concentration of 10 µmol · dm^{-3}. MDA was determined in plant hypocotyls three hours after starting the As treatment with As(V) in concentration of 10 µmol · dm^{-3}.

Arsenic speciation by HPLC-ICP-MS

The chemical speciation of As was performed with an HPLC-ICP-MS system. The operating conditions of the ICP-MS instrument were the following: the RF power was set to 1200 W. The plasma, the auxiliary and the nebuliser argon gas flow rate were 16.0, 0.8 and 1.1 dm^3 · min^{-1}, respectively. Meinhard nebuliser was used for sample introduction. The sampler and skimmer cones, with orifice diameter of 1.0 and 0.4 mm, respectively, were made of Ni. Medium resolution ($R = 4000$) was used for As determination. Peak area integration mode was applied for the calculations of the results. A Hamilton 10 µm PRP-X100 column of 250 × 4.1 mm equipped with a pre-column of 4.6 × 4.1 mm and 20 mmol · dm^{-3} $NH_4H_2PO_4$ (pH = 5.6 with NH_3) as mobile phase were used for the anion-chromatographic measurements [4]. Flow rate was 1.5 cm^3 · min^{-1}. Througout the experiments deionised Milli Q water was used. The As(III) stock solution in concentration of 0.1 mol · dm^{-3} was prepared from arsenic(III) trioxide (Sigma Aldrich) by its dissolution in 1 mol · dm^{-3} KOH followed by acidification with 1 mol · dm^{-3} HCl similarly to Quaghebeur *et al.* [5], and then it was kept at 4°C. The As(V) stock solution was prepared from potassium dihydrogen arsenate (Sigma Aldrich) and acidified with HNO_3 Suprapur (Merck). DMA was used as cacodylic acid (Fluka).

TXRF spectrometry for determination of arsenic, potassum and iron

The roots and the second leaves of the control and contaminated plants were dried at 80°C and digested in nitric acid applying a microwave-assisted digestion procedure. The concentrations of

As, Fe and K were determined by total reflection X-ray fluorescence (TXRF) spectrometry. Twenty microlitres of each solution were dropped onto the quartz carrier plate and dried at 80°C on a ceramic hot plate in a clean box. For excitation and detection of the fluorescent radiation, a Mo-microfocus X-ray tube and Si(Li) detector were used, respectively. The integration time amounted to 500 s. For calibration, Ga as internal standard was added to the solutions in concentration of 1 μg · cm^{-3}.

Malonedialdehide analysis

The weighed hypocotyls of control and As-treated plants were cut in three parts (upper third, central and lower third), placed into Eppendorf vials and frozen in liquid nitrogen before analyses. Samples were homogenised in 1% trichloracetic acid (TCA) and centrifuged at 4°C for 10 min (10000 rpm). A mixture containing 1% thiobarbituric acid 20% TCA was added to the supernatant. The resulted solution was incubated at 100°C for 30 minutes and then was placed into a Shimadzu UV-2101 spectrophotometer. The absorbency of the solutions was determined at 532 nm.

RESULTS AND DISCUSSION

Characterisation of lipid peroxidase activity in plant hypocotyls by malonedialhide analysis

In the case of plants treated with 10 μmol · dm^{-3} As(V) and 10 μ mol · dm^{-3} Fe(III)chloride, five days after the arsenic treatment began, only the roots loss their turgor. If As(V) treatment started on the 7th and 9th day for plants having two cotyledons, the plant hypocotyls and leaves also lost their turgor. The hypocotyl growth reduction, determined on the 14th day of the As(V) treatment, registered an 87-90% decrease *(fig. 1)*. If the experiments were repeated by changing Fe(III)chloride for Fe(III)ascorbate, the reduction growth was about 20%. As a drastically decrease in the hypocotyl growth was experimented when the plants As(V) treatment started 7 days after they had two cotyledons, it was interesting to investigate their hypocotyls by cutting them into three parts, which underwent to MDA determination. The MDA concentrations of these samples were higher than those of the control plants, indicating lipid peroxidation activity. This enzymatic activity is usually related to free radical formation in the plant. Moreover, the MDA concentration of the hypocotyls of plants whose iron supply was Fe(III)ascorbate were similar to those of the control hypocotyls.

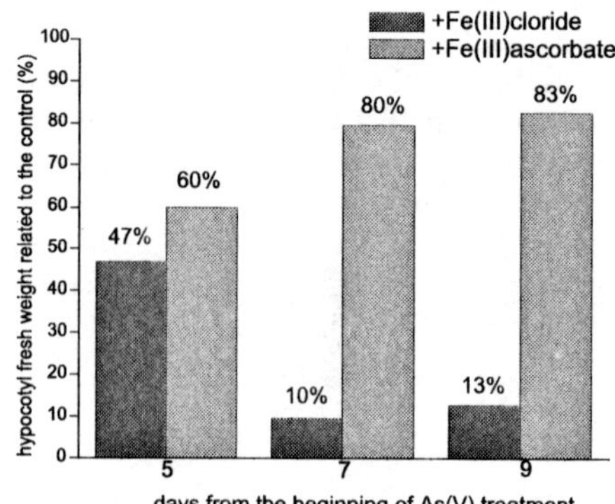

Fig. 1. Effect of 10 μmol · dm^{-3} As(V) treatment on the fresh hypocotyl weight (mg) related to the corresponding control values, started on the 5th, 7th or 9th days after that the plants developed two hypocotyls. Fresh hypocotyl masses were weighed on the 14th day of the treatment for 5 plants.

TXRF analyses of roots and leaves

The transport rates of As and Fe to the shoots were correlating in the sense that they were accumulated in the roots of the plants. Moreover, the K concentration of the roots of the treated plants decreased to about half of the corresponding values of the control plants *(table 2)*. As K is known to be a regulator of the water regime, this result also supports the turgor loss of the plants.

Table 2. Amounts of As and nutrient elements related to the dry weight (DW) in leaves and roots of cucumber plants in case of 10 µmol · dm^{-3}As(V) treatment

		Leaves		Roots	
		control	+As(V)	control	+As(V)
	c_{PO4} (µmol · dm^{-3}	concentration (mg · g^{-1} DW) (SD			
As	10.0	n.d.	0.106 ± 0.06	n.d.	0.871 ± 0.031
Fe	10.0	0.349 ± 0.022	0.073 ± 0.003	1.639 ± 0.109	7.147 ± 0.119
K	10.0	28.45 ± 1.22	19.88 ± 1.13	75.65 ± 2.15	38.25 ± 1.94

n.d. = not detectable

Arsenic speciation in xylem saps

Xylem sap could not be collected from plants treated with 10 µmol · dm^{-3} As(V), thus the As(V) concentration had to be lowered to 2 µmol · dm^{-3}. In order to exclude the competition between arsenate and phosphate, their ratio was set to 1:1. However, seedlings showed severe phosphate deficiency at 2 µmol · dm^{-3} PO_4^{-3} concentration. This inconvenience could be eliminated at a 250 µmol · dm^{-3} phosphate concentration. Reduction of As(V) to As(III) did not occur in the nutrient solutions. Three As species - As(III), DMA and As(V) - could be identified in the sap samples *(fig. 2)* with an anion-exchange HPLC column, however it can be stated that As(V) and DMA could be detected only in traces. Arsenite was the predominant arsenic species in the xylem saps and the following concentration order was determined: As(III) > As(V) ≈ DMA.

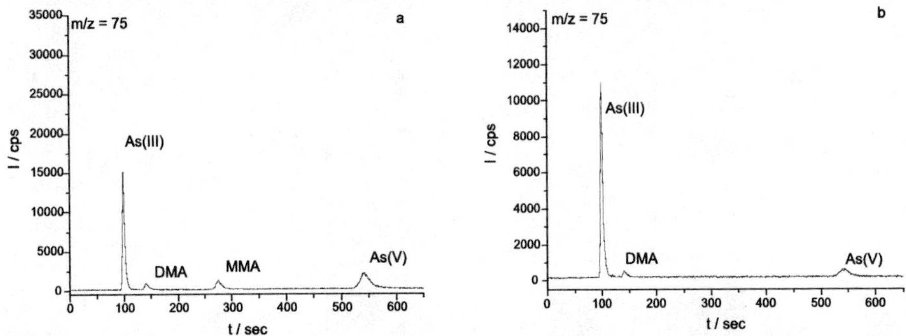

Fig. 2. HPLC ICP-MS chromatogram of a standard solution containing As(III), MMA, DMA and As(V) in concentration of 12, 1, 3 and 7 ng · cm^{-3}, respectively (a), and of a xylem sap of cucumber plants in case of 2 (mol · dm^{-3} As(V) treatment (b)

These results showed that arsenate reduction occurred inside the roots. This phenomenon is in concordance with the lipid peroxidase activity and with the fact that the semipermeability of the membranes had been destroyed.

CONCLUSIONS

On basis of the analytical data, the following conclusions can be drawn: in plants treated with arsenate in concentration of 10 $\mu mol \cdot dm^{-3}$ As(V), As(V) was reduced in the roots to As(III) causing turgor loss in the roots, hypocotyls and leaves depending on the development stage of the cucumber plants. Perturbation in the water regime of the plants was demonstrated from chemical point of view by the K decrease in the roots. Moreover, the malonedialdehide concentration of the hypocotyls indicated lipid peroxidation, which may be in connection with the As(V) $\rightarrow$ As(III) reduction by free radical formation. Fe(III)ascorbate protected the plant hypocotyls from turgor loss.

REFERENCES

1. Varsányi I, Godre Z, Bartha A. Arsenic in Drinking water and mortality in the Southern Great Plain, Hungary. *Environmental Geochemistry and Health* 1991; 13:14-22.
2. Meharg AA, Hartley-Whitaker J. Arsenic uptake and metabolism in arsenic resistant and nonresistant plant species. *New Phytol* 2002; 154:29-43.
3. Meharg AA, Macnair MR. Polymorphism and physiology of arsenate tolerance in Holcus Lanatus L from an uncontaminated site. J Exp Bot 1992; 43:519-524.
4. Gallagher PA, Wei XY, Shoemaker JA, Brockhoff CA, Creed JT. Detection of arsenosugars from kelp extracts via IC-electrospray ionization MS-MS and IC membrane hydride generation ICP-MS. *J Anal Atom Spectrom* 1999; 14:1829-1834.
5. Quaghebeur M, Rengel Z, Smirk M. Arsenic speciation in terrestrial plant material using microwave-assisted digestion, ion chromatography and inductively coupled plasma mass spectrometry. *J Anal At Spectrom* 2003; 18:128-134.

Metal Ions in Biology and Medicine: vol. 9. Eds Maria Carmen Alpoim, Paula Vasconcellos Morais, Maria Amélia Santos, Armando J. Cristóvão, José A. Centeno, Philippe Collery.
John Libbey Eurotext, Paris © 2006 pp. 163-1.

Effect of activate sludge addition on the microbial activity of soil

Bruno de Jesus[1], R. Branco[1], T. Natal da Luz[2], J.P. Sousa[2] and P.V. Morais[1]

[1]*Instituto do Ambiente e Vida, 3004-517 Coimbra, Portugal.*
[2]*Departamento Zoologia, Faculdade de Ciências e Tecnologia da Universidade de Coimbra, 3004-517, Coimbra, Portugal.*

Urban residues like activated sludge from wastewater treatment plants are being used as fertilizers or soil correctors. However, sewage sludge can also contain contaminants, such as heavy metals, organic compounds and human pathogens, which should be considered. The application of sewage sludge can either stimulate soil microbial activity, due to an increase in available carbon and nutrients, or inhibit activity, due to the presence of heavy metals and other pollutants. Therefore, the behavior of the microbial population depends on the quality and amount of the residues that are added to the soil. The addition of organic material can lead to an increase in the microbial populations activity and diversity in the soil and long-term tolerance of microbes to metals. An inhibition of microbial activity leads to reductions in ecological processes related to the cycling of nutrients and the turnover of organic matter. Generally, chromium is found in the environment in two stable states: Cr(III) and Cr(VI). The first is not very soluble and is immobilized by precipitation as hydroxides, and the later is toxic, soluble and easily transported to water resources. Microbial Cr(VI) reducing ability have been developed for remediation of Cr-contaminated water and soils.

This study aims to evaluate the effect of adding to soil sludges with different chemical and biological composition. In order to do it microcosms were constructed and sludges with 3 different chemical and biological compositions and at 4 different concentrations were added. Two of the sludges were from industrial origin and one them contained 980mg/Kg of Cr(VI). The third sludge was from a wastewater treatment plant receiving urban wastewater. During 8 weeks incubation we followed in each microcosm the changes in microbial diversity by ARDRA (Amplified Ribossomal DNA Restriction Analysis) profiling, the number of heterotrophic cultivated bacteria and β-glucosidase, usease, DHA and alkaline phosphatase enzymes activity. The number of heterotrophic cultivated bacteria was higher on soils with sludge addition compared to the control but the number was different and related with the sludge origin. The temporal fluctuations in the enzymatic activity were much less pronounced than for microbial biomass.

INTRODUCTION

The agricultural use of sewage sludge has been recommended, since it contains organic matter and is rich in macro and micronutrients [7]. Urban residues like activate sludge from wastewater treatment plants are usually used as fertilizers or soil correctors. However, sewage sludge can also contain contaminants, such as heavy metals, organic compounds and human pathogens, which should be considered. When sewage sludge is applied to soil, it causes alterations in the structure and functioning of the agroecosystem; one of the most sensitive components is the microbial community, which can be utilized as an indicator for changes in soil quality [5, 6].

The application of sewage sludge can either stimulate soil microbial activity, due to an increase in available carbon and nutrients, or inhibit activity, due to the presence of heavy metals and other pollutants [1, 2]. Therefore, the behavior of the microbial population depends on the quality and amount of residues that are added to the soil. An inhibition of microbial activity leads to reductions in ecological processes related to the cycling of nutrients and the turnover of organic matter [3, 8]. The diversity of environmental microbial communities has been studied using new techniques for describing different microbial populations [4, 2, 8]. However, as no one single method is currently available for exploring the whole bacterial community, a combination of methods is necessary to obtain a detailed view of its structure and diversity.

The aim of this study was evaluating the effect of adding to soil sludges with different chemical and biological composition. In order to do it we followed during 8 weeks incubation in soil microcosms the changes in microbial diversity by ARDRA (Amplified Ribossomal DNA Restriction Analysis) profiling, the number of heterotrophic cultivated bacteria and β-glucosidase, usease, DHA and alkaline phosphatase enzymes activity.

MATERIALS AND METHODS

Soil sampling and characterization

A field-collected reference soil from an agricultural field located outside the city limits of Coimbra, Portugal, was used. The choice of this soil was based on his use history, being free of pesticides and fertilizer applications for more than 5 years.

The reference soil was previously sieved (5mm mesh) and defaunated (with freeze-thawing cycles) before to be mixed with the test sludges. Its microbial community was re-established by inoculating the bulk soil with an elutriate of a fresh sample of the reference soil. The soil parameters measured were the soil pH (1M KCl 1:6 v:v), the water holding capacity (ISO 11267, Annex C), the cation exchange capacity (ISO 11260), the organic matter content (loss on ignition at 500°C for 6h), the soil texture (LNEC-E 239) and the metals in bulk soil.

Sewage samples

Sewage sludge was obtained from: 1) the biological municipal Wastewater Treatment Plant, in Coimbra, Portugal, which treats home sewage (Sludge C); 2) the biological and secondary Wastewater Treatment Plant treating industrial sewage from a chromate industry (Ceira, Portugal) (Sludge T); 3) the biological and secondary Wastewater Treatment Plant treating industrial sewage from food industry (Mira, Portugal) (Sludge M). The most important characteristics of these sludges are presented in *table 1*, determined according to EPA SW-846-3051.

Microcosms construction

The experiments were carried out in microcosms containing reference soil. All sewage sludges were mixed with the reference soil in five different doses according to the usual doses applied in fertilization assays and concerning the legal limits of the application. Thus, 0, 6, 15, 25 and 45T/ha of dry matter of each sewage sludge were the doses used for these tests.

Samples for microbial parameters (soil enzymes and CFU's) were taken from each treatment after 12h, 1, 4 and 8 weeks. ARDRA profiles were performed for each sludge use.

RESULTS

The amount of total nitrogene (%) in microcosms with sludge C was 0.1, 0.11, 0.13 and 0.17; in microcosms with sludge M was 0.09, 0.1, 0.1 and 0.14; and in microcosms with sludge T was 0.08, 0.09 0.09 and 0.09 for amend concentrations of 6T/ha, 15T/ha, 25T/ha and 45T/ha, respectively. The ARDRA profiles were different between sludges indicating different microbial communities' composition *(fig. 1)*. The same results were obtained with the two different restriction enzymes used.

Table 1. Total heavy metal concentrations, ph and organic matter content of the test sludges used in this study and the upper limit values of the heavy metals according to EU Directive 86/278/CEE.

	Reference soil	**Sludge C**	**Sludge M**	**Sludge T**	**Higher Limits** (EU Directive 86/278/CEE)
pH (1M KCl)	7.9	6.9	8.6	7.7	
WHC (%)	46				
CEC (meq/Kg)	90.4				
Soil texture	Loamy sand				
Organic matter (%)	2.9	48.7	5.7	42.0	
Nitrogen total (%)	0.06	-	-	-	
Metals (mg/Kg)					
Mercury	n.d	n.d.	0.3	0.07	18
Cadmium	<2.8	3.2	<0.5	<QL	20
Copper	12	436	66	42	1000
Chromium	11	121	74	4790	1000
Nickel	<14	39	33	58	300
Lead	61	145	19	3.5	750
Zinc	96	1731	350	900	2500

n.d. Not determined
QL - not detected or if present in concentrations under the quantification limit

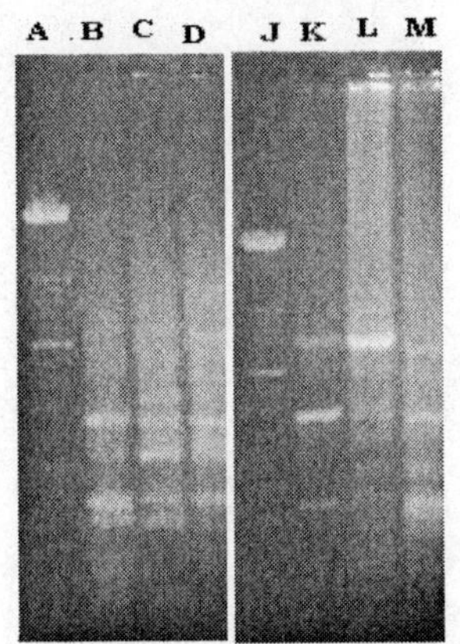

Fig. 1. Restriction pattern of sludge T (B), sludge C (C) and sludge M (D) digested with restriction enzyme *cfo*I and restriction patterns of the same sludges (K, L, M) digested with restriction enzyme *Del*I. A and J molecular weigh markers.

The temporal variation observed in the number of heterotrofic cultivable bacteria (CFU) and enzymes activity in the soil amended with sludge C are described in *fig. 2*. The addition of sludge to the soil increased the number of CFU proportionately to the quantity of sludge added but after 8 weeks the number of CFU was similar to the control. The enzyme activities were decreased by sludge addition to the soil but after 8 weeks only β-glycosidase activity was slight lower then the control.

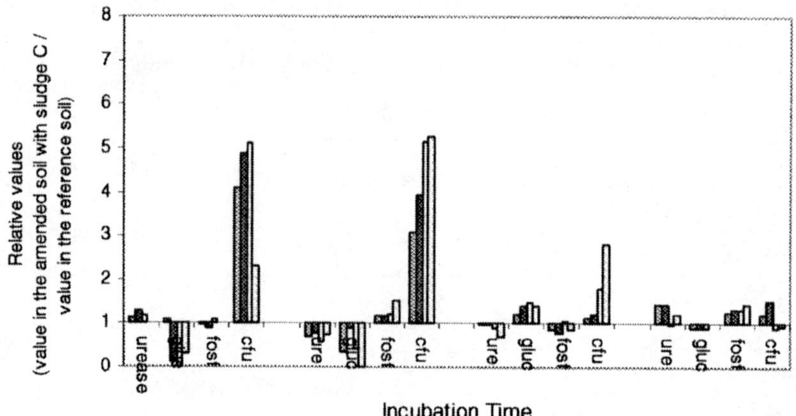

Fig. 2. Relative values (value in the amended soil with sludge C / value in the reference soil) for the urease activity, β-glucosidade, alkaline phosphatase and the number of heterotrophic bacteria (CFU) found in the sludge C amended microcosms with 6T/ha (dark blue), 15T/ha (purple) 25T/ha (yellow) and 45T/ha (light blue), during the incubation period (12h, 1, 4 and 8 weeks).

Figure 3 described the variation between the parameters observed in the soil and after soil amended with slugde T during 8 weeks incubation period. Sludge addition increased CFU number in the soil immediately after addition (12h) but did not change the enzymatic activity in the soil. After 1 week all the parameters in the microcosms with sludge were similar or slightly lower when comparing to the control.

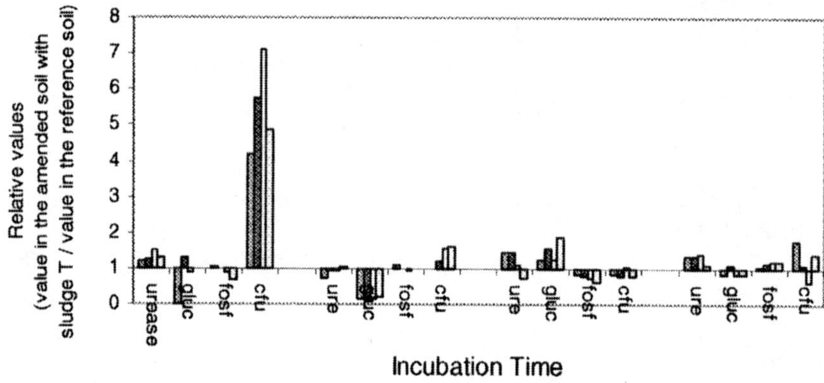

Fig. 3. Relative values (value in the amended soil with sludge T / value in the reference soil) for the urease activity, β-glucosidade, alkaline phosphatase and the number of heterotrophic bacteria (CFU) found in the sludge T amended microcosms with 6T/ha (dark blue), 15T/ha (purple) 25T/ha (yellow) and 45T/ha (light blue), during the incubation period (12h, 1, 4 and 8 weeks).

The addition of increasing concentrations of sludge M to the soil increased slightly the enzymatic activity in the soil and increased dramatically the number of CFU (35 fold) *(fig. 4)*. The increase in CFU number was directly proportional to the amount of sludge added. After 8 weeks all the parameters in the microcosms amend with sludge were higher then in the control soil.

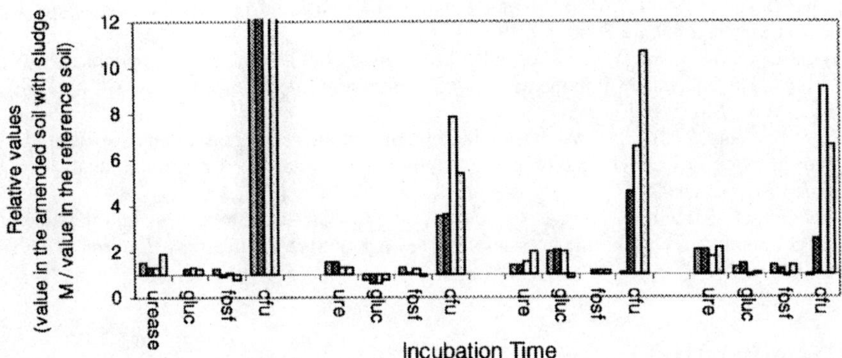

Fig. 4. Relative values (value in the amended soil with sludge M / value in the reference soil) for the urease activity, β-glucosidade, alkaline phosphatase and the number of heterotrophic bacteria (CFU) found in the sludge M amended microcosms with 6T/ha (dark blue), 15T/ha (purple) 25T/ha (yellow) and 45T/ha (light blue), during the incubation period (12h, 1, 4 and 8 weeks)

DISCUSSION

Knowledge about the changes in composition and activity of microbial communities in contaminated soils is of particular interest to predict the soil response to contaminants. When comparing the β-glucosidase activity in the different sludge amend microcosms used in this experiment we can see that after 8 weeks incubation the activity was increased only when sludge M was used. β-glucosidase activity has been suggested as a sensitive indicator of the effect of improved uncultivated managements on site degradation (9). Surprisingly, sludge M had a lower amount of organic matter compared to the other sludges and the same percentage of nitrogen. Therefore, the effect observed could probably be related to the lower amount of contaminants or to the presence of a higher number of active microorganisms. Although sludge T contained 4 times the amount of chromium allowed by EC directive it did not affect either the soil enzyme activity or the CFU numbers after an incubation period. In conclusion, we can say that the temporal fluctuations found in the enzymatic activity were much less pronounced than for microbial biomass, which fluctuated highly, furthermore both observed effects were dependent on sludge origin.

REFERENCES

1. Bååth, E. Effects of heavy metals in soil on microbial process and population: a review. *Water Air Soil Pollut.* 1989, 47, 335-379.
2. Bååth, E. M. Diaz-Ravina, Å. Frostegård, and C. D. Campbell. Effect of metal-rich sludge amendments on the soil microbial community. *App. Environ. Microbiol.* 1998, 64:238-245.
3. Barkay, T., Shearer, D.F. and Olson, B.H. Toxicity testing in soil using microorganisms (Dutka, B.J. and Bitton, G., Eds.), *Toxicity Testing Using Microorganisms* 1986, vol. 2, pp. 133-155. CRC Press, Boca Raton, FL.
4. Branco, R., A-P Chung., A. Veríssimo, and P. V Morais. Impact of chromium contaminated wastewaters in the microbial community of a river. *FEMS Microbial. Ecol* 2005 54: 35-46.
5. Dick, R.P. Soil enzyme assays as indicators of soil quality. In: Doran, J.W.L., Coleman, D.C., Bezdicek, D.F., Stewart, B.A. (Eds.), *Defining Soil Quality for a Sustainable Enviroment.* Soil Science Society of America, Madison, WI, Soil Sci. Soc. Am. (Special Publication no. 35) 1994, pp. 107-124.
6. Giller, K.E., Witter, E., McGrath, S.P. Toxicity of heavy metals to microorganisms and microbial process in agricultural soils: a review. *Soil Biol. Biochem.* 1998, 30, 1389-1414.
7. Melo, W.J., and O.M. Marques. Potencial do lodo de esgoto como fonte de nutrientes para as plantas.

In: Bettiol, W., Camargo, O.A. (Eds.), *Impacto ambiental do uso agricola do lodo de esgoto*. Jaguariuna, SP, Embrapa Meio Ambiente 2000, pp. 193-142.

8. Muyzer, G., E. C. Waal, and A. G. Uitterlinden Profiling of complex microbial populations by denaturant gel electrophoresis analysis of polymerase chain reaction-amplified genes for 16S rRNA. *App. Environ. Microbiol.* 1993, 59:695-700.
9. Smit, E., P. Leeflang, and K. Wernars Detection of shifts in microbial community structure and diversity in soil caused by copper contamination using amplified ribosomal DNA restriction analysis. *FEMS Microb. Ecol.* 1997, 13:249-261.
10. Witter, E., Gong, P., Bååth, E. and Marstorp, H. A study of the structure and metal tolerance of the soil microbial community six years after cessation of sewage sludge applications. *Environ. Toxicol. Chem.* 2000, 19, 1983-1991

ACKNOWLEDGEMENTS

This research was funded by Fundação para a Ciência e Tecnologia (FCT), Portugal, under POCTI and FEDER programs, contract POCTI/BSE/42414/2001. R. Branco was supported by a Ph.D. scholarship from FCT (SFRH/BD/10737/2002).

Metal Ions in Biology and Medicine: vol. 9. Eds Maria Carmen Alpoim, Paula Vasconcellos Morais, Maria Amélia Santos, Armando J. Cristóvão, José A. Centeno, Philippe Collery.
John Libbey Eurotext, Paris © 2006 pp. 169-1.

Comparative effects of NH_4VO_3 on detoxication enzymes and redox state of wine *Saccharomyces*

Ferreira, R.[1,2]; Alves-Pereira, I.[1,2]; Magriço, S.[2]; Ferraz-Franco, C.[2]

[1]*Instituto de Ciências Agrárias Mediterrânicas (ICAM), Universidade de Évora, Apartado 94, 7002-554 Évora, Portugal, raf@uevora.pt*

[2]*Departamento de Química, Universidade de Évora, Apartado 94, 7002-554 Évora, Portugal*

The aims of this work was to compare the effects of NH_4VO_3, a pentavalent salt of vanadium, on cell viability, GST (EC 2.5.1.18) and γ-GT (EC 2.3.2.2) activities, and redox state of wild wine yeast *Saccharomyces cerevisiae* UE-ME3 and *Saccharomyces chevalieri* UE-ME1. Our results show that *S. cerevisiae* was more tolerant to NH_4VO_3 than *S. chevalieri* cells, which do not survive for concentration higher than 7.5 mM in culture medium, while *S. cerevisiae* cells remain viable in presence of 75 mM of ammonium metavanadate. In addition, we observed that values of GST activities and GSH/GSSG ratio in *S. cerevisiae* are higher than *S. chevalieri*, a good sign of strong antioxidant response has occurred in *S. cerevisiae*. Conversely the γ-GT activities level determined in *S. cerevisiae* were lower than in *S. chevalieri*. The ammonium metavanadate salt caused a significantly decrease ($p<0,01$) of GST and γ-GT activities in both yeast and a decrease of GSH/GSSG in *S. cerevisiae*. These facts suggest that ammonium metavanadate disturb the detoxycation capacity and protection mechanisms against oxidative stress of both yeast species mainly on *S. chevalieri*.

INTRODUCTION

The incomplete reduction of oxygen to water during respiration leads to the formation of reactives oxygen species (ROS) such as the superoxide anion radical, hydrogen peroxide and the hydroxyl radical. Consequently, aerobic organisms have to maintain a reduced cellular redox environment in the face of the prooxidative conditions of aerobic life (1, 2, 3, 4). ROS are also produced by others processes like β-oxidation of fatty acids or exposition to metals, and drugs, when present in high levels, disturb the cell redox status and bring toxic damages to lipids, proteins, and DNA, which in several cases lead to cell death (4). All organisms have evolved protective mechanisms and programmed responses to limit cellular damages from exposure to toxic compounds in their environment. Glutathione *S*-transferases (GST), a family of evolutionarily conserved enzymes, play an important role in detoxication of many electrophilic xenobiotic, catalyzing its conjugation with glutathione and producing compounds that are generally less reactive and more water soluble and removing them from the cell via membrane-based glutathione conjugate pumps (5, 6). In other hand GST have long been suspected to be important in protecting cells from oxidative stress by detoxifying some of the secondary ROS produced when ROS react with cellular constituents (5, 6). Interestingly, other researcher has established that GST may have a wider role in the response to cellular stress beyond their enzymatic activity (7, 8). Glutathione (GSH; γ-glutamyl-l-cysteinylglycine) is present in high concentration in most living cells from microorganisms to man, and has been shown to play numerous roles, in particular in the yeast *S. cerevisiae*, where it may account for 1% of the cell dry weight (9). In this yeast, GSH catabolism appears to be mediated by γ-glutamyl transpeptidase (γ-GT), and cysteinylglycine dipeptidase, vacuolar-membranebound enzymes (10), which leads to the formation of glutamate, cysteine and glycine (11, 12). *Saccharomyces cerevisiae* cells disrupted for glutathione biosynthesis exhibit reduced tolerance to a wide range of stress conditions (13, 14, 15, 16) and undergo apoptosis at a high rate relative to the parental cells (17). Conversely, exogenous administration of glutathione rescues the accelerated aging of *S. cerevisiae* cells in elevated oxygen environment (18). Its use/degradation necessitate vacuolar compartmentalization and cleavage of the γ-glutamyl linkage via the specific action of γ-GT (19, 20). There are thousands of millions of types of yeast. Of those, only 250 will produce fermentation, and of those, only 24, including *Saccharomyces cerevisiae* and *Saccharomyces chevalieri* are "good" yeast for winemaking presented at different phases of fermentation process. Considering that capacity of wine fermentation is greatly influenced by the yeast resistance to the stress conditions, including the oxidative stress (21) we select this good fermentation yeast to evaluate de effects of vanadium, a soil and wine cellar contaminant, on eukaryotic antioxidant responses.

MATERIALS AND METHODS

Microorganisms and growth conditions

The eukaryotic model used was the wine yeast *Saccharomyces cerevisiae* UE-ME3 and *Saccharomyces chevalieri* UE-ME1, strains isolated from regional wine (Alentejo-Portugal) belonging to the Enology laboratory collection of Évora University. The isolated colonies of strains were stored in glycerol (30%, w/v) at -80°C.

Exponential-phase cells were harvest and suspended in mineral medium with vitamins, oligoelements and 2% (w/v) of glucose (22), containing ammonium metavanadate in a range from 0.25 to 200 mM at 28°C during 200 minutes. Samples from each treatment were used to determine cfu and generate the respective dose-response curves.

For enzymatic assays and glutathione contents determination, exponential-phase cells were harvest and inoculated in agar plate enriched mineral medium with vitamins, oligoelements and 2% (w/v) of glucose (22), and incubated during 72 hours at 28°C in the absence or presence of 25 and 75 mM NH_4VO_3 *(S. cerevisiae)* or 0.25, 0.75, 2.5 7.5 mM NH_4VO_3 *(S. chevalieri).*

Enzymatic assays

Cells growing in agar plate enriched mineral medium were harvest, disrupted with glass beads and the post-peroxissomal supernatants obtained by differential centrifugation were used for determination of GST (EC 2.5.1.18) and γ-GT (EC 2.3.2.2) activities according to Habig (23) and Szas (24) methods, respectively. All enzymatic measurements were carried out with a double beam spectrophotometer, Hitachi-U2001.

Protein and glutathione determination

Protein determination was realized according to Lowry (25) method using BSA as standard.

The post-peroxissomal supernatant were used for determination of intracellular glutathione contents and GSH/GSSG ratio calculation according Anderson (26).

Statistical analysis

All the experiments were repeated at least five times independently and the data presented are mean values performed in five experiments ± S.D. The statistical analysis of results were realized by ANOVA I and Tukey tests were carried out to determine significant differences ($p < 0.01$) between the enzymatic activities of cells growing in the absence or presence of NH_4VO_3 (27).

RESULTS

Our results shows that in cultures of *S. cerevisiae* UE-ME3 after 200 min of treatment with 25 mM and 75 mM of ammonium metavanadate were found 19% and 12% of viable cells, respectively, when assessed by cfu. Conversely, in *S. chevalieri* UE-ME1 growing 200 min in presence of 7,5 mM ammonium metavanadate only were found 5% of viable cells *(fig. 1)*. These results point us the effects of NH_4VO_3 on the cell-proliferative capacity more pronounced in *S.chevalieri* than in *S.cerevisiae*.

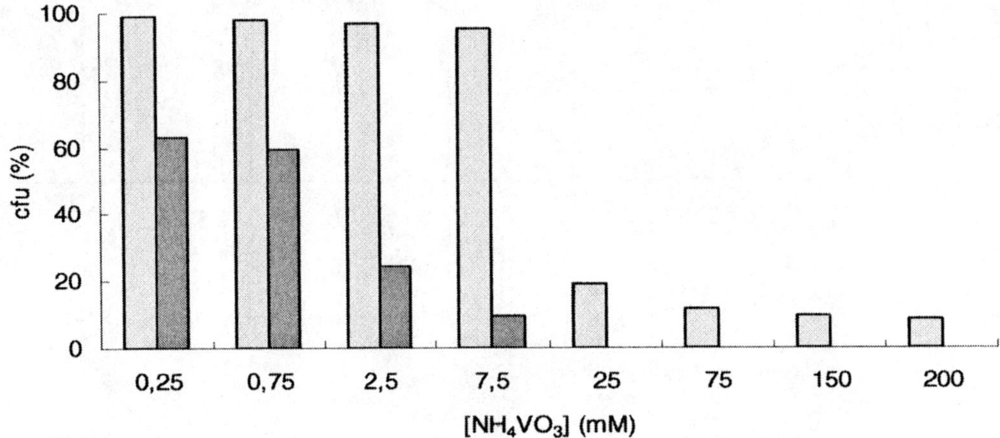

Fig. 1. Relative survival (cfu) of *Saccharomyces cerevisiae* UE-ME3 ▒ and *Saccharomyces chevalieri* UE-ME1 ■ growing for 200 min in the absence or presence of 0.25, 0.75, 2.5, 7.5, 25, 75, 150 and 200 mM of NH_4VO_3. Each bars represents mean value of three replicates, 100% corresponds to cfu at time zero.

The results of *figure 2* shows in *S. cerevisiae* GST activity values approximately 50 fold more elevated than the GST activity determined in *S. chevalieri*. We also observed that NH_4VO_3, a pentavalent salt of vanadium caused a significantly ($p<0,01$) decrease of GST activities in both yeast species, which in case of *S. chevalieiri*, this effect depend on concentration of ammonium metavanadate in culture medium. The decrease observed of GST activity in presence of transition metal salt could disturb the detoxycation capacity of yeast *Saccharomyces* cells by conjugation of xenobiotics with glutathione tripeptide, particularly in the case of *S.chevalieri*, affecting its surviving capacity.

In addition we observed, *figure 3*, that γ-GT activity values in *S. cerevisiae* were 4 fold smaller than γ-GT activity values determined in *S. chevalieri*. In both species, the NH_4VO_3 caused a significantly ($p<0,01$) decrease of γ-GT activity which depend on ammonium metavanadate concentration, in culture medium. These results suggest that ammonium metavanadate could affect the vacuolar transport and metabolism of GSH in *Saccharomyces* yeast, particularly in the case of *S.chevalieri*.

Finally, in this work we observed that GSH/GSSG ratio determined in *S. cerevisiae* were 15 fold more elevated than which were determined in *S. chevalieri*. In presence of ammonium metavanadate occur increases of oxidant status of *S. cerevisiae* cells confirmed by a decrease of GSH/GSSG ratio a marker of oxidative stress induction in *S. cerevisiae*. Moreover, in the *S. chevalieri* UE-ME1 the effect observed suggest an upregulated synthesis of GSH, which point to an eventual adaptative response to stress conditions caused by ammonium metavanadate. However, this response seems not enough to support the cell surviving, since the ratio values are always lower than which determined in *S.cerevisiae*, *figure 4*.

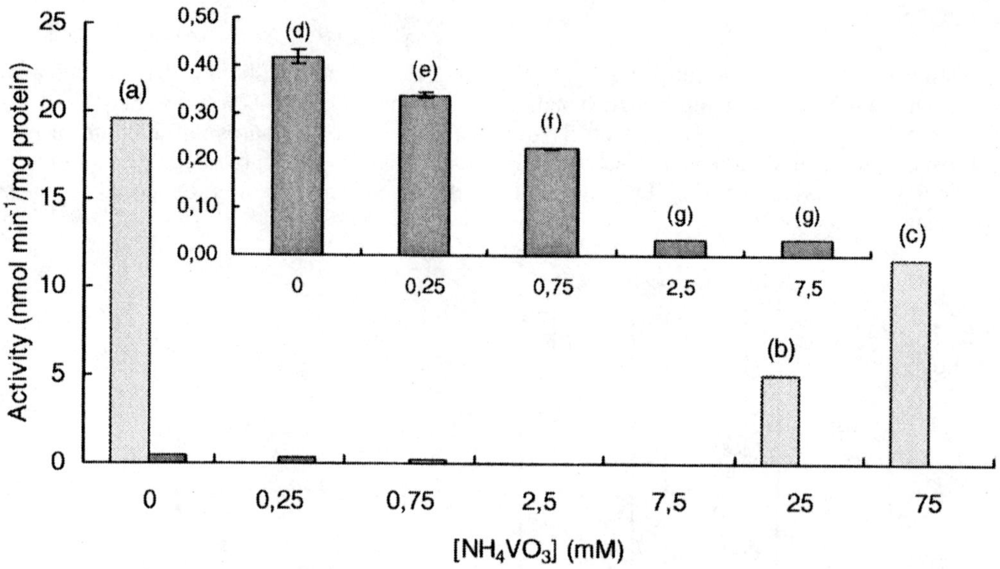

Fig. 2. Effect of NH_4VO_3 on the GST activity of wine *Saccharomyces cerevisiae* UE-ME3 and *Saccharomyces chevalieri* UE-ME1 cell extracts. Each bar represents the mean ± SD of five replicates (bars with no common letter are significantly different, $P < 0{,}01$).

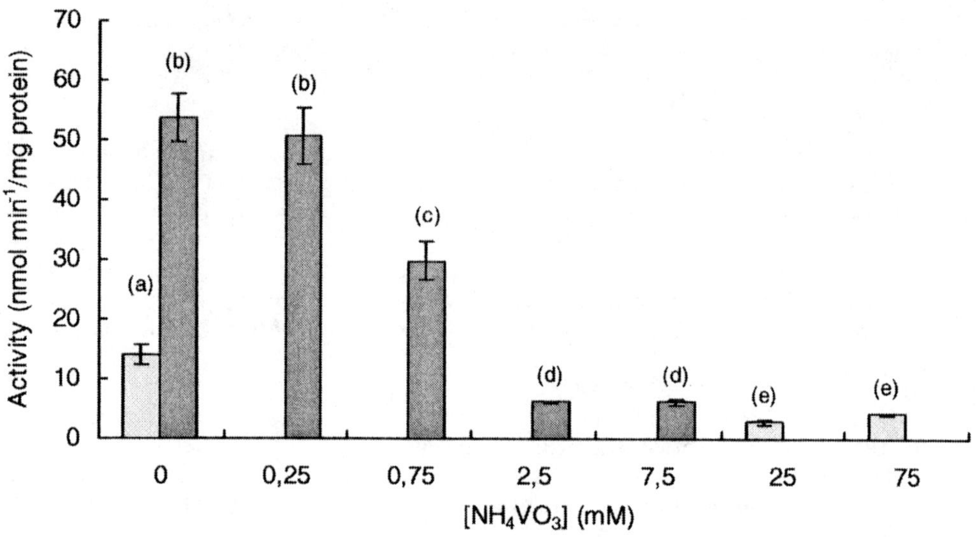

Fig. 3. Effect of NH_4VO_3 on the γ-GT activity of wine *Saccharomyces cerevisiae* UE-ME3 and *Saccharomyces chevalieri* UE-ME1 cell extracts. Each bar represents the mean ± SD of five replicates (bars with no common letter are significantly different, $P < 0{,}01$).

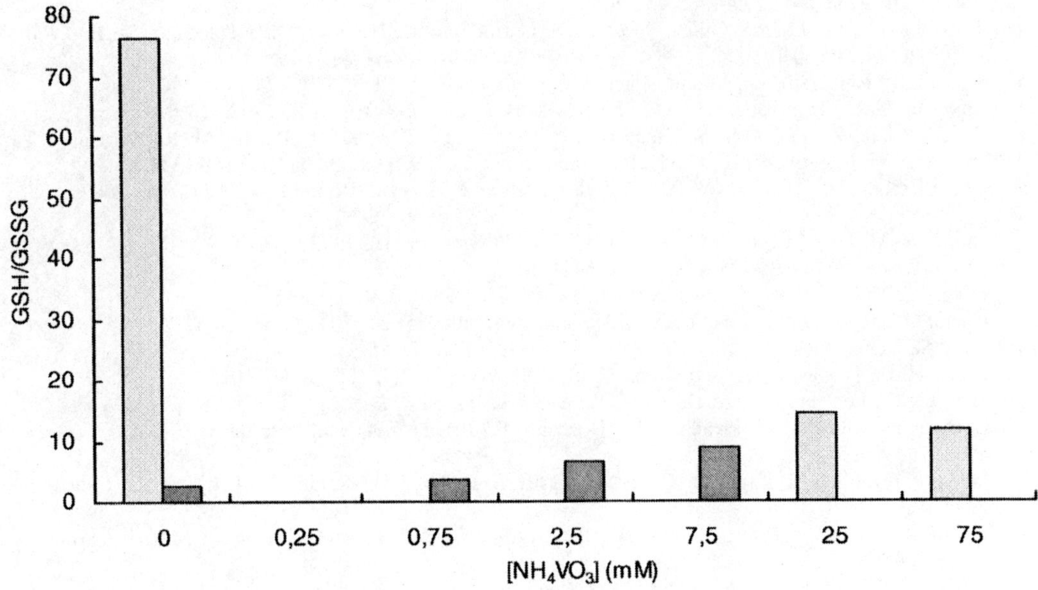

Fig. 4. Effect of ammonium metavanadate on the yeast's intracellular GSH/GSSG ratio in *Saccharomyces cerevisiae* UE-ME3 ▒ and *Saccharomyces chevalieri* UE-ME1 ■.

DISCUSSION

Considering that *S. cerevisiae* cells remain viable in presence of 75 mM of ammonium metavanadate and *S. chevalieri* cells do not survive to concentration higher than 7.5 mM in culture medium we conclude that *S. cerevisiae* was more tolerant to NH_4VO_3 than *S. chevalieri*. In addition, the more elevated values of GST activities and GSH/GSSG ratio determined in *S. cerevisiae*, suggest that this yeast species have antioxidant defenses more strong than *S. chevalieri* despite the γ-GT activity determined in *S. cerevisiae* were lower than which were determined in *S. chevalieri*. The observed decrease of GST and γ-GT activities, caused by pentavalent salt of vanadium, in both yeast species studied, suggest that NH_4VO_3, probably disturb its detoxycation capacity and vacuolar transport of aminoacids as well as protection mechanism against oxidative stress. The increase of oxidant conditions of *S. cerevisiae* cells growing in presence of elevated concentration of NH_4VO_3, expected by the decrease of GSH/GSSG ratio, advise ammonium metavanadate as inductor of oxidative stress in *S.cerevisiae*. In other hand, the increase of reduced redox status of the *S. chevalieri* cells growing in presence of little concentration of NH_4VO_3, could be considered as adaptative response to the oxidative stress by this yeast species, but this response isn't enough to support cell surviving of this species in presence of heavy metal vanadium. In conclusion, we consider that *S cerevisiae*, a good fermentation yeast is more tolerant to vanadium in aerobic conditions than *S. chevalieri*, because to have, probably, more strong antioxidant and xenobiotics metabolization/elimination mechanisms.

REFERENCES

1. Halliwell, B., and Gutteridge, J. M. C. 1989 Free Radicals in Biology and Medicine, Clarendon Press, Oxford.

2. Storz, G., Tartaglia, L. A., Farr, S. B., and Ames, B. N. *Trends Genet.* 1990; 6: 363-368.
3. Halliwell, B. *Nutr. Rev.* 1994; 52: 253-265.
4. Lee, J., Godon, C., Lagnie, Gilles, Spector, D., Garini Jerome, Labarre J. and Toledano, M. B. *J.Biol Chem* 1999; 274: 16040-16046.
5. Hubatsch, I., Ridderstrom, M., and Mannervik, B. *Biochem. J.* 1998; 330: 175-179.
6. Danielson, U. H., Esterbauer, H., and Mannervik, B. *Biochem. J.* 1987; 247: 707-713.
7. Adler, V., Yin, Z., Fuchs, S. Y., Benezra, M., Rosario, L., Tew, K. D., Pincus, M. R., Sardana, M., Henderson, C. J., Wolf, C. R., Davis, R. J., and Ronai, Z. *EMBO J.* 1999; 18: 1321-1334.
8. Veal, Elizabeth A., Toone, W. Mark, Jones Nic, and Morgan, Brian A. *J.Biol.Chem.* 2002; 277: 35523-35531.
9. Penninckx, M. J. and Elskens, M. T. *Adv. Microb. Physiol.* 1993; 34: 239-301.
10. Jaspers, C. and Penninckx, M. *Biochimie.* 1984; 66: 71-74.
11. Mehdi, K., Thierie, J. and Penninckx, M. J. *Biochem. J.* 2001; 359: 631-637.
12. Jaspers, C., Gigot, D. and Penninckx, M. *Phytochemistry* 1985; 24: 703-707.
13. Izawa, S., Inoue, Y., and Kimura, A. *FEBS Lett.* 1995; *368*: 73-76.
14. Turton, H. E., Dawes, I. W., and Grant, C. M. *J. Bacteriol.* 1997; 1*79*: 1096-1101.
15. Grant, C. M., Perrone, G., and Dawes, I. W. *Biochem. Biophys. Res. Commun.* 1998; 253: 893-898.
16. Maris, A. F., Kern, A. L., Picada, J. N., Boccardi, F., Brendel, M., and Henriques, J. *A. Curr. Genet.* 2000; 37: 175-182.
17. Madeo, F., Frohlich, E., Ligr, M., Grey, M., Sigrist, S. J., Wolf, D. H., and Frohlich, K. U. J. *Cell Biol.* 1999; 145: 757-767.
18. Nestelbacher, R., Laun, P., Vondrakova, D., Pichova, A., Schuller, C., and Breitenbach, M. *Exp. Gerontol.* 2000; 35: 63-70.
19. Mehdi, K., Thierie, J., and Penninckx, M. J. *Biochem. J.* 2001; 359: 631-637.
20. Perrone, G. G., Grant, C. M., and Dawes, I. W. *Molecular Biology of the Cell.* 2005; 16: 218-230.
21. Carrasco, P., Querol A.and del Olmo M. *Arch Microbiol.* 2001; 175: 450-457.
22. Van Uden, N. *Arch. Microbiol.* 1967; 58: 155-168.
23. Habig, W. H., Pabsy, M. J. and Jakoby, W. B. *J. Biol. Chem.* 1974; 249: 7130-7139.
24. Szas, G. *Clin. Chem* 1976; 22: 2051-2055.
25. Lowry, O. H., Rosenbrough, N. J., Farr, L. and Randall, R.J. *J. Biol. Chem.* 1951; 193: 265-275.
26. Anderson, M.E. *Methods in Enzymology Analysis* (Bergmeyer HU, ed) 1985, Academic Press, New York.
27. Sokal, R. R. and Rohlf, F. J. 1997 Biometry. W. H. Freeman, New York.

Metal Ions in Biology and Medicine: vol. 9. Eds Maria Carmen Alpoim, Paula Vasconcellos Morais, Maria Amélia Santos, Armando J. Cristóvão, José A. Centeno, Philippe Collery.
John Libbey Eurotext, Paris © 2006 pp. 175-1.

Bioaccumulation of metals in the Genus *Cinachyra (Porifera)* from the Mid-Atlantic Ridge

Gomes, T. C. M.; Serafim, M. A.; Company, R. S. & Bebianno, M. J.

Centre for Marine and Environmental Research, Faculty of Marine and Environmental Sciences, University of Algarve, Campus de Gambelas, 8005-139 Faro, Portugal, +351 289 800 953 (telephone), +351 289 818 353 (fax) tania_g@portugalmail.com; aserafim@ualg.pt, rcompany@ualg.pt, abebian@ualg.pt

Hydrothermal vents are one of the most extreme habitats of the deep sea, characterized by high pressure and temperature, as well as high concentrations of sulphides, methane and metals. The vent environments are metal-rich due to the presence of metal sulphides, e.g., iron, nickel, copper, zinc, cadmium and mercury, following discharge of vent waters, enriched with metals through leaching out of magmatic rocks. Sponges are one of the filter feeders that can be found on these extreme environments, although the information about these animals in hydrothermal vents is still scarce, as well as their relationship with metal concentrations.

The aim of the present study was to determine metal and metallothionein concentrations in marine sponges from the genus *Cinachyra* from Monte Saldanha hydrothermal vent.

After homogenisation of the sponge tissues, metal concentrations (cadmium, copper, zinc, nickel, iron, manganese, silver and vanadium) in total and subcellular fractions (insoluble and soluble) were determined by atomic absorption spectrophotometry, and metallothionein levels were determined by differential pulse polarography.

The results indicate that essential metals, essentially iron and zinc, are the most abundant metals in these sponges, while cadmium and silver are the less common. So, the pattern of accumulation of metals analysed was: Zn>Fe>Mn>Ni>V>Cu>Cd>Ag. In what concerns their subcellular distribution, cadmium and zinc showed similar distribution between the two fractions. As for manganese and silver, the insoluble fraction was generally more important than the soluble fraction, while for nickel, the soluble fraction was clearly the most significant. The metallothionein concentration in the genus *Cinachyra* is 224.47 ± 75.04 $\mu g.g^{-1}$ d.w.

These findings demonstrate that the high metal concentrations found in these sponges may be due to the enrichment of metals in the hydrothermal ecosystem, and that the pattern of accumulation of many of these metals reflects the dissolved metal concentrations in the surrounding environment.

The different distributions between soluble and insoluble fractions obtained, for each metal, illustrates the ability of these sponges to regulate their intracellular metal levels by different mechanisms of detoxification or accumulation in non-toxic forms. The presence of metallothioneins may most likely be one of them.

INTRODUCTION

The hydrothermal environment is characterized by high pressure and temperature, low pH, anoxia, as well as high concentrations of sulphides, methane and heavy metals. Hydrothermal activity occurs at seafloor spreading centers worldwide, originating from the penetration of seawater into cracked crustal basalt and its subsequent heating by magma chambers and hot rock reservoirs [1, 2].

Deep-sea hydrothermal communities live in the interfacial zone where hydrothermal fluids mix turbulently with bottom seawater. This instable environment provides a cyclical access to metal-rich vent waters, e.g., iron, nickel, copper, zinc, cadmium and mercury, enriched through leaching out of magmatic rocks [2, 3].

Biological communities can survive in this toxic environment due to their ability to regulate intracellular metal levels by excretion or accumulation in non-toxic forms. One of the detoxification processes that have been identified within hydrothermal organisms is the binding to specific and soluble ligands such as metallothioneins (MT) [4].

Sponges are one of the filter feeders that exist on hydrothermal environments [3], although the information about these animals is still scarce, as well as their relationship with metal concentrations.

So, the aim of the present study was to determine metal and metallothionein concentrations in marine sponges from the genus *Cinachyra* from Monte Saldanha hydrothermal vent, and study the relationships between metals and their subcelular distribution.

MATERIAL AND METHODS

Sponges from the genus *Cinachyra* were collected in the Mid-Atlantic Ridge hydrothermal vent Monte Saldanha *(fig. 1)* in the summer 2002 during the SEAHMA cruise and immediately frozen in liquid nitrogen.

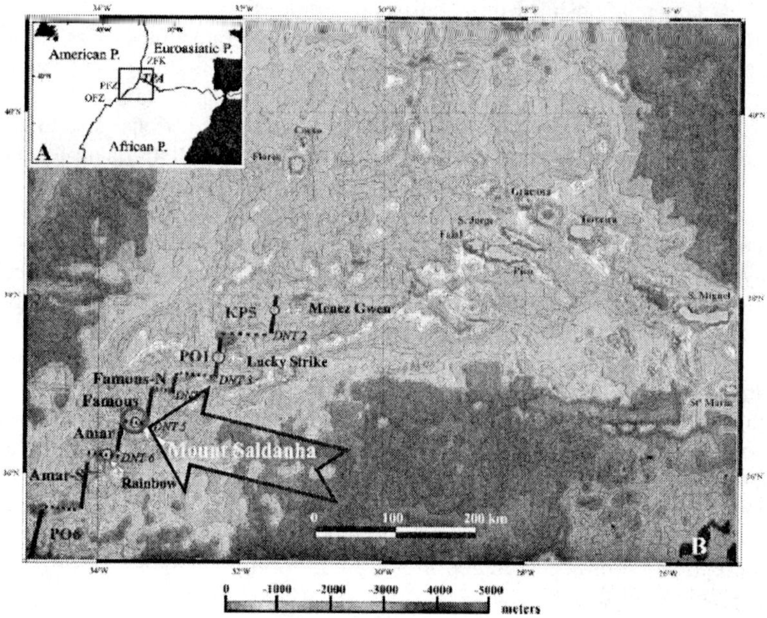

Fig. 1. Bathymetric map showing Mount Saldanha hydrothermal vent in the Mid-Atlantic Ridge, adapted from [5].

To characterize metal-binding compounds, sponge tissues were homogenised in three volumes of a Tris-HCl buffer (20 mM pH=8.6), and centrifuged at 30 000 *g* for 45 minutes (4°C) to separate the soluble and insoluble fractions. The soluble fraction was heat-treated at 80°C for 10 minutes, and centrifuged at 30 000 *g* for another 45 minutes (4°C) to separate the soluble heat-stable thiolic compounds (including MT).

MT analysis

The quantification of metallothionein (MT) was performed on aliquots of the heat-treated cytosol by Differential Pulse Polarography, according to the method developed by [6]. Standard addition method was used for calibration with rabbit liver MT-1 (Sigma), in the lack of a sponge MT standard. The results were expressed in μg $MT.g^{-1}$ dry weight.

Metal analysis

Metal analysis was performed on dried samples of the homogenate, insoluble fraction and heat-treated cytosol (soluble fraction), after a wet digestion in a microwave oven with 2 ml of nitric acid and 0.5 ml of H_2O_2. After digestion, metal levels were determined by flame (Zn, Fe) or graphite furnace atomic absorption spectrophotometry (Cd, Cu, Ni, Mn, Ag, V). Results are expressed on a dry tissue weight basis.

Statistics

The data was analysed to detect existent relationships between metal fractions, using linear regression ($p<0.05$).

RESULTS

Metallothionein concentration and metal distribution between soluble and insoluble fractions

Table 1 express metallothionein in the heat-treated cytosol and total metal concentrations in the homogenate of the sponges from the Genus *Cinachyra*. Essential metals, basically iron and zinc, are the most abundant in these sponges, while cadmium and silver are the less accumulated. Metal concentrations in the sponges resulted in a pattern of decreasing order: Zn>Fe>Mn>Ni>V>Cu>Cd>Ag.

MT in the heat-treated cytosol from the genus *Cinachyra* is 224.47 ± 75.04 $\mu g.g^{-1}$ d.w.

Table 1. MT ($\mu g.g^{-1}$ d.w.) and total metal concentrations ($\mu g.g^{-1}$ d.w. and $mg.g^{-1}$ d.w.) in sponges from the Genus *Cinachyra* collected in Mount Saldanha hydrothermal vent.

	Metal concentrations								MT
	$\mu g.g^{-1}$ d.w.				$mg.g^{-1}$ d.w.				μg.g-1 d.w.
	Cd	**Cu**	**V**	**Ag**	**Zn**	**Mn**	**Fe**	**Ni**	
m	2.045	18.400	76.267	0.621	6.463	0.667	3.873	0.373	224.47
s	0.730	8.534	60.367	0.159	2.186	0.464	2.322	0.147	75.04

m-median; s-standard deviation; d.w. - dry weight

The influence of increasing concentrations of total accumulated metals on their distribution between soluble and insoluble fractions has only been observed for cadmium, zinc, manganese, nickel and silver *(fig. 2)*. In the case of cadmium and zinc, there is a nearly equal distribution between the two fractions *(figs. 2A and B)*, for manganese and silver, the insoluble fraction was generally more important than the soluble fraction throughout the range of total metal concentrations *(figs. 2C and D)*, while for nickel, the soluble fraction was clearly the most significant *(fig. 2E)*.

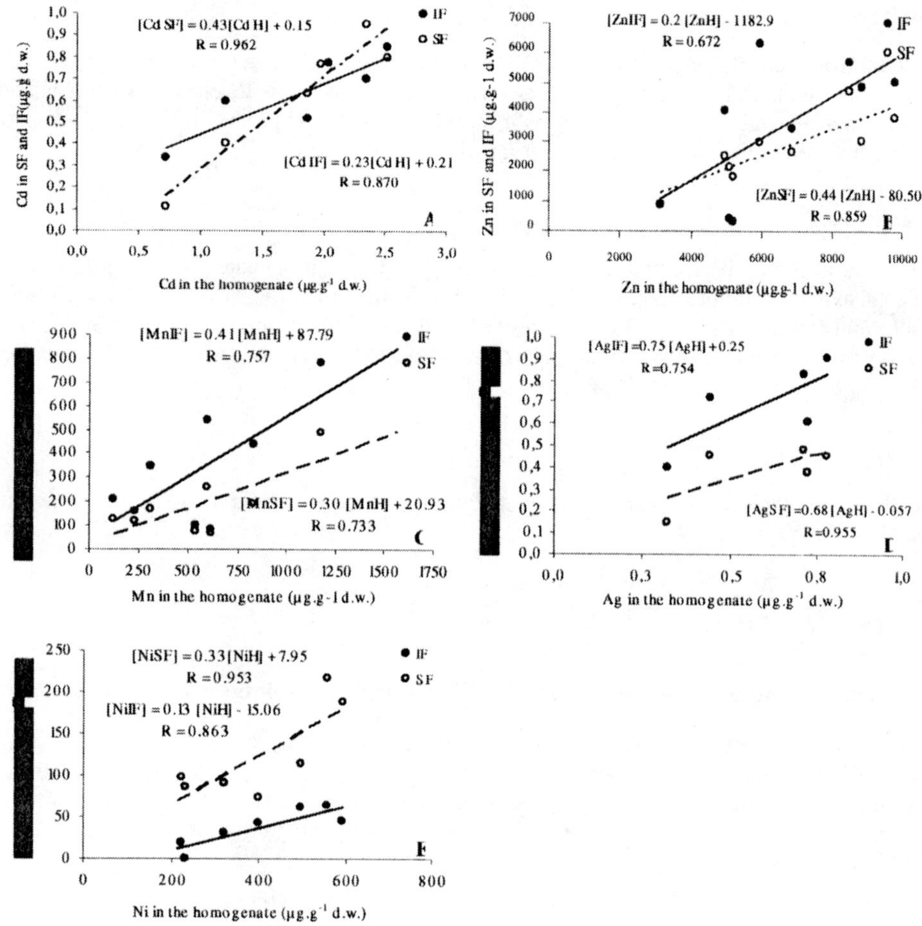

Fig. 2. Relations between total metal concentrations and subcelular fractions (soluble and insoluble, µg.g-1 d.w.) of the sponges from the Genus *Cinachyra* from Monte Saldanha hydrothermal vent. ● Insoluble Fraction ○ Soluble Fraction

DISCUSSION

In the sponges from the Genus *Cinachyra* essential metals, essentially Fe and Zn are the most abundant, while Cd and Ag are the less abundant. In hydrothermal fluids Fe and Mn are the most abundant transition metals in the Mid-Atlantic Ridge hydrothermal fluids. The enrichment of these two metals is usually associated with enrichment of other transition metals, potentially toxic. Zn and Cu are intermediately abundant in proportions ranging between 1 and 10% of the iron content, while several others transition metals (e.g. Cd, Pb, Ag and Sb) range from a few nanomoles per kilogram to a few tens of nanomoles per kilogram of fluid [3, 7].

So, our findings demonstrate that high metal concentrations in these sponges may be due to the enrichment of metals in the hydrothermal ecosystem, and the pattern of accumulation of many of these metals reflect the dissolved metal concentrations in the surrounding environment. In fact, previous studies on accumulation of metals in marine sponges from coastal areas showed that accumulation of dissolved metals in sponges is directly related with the dissolved metals in the medium, reflecting the degree of contamination of the nearby water [8, 9, 10, 11].

The distribution of metals in the subcelular fractions showed that Cd, Zn, Mn, Ag and Ni concentrations in the soluble fraction increased with increasing total concentrations. The result obtained for Zn is consistent with the findings reported by [12], in *Spongia officinalis* from the French Mediterranean coast, but inconsistent for Ag, where the percentage was similar in the insoluble and insoluble fractions.

Analyses of cleaned skeletons and whole sponges from coastal areas indicate that the preferential sites for metal accumulation within sponges are the living tissue, skeleton and gemmules [9, 13, 14]. In fact, previous findings in *Spongia officinalis* showed that Cu is equally distributed between the skeleton and the living tissue; Ni, Hg, Mn and Cd are mainly in the living tissue; while others like Fe, Zn, Pb and V are fixed in the skeleton. Among the metals fixed on the skeleton, Fe can reach up to 7.5% of the skeleton dry weight [14]. The distribution between soluble and insoluble fractions of each metal illustrates the ability of these sponges to regulate their intracellular metal levels by different mechanisms of detoxification or accumulation in non-toxic forms. The presence of some metals in the soluble fraction of sponges is important because the cytosol is a metabolically active compartment, and metals can bind to proteins like MTs.

The studies of metal effect in sponge populations lead to the hypothesis that their capacity to link to metals is possible because of presence of proteins like metallothioneins [15]. MT concentrations in the sponges from the Genus *Cinachyra* are 224.47 ± 75.04 μg.g^{-1} d.w. The presence of MTs has also been reported in several sponge species from coastal areas, *Spongia officinalis* [12], *Suberites domuncula* [15] and *Microciona prolifera* [16]. The different concentrations found in all these sponges may be related to the metal concentration that can be found in their tissues. Sponges from polluted sites (like *Spongia officinalis*) have higher MT (4.9 ± 0.8 mg.g^{-1} d.w., 3.9 ± 0.5 mg.g^{-1} d.w. and 4.7 ± 1.3 mg.g^{-1} d.w.) [12], while those from non polluted areas (like *Microciona prolifera*) have lower values (10.01 ± 1.053 μg.g^{-1} d.w.) [16]. However, the relationship between metals and MTs is difficult to explain, although some studies reported relationships between some metals and MT, hypothesising that they can be potential inducers of MTs [12]. Nevertheless, there is a need for more studies to identify the biological significance between metals and MTs in this hydrothermal vent genus, as well as the characterization of their MTs and the mechanism of detoxification used to support these extreme conditions.

REFERENCES

1. Ruelas-Inzunza J., Soto L. A., Páez-Osuna F. Heavy-metal accumulation in the hydrothermal vent clam *Vesicomya gigas* from Guaymas basin, Gulf of California. *Deep-Sea research I* 2003; 50: 757-761.
2. Cosson R. P., Vivier J. P. Interaction of metallic elements and organisms within hydrothermal vents. *Cahiers Le Biologie Marine* 1997; 38: 43-50.
3. Desbruyères D., Almeida A., Biscoito M., Comtet T., Khripounoff N, Sarradin P. M., Segonzac M. A review of the distribution of hydrothermal vent communities along the northern Mid-Atlantic Ridge: dispersal vs. environmental controls. *Hydrobiologia* 2000; 440: 201-216.
4. Rousse N., Boulegue J., Cosson R. P., Fiala-Medioni A. Bioaccumulation dês métaux chez le mytilidae hydrothermal *Bathymodiolus* sp. de la ride médio-atlantique. *Oceanologica acta* 1998 ; 21(4): 597-607.
5. Dias A., Barriga F. J. A. S. Mineralogy and geochemistry of hydrothermal sediments from the serpentine-hosted Saldanha hydrothermal field. *Marine Geology* 2006; 225: 157-175.
6. Bebianno M.J., Langston W.J. Quantification of metallothioneins in marine invertebrates using differential pulse polarography. *Portugaliæ Electrochimica Acta* 1989; 7: 59-64.
7. Douville E., Charlou J. L., Donval J. P., Knoery J., Fouquet Y., Bienvenu P., Appriou P. Trace elements in fluids from the new Rainbow hydrothermal field (36° 14' N, MAR): a comparison with other Mid-Atlantic fluids. *Eos Tran Am Geophys Union* 1997; 78 (46): 832.
8. Hansen I. V., Weeks J. M., Depledge M. H. Accumulation of copper, zinc, cadmium and chromium by the marine sponge *Halichondria panicea* pallas and the implications for biomonitoring. *Marine Pollution Bulletin* 1995; 31: 133-138.
9. Richelle-Maurer E., Degoudenne Y., de Vyver G. Van. Some aspects of heavy metal tolerance in fresh-

water sponges. In: Van Soest R. W. M., Van Kempen T. M. G., Braekman J. C., eds. *Sponges in Time and Space*. Netherlands: A. A. Balkema, 1994: 351-354.
10. Richelle E., Degoudenne Y., Van de Vyer G., Dejonghe L. Experimental and field studies on effect of selected heavy metals on three freshwater sponge species: *Ephydatia fluviatilis, Ephydatia muelleri & Spongilla lacustris. Arch hydrobiol* 1995 ; 135: 209-231.
11. Pérez T., Longet D., Schembri T., Rebouiloon P., Vacelet J. Effects of 12 years' operation of a sewage treatment pant on trace metal occurrence within a Mediterranean commercial sponge (*Spongia officinalis*, Demospongiae). *Marine Pollution Bulletin* 2005; 50: 301-309.
12. Berthet B., Mouneyrac C., Pérez T., Amiard-Triquet C. Metallothionein in sponges *(Spongia officinalis)* as a biomarker of metal contamination. *Comp Bioch Phys* 2005; 141: 306-313.
13. Vacelet J., Verdenal B., Perinet G. The iron mineralization of *Spongia officinalis* L. (Porifera, Dictyoceratida) and its relationships with the collagen skeleton. *Biology of the cell* 1988; 62: 189-198.
14. Verdenal B., Diana C., Arnoux A., Vacelet J. Pollutant levels in mediterranean commercial sponges. In: Rutzler K., ed. *New perspectives in sponge biology*. Washington D. C.: Smithsonian Institution press, 1990: 516-524.
15. Schröeder H. C., Shostak K., Gamulin V., Lacorn M., Skorokhod A., Kavsan V., Müller W. E. G. Purification, cDNA cloning and expression of a cadmium-inducible cysteine-rich metallothionein-like protein from the marine sponge *Suberites domuncula. Marine Ecology Progress Series* 2000; 200: 149-157.
16. Philp R. B. Cadmium content of the marine sponge *Microciona prolifera*, other sponges, water and sediment from the eastern Florida panhandle: possible effects on *Microciona* cell aggregation and potential roles of low pH and low salinity. *Comparative Biochemistry and Physiology Part C*. 1999; 124: 41-49.

Metal Ions in Biology and Medicine: vol. 9. Eds Maria Carmen Alpoim, Paula Vasconcellos Morais, Maria Amélia Santos, Armando J. Cristóvão, José A. Centeno, Philippe Collery.
John Libbey Eurotext, Paris © 2006 pp. 181-1.

Temporal trend in metal levels in soils and vegetation near a municipal solid waste incinerator. Human health risks.

Mari M, Ferré-Huguet N, Nadal M, Schuhmacher M, Domingo JL*

*Laboratory of Toxicology and Environmental Health, School of Medicine, "Rovira i Virgili" University, San Lorenzo 21, 43201, Reus, Catalonia, Spain. * joseluis.domingo@urv.net*

INTRODUCTION

Municipal solid wastes typically contain metals such as mercury (Hg), lead (Pb), copper (Cu), zinc (Zn), manganese (Mn), chromium (Cr) or cobalt (Co), among others. Toxic metals may appear in the effluents of different combustion processes, and consequently may be emitted by municipal solid waste incinerators (MSWIs) and hazardous waste incinerators (HWIs). Since 1991, a MSWI has been operating in Tarragona (Catalonia, Spain). In 1994, a wide surveillance program was initiated in order to provide information on the environmental impact and the health risks of metals, and dioxins and furans (PCDD/Fs) in the surroundings of the MSWI [1, 2]. Soils and herbage were chosen as indicators of long-term and short-term environmental pollution, respectively. With respect to metals, according to the results, the impact of the MSWI was not relevant in comparison to other potential emission sources located in the same area.

In 2002, a 4-year environmental surveillance program was again started. During this period, soil and herbage samples were periodically monitored for metals and PCDD/Fs. In this paper, the levels of metals in soils and herbage collected in the vicinity of the MSWI between 2002 and 2005 are reported. They are compared with the concentrations found in the 1999 survey. Moreover, the potential health risks for the local population potentially exposed to metals were also assessed and are here reported.

MATERIALS AND METHODS

Sampling

Between 2002 and 2005, herbage (*Pipatherum paradoxum* L.) and soil samples were alternatively collected in the vicinity of the MSWI. Twenty-four sampling locations were chosen, considering different distances (250, 500, 750, 1000, 1250 and 1500 m) and wind directions (NE, NW, SE and SW) from the MSWI stack. Herbage was sampled in 2002 and 2004, while soils were taken in 2003 and 2005. Herbage samples were obtained by cutting at about 5 cm from the ground, properly stored in a double-aluminum fold, and dried at room temperature until analyses. In turn, soil samples were taken from the upper 3 cm and stored in polyethylene bags. They were dried at room temperature until constant weight. Subsequently, they were sieved through a 2-mm mesh screen to get a homogeneous grain distribution. Further details about sampling were previously reported [3-5].

Analytical procedure

Approximately 0.50 g of dried soil or herbage samples were treated with 5 ml of nitric acid (Suprapur, 65% purity, E. Merck, Darmstadt, Germany) in teflon bombs. Samples were digested following the same methodology used in previous surveys [4]. The concentrations of As, Be, Cd, Cr, Hg, Mn, Pb, Tl and V in soils were determined by inductively coupled plasma spectrometry (ICP-MS, Perkin Elmer Elan 6000), while atomic absorption spectrophotometry with graphite furnace atomization (AAS, Varian spectrophotometer, Spectra A-30) was used to determine the levels of Ni. In turn, the levels of As, Be, Cd, Hg, Mn, Pb and Tl in herbage were determined by ICP-MS, whereas those of Cr, Ni and V were analyzed by AAS-GF [6, 7]. The analytical procedures were checked by using triplicates, controls and standards. The limits of detection in soils were the following: 0.1 µg/g for As, 0.25 µg/g for Be, Cr and V, 0.03 µg/g for Mn, Cd, Pb and Tl, 0.01 µg/g for Ni, and 0.05 µg/g for Hg. In herbage, the detection limits were 0.02 µg/g for Pb, Mn, Cr and Cd, 0.01 µg/g for Ni, 0.1 µg/g for As, 0.03 µg/g for Tl and V, 0.05 µg/g for Hg, and 0.25 µg/g for Be.

Health risks and statistics

The estimation of risks to metals for the local population was carried out by two pathways: ingestion and inhalation [8, 9]. For calculations, when an element showed a value under its detection limit, the metal concentration was assumed to be one-half of that limit of detection (ND = 1/2 LOD). Statistical significance was computed by one way analysis of variance (ANOVA) followed by Student's t-test or by the Kruskal-Wallis test. Probabilities of 0.05 or lower were considered as significant. Statistical analysis was carried out using the SPSS-13.0 Statistical Software Package.

RESULTS AND DISCUSSION

Environmental monitoring program

The mean concentrations of the analyzed elements in soil and herbage samples collected in the vicinity of the MSWI of Tarragona in various surveys between 1999 and 2005 are summarized in *table 1*. The temporal variation (percentages) between the samplings is also shown. In soils, the highest concentrations corresponded to Mn and Pb. With respect to the temporal trends, the levels of As, Cr, Hg, Mn, Ni, Tl and V showed a significant reduction between 1999 and 2005. Only Cd and Pb concentrations notably increased during this period, but not in a significant way.

When the 2005 levels were compared to those corresponding to the immediately previous survey (2003), a significant reduction was observed for As, Cr, Mn, Ni, Tl and V concentrations in soils collected near the MSWI. In contrast, the increased concentrations noted for some elements did not reach the level of statistical significance ($p<0.05$). In any case, the current (2005) concentrations were similar (or even lower) to those found in previous surveys performed near the HWI of Tarragona [10, 11], as well as in other industrial areas of Catalonia [7, 12]. Moreover, the levels here found are in the low part of the range of those reported by a number of authors in various soils worldwide [13-16].

In all surveys, the levels of Be and Tl in herbage were below their respective analytical detection limits (0.25 and 0.03 µg/g, respectively), while the highest levels corresponded also to Mn *(table 1)*. Between 1999 to 2004, the concentrations of all analyzed elements significantly diminished ($p<0.001$). Because of the ban on the use of leaded gasoline [17], the content of Pb in herbage samples reflected an important reduction. The differences found between different surveys in metal concentrations in herbage samples would be probably due to the heterogeneity of the samples rather than to the potential differences in the atmospheric concentrations of metals in the area under study. On the other hand, although in the period 2002-2004 some metals (i.e., Cr, Mn, Ni, Pb) showed lower concentrations in herbage, the level of statistical significance for these decreases was only reached by Pb ($p<0.01$). The levels of As, Cd and Hg in 2004 were higher than those found in the previous survey (2002). However, V concentrations showed a significant increase between both surveys (75.2%, p<0.001). Anyhow, the 2005 metal concentrations in herbage samples collected near the MSWI of Tarragona seemed to be similar or even lower than those reported by a number of authors in different vegetal species [18, 19].

Table 1. Metal concentrations (µg/g ± SD) in soil and herbage samples collected near the MSWI of Tarragona (Catalonia, Spain).

Soil	1999	2003	2005	%1999-2005	%2003-2005
As	5.56 ± 3.45	5.99 ± 1.26	1.71 ± 0.62	-69.24**	-71.45***
Be	0.33 ± 0.12	0.34 ± 0.15		ND	--- ND
Cd	0.15 ± 0.06	0.20 ± 0.11	0.22 ± 0.09	46.67	10.00
Cr	11.30 ± 4.25	14.99 ± 5.67	4.57 ± 2.44	-59.55**	-69.51***
Hg	0.06 ± 0.02	0.03 ± 0.02	0.03 ± 0.01	-50.00**	-16.67
Mn	223.96 ± 72.13	241.2 ± 56.01	158.70 ± 45.49	-29.15**	-34.20***
Ni	8.75 ± 2.87	10.84 ± 6.17	2.06 ± 0.64	-76.49**	-81.03***
Pb	25.68 ± 21.44	29.7 ± 14.54	33.74 ± 34.76	31.28	13.75
Tl	0.06 ± 0.02	0.12 ± 0.04	0.02 ± 0.01	-66.48**	-83.24***
V	16.00 ± 4.20	20.48 ± 5.10	7.55 ± 1.83	-52.84**	-63.16***
Herbage	**1999**	**2002**	**2004**	**%1999-2004**	**%2002-2004**
As	0.13 ± 0.01	0.08 ± 0.05	0.09 ± 0.04	-34.65**	13.87
Be	ND	ND	ND	---	---
Cd	0.03 ± 0.02	0.02 ± 0.01	0.02 ± 0.02	-39.26***	3.54
Cr	0.27 ± 0.15	0.69 ± 1.32	0.01 ± 0.00	-96.78***	-98.73
Hg	0.10 ± 0.00	0.03 ± 13.45	0.03 ± 0.00	-66.62***	6.72
Mn	36.20 ± 1.32	31.54 ± 10.97	28.12 ± 13.57	-12.87***	-10.86
Ni	1.02 ± 0.65	0.77 ± 2.78	0.40 ± 12.74	-61.00***	-48.20
Pb	1.22 ± 0.92	0.73 ± 0.42	0.48 ± 0.37	-60.66***	-34.03**
Tl	ND	ND	ND	---	---
V	0.60 ± 0.34	0.22 ± 0.15	0.39 ± 0.19	-35.07	75.20***

ND = not detected. Asterisks indicate significant differences at: * p<0.05; ** p<0.01; *** p<0.001.

Human health risk assessment

The Hazard Quotient (HQ) was calculated by comparing the predicted exposure through ingestion and the oral reference dose for each element. The values of HQ for adults and children living in the vicinity of the MSWI are depicted in *figure 1*. The maximum HQ corresponded to V in 2005 with levels of $1.49 \cdot 10^{-2}$ and $2.78 \cdot 10^{-2}$ for adults and children, respectively. However, the quotient was below the safety level of 1. Similar results were also found in recent investigations performed in a petrochemical zone and close to a HWI, which are both located near the MSWI here evaluated [11, 12].

The non-carcinogenic risks for As, Be, Cd, total Cr, Hg, Mn, Ni, Tl and V in soils are shown in *figure 2A*. These risks were calculated by comparing the metal concentrations in soil with the Preliminary Remediation Goals (PRG) developed by the US EPA [20], which are considered as safe levels for people. Although V and Mn showed the highest risks, their values were clearly below the safe level of 100%.

The carcinogenic risk for the population living near the MSWI is summarized in *table 2*. Cancer risk was calculated by using the daily intake through ingestion and inhalation as well as the corresponding slope factors. Considering a maximum acceptable risk of 10^{-6}, only As ingestion and inhalation, as well as Cr inhalation exceeded this value. However, it is important to remark that the threshold value for As has been often exceeded in soil samples from a number of countries [11]. In turn, inhalation of Cr might mean some risk because it was conservatively assumed that Cr^{6+} was 1/6 of total Cr. Consequently, the maximum allowed level may be easily exceeded.

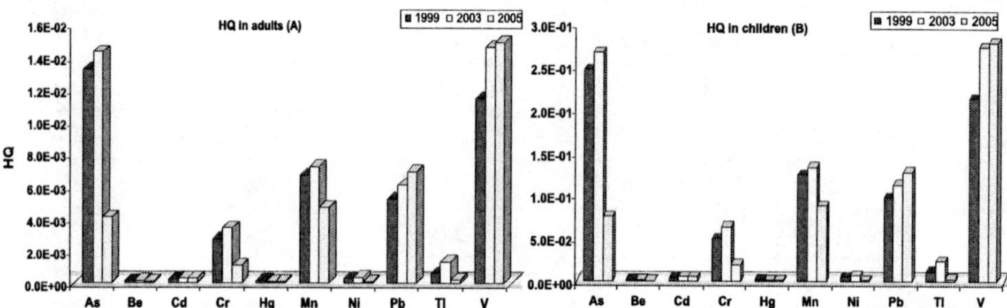

Fig. 1. Hazard quotients for adults (A) and children (B) living near the MSWI of Tarragona (Catalonia, Spain).

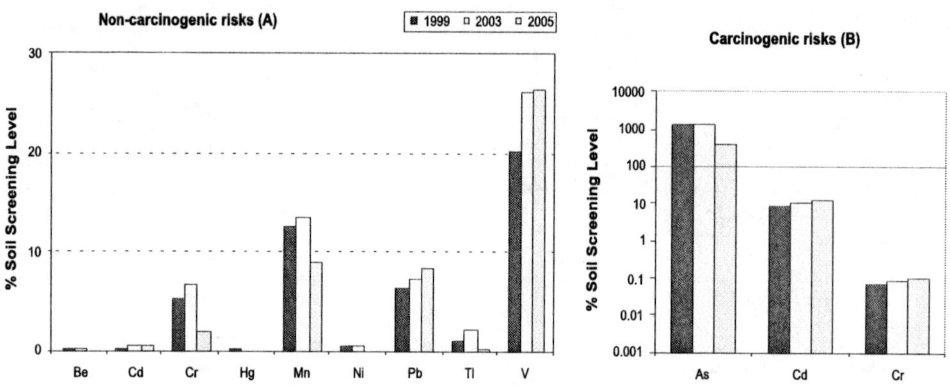

Fig. 2. Non-carcinogenic (A) and carcinogenic (B) risks for the population living near the MSWI of Tarragona (Catalonia, Spain). Comparison between the metal concentrations in soils and the Preliminary Remediation Goals.

To assess carcinogenic risks, the metal concentrations in soil samples corresponding to the period 1999-2005 were compared to the PRG for As, Cd and Cr [20] *(fig. 2B)*. The carcinogenic risks for Cd and Cr were clearly below 100%, while As levels in soils were approximately 10 times higher than the cancer endpoint in the PRG (0.39 µg/g). Soil screening levels for As were 1430, 1540 and 440%, in 1999, 2003 and 2005, respectively. Although in soil samples As concentration was higher in the last survey (2005), this level was lower than those found in the previous survey. It means an important decrease of the carcinogenic risk. Similar results were shown in studies performed in a petrochemical area and a HWI near to the MSWI here examined [11, 12].

Table 2. Risk of cancer due to oral and inhalation exposures to metals from soils of the levels for adults and children living in the vicinity of the MSWI of Tarragona (Catalonia, Spain).

		Adults				Children			
		CSF (kg day/mg)	1999	2003	2005	CSF (kg day/mg)	1999	2003	2005
Oral	As	1.5	2.6E-06	2.8E-06	7.9E-07	15.0	9.5E-06	1.0E-05	2.9E-06
Inhalation	As	15.1	2.6E-05	2.8E-05	7.9E-06	6.5	4.1E-05	4.4E-05	1.3E-05
	Be	8.4	8.5E-07	8.7E-07	3.3E-07	3.6	1.4E-06	1.4E-06	5.3E-07
	Cd	6.3	3.0E-07	3.9E-07	4.2E-07	2.7	4.7E-07	6.2E-07	6.7E-07
	Cr	42.0	1.5E-04	1.8E-04	5.9E-05	18.0	2.3E-04	3.0E-04	9.4E-05

CSF: Cancer Slope Factor for oral (ingestion) and inhalation exposure.

In summary, the relatively low metal concentrations in soils and herbage here found indicate that the MSWI of Tarragona is not a relevant source of metals for the surrounding environment. However, as it has been suggested in previous investigations carried out in the vicinity of various MSWIs, metal contamination resulting from these facilities is rather difficult to detect in environments with other metal pollution sources [1, 7, 16, 21]. With respect to the human health risks, the presence of the MSWI here assessed should not mean, in principle, significant non-carcinogenic or carcinogenic risks for the population living in the surroundings. However, as it has been concluded in previous investigations carried out in the same sampling area [11, 12], some efforts should be focused on reducing the environmental levels of As and Cr in the industrial zone of Tarragona.

REFERENCES

1. Llobet JM, Granero S, Schuhmacher M, Domingo JL. Temporal variation in metal concentrations in soils and vegetation in the vicinity of a municipal solid waste incinerator. *Toxicol Environ Chem* 1999; 71: 63-73.
2. Schuhmacher M, Domingo JL, Granero S, Llobet JM, Eljarrat E, Rivera J. Soil monitoring in the vicinity of a municipal solid waste incinerator: Temporal variation of PCDD/Fs. *Chemosphere* 1999; 39: 419-29.
3. Schuhmacher M, Xifro A, Llobet JM, de Kok HAM, Domingo JL. PCDD/Fs in soil samples collected in the vicinity of a municipal solid waste incinerator: human health risks. *Arch Environ Contam Toxicol* 1997; 33: 239-46.
4. Schuhmacher M, Granero S, Xifro A, Domingo JL, Rivera J, Eljarrat E. Levels of PCDD/Fs in soil samples in the vicinity of a municipal solid waste incinerator. *Chemosphere* 1998; 37: 2127-37.
5. Domingo JL, Schuhmacher M, Llobet JM, Muller L, Rivera J. PCDD/F concentrations in soil and vegetation in the vicinity of a municipal waste incinerator after a pronounced decrease in the emissions of PCDD/Fs from the facility. *Chemosphere* 2001; 43: 217-26.
6. Meneses M, Llobet JM, Granero S, Schuhmacher M, Domingo JL. Monitoring metals in the vicinity of a municipal waste incinerator: temporal variation in soils and vegetation. *Sci Total Environ* 1999; 226: 157-64.
7. Llobet JM, Schuhmacher M, Domingo JL. Spatial distribution and temporal variation of metals in the vicinity of a municipal solid waste incinerator after a modernization of the flue gas cleaning systems of the facility. *Sci Total Environ* 2002; 284: 205-14.
8. Abrahams PW. Soils: their implications to human health. *Sci Total Environ* 2002; 291: 1-32.
9. Granero S, Domingo JL. Levels of metals in soils of Alcala de Henares, Spain: human health risks. *Environ Int* 2002; 28: 159-64.
10. Llobet JM, Schuhmacher M, Domingo JL. Observations on metal trends in soil and vegetation samples

collected in the vicinity of a hazardous waste incinerator under construction (1996-1998). *Toxicol Environ Chem* 2000; 77: 119-29.
11. Nadal M, Bocio A, Schuhmacher M, Domingo JL. Monitoring metals in the population living in the vicinity of a hazardous waste incinerator: levels in hair of school children. *Biol Trace Elem Res* 2005; 104: 203-13.
12. Nadal M, Schuhmacher M, Domingo JL. Metal pollution of soils and vegetation in an area with petrochemical industry. *Sci Total Environ 2004*; 321: 59-69.
13. Loska K, Wiechula D, Korus I. Metal contamination of farming soils affected by industry. *Environ Int* 2004; 30: 159-65.
14. Chen TB, Zheng YM, Lei M, Huang ZC, Wu HT, Chen H, Fan KK, Yu K, Wu X, Tian QZ. Assessment of heavy metal pollution in surface soils of urban parks in Beijing, China. *Chemosphere* 2005; 60: 542-51.
15. Ruiz-Cortés E, Reinoso R, Díaz-Barrientos E, Madrid L, Concentrations of potentially toxic metals in urban soils of Seville: Relationship with different land uses. *Environ Geochem Health* 2005; 27: 465-74.
16. Rimmer DL, Vizard CG, Pless-Mulloli T, Singleton I, Air VS, Keatinge ZA. Metal contamination of urban soils in the vicinity of a municipal waste incinerator: One source among many. *Sci Total Environ*; in press.
17. Belles, M, Rico A, Schuhmacher M, Domingo JL, Corbella J. Reduction of lead concentrations in vegetables grown in Tarragona Province, Spain, as a consequence of reduction of lead in gasoline. *Environ Int* 1995; 21: 821-25.
18. Schuhmacher M, Agramunt MC, Bocio A, Domingo JL, de Kok HAM. Annual variation in the levels of metals and PCDD/PCDFs in soil and herbage samples collected near a cement plant. *Environ Int* 2003; 29: 415-21.
19. Bosco ML, Varrica D, Dongarra G. Case study: Inorganic pollutants associated with particulate matter from an area near a petrochemical plant. *Environ Res* 2005; 99: 18-30.
20. US EPA. Preliminary Remediation Goals; 2004. Available at www.epa.gov/region09/waste/sfund/prg/index.html.
21. Capuano F, Cavalchi B, Martinelli G, Pecchini G, Renna E, Scaroni I, Bertacchi M, Bigliardi G. Environmental prospection for PCDD/PCDF, PAH, PCB and heavy metals around the incinerator power plant of Reggio Emilia town (Northern Italy) and surrounding main roads. *Chemosphere* 2005; 58: 1563-69.

ACKNOWLEDGEMENTS

This study was financially supported by SIRUSA, Tarragona, Spain.

Metal Ions in Biology and Medicine: vol. 9. Eds Maria Carmen Alpoim, Paula Vasconcellos Morais, Maria Amélia Santos, Armando J. Cristóvão, José A. Centeno, Philippe Collery.
John Libbey Eurotext, Paris © 2006 pp. 187-1.

Rhizofiltration of uranium from contaminated mine waters

Paulo, C.[(1)]; Pratas, J.; Rodrigues, N.

(1) Earth Sciences Department, Faculty of Sciences and Technology of the University of Coimbra, Largo Marquês de Pombal, 3000-272 Coimbra, Portugal. carlos.januario@gmail.com

ABSTRACT

This study presents the preliminary results of a prototype phyto-system, based on rhizofiltration, to reduce the uranium concentration in waters emanating from mine effluents. The species *Callitriche stagnalis* Scop., *Potamogeton natans* L. and *Potamogeton pectinatus* L. of the vegetable community of the uraniferous region of Beiras were selected because they are autochthonous and they show high accumulation levels.

The installed prototype consists of a closed circuit of channels. The system was initially contaminated with 500 µg/L of U as uranyl. The performance of this system was very effective. The uranium concentration in the water dropped to 220 µg/L in 24 hours and after two weeks it had decreased to 72.3 µg/L. The concentration in C. stagnalis increased from 0.98 to 1567 mg/kg, in P. natans increased from 3.46 to 270.9 mg/kg and in P. pectinatus increased from 2.63 to 1588 mg/kg. The results show the effectiveness of these plants to remove uranium from the water.

INTRODUCTION

Numerous old uranium mines of the Beiras region, Portugal, still represent a high environmental health risk due to the radioactivity of their residues. The recorded concentration of uranium in the waters of their vicinity varies from 30 µg/L to 1000 µg/L.

The selection of an environmental remediation methodology must be based on several criteria such as characteristics of the contaminated area, nature of the pollutants, their bioavailability and efficiency of the technology. Research efforts are searching less expensive and more environmental friendly methodologies. Phytoremediation techniques are being proposed as viable alternatives to traditional remediation methodologies which often are inefficient in dealing with large quantities of residues with low to medium contamination. The phytoremediation techniques derive from the natural capacity of the plants to accumulate metals and/or organic compounds. Their direct use is possible to remediate *in situ* contaminated soils, mud, sediments, and waters [1, 2, 3].

The metal accumulation capacity of aquatic plants has been known for some time and it suggests the possibility of using them in specific phyto-systems based on phytoremediation techniques such as rhizofiltration [4]. This technique is particularly suited for the decontamination of aqueous substrates. It can target metals like Pb, Cd, Ni, Cu, Cr, V, organic compounds and also radionuclides like U, Cs and Sr [3, 5]. Usually, this technique involves the hydroponic culture of plants in the contaminated system. Once the plants have successfully accumulated and stored the metals in their tissues, they must be harvested and then they have to be safely disposed [3, 5, 7]. Several aquatic plant species have been identified as natural hyperaccumulators of heavy metal and as a result they might prove useful on rhizofiltration methods. To name but a few *Eichhornia crassipes* (Mart.) Solms (U), *Lemna gibba* L. (As, U), *Azolla pinnata* R. Brown (Pb, Zn), *Myriophyllum aquaticum* (Vell.) Verdc. (Cu, Fe, Hg and Zn), *Ludwigina palustris (L.) Ell.* (Cu, Fe, Hg and Zn), *Ceratophylum demersum* L. (Cu, Cr, Fe, Mn and Pb) and *Mentha aquatica* L. (Cu, Fe, Hg and Zn) [2,

6, 8, 9, 10]. The use of hydrophyte species as biofilters of U and other radionuclides is not a new procedure. Pioneer studies seem to have been those of Timofeeva-Ressovskaia in the early fifties involving the development of a pilot phyto-system for depleted uranium rhizofiltration. This system was characterised by a cascading sequence of ponds. The contaminated water had to flow slowly through them. The system has been reported to have an efficiency of 99.3% of depleted uranium removal according to Dushenkov, S. [11].

Later, different U phyto-systems were developed and several aquatic species were identified as having practicable use. These were the cases of *Eichhornia crassipes* (Mart.) Solms, *Lemna gibba* L., *Lemna minor* L., *Callitriche stagnalis* Scop. [10, 12, 13, 14]. These systems are advantageous where continuous metal removal is necessary because the continuous growth of the biological material provides new opportunities for metal sequestration [2].

In spite of the advantages the rhizofiltration techniques are more prone to failure than other methods with similar costs. The dependence on temperature (which affects growth), the maintenance of the hydroponic solution, the difficulty in reproducing laboratory results in the field and, in most cases, the use of foreign plants, all these factors make rhizofiltration susceptible to failure [3, 7]. Some authors consider that fresh water plants are not very efficient in removing heavy metals from the water because they have a slow growth rate and a small rooting system in contrast with some terrestrial plants [15].

Therefore the selection of the adequate species for phyto-system composition represents an important step on the development of a rhizofiltration application. Our ongoing study aims to develop phyto-systems, based on rhizofiltration, with the ability to reduce uranium concentration in waters emanating from the mine effluents.

To minimize the rhizofiltration disadvantages several hydrophytes species of the vegetable community of the uraniferous region of Beiras were previously analysed to assess their uranium accumulation potential [14]. The endemicity and geographic distribution of aquatic species were established on the study area as important factors for future *in situ* applications. It was intended to exclude the invader factor so, in a previous study, we selected the species *Callitriche stagnalis* Scop. taking into account its surface distribution and its high Biological Absorption Coefficient (BAC) ($8,14 \times 10^3$). Even tough *Potamogeton natans* L. and *Potamogeton pectinatus* L. were not as common as *C. Stagnalis* they were also selected based on their ability to accumulate uranium.

The objective of the present study is to test the potential of these three species for the decontamination of uranium contaminated surface waters of former uranium mines. The preliminary results obtained in the laboratory with a prototype phyto-system are described.

MATERIAL AND METHODS

The following sub-sections describe the prototype setup, the species and the analytical procedures.

Rhizofiltration prototype

The installed prototype consists of 70 L of water flowing in a closed circuit of channels *(fig. 1)*. A modified hydroponic solution of Murashige-Skoog without PO_4 has been added to the water. The alteration on the solution was made because there was the possibility of the formation of uranium phosphate and, as a result, the uranyl bioavailability would have decreased [16]. Initially the system was contaminated with 500 µg of U/L as uranyl and the measured solution pH was 6,55. The water was then continuously pumped from tank 1 to tank 2 and a closed circuit established *(fig. 1)*.

In order to have a clean set up the plants were collected in a non-uraniferous area (Ribeira de Alveite, Poaires, Centre of Portugal, a sedimentary basin with no significant radionuclides). The initial biomass was about ninety grams.

Samples of the plants and of the water were then collected at the beginning of the test and after 1, 2, 7, and 15 days of continuous circulation. During this experimental period the atmospheric conditions and water temperature remained constant.

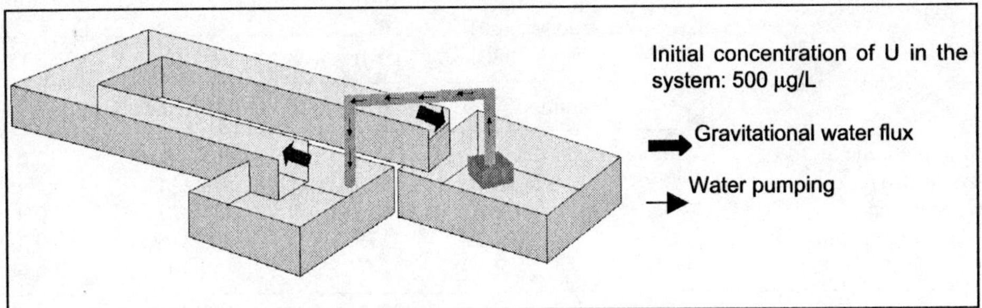

Fig. 1. Laboratory set up (Dimensions: about 3 m by 1 m

Uranium determination

A "Fluorat-02-2M" analyzer (built by Lumex, Russia) has been used for the determination of the mass concentration of uranium in the water and plant samples. In this device, the concentration of uranium in solution is deducted from the measured intensity of the delayed fluorescence of the uranyl-ions (λ=530 nm).

The water samples were filtered and acidified and then they were analysed by standard fluorometric analysis. For quality control of the results, a certified reference water produced by the National Water Research Institute of Canada (reference TMDA-62) has been used.

The plants were cleaned in running water and then they were dried in an oven at 60 °C. Following that they were ground and crushed for later chemical analysis. Fluorometry was the methodology adopted for the determination of the uranium content in the plants, as described in the work of Huffman, Jr. and Riley, 1970, and Van Loon and Barefoot, 1989 [17, 18]. Certified Virginia tobacco leaves (reference CTA-VTL-2, Polish certified reference material) have also been analysed to assure the quality of the analytical results.

RESULTS AND DISCUSSION

The variation of the uranium concentration measured in the plants and in the water during this exercise is shown in *table 1*. These results indicate that the system was performing very effectively. After two weeks the uranium concentration in the water had decreased to 72.32 µg/L *(fig. 2)*. It must be pointed that the water pH remained between 6 and 7 throughout the entire experience and this does not correspond to the pH of maximum bioavailability of uranyl [20]. The plants used in this phyto-system acted as U biofilters. The kinetics of U uptake by the plant species is very fast. After 24 hours the U concentration in *C. stagnalis* increased from 0.98 to 144.71 mg/kg, in *P. natans* increased from 3.46 to 270.9 mg/kg and in *P. pectinatus* increased from 2.63 to 1588 mg/kg *(fig. 3)*. The final values were 1567.08 mg/kg in *C.stagnalis*, 270.92 mg/kg in *P.natans* and 1588.02 mg/kg in *P. pectinatus*. The results demonstrate the effectiveness of these plants to remove uranium from the water *(table 1)*.

Table 1. Variation of uranium concentration in water and plants.

	Uranium Concentration in water (µg/L)				
Sample collection	Initial	1 d	2 d	7 d	15 d
Water	500	220	162.2	79.44	72.32
	Uranium Concentration in plants (mg/kg dried weight)				
Sample collection	Initial	1 d	2 d	7 d	15 d
Callitriche stagnalis	0.98	144.71	256.27	1082.90	1567.08
Potamogeton natans	3.46	97.45	205.01	239.79	270.92
Potamogeton pechinatus	2.63	675.35	755.79	1132.92	1588.02
Water U reduction (%)	0	56	67.56	84.11	85.54

Although we can consider the species tested in this phyto-system as U hyperaccumulators, their accumulation capacity reflects different toxicity responses. The *C. stagnalis* proved to be more tolerant to uranium contamination and *P. natans* the most sensitive. In this species the U uptake stabilized after 2 days in contrast with the others *(fig. 3)*. This behaviour is related to the toxicity level of each species, a factor which has not been determined in this study.

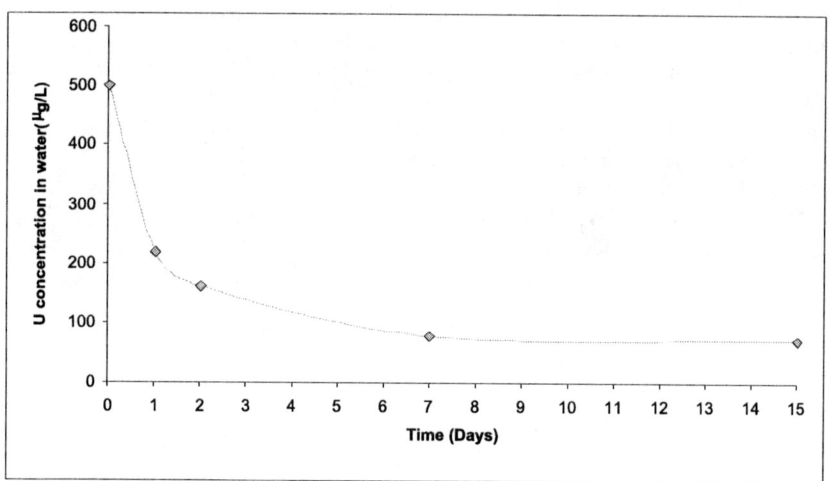

Fig. 2. Uranium concentration in water during the phyto-system activity

At the end of the experiment the concentration of U in the water was 72.32 µg/L or a reduction of 85.54% compared to the initial value. These results seem to indicate an exponential decay process. A mathematical exercise, with the logarithms of the values and the Excel function PROJ.LIN (in the English version corresponds to the function LINEST), provided the following function: $C_{water} = C^{0}_{water} \times e^{-kt}$ with C^{0}_{water} of about 250 µg/L and k about -0,2 day^{-1} (here we were testing an exponential decay process). Another trial-and-error exercise provided a better fit with a rectangular hyperbolic curve like $C_{water} = C_{initial} - \frac{C_{initial} \times t}{K + t}$, with $C_{initial}$ = 500 µg/L and K = 1 day (this curve reminds a "mirror" Michaelis-Menten equation, notice that for $t=K$, $C_{water} = 0,5 \times C_{initial}$). Naturally the data are insufficient and we do not attempt to draw statistically significant conclusions.

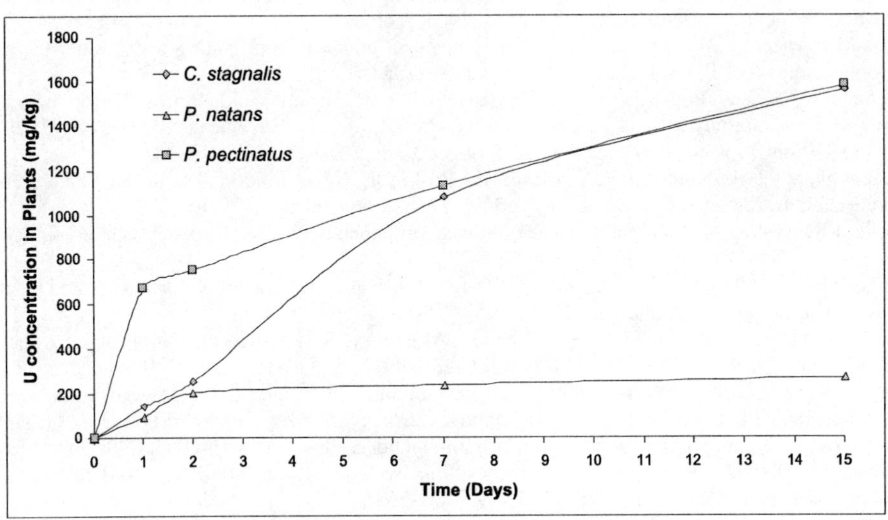

Fig. 3. Uranium uptake by plant biomass

CONCLUSIONS

The advantage of the phyto-system proposed in this study is related to the high tolerance of the species tested to U contamination and with their abundance and endemicity in the Portuguese rivers which prevent the invader factor for an *in situ* application. In fact, the endemic character of these species represents a very important factor for the establishment of this technology taking into account the sociability relationships with other aquatic species and their ecosystems adaptation.

The aquatic plants tested in the uranium rhizofiltraton prototype showed a high ability for U accumulation and, therefore, they can be useful choices for future *in situ*a pplications. The results described show a reduction of U concentration, in the water, from 500 to 72.32 µg/L of U thus representing an efficiency of 85.54%. The concentration in C. stagnalis increased from 0.98 to 1567 mg/kg, in P. natans increased from 3.46 to 270.9 mg/kg and in P. pectinatus increased from 2.63 to 1588 mg/kg. All these species showed a rapid U uptake.

It is our belief that a combination of several species, resembling the natural environment, can prove more effective than the usual mono-specific culture option.

To sum up the results show the effectiveness of the selected plants to remove uranium from the water. They are a promising choice for the remediation of low to medium uranium contaminated waters. However to assess the real phytotechnological potential of the proposed system, and before an *in situ* application, laboratory tests are needed to determine the toxicity level, the biomass productivity and what enhancement strategies of uranium uptake can be used. For instance, adding citric acid to the phyto-system can be an option for maximizing the uranyl bioavailability and, as consequence, the U accumulation by plants [19, 20].

The issue of the final disposal of the generated residues also has to be addressed.

REFERENCES

1. Watanabe, M. E. Can bioremediation bounce back?. Nature Biotechnology 2001;19, 1111-1115.
2. Kamal, M., Ghaly, A.E., Mahmoud, N., Coté, R. Phytoaccumulation of Heavy Metals by aquatic. Environ international, Elsevier. 2004; 29; 1029-1039.

3. Prasad, M.N.V; Freitas, H. Metal Hyperaccumulation in plants - Biodiversity prospecting for phytoremediation technology. Elec J Biotech (online). 2003; Vol. 6; No. 3.
4. Kalin, M.; Wheeler, W.N.; Meinrath, G. The removal of uranium from mining waste water using algal/ microbial biomass. J Environ Radio, Elsevier. 2005; 78; 151-177.
5. Saxena, P.K.; KrishnaRaj, S; Dan, T.; Perras, M.R.; Vettakkorumakankav, N.N. Phytoremediation of Heavy Metal Contaminated and Polluted soils. In Prasad, M.N.V; Hagemeyer ed. Heavy Metals Strees in Plants - From Molecules to ecosystems. Springer-Verlag, Berlin 1999; 157-181.
6. Dushenkov, V. et al.; Kumar, P.B.A.; Motto, H.; Raskin, I. Rhizofiltration: The use of Plants to remove heavy metals from aqueous streams. Environ Sci Tech. 1999; N° 29, 1239-1245.
7. Brooks, R.R. (1998) - Plants that hyperaccumulate heavy metals. Wallingford, CAB International. 1998, 384.
8. Rai, U.; Sinha, S.; Tripathi, R.; Chandra, P. Wastewater treatability potential of some aquatic macrophytes: Removal of Heavy metals. Ecol Eng. 1995; 5; 5-12.
9. Zhu, Y.L.; Zayed, A.M.; Quian, J.H.; De Souza, M.; Terry, N. Phytoaccumulation of trace metals by wetland plants: II. Water hyancinth. J Environ Qual. 1999; 28, 339-344.
10. Mkandawire, M.; Dudel, E.G. Accumulation of arsenic in *Lemna gibba L.* (duck-weed) in tailing waters of two abandoned uranium mining sites in Saxony, Germany, Sci Total Enviro. 2005; 336; (1-3); 81-89.
11. Dushenkov, S. Trends in phytoremediation of radionuclides. Plant and soil. 2003; 249; 167-175.
12. Bhainsa, K., D'souza, S. Uranium (VI) Biosorption by Dried Roots of Eichhornia Crassipes (Water Hyacinth). J Environ Sci Health. 2001; A36(9); 1621-1631.
13. Mkandawire, M.; Dudel, E.G.; Müller, C. Possible mineralization of Uranium in Lemna gibba G3. in Uranium Mining Areas of Portugal. *in* Merkel, B.; Hasche-Berger, A. ed. Uranium in the Environment: mining Impact and consequences. Springer-Verlag.Berlin, 2005; 496-505.
14. Pratas, J.; Rodrigues, N.; Paulo, C. Uranium accumulator plants from the centre of Portugal - their potential to phytoremediation. in Uranium Mining Areas of Portugal. *in* Merkel, B.; Hasche-Berger, A. ed. Uranium in the Environment: mining Impact and consequences. Springer-Verlag.Berlin, 2005; 477-482.
15. Dushenkov, S., Vasudev, D., Kapulnik, Y., Gleba, D., Fleisher, D, Ting, K.C., Ensley, B. - Removal of Uranium from Water Using Terrestrial Plants. Environ Sci Tech 1997; 31; 3468-3474.
16. Eapen, S.; Seseelan, K.; Tivarekar, S.; Kotwal, S; Mitra, R. Potential for rhizofiltration of uranium usin hairy roots cultures of *Brassica juncea* and *Chenopodium amaranticolor*. Environ Res. 2003; 9; 127-133.
17. Huffman, Jr. C., Riley, L.B. The Fluorimetric Method - Its use and precision for de-termination of uranium in the ash of plants. U.S. Geol. Survey Prof. Paper. 1970; 700-B; 181-183.
18. Van Loon, J.C.; Barefoot, R.R. Analytical Methods for Geochemical Exploration. Academic Press, Inc. 1989; 344.
19. Ebbs, S., Brady, D., Kochian, L. Role of Uranium speciation in the uptake and translocation of uranium by plants. J Exp Bot. 1998; Vol.49; No.324; 1183-1190.
20. Chang, P.; Kim; K., Yoshida, S.; & Kim; S. Uranium accumulation of crop plants enhanced by citric acid. Environ Geoche Health. 2005; 27; 529-538.

ACKNOWLEDGMENTS

This work has been funded by a grant of the Portuguese Foundation of Science and Technology (Project POCI/ECM/60750/2004).

Metal Ions in Biology and Medicine: vol. 9. Eds Maria Carmen Alpoim, Paula Vasconcellos Morais, Maria Amélia Santos, Armando J. Cristóvão, José A. Centeno, Philippe Collery.
John Libbey Eurotext, Paris © 2006 pp. 193-1.

Organic matter effect on phytoremediation of cadmium contaminated soils

Pinto, A. P.[1], Gonçalves, M. L.S.[2], Mota, A. M.[2]

[1]*Departamento de Química, Universidade de Évora, Colégio Luis António Verney, R. Romão Ramalho nº 59, 7000 Évora, Portugal. app@uevora.pt*
[2]*Departamento de Engenharia Química, Instituto Superior Técnico, Av. Rovisco Pais, 1049-001 Lisboa, Portugal.*

ABSTRACT

Phytoremediation refers to clean-up of polluted sites, terrestrial as well as aquatic environments, from heavy metal and organic contaminants by plants. A good phytoremediator plant should ideally have high and fast biomass production, and ability to translocate the pollutants into the shoot. In the last few years, great efforts have been directed to the search of hyperaccumulator plants and the study of their tolerance mechanisms. Due to its high toxicity to bioorganisms and its high solubility in water, cadmium (Cd) is one of the most problematic heavy metal pollutants. Cadmium is considered biologically as a non-essential trace metal, although at low concentration it was found to have stimulatory effects on plants growth and on some physiological functions.

The *in situ* phytoextraction of Cd from soils can only be achieved using plants that are both tolerant to high concentrations and able to extract sufficient amounts of the metal. However, very few plant species are capable of remediating Cd polluted soils in a reasonable time frame. The aim of this study was to investigate Cd phytoextraction ability with high production plant as sorghum. A stimulatory effect of Cd was observed on sorghum biomass for low metal concentrations ($\leq$ 4,5 mg Cd kg^{-1} of soil), suggesting a hormesis phenomenon. The pot study conducted with 2 to 70 mg Cd kg^{-1} of soil, indicated that phytoremediation is feasible when the soil is moderately contaminated with Cd ($\leq$ 9 mg Cd kg^{-1} of soil). In this concentration range, the addition of organic matter (35 or 70 g of OM kg^{-1} of soil) did not improve significantly the phytoextraction capacity of sorghum. For polluted soils with high Cd concentrations (35 mg Cd kg^{-1} soil), the addition of organic matter induced a significant increase on the phytoextraction capacity.

These findings have important implications for phytoremediation and human health risk assessment.

MATERIALS AND METHODS

Experimental set up

Pot culture experiments were conducted using a sandy soil treated (spiked) with cadmium nitrate [$Cd(NO_3)_2$]. For comparison an unamended control soil was also used. The solution of $Cd(NO_3)_2$ was uniformly mixed with air dried soil previously sieved (< 2 mm), and placed in pots (5 kg); the final Cd soil concentration was 2, 4.5, 9, 18, 35 and 70 mg Cd kg^{-1} (ppm), respectively. The soil presented a pH of 5.3, 3 g of organic carbon kg^{-1}, 930 g of sand kg^{-1} and 17 g of clay kg^{-1}. A dry Irish peat moss was added to provide organic matter (OM), which presented 1280 mg of dissolved organic carbon (DOC) kg^{-1} of peat. It was assumed that DOC in soil solution solely consisted of fulvic acids, having a carbon content of 80%. Three treatments were used: i) without

OM addition; ii) with addition of 35 or 70 g of OM per kg of soil. Ten seeds of *Sorghum bicolor* (L.) Moench. x *Sorghum sudanense* (cv. "Grazer N2") were sown in the soil to germinate, but only 6 uniform plants were allowed to grow in each pot, at an uniform distance apart. The treatments were completely randomised with three replicates. Plants were grown in a greenhouse, under natural light and ambient temperature.

Plant growth and harvesting

Plants were harvested after 20, 40 and 60 days without damaging the roots. They were rinsed in distilled water to remove dust and soil mineral particles and were separated into leaves and roots. Dry biomass (oven dried at 60 °C for 48 h), of roots and shoots were measured.

Cadmium analysis

Dried samples were ground into a fine powder using a mortar. Cd analysis was performed by atomic absorption with flame or graphite furnace, after digesting the samples in an acidic mixture [1].

Statistical analysis

All analytical determinations were performed in triplicate. All data were analysed by analysis of variance (ANOVA) for a one or two-factor factorial experiment. The Least Significant Difference (LSD) was used to compare means. The minimum level of significance was set at $p = 0.05$.

RESULTS AND DISCUSSION

Plant growth

Indicating the toxic level, the selected plants failed to grow at 70 mg Cd kg^{-1} soil, but they are capable of extraction up to 35 mg Cd kg^{-1} soil. Cadmium treatment resulted in increases of 10% on the root biomass of sorghum grown with 2 mg Cd kg^{-1} of soil, after 40 days (data not shown). For 4.5 mg Cd kg^{-1} of soil, the sorghum root biomass was 35% greater than for the control, after 60 days of growth *(fig. 1)*. This result suggests a biostimulation (hormesis) phenomen, as previously observed in nutrient solution experiments [2, 3].

Reductions of 82 and 70% were observed on the biomass of sorghum roots and shoots, respectively, in the presence of 35 mg Cd kg^{-1} of soil, at the end of the experiment *(fig. 1)*. Indeed, since the root is the first compartment to be in contact with Cd, it is more rapidly affected by the increase of metal concentration in soil.

In heavily contaminated soils ($\geq$ 35 mg Cd kg^{-1} of soil), the addition of OM led to a very significant increase ($p < 0.01$) on the root and shoot biomass *(fig. 1)*. The advantage of the organic matter addition to the heavily contaminated soils was the higher biomass production obtained, which led to an increase in the extracted Cd. A combination of soils with natural organic amendments and plants of high biomass with sufficient metal tolerance may enlarge the efficiency of phytoextraction.

Plant metal uptake

Cd bioavailability depends on organic matter content, redox potential, soil pH, and rhizosphere chemistry. The accumulation and extraction of Cd by plants, calculated on a dry weight basis, is reported only for 60 days of growth. As presented in *figure 2*, cadmium concentrations in the sorghum tissues (roots and shoots) markedly increased with rising Cd concentrations in soil. Cd concentration in sorghum roots was in general greater than in shoots, i.e. roots acted as a barrier to cadmium transport to shoots.

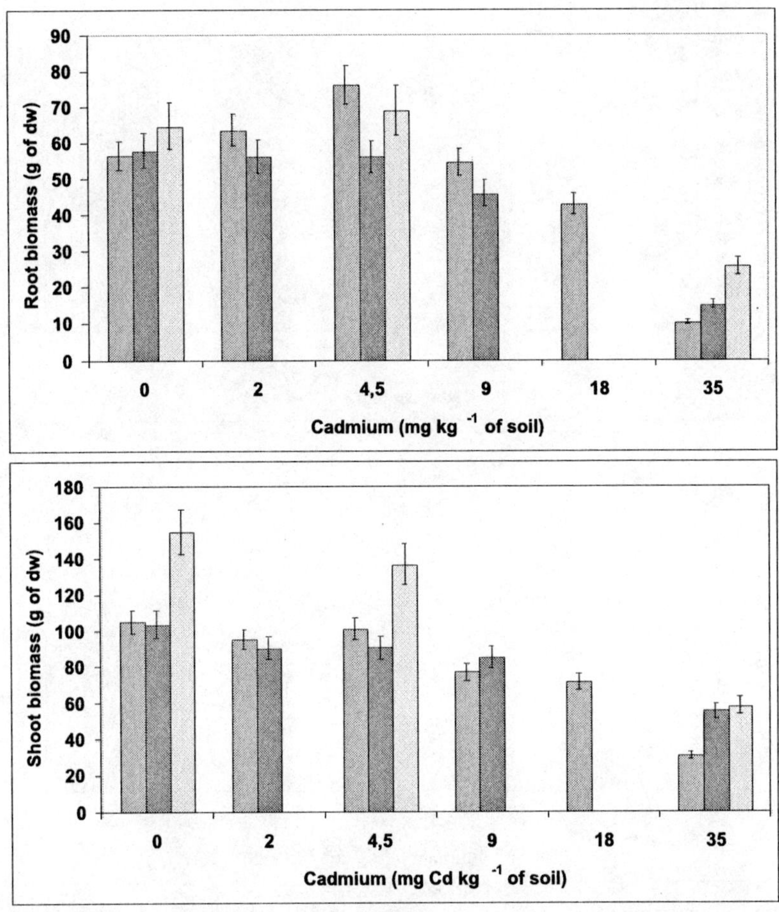

Fig. 1. Root and shoot biomass of sorghum after 60 days of growth in a soil with different levels of Cd, without OM addition (▒), and with addition of 35 g (■) or 70 g (░) of OM kg^{-1} of soil. Average ± SE of triplicates (n=3).

The highest Cd concentration was observed in the roots treated with 35 mg Cd kg^{-1} of soil (808 mg Cd kg^{-1} d.w.), which is about 5 times higher than the concentration in shoots.

The shoot concentrations ranged from approximately 24 mg Cd kg^{-1} to 156 mg Cd kg^{-1} *(fig. 2)*, for soil contamination between 2 and 35 mg Cd kg^{-1}. Although cadmium concentration in plant tissues increased with soil Cd level, the Cd content decreased for the highest Cd level, due to a significant decrease on the biomass production. The organic matter addition to heavily contaminated soils decreases Cd uptake in terms of concentration *(fig. 2)*, but not in terms of content, due to the increase of biomass in the presence of OM.

Cadmium extraction

Because of its high biomass production sorghum may have a significant potential for phytoextraction. The potential for phytoextraction depends on three variables: plant biomass, soil mass that requires remediation and bioconcentration factor [4]. Sorghum Cd extraction was evaluated through the calculation of the Cd removed from the soil by one crop (% of total soil Cd) = Bioconcentration factor × (Shoot Biomass / Soil mass in the rooting zone) × 100, where the

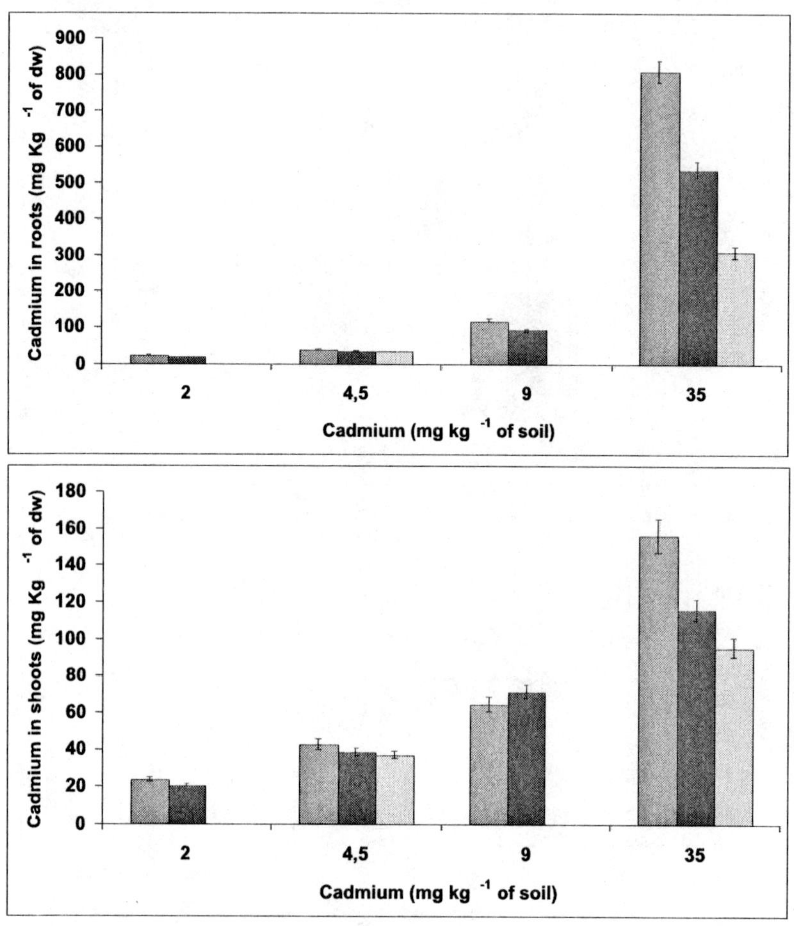

Fig. 2. Cadmium concentration (mg Cd kg^{-1} of dw) in roots and shoots after 60 days of growth in a soil with different levels of Cd, without organic matter addition (▒) and with addition of 35 g (■) or 70 g (░) of OM kg^{-1} of soil. Average ± SE of triplicates (n=3).

bioconcentration factor is given by the ratio between the shoot metal concentration and the soil metal concentration. The potential of sorghum for soil Cd phytoextraction, determined from our experiments, is presented in *figure 3*. From this figure it can be seen that (i) sorghum has a large phytoextraction capacity for Cd concentrations ≤ 9 mg Cd kg^{-1} in soils; (ii) the capacity of soil cleaning decreases with the increase of soil Cd concentration. This reduction was accompanied by a decrease on the biomass production, which limits the ability of sorghum to clean the soil. The total extraction by shoots at 35 mg Cd kg^{-1} soil showed a sharp drop in this species. The higher sorghum Cd extraction in the presence of OM for high Cd levels, makes the addition of OM an important factor for phytoextraction at toxic levels of Cd. In the presence of OM and for 35 mg Cd kg^{-1}, an increase higher than 30% was observed in the Cd removed by sorghum shoots. However, even so the phytoextraction capacity remained much lower than those observed for Cd soil concentrations ≤ 9 mg Cd kg^{-1}, in the presence or absence of OM.

Figure 4 shows that, for an initial concentration of 4.5 mg Cd kg^{-1} of soil, it would be necessary two successive crops to achieve the acceptable target of 3 mg Cd kg^{-1} [4], which could take place in a single year. For initial concentrations of 9 and 18 mg Cd kg^{-1} of soil, 8 and 16 successive crops of sorghum (4 and 8 years) would be needed, respectively. Thus, phytoextraction of Cd using sorghum could restore soil health to moderately Cd contaminated land within realistic time scales, providing a green technology and an economic return from the crop during the clean-up step.

It should be noticed that to calculate the real phytoextraction capacity of sorghum, studies under field conditions are necessary to evaluate the potential of this plant species more accurately.

The interest in Cd phytoextraction is due to its high toxicity to bioorganisms associated to its high solubility in water [5].

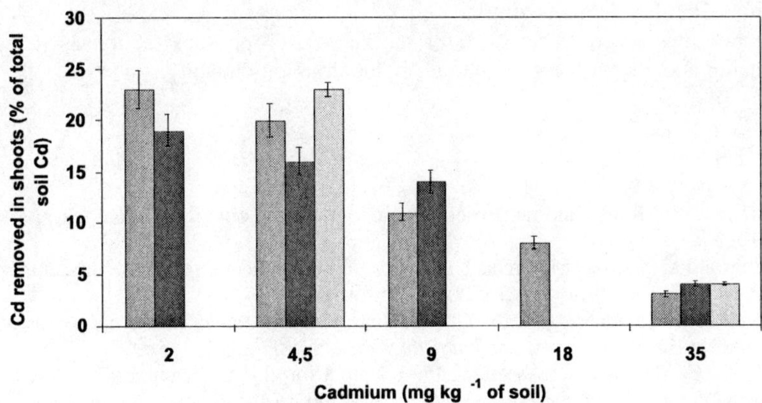

Fig. 3. Cd removed in shoots of sorghum after 60 days of growth in a soil with different levels of Cd, without organic matter addition (▒), with addition of 35 g (■) or 70 g of peat kg^{-1} of soil (░). Average ± SE of triplicates (n=3).

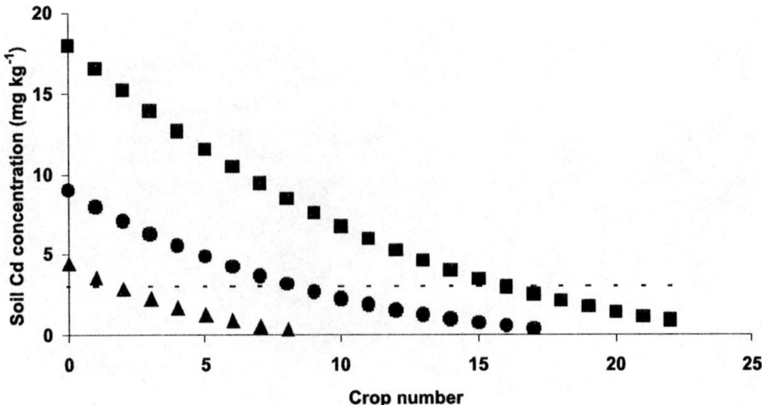

Fig. 4. Calculated concentrations of Cd in the soil after successive crops of sorghum, based on experiments of 60 days. The horizontal line represents the adopted target for remediation.

CONCLUSIONS

A stimulating effect of Cd was observed on sorghum root biomass for low metal concentrations in soil (<9 mg Cd kg^{-1}). This result is consistent with reported effects on specific processes at low Cd concentrations.

Organic matter did not influence significantly the shoot/root Cd concentration ratio in low or moderately Cd contaminated soils, but increased that ratio in more than 60% for heavily contaminated soils, which is advantageous to phytoextraction. However, even so the fitoextraction capacity remained too small compared to the values obtained for Cd soil concentrations $\leq$ 9 mg Cd kg^{-1}, in the presence or absence of OM.

In our results *Sorghum bicolor* (L.) Moench. × *Sorghum sudanense* presented maximum extraction for Cd levels < 9 mg Cd kg^{-1} of soil due to the higher biomass produced. It was shown that soils contaminated with 4.5, 9 and 18 mg Cd kg^{-1} of soil could be cleaned with sorghum in a period of 1, 4 and 8 years, respectively, in order to attain the target of 3 mg Cd kg^{-1} of soil. In field conditions the biomass produced is expected to be higher, which implies lower extraction times if Cd bioavailability remains similar.

This study provides a promising start for biomass-based phytoextraction as it includes high biomass producing species with a reasonable phytoextraction capacity.

REFERENCES

1. Souza JF, Rauser WE. Maize and radish sequester cadmium and zinc in different ways. *Plant Sci* 2003; 165: 1009-1022.
2. Arduini I, Masoni A, Mariotti M, Ercoli L. Low cadmium application increase miscanthus growth and cadmium translocation. *Environ Exp Bot* 2004; 52: 89-100.
3. Pinto AP, Mota AM, Varennes A, Pinto FC. Influence of organic matter on the uptake of cadmium, zinc, copper and iron by sorghum plants. *Sci Total Environ* 2004; 326: 237-245.
4. Zhao FJ, Lombi E, McGrath SP. Assessing the potential for zinc and cadmium phytoremediation with the hyperaccumulator *Thlaspi caerulescens. Plant Soil* 2003; 249: 37-43.
5. Ghosh M, Singh SP. A comparative study of cadmium phytoextraction by accumulator and weed species. *Environ Pollut* 2005; 133: 365-371.

Metal Ions in Biology and Medicine: vol. 9. Eds Maria Carmen Alpoim, Paula Vasconcellos Morais, Maria Amélia Santos, Armando J. Cristóvão, José A. Centeno, Philippe Collery.
John Libbey Eurotext, Paris © 2006 pp. 199-1.

Effect of manganese addition to substrate of mushroom *(Agaricus bisporus)*

László Rácz[1], József Rácz[2], Gyula Záray[3]

[1]*Department of Chemistry, Eszterházy Károly Teacher Training College, H-3300 Eger, Hungary, rleger@gemini.ektf.hu*

[2]*Korona Mushroom Society, H-3395 Demjén, Hungary*

[3]*Department of Analytical Chemistry, Eötvös University, P.O. Box 32, H-1518 Budapest, Hungary*

INTRODUCTION

Manganese is an essential microelement for plants, animals and humans, being an important component and activator of several enzyme systems. Plants take manganese from soil solution as Mn(II) ions, however, the uptake of manganese depends on the pH and organic material content. It is well known from the literature [1] that for the proper functioning of different enzymes (e.g. peptidases, dehydrogenases, certain decarboxylases, phosphorylases) the presence of manganese is indispensable. Recently the role of manganese in the enzymatic decomposition of lignin was also demonstrated [2]. The degradation of cellulose and the lignin content of straw during a 70-day-long cultivation period of mushrooms show different pictures [3]. The cellulose and hemicelluloses contents decrease more rapidly than the lignin content. In order to increase the degradation of lignin and thereby to provide a more usable carbon source for mushrooms, the addition of manganese to the substrate seemed to be a promising way. However, it was necessary to study the uptake of manganese and its effect on the uptake of other essential elements. This paper summarizes the most important results of experiments related to manganese addition.

MATERIALS AND METHODS

Cultivation of mushrooms: 1 liter $MnCl_2$ solutions in 5 different concentrations were added to 5 polyethylene sack each. All the sacks contained 20 kg thermally treated substrate. Then the content of the 25 sacks were homogenized one by one. The added amounts of manganese into the sacks were 0.91, 2.28, 4.55, 9.1 and 18.2 g resulting in a concentration of 20, 50, 100, 200 and 400 mg/kg, respectively. In case of the 5 control (untreated) samples only 1 liter water was added. Into each sack 150 cm^3 of K-23 grain spawn was introduced and the substrate was mixed again. The control and the manganese treated substrata were stored in a cellar with regulated humidity. The first harvests of mushrooms were carried out following a 21-day growing period.

Sample preparation and analytical methods: Three fruit bodies were taken from three sacks containing the same substrate. These mushrooms were cut in eight pieces by plastic knife. From the 24 pieces about 20 g was selected and dried at 150 °C. After grinding in a Retsch mill the samples were sieved and the fractions of less than 60 µm were separated for analysis. 400 mg each sample was digested in a mixture of 2 cm^3 cc. HNO_2 and 2 cm^3 H_2O_2 (30% w/w) at 160 °C for 3 hours applying closed teflon bombs. The clear solutions were filled up to 25 cm^3 with bidistilled water. The analytical measurements were carried out by inductively coupled plasma atomic emission spectrometry using a Spectroflame equipment (Spectro GmbH, Kleve, Germany).

RESULTS AND DISCUSSION

On basis of our laboratory experiments it was demonstrated that the yield of mushrooms can be increased by addition of manganese to the substrate *(table 1)*. The highest increment was achieved at manganese concentration of 100 mg/kg and amounted to abut 16%. However, it was questionable that manganese has any influence on the uptake of other essential or even toxic elements and how changes its uptake at elevated concentrations in the substrate. As the data of *table 2* show the concentrations of Al, Cd, Cr, Cu in the mushrooms practically were not influenced by manganese addition, since their concentrations changed within the standard deviation ranges. However, the concentration of Fe and Ni decreased by about 15%, while the uptake of manganese increased by 10%. These concentration changes are negligible from the point of plant physiological processes in the mushrooms.

Table 1. Yield of mushrooms cultivated on substrata containing manganese in different concentrations and harvested after 21, 30 and 38 days

Number of days	kg mushroom/100 kg substrata					
	Control	Mn 20 mg/kg	Mn 50 mg/kg	Mn 100 mg/kg	Mn 200 mg/kg	Mn 400 mg/kg
21	8.3	8.8	9.1	10.6	10.2	10.0
30	10.0	9.2	10.9	10.7	10.8	11.1
38	5.2	4.8	5.1	6.1	6.1	5.6
Total	23.5	22.8	25.1	27.4	27.1	26.7
Deviation from control%	-	-3.0	+7.2	+16.6	+15.3	+13.2

Table 2. Concentration of elements in dried mushrooms cultivated in control and manganese treated substrata (100 mg Mn/kg)

	Concentration mg/kg							
	Al	Cd	Cr	Cu	Fe	Mn	Ni	Zn
Control substrate	9.1 ±0.3	0.4 ±0.1	3.8 ±0.2	38.1 ±2.2	57.2 ±2.4	4.0 ±0.3	3.1 ±0.2	45.7 ±2.7
Mn-treated substrate	8.7 ±0.4	0.3 ±0.1	3.9 ±0.3	38.9 ±1.8	48.3 ±2.1	4.4 ±0.2	2.6 ±0.2	47.5 ±2.4

The manganese treatment of substrate was also applied in industrial scale experiments. The yield of mushrooms increased in similar ratio as in case of the laboratory scale experiments *(table 3)*.

Table 3. Yield of mushrooms cultivated on control and manganese treated substrata (100 mg Mn/1 kg substrate) in industrial-scale experiments

	kg mushroom/100 kg substrate		
	harvested after 21 days	harvested after 30 days	harvested after 38 days
Control substrate	10.1 ± 0.9	8.6 ± 0.8	5.4 ± 0.5
Mn treated substrate	10.9 ± 1.0	10.2 ± 0.9	6.0 ± 0.7

Since the addition of manganese to the substrate resulted in higher yield of mushrooms without any critical changes in the elemental composition, this simple technology can be recommended for the producers of Agaricus bisporus.

REFERENCES

1. Jakucs, E. The role of fungi in degradation of cellulose and lignin, Mycological Acta (1990) 1-3, 13-36.
2. Bonnen, A. M., Anton, L.H., Orth, A. B. Lignine-Degrading Enzymes of Commercial Button Mushroom (Agaricus bisporus), Appl. and Environ. Microbiol. (1994) 60, 960-965.
3. Durrant, A. J., Wood, D. A., Cain, R. B. Lignocellulose biodegradation by Agaricus bisporus during solid substrate fermentation, J. General Microbiol. (1991) 137, 751-755.

V MICROORGANISMS

Metal Ions in Biology and Medicine: vol. 9. Eds Maria Carmen Alpoim, Paula Vasconcellos Morais, Maria Amélia Santos, Armando J. Cristóvão, José A. Centeno, Philippe Collery.
John Libbey Eurotext, Paris © 2006 pp. 205-1.

Identification of genes involved in oxyanions resistance in *Ochrobactrum tritici* 5bvl1 by transposon mutagenesis

Rita Branco[1] and Paula Vasconcellos Morais[1,2]

[1]*Instituto Ambiente e Vida, 3004-517 Coimbra, Portugal*
[2]*Departamento de Bioquímica, Faculdade de Ciências e Tecnologis da Universidade de Coimbra, 3001-401 Coimbra, Portugal*

Heavy metals and metalloids are usually toxic in excess therefore the ability of microrganisms to tolerate and transform the toxic elements to the non-toxic forms has considerable importance for detoxification and bioremediation of contaminated sites. Strain 5bvl1 isolated from a chromium-contaminated environment, and previously identified as *Ochrobactrum tritici*, was exposed to several concentrations of different oxyanions. This strain was resistant to several of the metal ions tested in addition to chromate [Cr(VI)], namely, selenate [Se(IV)], selenite [Se(III)], arsenate [As(V)] and tellurite [Te(III)]. The aim of this work was to locate genes for oxyanions resistance in strain 5bvl1 using transposon insertion mutagenesis. Thousands of mutants selected after conjugation of strain 5bvl1 with *E.coli* S17-1 (pSUP5011) were screened on plates supplemented with Cr(VI). From these transconjugants, two colonies, called E117 and Q152, showed an increased susceptibility to this heavy metal. The ability of mutant E117 to resist to Cr(VI) was clearly affected, while mutant Q152 showed an intermediate chromate-sensitive phenotype. The regions interrupted by transposon were obtained by inverse PCR (IPCR) and sequence analysis of these fragments identified two genes, named *chr*A and *ruv*B, in mutants E117 and Q152, respectively. The gene *ruv*B encodes a helicase RuvB involved in DNA replication, recombination and repair. This work also allowed the detection of an additional gene, *tel*B, which it is normally involved in resistance to tellurite. However, during this study was not possible to associate the presence of this gene with tellurite resistance.

INTRODUCTION

Of the various toxic heavy metals discharged into the environment through various industrial wastewaters, constituting one of the major causes of environmental pollution, chromium is one of the most toxic and has become a serious health concern. Extensive use of chromium, e.g., in electroplating, tanning, textile dyeing and as a biocide in power plant cooling water, results in discharge of chromium-containing effluents. The effluents from these industries contain Cr(VI) and Cr(III) at high concentrations. While Cr(VI) is known to be toxic to both plants and animals, a strong oxidizing agent and a potential carcinogen, Cr(III) is generally only toxic to plants at very high concentrations and is less toxic or non-toxic to animals. Chromate exerts diverse toxic effects on bacteria, including competitive inhibition of sulphate transport as well as DNA and protein damage after Cr(VI) intracellular reduction to the Cr(III) species, a process generating reactive oxygen species (ROS) [1]. Mechanisms for bacterial resistance to chromate are varied and may be conferred by genes located in chromosomes or in plasmids.

With the development of a broad host range of delivery system, the tn5 transposon and its derivatives have become popular tools to study molecular genetics of Gram-negative bacteria [2].

However, identification of tn5 disrupted genes required restriction with enzymes that did not cut within the large transposon. So, this method was restrictive, since the use of many of those enzymes resulted in fragments flanking the tn5 which were too long to amplify and difficult to clone. This problem was solved by adapting the inverse PCR method to utilize restriction enzymes that cut the transposon at least once. This allows the design of an outward extending primer with respect to the endonuclease site of the transposon. This primer used in conjugation with a primer complementary to the inverted terminal repeats can be used to amplify DNA flanking one side of the transposon.

MATERIAL AND METHODS

Determination of heavy metal resistance of strain *O. tritici* 5bvl1

For determining the resistance of strain *O. tritici* 5bvl1 to some oxyanions, bacterial suspensions were transferred to solid MMT medium [3] plates supplemented with increasing concentrations of chromate [Cr(VI)], arsenate [As(V)], arsenite [As(III)], selenate [Se(IV)], selenite [Se(III)], antimonite [Sb(III)] and tellurite [Te(III)]. The resulting plates were incubated at 30 °C for 5 days.

Transposon mutagenesis and screening

Transposon insertion mutants were generated by mobilization of the suicide plasmid pSUP5011 from the donor strain *E. coli* S17-1 to the recipient strain 5bvl1. In this procedure, the tn5::Kan^r transposon is transferred from *E. coli* to strain 5bvl1 (Tc^r) where the transposon randomly inserts into the DNA, thus generating a library of insertion mutants. The strain 5bvl1 was grown overnight in LB at 30 °C with shaking and the donor *E. coli* strain was grown at 37°C to exponential phase. A 2:1 proportion of donor and recipient cells was mixed on nylon filters, placed on LB agar plates, and incubated overnight at 30°C. The bacteria were suspended in LB and dilutions were spread on plates containing Kanamycin (750 µg/ml) and tetracycline (10 µg/ml). Transconjugants were picked to LB plates with 2 mM chromate and after 36 h incubation at 30°C, clones unable to grown on 2 mM chromate were recovered from the plates and chosen as chromate-sensitive mutants (Cr^s).

Confirmation of transposon mutagenesis by southern hybridization

To confirm the mutants transposon insertion, Southern blot analysis was performed as described previously [4]. Purified DNAs (10 µg) of mutants were subjected to digestion with restriction enzymes (*Sph*I, *Sal*I and *BamH*I) and electrophoresed on agarose gel [0.8% (w/v)]. DNA was capillary transferred for approximately 16 h to a nylon membrane in 0.4N NaOH, 1M NaCl buffer following neutralization. DNA probe for tn5 were amplified by PCR using specific primers (tn5f and tn5r), which resulted in a 4Kbp-fragment that was cut from agarose gels and purified. This probe was labelled with dioxigenin-dUTP nonradioactive (Roche) and the subsequent prehybridization and hybridization with membrane were performed at 55 °C using DIG High Prime DNA Labelling and Detection Starter Kit II, following the manufacturer's instructions. The membrane was washed twice with 2× SSC-0.1% SDS at room temperature and twice with 0.2× SSC-0.1% SDS for 15 min at 68°C by constant agitation. Membrane was autoradiographed after incubation at 37°C for 45 min.

DNA procedures

Templates for inverse PCR (IPCR) were prepared from about 1µg of total DNA digested with enzymes that cut once inside the tn5 transposon. The digested DNAs were ligated overnight at 14°C in a total volume 50 µl with T4 DNA ligase. DNA flanking the tn5 insertion was amplified by PCR with specific primers, designed from the transposon inverted repeats.

RESULTS

Strain *O. tritici* 5bvl1 was resistant to high concentrations of Cr(VI), Se(IV), Se(III) and As(V) but only at low concentrations of As(III), Sb(III) and Te(III).

Mutants 5bvl1-Kan^r, obtained by random mutagenesis using the tn5::Kan^r transposon, were selected after conjugation of strain 5bvl1 with *E. coli* S17-1 (pSUP5011). The resulting collection of 4000 colonies was then screened on LB plates containing chromate. Four clones showing higher chromate sensitivity, as compared to the wild type strain, were selected. After the chromate susceptibility tests in liquid medium, two mutant strains were chosen for further analysis: the E117 mutant, which was clearly sensitive to chromate and the Q152 mutant, with an intermediate chromate-sensitive phenotype *(fig. 1)*. Southern blot analysis of *Sph*I, *Sal*I and *BamH*I digested E117 and Q152 DNA confirmed that tn5 insertion had occurred in both mutants but at different positions. Also, hybridisation of *Sph*I digested DNA E117, showed more than two expected signs, indicating that probably two tn5 insertions had occurred. Tn5 probe hybridisation to DNA digested with *Sph*I and *Sal*I showed that these were potential enzymes for IPCR whereas *BamH*I yielded fragments too long for IPCR amplification.

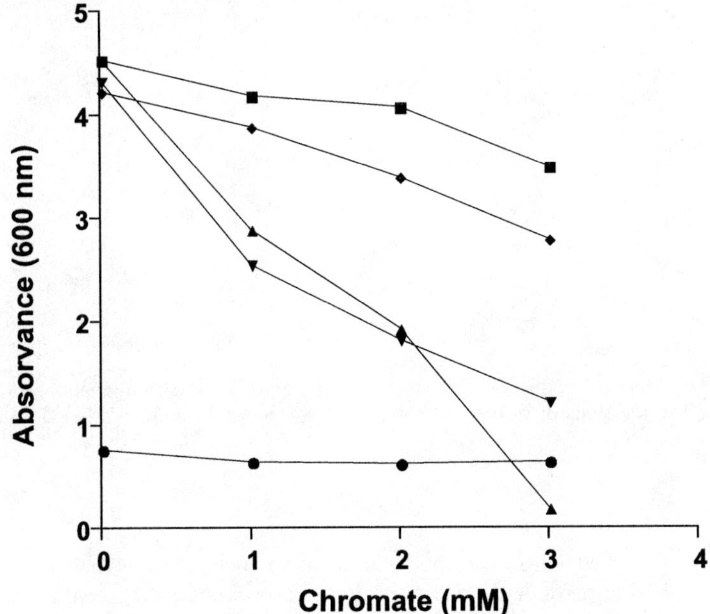

Fig. 1. Susceptibility to chromate of *O. tritici* 5bvl1 and mutants. Cultures were grown in LB medium for 24 hours at 30 °C. Wild type strain (■), E117 (▲), Q152 (▼), O116 (◆) and V17 (●).

To identify the affected genes in the Cr^s mutant strains, the regions interrupted by the transposon were amplified by IPCR using primers corresponding to sequences from the ends and the middle of the transposon. From *Sal*I digested E117 DNA, one IPCR product for left side was obtained, whereas for Q152 these enzymes did not result leading to the test of other enzymes. When the Q152 DNA digested with *Nco*I was subjected to IPCR, a unique small fragment for right side was amplified. These fragments were cloned into the pGem T-Easy and then sequenced using a vector-specific primer. The data obtained were then submitted to NCBI Blast analyses. These analyses established that the genes interrupted were *chr*A in E117 and *ruv*B in Q152 *(fig. 2)*.

Total DNA from E117 mutant was also digested with *Sph*I and resulting digestion was cloned into the *Sph*I site of pUC18 vector. Ligation mixtures were transferred to competent *E. coli* cells, and transformants were selected on Ampicillin plates. Then, we identified the plasmid with the transposon insertion by PCR with vector primer and transposon specific primer. This plasmid was sequenced and one gene *tel*B was identified by homology.

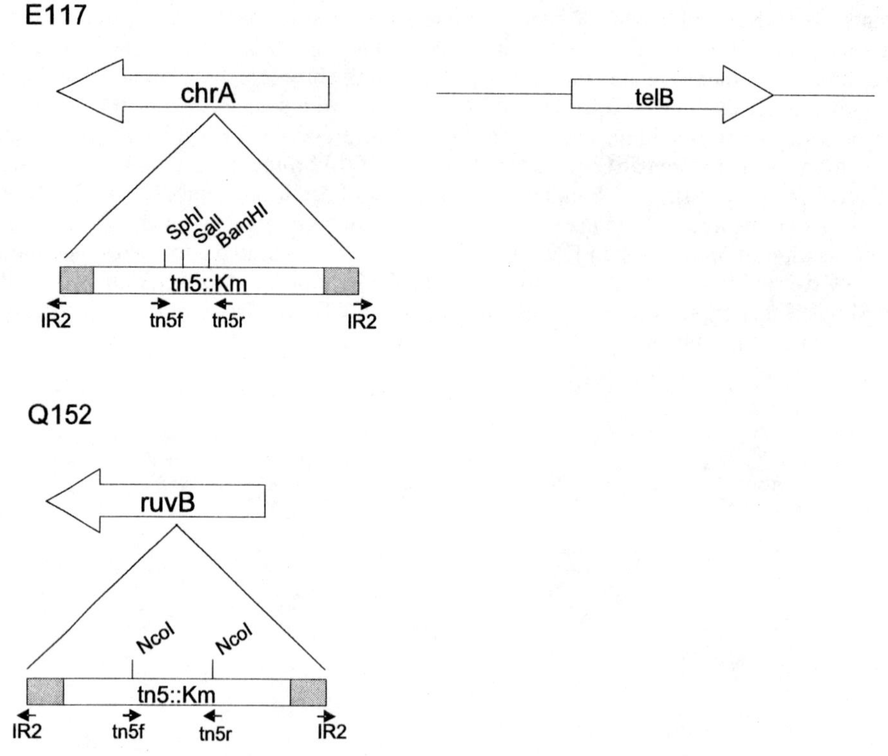

Fig. 2. Location of the transposon insertions in strains E117 and Q152. Restriction sites *Sph*I, *Sal*I, *Nco*I and *BamH*I are shown. The locations of primers IR2, tn5f and tn5r are indicated.

DISCUSSION

The procedure described here is a simple alternative method to isolate DNA flanking tn5 insertions. This method is particularly useful in those cases when a fragment of suitable size for cloning or IPCR cannot be generated using enzymes that do not cut within tn5 [5]. These IPCR products can be used to quickly obtain sequence information on the region of insertion of the transposon.

O. tritici 5bvl1 mutants characterized in this work were mutated in the *chr*A or *ruv*B genes, corresponding to putative chromate efflux protein ChrA and helicase RuvB, respectively. In mutant Q152, with the *ruv*B gene interrupted, the RuvABC complex probably does not form, thus blocking the migration of the Holliday junctions and prevent the repair of DNA damage [6]. The ROS species generated during Cr(VI) reduction to Cr(III) have been already associated to DNA damage and under these conditions bacteria need a repair system [6]. It seems that RuvB helicase is part of this repair system and will participate in the process of repair of DNA damages caused by the exposure of strain 5bvl1 to the toxic ion chromate and, most probably, also to the exposure other oxyanions.

In spite of strain 5bvl1 being unable to resist to high concentrations of tellurite, a gene that showed strong homology with the tellurite resistant gene -*tel*B- was found. This gene usually associated to other genes (*tel*ABCDE) has been already detected in a wide range of bacterial species, suggesting that these determinants provide some selective advantage in natural environments, which may be unrelated to the Te^r phenotype [7]. Perhaps the tellurite resistance genes are associated with protection from other forms of oxidative stress or agents causing damages.

REFERENCES

1. Cervantes, C., J. Campos-Garcia, S. Devars, F. Gutiérrez-Corona, H. Loza-Tavera, J. C. Torres-Guzmán, and R. Moreno-Sánchez. Interactions of chromium with microorganisms and plants. *FEMS Microbiol. Rev.* 2001; 25: 335-347.
2. Simon, R., U. Priefer, and A. Puehler. A broad host range mobilization system for in vivo genetic engineering: transposon mutagenesis in gram-negative bacteria. *Bio/Technology.* 1983; 1: 784-791.
3. Branco, R., M. C. Alpoim, and P. V. Morais. *Ochrobactrum tritici* strain 5bvl1- characterization of a Cr(VI)-resistant and Cr(VI)- reducing strain. *Can. J. Microbiol.* 2004; 50: 697-703.
4. Sambrook, J., E. F. Fritsch, and T. Maniatis. Molecular cloning: A laboratory manual, second edn. 1989. Cold Spring Harbor Laboratory Press. Cold Spring harbor, NY.
5. Martin, V. J., and W. W. Mohn. An alternative inverse PCR (IPCR) method to amplify DNA sequences flanking Tn5 transposon insertions. *J. Microbiol. Meth.* 1999; 35: 163-166.
6. Miranda, A. T., M. V. González, G. González, E. Vargas, J. Campos-Garcia, and C. Cervantes. Involvement of DNA helicases in chromate resistance by *Pseudomonas aeruginosa* PAO1. *Mut. Res.* 2005; 578: 202-209.
7. Toptchieva, A., G. Sisson, L. J. Bryden, D. E. Taylor, and P. S. Hoffman. An inducible tellurite-resistance operon in *Proteus mirabilis*. *Microbiology.* 2003; 149: 1285-1295.

ACKNOWLEDGEMENTS

This research was funded by Fundação para a Ciência e Tecnologia (FCT), Portugal, under POCTI and FEDER programs, contract POCTI/BSE/42414/2001. R. Branco was supported by a Ph.D. scholarship from FCT (SFRH/BD/10737/2002).

Metal Ions in Biology and Medicine: vol. 9. Eds Maria Carmen Alpoim, Paula Vasconcellos Morais, Maria Amélia Santos, Armando J. Cristóvão, José A. Centeno, Philippe Collery.
John Libbey Eurotext, Paris © 2006 pp. 210-1.

Plasma membrane sensitivity of phototrophic sulfur bacterium *Thiocapsa roseopersicina* to heavy metal ions

A. Yu. Ivanov[1], L. A. Khassanova[2,5], I.N. Gogotov[3], D. O. Safieva[4], J.-C. Etienne[5], Z.M. Khassanova[5,6]

[1]*Institute of Cell Biophysics RAS, Pushchino, 142290,*
[2]*Russian State University of Oil and Gas, 65, Leninsky prospect, Moscow, 119991, Russia; Russia;*
[3]*Institute of Basic Biological Problems RAS, Pushchino, 142290, Russia;*
[4]*Institute of Biochemical Physics RAS, 4, Kosygin street, Moscow, 117997, Russia;*
[5]*International Research Institute on Metal Ions, University of Reims, Champagne-Ardenne, BP 1039, 51687 Reims cedex2, France;*
[6]*Bashkir State Pedagogical University, 3a, October revolution street, Ufa, 450000, Russia*

ABSTRACT

The effect of heavy metals: Cu, Cd and Ni (10-200 μM) on the barrier properties of plasma membrane (PM) of phototrophic purple sulfur bacterium *Thiocapsa roseopersicina* was studied by the method of electroorientational spectroscopy (EO-spectroscopy). There was toxic effect of all three metal ions on *T. roseopersicina* cells. Time and concentration dependence of this toxic effect was observed.

The following order of metal toxicity for cell PM was obtained: $Cu^{2+} > Cd^{2+} > Ni^{2+}$.

INTRODUCTION

One of the main task of the environmental conservation is the search of effective refining technologies of industrial sewage from wastes, especially, from heavy metals. Integrated employment of biological and chemical methods permits to decrease environmental pollution by heavy metals significantly. A lot of microorganisms have abilities to accumulate a great quantity of heavy metals by their biomass, also they can transform the high toxic metal ions in slightly or non soluble complexes or precipitates of free metals (Gogotov, 2002). It was shown that some microorganisms, contained a hydrogenases, have capacity to recover metal ions till free metal forms at H_2 presence. Phototrophic microorganisms, particularly purple sulfur bacterium *T. roseopersicina*, is perspective object for this kind of investigations because of their recovery properties. As microorganisms themselves and as an extracted from microorganisms hydrogenases recover Ni^{2+}, Pb^{2+}, Pd^{2+}, Pt^{2+}, Ru^{3+} till metal form (Zadvorny et al, 2000). However recovering Cd^{2+}, Co^{2+} and Cu^{2+} was not observed.

It is well known that ions of heavy metals (Cd^{2+}, Cu^{2+}, Co^{2+}, Ni^{2+} etc.) can toxically influence on cell barrier properties of different microorganisms (De Filippe L.F. 1979; Geier B.M. et al, 1987; Khassanova, 1996; Ivanov et al, 1997). The aim of our study is to widen understanding of processes, which have place at metal recovery in whole cells. In this work we have been investigated the influence of some heavy metals Cu^{2+}, Cd^{2+} and Ni^{2+} on barrier properties of cell PM of purple sulfur bacterium *T. roseopersicina*.

MATERIALS AND METHODS

The clean culture of phototrophic purple sulfur bacterium *Thiocapsa roseopersicina (BBS strain)* from the "Collection of Institute of Basic Biological Problems RAS" was studied. *T. ro-*

seopersicina cells were grown in a modified Pfennig medium (Bogorov, 1974) in photoheterotrophic conditions. For experiments cells were precipitated, twice washed with distilled water and stored in a dense suspension (10^{10} cells/ml) for 3h at +4°C.

Water solutions of heavy metal salts in need concentrations and control solution with sodium chloride (0,1 MM) were prepared. For copper solutions pH was 7,0; for nickel and cadmium solutions pH was 8,2. Aqueous media with appropriate pH and electroconductivity were prepared on a distilled water by using 0,01n HCl and 0,01 M *tris* solutions. The pH value, chosen for each metal, corresponded to the maximal metal toxicity for cell PM (Ivanov et al., 1997). Bacterial suspensions with optical density D = 0,15 (540 nM, cuvette 1 sm) were incubated with heavy metal ions at +20°C for 15, 60 and 420 min. After incubation cells precipitated and transfer to measurement media with pH 5,4 and specific electroconductivity 0,0025 Sm/m. Decreasing of pH measurement media allowed better to detect cell PM damages by heavy metals.

EO-spectra of cells were obtained by measuring the relative change in cell suspension optical density due to orientation of cells in an uniform alternating electric field of a fixed frequency (f) within 100 Hz - 5 MHz at field intensity 24 and 60 V/sm. Experimental equipment, analysis details and interpretation of EO measurement were described earlier (Miroshnikov et al., 1986). The cell PM damage was judged from the course of the high-frequency decline of their EO-spectra by calculating the ratio β (beta) value of the EO effect (EOE) of cells at a field frequency of 5MHz to that at 0,5 MHz (Fomchenkov et al., 1986): $\Delta\beta/\beta_\kappa = (\beta_o - \beta_\kappa)/\beta_\kappa$, where β_o and β_κ - EO-spectrum values for treated and control cells consequently. The negative values of $\Delta\beta/\beta_\kappa$ testify to cell PM damages: when this negative $\Delta\beta/\beta_\kappa$ value is higher it means that the cell damage is stronger. All measurements were made at +25°C. The following salts of heavy metals were used: $NiCl_2 \times 6H_2O$, $CuCl_2 \times 2H_2O$, $CdSO_4 \times 8H_2O$ ("Reachim", Russia). For preparing of salt solutions distilled water with specific electroconductivity $1,3 \times 10^{-4}$ Sm/m was utilized.

RESULTS AND DISCUSSION

EO-spectra of intact and treated (60 min) by copper ions cells of *Thiocapsa roseopersicina* are shown in *fig. 1*. High frequency decline of EO spectra of copper treated cells displaced to the area of really lower frequencies. This character of change of high frequency region of cell EO-spectra at copper treatment testifies to the disturbance of barrier properties of cell PM.

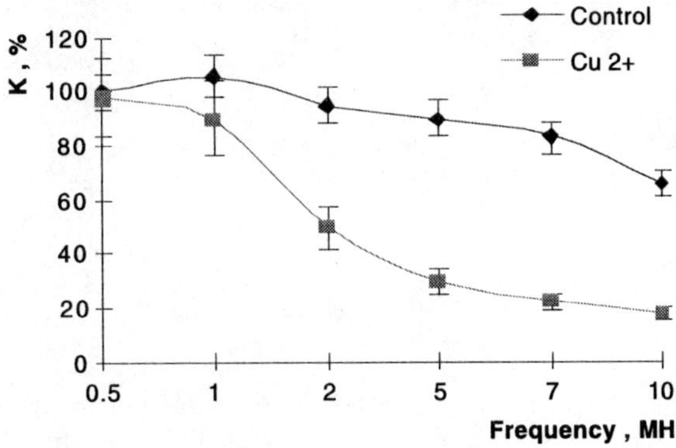

Fig. 1. EO-spectra of *Thiocapsa. roseopersicina* cells: control (1); incubated with copper ions 25 μM for 60 min (2). $K = (\Delta D_i / \Delta D_o) \times 100\%$, where ΔD_i is the change in optical density of cell suspension on switching of the electric field: ΔD_o is for the suspension of control cells at a field frequency of 0.5 MHz.

Analogous changes of EO-spectra of different bacterial cells were observed at cell damages caused injuring factors of various nature (Fomchenkov et al., 1986; Miroshnikov et al., 1986;

Ivanov et al., 1997). Because of disturbance of barrier properties of cell PM a significant part of free ions and low molecular compounds of cytoplasm are going out to the extra cellular media, where the concentration of ions is lower. As a result, the cell effective electroconductivity is slow down and this phenomenon lead to the shift of high frequency decline of EO-spectrum to lower frequencies (Miroshnikov et al., 1986).

From the analysis of EO-spectra in the area of high frequency decline it was determined the degree of injuring effect of Cu^{2+}, Cd^{2+} and Ni^{2+} cations on cell PM. *Fig. 2* and *fig. 3* demonstrate concentration and time dependence of change of $\Delta\beta/\beta_\kappa$ values for *Thiocapsa roseopersicina* cells, characterized a degree of cell PM damages by studying heavy metal cations. The following order of metal toxicity for cell PM was observed: $Cu^{2+} > Cd^{2+} > Ni^{2+}$, moreover the injuring metal effect depended on and on a time of exposure with heavy metal and on a metal concentration.

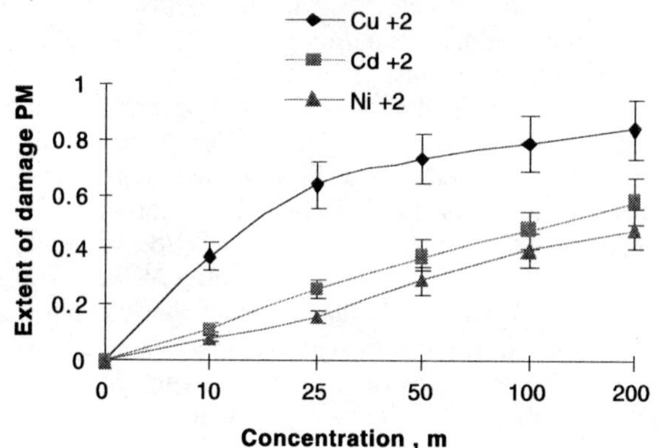

Fig. 2. $\Delta\beta/\beta_\kappa$ (extent of PM damage) of *Thiocapsa roseopersicina* cells, incubated 60 min with different concentrations of Cu^{2+}, Cd^{2+} and Ni^{2+}.

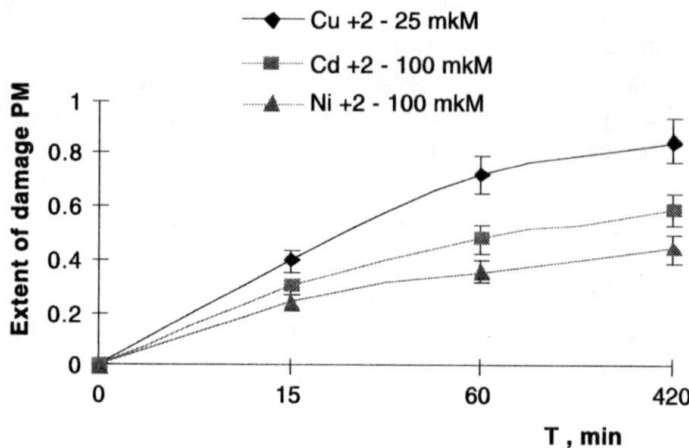

Fig. 3. $\Delta\beta/\beta_\kappa$ (extent of PM damage) of *Thiocapsa roseopersicina* cells, incubated with metal ions: Cu^{2+} (25 μM), Cd^{2+} (100 μM) and Ni^{2+} for different time.

Thus, investigation of influence of heavy metals on *T. roseopersicina* cells showed that copper, cadmium and nickel cations in low concentrations (10-200 μM) can disturb PM barrier properties. These data correspond to results of EO-spectroscopy of heavy metal effects on PM of different cells (Khassanova, 1996; Ivanov et al., 1997). However it is necessary to note that results on toxic effect of heavy metals on PM of *T. roseopersicina* cells were obtained in the solutions with low ionic force. The following research gives the definitive recommendations for recovery of studied metals by this phototrophic bacterium, therefor the additional investigations on influence of these metals on cell PM in the microorganism growth media are required.

REFERENCES

Bogorov L.V. Properties of *Thiocapsa roseopersicina* strain BBS isolated from the estuary of the White sea. *Microbiologiya* (Moscow). 1974, 43:326-332.

De Filippis L.F. The effect of heavy metals compounds on the permeability of *Chlorella* cells. *Z. Pflanzenphysiol.* 1979, 92:33-38.

Fomchenkov V.M. et al. Electric characteristics of bacterial cells measured when the barrier function of cytoplasmic membrane is disordered. *Microbiologiya* (Moscow). 1986, 55:754-759.

Geier B.M. et al. The effect of mercuric salts on the electrorotation of yeast cells and comparison with theoretical model. *Biochem. et Biophys. acta.* 1987, 900:825-831.

Gogotov I.N. et al. Biosorption of metal ions by microorganisms and their consortia with aqueous plants. *Metal Ions in Biology and Medicine.* V.7. Eds. L. Khassanova et al. John Libbey Eurotext, Paris. 2002, pp. 247-251.

Ivanov A. Yu. et al. Toxic effect of hydroxylated metal ions on the plasma membrane of bacterial cells. *Microbiologiya* (Moscow). 1997, 66:588-594.

Khassanova L. A. Electrophysical analysis and physiological-biochemical particularities of cell damages by heavy metal ions. Thesis (St. Petersburg). 1996.

Miroshnikov A. I., Fomchenkov V.M., Ivanov A. Yu. Electrophysical analysis and separation. Nauka (Moscow). 1986, 198 p.

Zadvorny O. A. et al. The effect of metal ions on hydrogenase of purple sulfur bacterium *Thiocapsa roseopersicina. Biochemistry (Russian edition)* 2000, 65:1525-1529.

Metal Ions in Biology and Medicine: vol. 9. Eds Maria Carmen Alpoim, Paula Vasconcellos Morais, Maria Amélia Santos, Armando J. Cristóvão, José A. Centeno, Philippe Collery.
John Libbey Eurotext, Paris © 2006 pp. 214-1.

Involvement of disulphide reductases in the response of *Campylobacter jejuni* to cadmium stress

Nadeem O. Kaakoush, George L. Mendz

School of Biotechnology and Biomolecular Sciences, The University of New South Wales, Sydney, NSW, Australia

ABSTRACT

Disulphide reductases and their substrates have many roles in cellular processes, including protection against reactive oxygen species and detoxification of xenobiotics, such as cadmium. This project studied the involvement of disulphide reductases in the response of the bacterium *Campylobacter jejuni* to cadmium stress. Growth-response curves were employed to investigate the effects of cadmium chloride on *C. jejuni*. The bacterium showed reduced growth in the presence of 0.3 mM cadmium chloride, and the metal ions were lethal at 1 mM concentration. Two-dimensional gel electrophoresis combined with tandem mass spectrometry analysis served to identify proteins differentially expressed in cells grown with and without 0.3 mM cadmium chloride. Thioredoxin reductase was downregulated in cells grown with cadmium ions; this result was confirmed by measuring enzyme activity using spectrophotometry. Proton nuclear magnetic resonance spectroscopy was employed to detect glutathione reduction activity in cell-free extracts of *C. jejuni*. Rates of glutathione reduction were measured in cells grown with and without 0.3 mM cadmium chloride. The rates were higher in cells grown in the presence of cadmium ions. Although cadmium inhibits the activity of thioredoxin reductase, many organisms respond by increasing the expression of this enzyme under cadmium stress. The data suggested, that unlike other organisms, in the presence of cadmium, *C. jejuni* downregulated thioredoxin reductase and upregulated enzymes which reduced disulphide substrates.

INTRODUCTION

Cadmium ions (Cd^{2+}) are a demonstrated potent carcinogen in animals, and cadmium is a toxic metal of significant environmental and occupational importance for humans. Disulphide reductases are essential enzymes in the antioxidant mechanisms of many bacteria, and have a role in protecting them from the toxic effects of heavy metals [1-3]. CXXC motifs and CXXC-derived motifs are present in the active sites of disulphide reductases [4], and could be involved in metal coordination and metal detoxication. For example, clusters of cysteines which are capable of coordinating zinc atoms are known as "zinc knuckles" or "zinc fingers" [4, 5].

The *Campylobacter* genus comprises a group of bacteria that can cause disease in humans and animals [6]. These bacteria have been isolated from laboratory and husbandry animals, pets, and birds. Most human diseases caused by organisms of this genus are due to *Campylobacter jejuni*, and only 1% of human campylobacteriosis cases are caused by other species [6]. Since little is known about the detoxication pathways of this microaerophilic bacterium, this study was performed to characterise the effects of cadmium ions on disulphide reductases of *C. jejuni*.

MATERIALS AND METHODS

Bacterial strain and growth conditions

Campylobacter jejuni NCTC 11168, isolated from humans, was grown on Campylobacter Selective Agar plates [7]. Liquid cultures were grown in vented flasks using 50 ml Brain Heart Infusion (Oxoid, VIC, Australia) supplemented with cadmium chloride (Sigma-Aldrich, NSW, Australia) at concentrations at 0%, 0.05%, 0.1%, 0.3%, 0.5% and 1%. Cells were tested for purity using phase contrast microscopy.

Preparation of cell-free protein extracts for two-dimensional electrophoresis

Chloramphenicol was added to bacterial suspensions to a final concentration of 128 μg/ml after 18 h of incubation. Cultures were centrifuged at 2879*g* for 25 minutes at 4 °C, and the pellet was washed with 0.2 M ice cold sucrose. This was repeated twice, the cell pellet was disrupted by thrice freeze-thawing, and resuspended in 1 ml TSU buffer (50 mM Tris pH 8.0, 0.1% SDS, 2.5 M Urea). Cell debris was removed by centrifugation at 14000*g* for 20 minutes at 4 °C. Protein concentrations were determined using the bicinchoninic acid method employing a microtitre protocol (Pierce, ILL, USA). Absorbances were measured using a Beckman Du 7500 spectrophotometer.

Two-dimensional and image analysis

One-hundred and ten μg of protein was suspended in 490 μl using a rehydration buffer consisting of 8 M urea, 100 mM dithiothreitol (DTT), 65 mM 3-[(3-cholamidopropyl)-dimethylammonio]-1-propanesulfonate (CHAPS), 40 mM Tris-HCl pH 8.0, 10 μl pH 4-7 IPG buffer (Amersham Biosciences, NSW, Australia). Nuclease buffer (10 μl) was added, and the mixture was incubated at 4 °C for 20 minutes. The sample was centrifuged at 14000*g* and 4 °C for 20 minutes, and the supernatant was loaded on to an 18 cm Immobiline DryStrip pH 4-7 (Amersham Biosciences), which was left to incubate for 20 h sealed at room temperature. Isoelectric focusing was performed using a flatbed Multiphor II unit (Amersham Biosciences) programmed for 2 h at 100 V; followed by 0.5 h at 500 V, 1500 V, and 2500 V; and a final 18 h step of 3500 V. Focused Imobiline DryStrips were equilibrated sequentially in two buffers of 6 M urea, 20% (w/w) glycerol, 2% (w/v) SDS, 375 mM Tris-HCl, the first containing 130 mM DTT, and the second containing 135 mM iodoacetamide (IA) (Sigma-Aldrich). Sodium dodecyl sulfate-polyacrylamide gel electrophoresis was performed on 11.5% acrylamide gels using the Protean II system (Bio-Rad, NSW, Australia) at 50 V for 1 h, followed by 64 mA until the dye reached the bottom of the gel. Gels were fixed individually in 0.2 l fixing solution (50% (v/v) methanol, 10% (v/v) acetic acid) for a minimum of 1 h, and were subsequently stained using a sensitive ammoniacal silver method.

Mass spectrometry identification of proteins

Excised gel slices were washed twice with 0.2 ml of 100 mM NH_4HCO_3 for 10 min, reduced with 50 μl of 10 mM DTT at 37 °C for 1 h, alkylated in 50 μl of 10 mM IA at 37 °C for 1 h, washed three times for 10 min with 0.2 ml milli-Q water, washed with 0.2 ml of 10 mM NH_4HCO_3 for 10 min, dehydrated in acetonitrile, and rehydrated in a buffer containing 10.5 ng μl^{-1} trypsin. After digestion for 14 h, peptides were extracted by washing the gel slice with 25 μl 1% formic acid for 15 min, followed by dehydration with acetonitrile. Digests were separated by nano-LC using an Ultimate/Famos/Switchos system. Samples (5 μl) were loaded on to a Micron C18 precolumn (500 μm × 2 mm) with buffer A (H_2O:CH_3CN (98:2 v/v) and 0.1% formic acid) at 25 μl min^{-1}. After a 4 min wash, the flow was switched into line with a PEPMAP C18 RP analytical column (75 μm × 15 cm) and eluted using buffer A to H_2O:CH_3CN (40:60, 0.1% formic acid) at 200 nl min^{-1} over 30 min. The nano electrospray needle was positioned ≈ 1 cm from the orifice of an API QStar Pulsar I tandem MS instrument. The QStar was operated in information-dependent acquisition mode. A time-of-flight mass spectrometry (TOF MS) survey scan was acquired (m/z 350-1700, 0.5 s), and the two largest precursors (counts >10) were selected sequentially by Q1 for tandem MS analysis (m/z 50-2000, 2.5 s). A processing script generated data suitable for submission to the database search programmes. Collision induced dissociation spectra were analysed using the Mascot MS/MS ion search tool (Matrix Science) with the following parameters: trypsin digestion allowing up to one missed cleavage, oxidation of methionine, peptide tolerance of 1.0 Da, and MS/MS tolerance of 0.8 Da. Protein searches were performed on the NCBI nr database.

Nuclear magnetic resonance spectroscopy

Proton nuclear magnetic resonance (^{1}H-NMR) free induction decays were collected using a Bruker DMX-600 spectrometer operating in the pulsed Fourier transform mode with quadrature detection as previously described [7]. Total disulphide reduction activities were measured in *C. jejuni* cell-free extracts with glutathione (GSSG) and NADH as substrates.

Spectrophotometry

Thioredoxin reductase activity was measured by dithiobis-2-nitrobenzoic acid (DTNB) reduction in the presence of NADPH using a Cary-100 UV-visible spectrophotometer. The reaction mixtures contained cell-free extracts and the appropriate substrates suspended in 50 mM TrisHCl, pH 7.2 buffer in a total volume of 1 ml, and were placed in 1 cm path-length cuvettes. The cell-free extracts were added just prior to measurement, and the change in absorbance at 412 nm over 2 minutes was recorded. The coefficient of molar absorbance for DTNB is 13.6×10^3 mol^{-1} cm^{-1} at 412 nm.

RESULTS

The effect of cadmium ions on the growth of *C. jejuni* was measured at five concentrations of these metal ions: 0.05, 0.1, 0.3, 0.5 and 1 mM. Two colony-forming unit (cfu/ml) counts were taken at 0 and 24 h from each culture. The bacteria grew approximately 1.5 log(cfu/ml) at 0 mM Cd^{2+} *(fig. 1). Campylobacter jejuni* showed increasing growth inhibition in the presence of 0.05 mM to 0.3 mM Cd^{2+}, and the cation was lethal at 1 mM concentration *(fig. 1)*. These data served to determine a concentration at which *C. jejuni* cells could be subjected to acute cadmium stress without completely inhibiting cell growth. At 0.3 mM Cd^{2+}, *C. jejuni* growth was significantly decreased but the cells were viable.

Campylobacter jejuni contains 33 putative disulphide reductases which have been identified bioinformatically [10]. Sequence analyses were performed on the disulphide reductases of *C. jejuni* to calculate the pI values of these proteins and determine their approximate positions on 2D-gels *(table I)*. This evaluation helped to map the spots corresponding to disulphide reductases on the gels. Thioredoxin reductase (TrxB) is a critical enzyme for redox regulation of protein function, signalling via thiol redox control, and bacterial defence against environmental stress. It has a pI of 5.6 and molecular weight of 33.1 kDa *(table I)*.

The response of cells grown with and without 0.3 mM cadmium was analysed via gel electrophoresis. *Figure 2* shows small sections of pI 4-7 gels. The circled spot was identified using tandem mass spectrometry analyses. Ten peptide sequences from the spot were matched to the enzyme TrxB from the *C. jejuni* strain 11168 genome. The larger than 2-fold downregulation of TrxB was confirmed using spectrophotometry. The activity of the enzyme was lower in cell-free extracts of cells grown with 0.3 mM cadmium than in extracts of cells grown without cadmium. The ratio of activities in cells grown with cadmium and cells grown without cadmium was approximately 1:4. This decrease in reduction rates was in agreement with the downregulation of protein expression observed in the gel analyses.

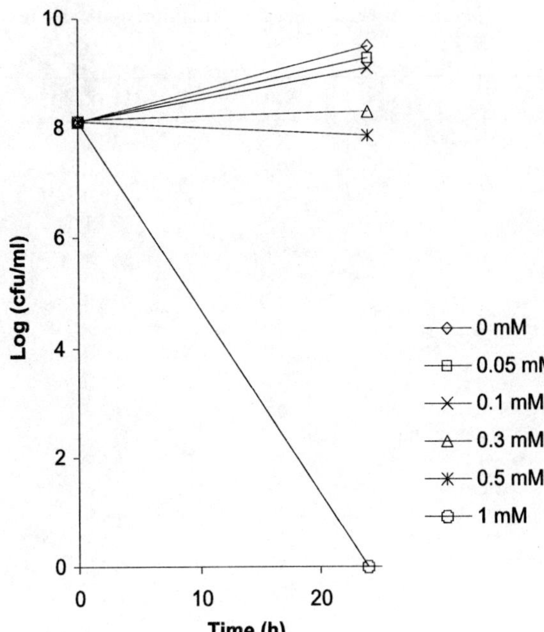

Fig. 1. Growth of *C. jejuni* in the presence of different concentrations of Cd^{2+}.

The measurement of disulphide reduction activities by ^{1}H-NMR spectroscopy was validated using several controls. Chemical reduction of GSSG was ruled out by observing no reduction in the absence of cell-free extracts. Negative controls of the assays showed that reduction of GSSG did not take place if NADH was not present. The enzymatic origin of the reactions was established by determining that no activity was present in suspensions of cell-free extracts which had been denatured by heating at 80 °C for 2 hours. The reduction rates for extracts of *C. jejuni* cells grown with or without cadmium were 170 and 54 nmole/mg/min, respectively.

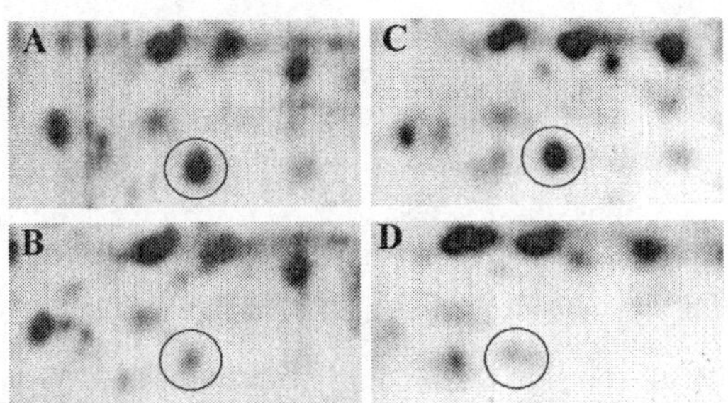

Fig. 2. Duplicates of 2D-gel sections of the *C. jejuni* proteome. Protein spots from gels of *C. jejuni* cells grown without cadmium (A, C), and in the presence of cadmium (B, D). The circled spots correspond to TrxB.

Table 1. Isoelectric point and molecular weight of disulphide reductases identified bioinformatically in *C. jejuni*.

ORF	Protein name	pI	MW (kDa)
CJ0017c	Putative ATP /GTP binding protein	8.6	56.8
CJ0058	Putative periplasmic protein	7.8	23.0
CJ0119	Hypothetical protein	6.0	19.9
CJ0146c	Thioredoxin reductase	5.6	33.1
CJ0147c	Thioredoxin	4.5	11.3
CJ0256	Putative integral membrane protein	8.3	59.3
CJ0262	Chemotaxis signal transduction protein	4.9	72.8
CJ0264c	Molybdopterin-containing oxidoreductase	8.5	93.3
CJ0280	Hypothetical protein	9.8	16.2
CJ0425	Putative periplasmic protein	5.4	15.6
CJ0535	2-oxoglutarate:acceptor oxidoreductase delta subunit	6.9	11.4
CJ0537	2-oxoglutarate:acceptor oxidoreductase beta subunit	8.0	31.2
CJ0559	Oxidoreductase	5.7	33.7
CJ0603c	Putative thiol:disulfide interchange protein	9.0	63.8
CJ0637c	Peptide methionine sulfoxide reductase	5.7	18.9
CJ0701	Putative protease	7.9	47.3
CJ0757	Putative heat shock regulator	5.2	30.9
CJ0865	Putative disulfide oxidoreductase	8.2	30.4
CJ0911	Putative periplasmic protein	8.4	21.8
CJ1006c	Hypothetical protein	8.6	47.1
CJ1019c	ABC transport system periplasmic binding	8.8	40.1
CJ1049c	Putative integral membrane protein	9.3	22.4
CJ1106	Possible periplasmic thioredoxin	5.3	23.0
CJ1112c	Hypothetical protein	6.8	13.4
CJ1168c	Putative integral membrane protein	8.9	22.6
CJ1278	Hypothetical protein	9.0	46.2
CJ1293	Possible sugar nucleotide epimerase	8.4	37.4
CJ1295	Hypothetical protein	6.0	49.9
CJ1380	Putative periplasmic protein	8.8	26.6
CJ1457c	Hypothetical protein	9.0	43.4
CJ1505c	Hypothetical protein	5.3	21.3
CJ1633	Hypothetical protein	7.6	36.8
CJ1665	Possible lipoprotein thioredoxin	7.6	18.9

DISCUSSION

Cadmium ions are very toxic even at low concentrations, but the basis for their toxicity is not fully understood. Several mechanisms have been proposed to explain how bacteria and lower eukaryotes protect themselves against cadmium toxicity. These include the enhanced expression of the low-molecular weight cysteine-rich protein metallothionein which sequesters cadmium, the accumulation of intracellular Zn^{2+}, the reduction of Cd^{2+} uptake, the binding of cadmium ions by other heavy metal-associated proteins, and the increase in intracellular disulphide content. The involvement of disulphide reductases, including TrxB, in cadmium detoxication has been demonstrated for several microorganisms. For example, *Saccharomyces cerevisiae* strains lacking thioredoxin and thioredoxin reductase are hypersensitive to cadmium [8].

To observe a change in *C. jejuni* growth, the bacterium required the presence of cadmium at micromolar concentrations *(fig. 1)*. This effect was comparable with those observed in other bacteria and yeast [8, 9]. The data confirmed that cadmium is highly toxic to microorganisms. The downregulation of the enzyme TrxB in *C. jejuni* cells grown with cadmium was unexpected, but this result was confirmed by spectrophotometry. Total disulphide reduction was measured to ascertain other responses of the bacteria to Cd^{2+} stress. An increase of approximately 4-fold in GSSG reduction was observed in cells grown with 0.3 mM cadmium. It was hypothesised that the bacterium expressed other disulphide reductases in response to the increased cadmium in the environment. Further studies are required to acquire a complete understanding of the molecular responses of *C. jejuni* to cadmium.

REFERENCES

1. Zegers I, Martins JC, Willem R, Wyns L, Messens J. Arsenate reductase from *S. aureus* plasmid pI258 is a phosphatase drafted for redox duty. *Nat Struct Biol* 2001; 8: 843-847.
2. Moore MJ, Miller SM, Walsh CT. C-terminal cysteines of Tn501 mercuric ion reductase. *Biochemistry* 1992; 31: 1677-1685.
3. Hayashi S, Abe M, Kimoto M, Furukawa S, Nakazawa T. The dsbA-dsbB disulfide bond formation system of *Burkholderia cepacia* is involved in the production of protease and alkaline phosphatase, motility, metal resistance, and multi-drug resistance. *Microbiol Immunol* 2000; 44: 41-50.
4. Rosato V, Pucello N, Giuliano G. Evidence for cysteine clustering in thermophilic proteomes. *TRENDS Genet* 2002; 18: 278-281.
5. Schwabe JW, Klug A. Zinc mining for protein domains. *Nat Struct Biol* 1994; 1: 345-349.
6. Moore JE, Corcoran D, Dooley JSG, Fanning S, Lucey B, Matsuda M, McDowell DA, Mégraud F, Millar BC, O'Mahony R, O'Riordan L, O'Rourke M, Rao JR, Rooney PJ, Sails A, Whyte P. *Campylobacter. Vet Res* 2005; 36: 351-382.
7. Kaakoush NO, Mendz GL. *Helicobacter pylori* disulphide reductases: role in metronidazole reduction. *FEMS Immunol Med Microbiol* 2005; 44: 137-142.
8. Vido K, Spector D, Lagniel G, Lopez S, Toledano MB, Labarre J. A proteome analysis of the cadmium response in *Saccharomyces cerevisiae. J Biol Chem* 2001; 276: 8469-8474.
9. Simonyte S, Cerkasin G, Planciuniene R, Naginiene R, Ryselis S, Ivanov L. Influence of cadmium and zinc on the mice resistance to *Listeria monocytogenes* infection. *Medicina (Kaunas)* 2003; 39: 767-772.
10. Kaakoush NO, Sterzenbach T, Miller WG, Suerbaum S, Mendz GL. Identification of disulphide reductases in Campylobacterales. *Arch Microbiol* 2006 (Submitted).

Metal Ions in Biology and Medicine: vol. 9. Eds Maria Carmen Alpoim, Paula Vasconcellos Morais, Maria Amélia Santos, Armando J. Cristóvão, José A. Centeno, Philippe Collery.
John Libbey Eurotext, Paris © 2006 pp. 220-1.

Bioleaching and chemical transformations of heavy metals and radionuclides mediated by soil microorganisms

Alexander A. Kamnev[1]*, Krisztina Kovács[2], Alexei G. Shchelochkov[1], Leonid A. Kulikov[3], Yurii D. Perfiliev[3], Erno Kuzmann[2] and Attila Vértes[2]

[1]*Laboratory of Plant-Bacterial Symbioses, Institute of Biochemistry and Physiology of Plants and Microorganisms, Russian Academy of Sciences, 410049 Saratov, Russia (E-mail: aakamnev@ibppm.sgu.ru)*
[2]*Research Group for Nuclear Techniques in Structural Chemistry, Hungarian Academy of Sciences; Department of Nuclear Chemistry, Eötvös Loránd University, Budapest-112, H-1518, Hungary*
[3]*Laboratory of Nuclear Chemistry Techniques, Department of Radiochemistry, Faculty of Chemistry, M.V. Lomonosov Moscow State University, Moscow, 119992, Russia*

ABSTRACT

Soil microorganisms are known to be involved in a range of biogeochemical processes leading to biomineralisation and a diversity of chemical transformations of soil minerals. In this study, various chemical and biological processes were investigated related to microbial activity in soil. It was found that some low-molecular-weight secondary bacterial and plant metabolites and related compounds (e.g. anthranilic acid, indolic substances including tryptophan and phytohormones of the auxin series excreted also by many soil microorganisms) can be involved in abiotic redox processes in acidic media which represent frequently occurring acidic soils. As a result, soil iron(III) can be reduced to iron(II) even under aerobic conditions. Products of auxin oxidation in the presence of iron(III) were found to be similar to those formed in the course of enzymatic and electrochemical oxidation under different conditions. Model studies showed that cobalt(II) is similarly rapidly sorbed by both live and dead bacterial cells in highly dilute solutions, with its further transformation within an hour in live cells.
Key words: heavy metals; bioleaching; soil microorganisms; iron(III) reduction; metal sorption

INTRODUCTION

Soil microflora is well documented to be an important active participant of biogeochemical processes leading to a diversity of chemical transformations of soil minerals. Some of diverse routes leading to bioleaching and biotransformation of minerals are represented by the following processes: microbial dissimilatory reduction of metal ions (e.g., Fe, Mn and many other less abundant redox-active metals) via different mechanisms; production of siderophores, carboxylic acids and other organics capable of binding and/or reducing metal cations, as well as contact interactions of microbial cells with metal complexes and solid compounds via microbial cell-wall biopolymers, sometimes with further involvement of metal ions in cellular metabolism or their inactivation via special intracellular mechanisms, etc. [1-6].

In this study, various chemical and biological processes were investigated related to microbial activity in soil involving some of their secondary metabolites and, on the other hand, some metal ions and their transformations. Using a complex of physicochemical techniques, it was shown that iron(III) can be reduced under aerobic conditions by a range of low-molecular-weight secondary bacterial and plant metabolites and related compounds (e.g. anthranilic acid, indolic substances including tryptophan and phytohormones of the auxin series excreted also by many soil microorganisms) with their concomitant oxidative degradation. In addition, emission Mossbauer spectroscopy (using the ^{57}Co radionuclide) was applied to the monitoring of primary cobalt(II) binding by live and dead bacterial cells and its further transformation in live cells.

EXPERIMENTAL

For ^{57}Fe transmission and ^{57}Co emission Mossbauer spectroscopic (EMS) studies, all standard preparation steps (including the use of the enriched ^{57}Fe stable isotope and the radioactive ^{57}Co nuclide, respectively), as well as methodological procedures were reported in detail earlier [7, 8]. Fourier transform infrared (FTIR) spectroscopic measurements were performed as described elsewhere [7, 9]. ^{1}H NMR spectra were obtained on a Bruker AC-300 spectrometer (300 MHz; internal standard - tetramethylsilane) in deuterated acetone solutions. Chromatography-mass spectrometry analysis was performed using an HP-5890 Series II+ spectrometer with an HP-5972 mass-selective detector (Hewlett-Packard) and an HP-5MS column (30 m $\times$ 0.25 mm; carrier: 5% diphenyl + 95% dimethylpolysiloxane); temperature range 60°C to 320°C; linear dynamic range 10^5. Soil bacterium *Azospirillum brasilense* Sp245 (The Collection of Cultures, IBPPM RAS, Saratov) was used in EMS studies.

RESULTS AND DISCUSSION

It is well known that bioavailability of iron, which is commonly abundant in most soils, is extremely low due to the very low solubility of ferric species that are most stable under aerobic conditions. Thus, iron(III) largely represented by oxyhydroxides of variable crystallinity is an essential component of many soil minerals. A variety of soil bacteria were documented to couple oxidation of soil organic matter, including organic pollutants, to dissimilatory reduction of many redox-active metals, primarily iron(III) and manganese(IV) [1, 3, 4]. As for iron(III), such processes can be realised via three most general mechanisms [1, 10]:

(1) contact reduction, when the bacterial cell attaches directly to the surface of iron(III)-bearing soil particle, with further reduction of iron(III) to iron(II) at the surface of the "parent" soil particle;

(2) chelator-assisted contact reduction, when iron(III) bound in a complex by a chelator in a soluble form is transported to the bacterial cell, with subsequent dissimilatory iron(III) reduction at the cell surface similar to the reduction step in the above-mentioned case;

(3) shuttle-assisted reduction involving specific compounds that serve as an electron shuttle between the bacterial cell and iron(III)-bearing mineral.

All the three mechanisms are clearly fundamentally different. Nevertheless, as for common features, the first two involve iron(III) reduction at the bacterial cell surface while mechanism (3) does not, which represents its main difference in the mode of electron transfer to iron(III). For mechanisms (2) and (3), the bacterial cell and the mineral (as an iron(III) source) need not be in contact as in the case of mechanism (1). Note that microbial dissimilatory reduction of Fe^{III} facilitates the release of traces of other metals often entrapped within ferric oxide minerals [8].

Besides the above-described directly biotic reduction of iron(III) by microbial cells, a range of secondary metabolites produced both by soil microorganisms and plant roots can abiotically reduce Fe^{III}. Our experiments using the powerful and sensitive ^{57}Fe Mossbauer spectroscopic technique showed that such low-molecular-weight organic substances as anthranilic (*o*-aminobenzoic) acid, indolic compounds including tryptophan, indole-3-acetic acid (a phytohormone of the auxin series produced by many soil microorganisms) and other auxins [7, 11, 12] can abiotically reduce Fe^{III} in acidic media (under pH 5) even under aerobic conditions.

In *fig. 1*, gradual iron(III) reduction to iron(II) by a series of indole-3-alkanoic acids in aqueous solutions is shown, as follows from Mossbauer spectroscopic measurements made after 15 min and 2 days of reaction at ambient temperature. Already 15 min after mixing iron(III) salt with an acid, iron(II) was readily detectable in the spectra of filtered and frozen solutions by its characteristic doublet with a large quadrupole splitting. After two days under these conditions, iron(II) dominated in all the solutions, except for indole-3-carboxylic acid (see *fig. 1,e*) for which the reduction rate was definitely lower than for the other indolic acids studied. It is noteworthy that for indole-3-acetic acid, practically full reduction is observed within 2 days, which corresponds to its more easily proceeding oxidative decarboxylation [13]. In all cases, the iron(II) doublet gave the following parameters: isomer shift, 1.38 to 1.40 mm s^{-1} (relative to alpha-Fe); quadrupole splitting, 3.3 mm s^{-1} (at T = 80 K), which corresponds to ferrous hexaaquo complex. Thus, the reduced iron ions in solution were most probably in the hydrated form not coordinated to the acids or their oxidation products.

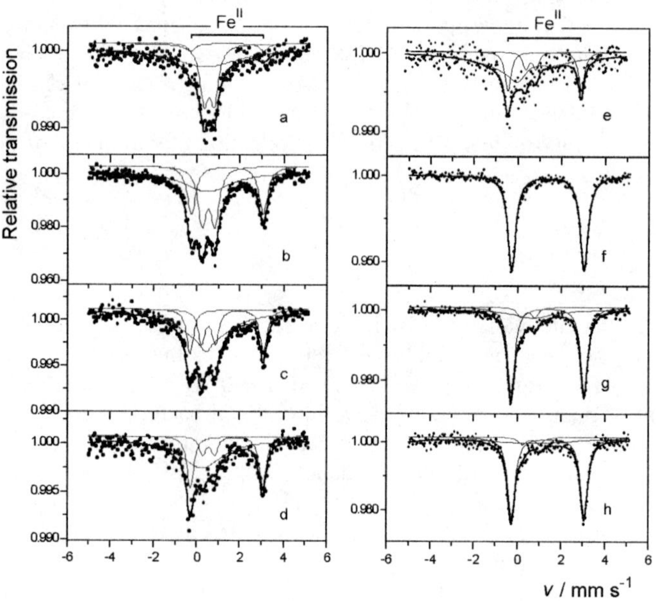

Fig. 1. Mossbauer spectra of $^{57}Fe^{III}$ nitrate and indole-3-alkanoic acid aqueous solutions filtered and rapidly frozen (at T = 80 K) 15 min (a-d) and 2 days (e-h) after mixing the reagents (pH 2-3). (a), (e) - indole-3-carboxylic acid; (b), (f) - indole-3-acetic acid; (c), (g) - indole-3-propionic acid; (d), (h) indole-3-butyric acid. The position of the Fe^{II} doublet is indicated in the upper plots by square brackets.

Raising the pH was found to result in a slower reduction, which, nevertheless, was still noticeable under pH 5 [11]. Since acidic soils are rather widely distributed (comprising over 30% of only arable territories [4], besides highly metal-polluted soils which often have lower pH), such abiotic reduction involving organic molecules of biotic origin may significantly contribute to Fe^{III} transformation in soil. Note that the resulting pool of iron(II) can further abiotically reduce toxic and mobile high-valent metals and metalloids [4] and contribute to reductive degradation of chlorinated and nitroaromatic organics [10].

Possible products of indole-3-acetic acid oxidation in the presence of Fe^{III} were investigated using FTIR spectroscopy, ^{1}H NMR and chromatography-mass spectrometry. The formation of oxindole-3-acetic acid was shown which formed a poorly soluble complex with Fe^{III} similar to that with indole-3-acetic acid [9]. From the reaction medium, using extraction with isobutanol and further chromatographic separation, two other oxidation products were isolated. One of the products gave an intensive FTIR band of carbonyl (1649 cm^{-1}), a couple of bands at 2925 and 2856 cm^{-1}

(aliphatic C-H stretching vibrations) and a band at 3403 cm^{-1} (N-H or O-H stretching vibrations). Its ^{1}H NMR spectrum in deuterated acetone showed a group of signals of the oxindole moiety (7.2-8.4 p.p.m.), a singlet of the >N-H proton (10.01 p.p.m.), a quadruplet (3.2-3.7 p.p.m.) of the proton in the position C3 of the oxindole moiety which split at neighbouring protons of the $-CH_3$ group. The latter three magnetically equivalent protons gave, in its turn, a doublet (split at the C3 proton) at 1.2 p.p.m. These data provided evidence for the formation of 3-methyl-2-oxindole as an oxidation product.

Traces of the other extracted product gave a number of signals in its mass spectrum which allowed the following fragmentation scheme to be assumed: $[M]^+$ 167 → (minus OH) → [M-17] 150 → (minus C=O) → [M-45] 122 → (minus NO_2) → [M-91] 76. This scheme suggests that the oxidation product was formed by oxidative splitting of the pyrrolin-2-one cycle. It was assumed that the product could be *o*-nitrobenzoic acid formed by oxidation of a possible intermediate, anthranilic acid, which did not accumulate in the reaction medium.

It should be noted that both oxindole-3-acetate and 3-methyl-2-oxindole, which formed in the course of chemical oxidation of indole-3-acetic acid in the presence of Fe^{III} (see above), had been reported among products of both enzymatic and electrochemical oxidation of indole-3-acetic acid [14, 15] at physiological pH, i.e. under different conditions and e^- transfer modes.

As mentioned above, both the microbially driven dissimilatory reduction of ferric oxide minerals and their abiotic reduction by bioorganics can result in release of other toxic metals entrapped within the ferric hydroxide matrix. In particular, it refers to the microbially mediated migration of radionuclides, e.g. ^{60}Co, from disposal sites (note that Co^{III} may also be used as an electron acceptor) [8]. In this study, cobalt(II) interaction with bacterial cells was monitored in model experiments using ^{57}Co EMS, a highly sensitive nuclear chemistry technique. The main EMS parameters (isomer shift and quadrupole splitting) were calculated from EMS spectra of aqueous bacterial suspensions rapidly frozen after various periods of time of contact with $^{57}Co^{II}$ traces *(fig. 2)*. In this plot, each "statistical point" represents a form (i.e., a microenvironment) of $^{57}Co^{II}$. It follows from *fig. 2* that both live cells (after 2 or 60 min of contact with $^{57}Co^{II}$) and dead cells, as well as the cell-free culture liquid have in each case two different forms of $^{57}Co^{II}$.

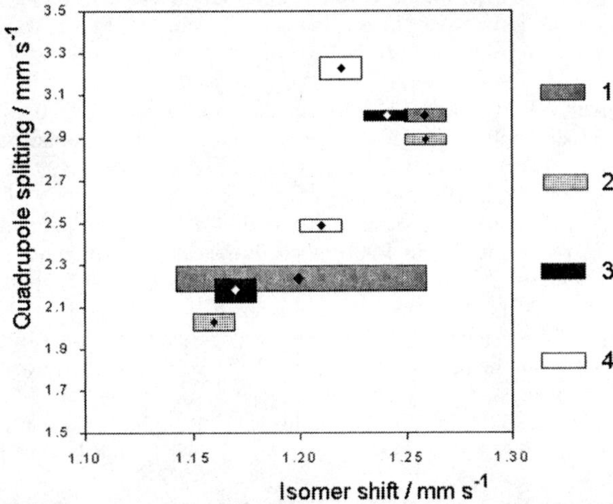

Fig. 2. Comparison of Mossbauer parameters - isomer shift (mm/s; relative to alpha-Fe) and quadrupole splitting (mm/s) - for different forms of [^{57}Co]-cobalt(II) in aqueous suspension of live cells of *Azospirillum brasilense* Sp245 rapidly frozen after (1) 2 min and (2) 60 min of contact with $^{57}Co^{II}$, (3) dead cells (hydrothermally killed at 95°C), and (4) cell-free supernatant liquid (measured at $T = 80$ K).

It can also be seen that the parameters of the two forms for 2-min-"treated" live cells (marked "1"; see *fig. 2*) are close to those for dead cells (marked "3"), the latter evidently reflecting purely chemical binding of $^{57}Co^{II}$. This mode of binding is therefore similar to the primary rapid binding by live cells, in line with the conclusions made in [5]. For 1-h-"treated" live cells (marked "2" in *fig. 2*), the parameters of both two forms are distinctly different reflecting ongoing metabolic transformations; whereas for the cell-free culture broth (marked "4"), the two Co^{II} forms differ from those in all other cell-bound samples. These model EMS studies, together with the literature data, reveal possible biotransformations of Co radionuclide traces that can result in its microbially mediated migration in soils and aquifers.

REFERENCES

1. Lloyd J.R. Microbial reduction of metals and radionuclides. *FEMS Microbiol. Rev.* 2003; 27: 411-25.
2. Faraldo-Gomez J.D., Sansom M.S.P. Acquisition of siderophores in Gram-negative bacteria. *Nature Rev. Mol. Cell Biol.* 2003; 4: 105-16.
3. Straub K.L., Schink B. Evaluation of electron-shuttling compounds in microbial ferric iron reduction. *FEMS Microbiol. Lett.* 2003; 220: 229-33.
4. Kamnev A.A. Phytoremediation of heavy metals: an overview. In M. Fingerman, R. Nagabhushanam (Eds.), *Recent Advances in Marine Biotechnology*. Vol. 8, *Bioremediation*. Science Publ., Enfield (NH), USA, 2003, pp. 269-317.
5. Jiang W., Saxena A., Song B., Ward B.B., Beveridge T.J., Myneni S.C.B. Elucidation of functional groups on Gram-positive and Gram-negative bacterial surfaces using infrared spectroscopy. *Langmuir* 2004; 20: 11433-42.
6. Rancourt D.G., Thibault P.-J., Mavrocordatos D., Lamarche G. Hydrous ferric oxide precipitation in the presence of nonmetabolizing bacteria: constraints on the mechanism of a biotic effect. *Geochim. Cosmochim. Acta* 2005; 69: 553-77.
7. Kamnev AA, Kuzmann E, Perfiliev YuD, Vanko Gy, Vertes A. Mossbauer and FTIR spectroscopic studies of iron anthranilates: coordination, structure and some ecological aspects of iron complexation. *J. Mol. Struct.* 1999; 482-483: 703-11.
8. Kamnev A.A. Application of emission (^{57}Co) Mossbauer spectroscopy in bioscience. *J. Mol. Struct.* 2005; 744-747: 161-67.
9. Shchelochkov A.G., Kamnev A.A., Tarantilis P.A., Polissiou M.G. Spectroscopic study of iron(III) complexes with some indole derivatives. In L. Khassanova, Ph. Collery, I. Maymard, Z. Khassanova, J.-C. Etienne (Eds.), *Metal Ions in Biology and Medicine*, Vol. 7. John Libbey Eurotext, Paris, 2002, pp. 37-40.
10. Kamnev A.A., Antonyuk L.P., Ignatov V.V. Biodegradation of organic pollution involving soil iron(III) solubilized by bacterial siderophores as an electron acceptor: possibilities and perspectives. In R. Fass, Y. Flashner, S. Reuveny (Eds.), *Novel Approaches for Bioremediation of Organic Pollution*, Kluwer Acad. / Plenum Publ., New York, 1999, pp. 205-217.
11. Kamnev A.A., Kuzmann E. Some rhizobacterial metabolites of non-siderophore nature as possible solubilizing agents for soil ferric species. In P. Carmona, R. Navarro, A. Hernanz (Eds.), *Spectroscopy of Biological Molecules: Modern Trends. Annex.* UNED Press, Madrid, 1997, pp. 85-6.
12. Kovacs K., Kamnev A.A., Mink J., Nemeth Cs., Kuzmann E., Megyes T., Grosz T., Medzihradszky-Schweiger H., Vertes A. Mossbauer, vibrational spectroscopic and solution X-ray diffraction studies of the structure of iron(III) complexes formed with indole-3-alkanoic acids in acidic aqueous solutions. *Struct. Chem.* 2006; 17: in press.
13. Savitsky P.A., Gazaryan I.G., Tishkov V.I., Lagrimini L.M., Ruzgas T., Gorton L. Oxidation of indole-3-acetic acid by dioxygen catalysed by plant peroxidases: specificity for the enzyme structure. *Biochem. J.* 1999; 340: 579-83.
14. Gazaryan I.G., Chubar T.A., Mareeva E.A., Lagrimini L.M., Van Huystee R.B., Thorneley R.N.F. Aerobic oxidation of indole-3-acetic acid catalysed by anionic and cationic peanut peroxidase. *Phytochemistry* 1999; 51: 175-86.
15. Hu T., Dryhurst G. Electrochemical and peroxidase O_2-mediated oxidation of indole-3-acetic acid at physiological pH. *J. Electroanal. Chem.* 1997; 432: 7-18.

ACKNOWLEDGEMENTS

This work was supported in part by NATO (Grants LST.CLG.977664, LST.NR.CLG.981092, CBP.NR.NREV.981748), the Russian Academy of Sciences' Commission (Grant No. 205 under the 6th Competition-Expertise of research projects), as well as under the Agreements on Scientific Cooperation between the Russian and Hungarian Academies of Sciences for 2002-2004 and 2005-2007.

Metal Ions in Biology and Medicine: vol. 9. Eds Maria Carmen Alpoim, Paula Vasconcellos Morais, Maria Amélia Santos, Armando J. Cristóvão, José A. Centeno, Philippe Collery.
John Libbey Eurotext, Paris © 2006 pp. 226-1.

Electrophysical analysis of Cr(III) and Cr(VI) influence on sulfate reductive bacterium *Desulfobacterium sp.63*

L. A. Khassanova[1,6], A. Yu. Ivanov[2], Z.M. Khassanova[3,6], I.N. Gogotov[4], Yu. A. Frank[4], D. O. Safieva[5], J.-C. Etienne[6]

[1]*Russian State University of Oil and Gas, 65, Leninsky prospect, Moscow, 119991, Russia;*
[2]*Institute of Cell Biophysics RAS, Pushchino, 142290, Russia;*
[3]*Bashkir State Pedagogical University, 3a, October revolution street, Ufa, 450000, Russia;*
[4]*Institute of Basic Biological Problems RAS, Pushchino, 142290, Russia;*
[5]*Institute of Biochemical Physics RAS, 4, Kosygin, Moscow, 117997, Russia;*
[6]*International Research Institute on Metal Ions, University of Reims, Champagne-Ardenne, BP 1039, 51687 Reims cedex2, France.*

ABSTRACT

The effect of Cr(III) and Cr(VI) (25 - 100 μM) on the permeability of plasma membrane (PM) and cell surface electric properties of *Desulfobacterium sp.63* was investigated by the method of electroorientational spectroscopy (EO-spectroscopy). Bacterial interaction with Cr(III) cations decreased cell surface polarization and increased cell PM permeability, Cr(VI) as CrO^{2-}_4 anions influenced only on the PM barrier properties. Chromium toxic effect on cell PM depends on metal concentration and time of exposure with metal ions and was higher in case of Cr(III).

INTRODUCTION

The toxic effects of heavy metals on cell barrier properties were observed for different biological objects (De Filippe L.F. 1979; Ivanov et al., 1992, 1997; Geier B.M. et al., 1987; Khassanova, 1996). EO-spectroscopy is using as an express method to detect cell damages by heavy metals (Miroshnikov et al., 1986). This method demonstrates changes of cell electrophysical properties (cell surface polarization, electric properties of PM and cytoplasm) under the heavy metal's influence (Ivanov et al., 1992; Khassanova, 1996). There are a few works devoted to investigations of chromium toxic effects on cell barrier properties (Khassanova, 1996). Electrophysical analysis of chromium interaction with sulfate reductive bacterium *Desulfobacterium sp.63*, which can be used for chromium recovery, is absent. Therefor the method of EO-spectroscopy was used for investigations of Cr(III) and Cr(VI) influence on the electrophysical properties of *Desulfobacterium sp.63* cells.

MATERIALS AND METHODS

The clean culture of sulfate reductive bacterium *Desulfobacterium sp.63* was obtained from the coastal sediments of the Black Sea. *Desulfobacterium sp.63* cells were grown in a mineral medium (Pfennig et al., 1981) at +28°C in the strict anaerobic conditions for 6 days, as an organic substrate lactate was used (Karnachuk, 1995). To adapt of *Desulfobacterium sp.63* to chromium ions bacterial cells were cultivated in the medium with 40 mg/l Cr(VI) and reinoculated with growing concentrations of $K_2Cr_2O_7$ salt. After that cells were precipitated, washed with distilled water and stored in a dense suspension throughout the experiment (1-2 h) at +20°C. Prior to the experiments cell suspension was prepared in Tris-HCl medium with specific electroconductivity

0,0042 Sm/m, pH 7,0-7,2 and optical density $D_{1.0} = 0.2$. Then the chromium salt solutions of an essential concentrations were introduced to cell suspensions and incubated at room temperature for 15 and 45 min. Before measurements the specific electroconductivity of suspensions was adjusted to 0,0055 Sm/m with 0,01 M sodium chloride solution. Inactivation of bacterial cells was carried out by heat treatment at +70°C on the water bath for 15 min.

EO-spectra of cells were obtained by measuring the relative change in cell suspension optical density due to orientation of cells in an uniform alternating electric field of a fixed frequency (f) within 100 Hz - 5 MHz at field intensity 24 and 60 V/sm. Experimental equipment, analysis details and interpretation of EO measurement were described earlier (Miroshnikov et al., 1986). The cell PM damage was judged from the course of the high-frequency decline of their EO-spectra by calculating the ratio β (beta) value of the EO effect (EOE) of cells at a field frequency of 5MHz to that at 0,5 MHz (Fomchenkov et al., 1986): $\Delta\beta/\beta_\kappa = (\beta_o - \beta_\kappa)/\beta_\kappa$, where β_o and β_κ - EO-spectrum values for treated and control cells consequently. The negative values of $\Delta\beta/\beta_\kappa$ testify to cell PM damages: when this negative $\Delta\beta/\beta_\kappa$ value is higher it means that the cell damage is stronger. All measurements were made at +25°C. The following salts of heavy metals were used: $CrCl_3 \times 10\ H_2O$ and $K_2Cr_2O_7$ ("Reachim", Russia). For preparing of salt solutions distilled water with specific electroconductivity $1{,}3 \times 10^{-4}$ Sm/m was utilized.

RESULTS AND DISCUSSION

EO-spectra of *Desulfobacterium sp.63*: native cells, cultivated without chromium (curve - C-Cr(VI)), heat inactivated cells, cultivated without chromium (curve - Inact) and native cells cultivated with 40 mg/l Cr(VI) (curve - C+Cr(VI)) are presented in *fig. 1*. It can be seen the following EO-spectra peculiarities: growing of EOE in the area of low frequency; middle frequency minimum; high frequency maximum and subsequent EOE decline. The low frequency EOE rise induced by relaxation of double electric layer (DEL) polarization on the cell surface and their value is determined by cell surface electric properties. High frequency maximum of EO-spectrum is conditioned by structural polarization and EOE value, mainly stipulates by the correlation of cell and medium electric conductivity. High frequency EOE depends on electric conductivity of cytoplasm and can describe the PM barrier properties of cells (Miroshnikov et al., 1986).

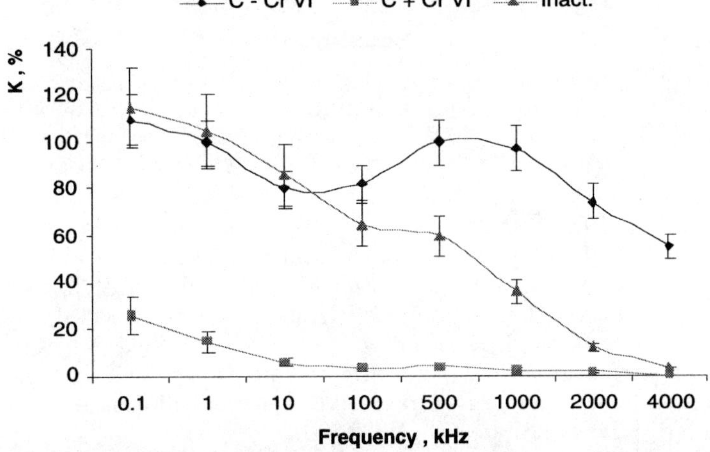

Fig. 1. EO-spectra of *Desulfobacterium sp.63*: native cells, cultivated without chromium (curve - C-Cr(VI)), native cells cultivated with 40 mg/l Cr(VI) (curve - C+Cr(VI)) and heat inactivated cells, cultivated without chromium (curve - Inact). $K = (\Delta D_i / \Delta D_o) \times 100\%$, where ΔD_i is the change in optical density of cell suspension on switching of the electric field: ΔD_o is for the suspension of control cells at a field frequency 0,5 MHz.

EOE for cells cultivated with Cr(VI) had low value practically in all diapason of frequencies *(fig. 1)*. That kind of spectrum (curve - C+Cr(VI)) is usually typical for cell suspensions with high concentrations of aggregates.

The microscopic control confirmed the presence of big cell aggregates in the investigated suspension. EO-spectrum of heat inactivated cells of *Desulfobacterium sp.63*, cultivated without chromium (curve - Inact) is shown in *fig. 1*, which demonstrated the change of high frequency region of EO-spectra of cells with disturbance of PM permeability. Heat inactivation of cells lead to decrease of high frequency maximum and their displacement in the area of lower frequencies. Similar character of EO-spectra changes in high frequency area was shown earlier for bacterial cell damages caused by different physicochemical factors (Fomchenkov et al., 1986; Ivanov et al., 1997; Khassanova, 1996, Miroshnikov et al., 1986).

Because of low EOE value of *Desulfobacterium sp.63* cells cultivated with Cr(VI) all further experiments carried out on the bacteria, growing without chromium.

The influence of two chromium forms: Cr(III) and Cr(VI) on the character of cell EO-spectra changes is shown in *fig. 2*. The cell treatment by Cr(III) (curve - Cr(III)) decreased EOE in high frequency area and moreover lead to the change of high frequency part of EO-spectra typical for cells with PM damages. Presence in suspension Cr(VI) in anion form (CrO^{2-}_4) was changed only cell EO-spectra (curve - Cr(VI)) in the area of high frequency decline of EOE.

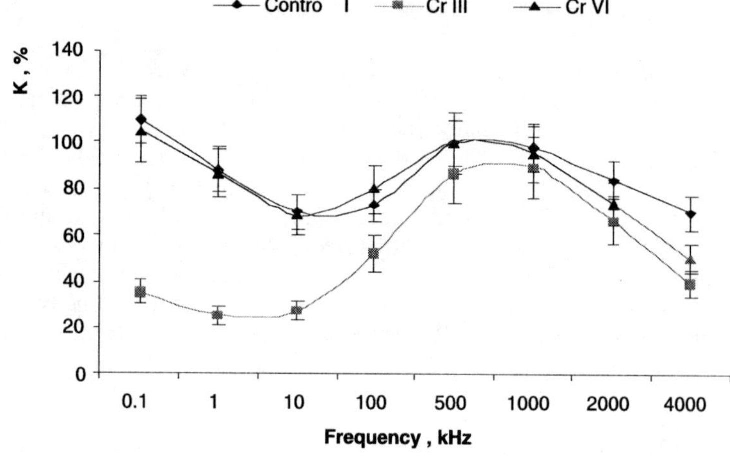

Fig. 2. EO-spectra of *Desulfobacterium sp.63*: native cells, cultivated without chromium (curve - control), native cells treated by 50 μM Cr(III) during 15 min (curve - Cr(III)) and native cells treated by 50 μM Cr(IV) during 15 min (curve - Cr(IV)). $K = (\Delta D_i / \Delta D_o) \times 100\%$, where ΔD_i is the change in optical density of cell suspension on switching of the electric field: ΔD_o is for the suspension of control cells at a field frequency 0,5 MHz.

EO-spectra analysis of *Desulfobacterium sp.63* cells in the area of high frequency decline of EOE gives possibility to determine the degree of damage effect of cell PM by two forms of chromium: Cr(III) and Cr(VI). Concentration and time dependence of $\Delta\beta/\beta_\kappa$ value changes demonstrated the degree of cell PM damages by Cr(III) and Cr(VI) are presented in *fig. 3* and *fig. 4*. The analysis of these dependence shows that the degree of cell PM damages by Cr(III) and Cr(VI) was significantly higher in case of bacteria treated by chromium in cationic form and depended on metal concentration and exposure time. The $\Delta\beta/\beta_\kappa$ value of cell damaged by chromium was compared with $\Delta\beta/\beta_\kappa$ value of heat treated cells *(fig. 4)*.

It is known, that under certain pH values metal cations are hydrolyzed in diluted solutions (Nazarenko et al., 1979). Water media with pH 5-8 is such area for Cr(III) cations. In these conditions Cr(III) cations pass from divalent hydroxylated form $CrOH^{2+}$ to monovalent hydroxylated form $Cr(OH_2^+)$. Because of decrease of hydrate envelope, a hydroxylated monovalent forms of metal cations have high adsorption properties. Earlier it was shown for different groups of microorganisms (Collins et al., 1992; Khassanova, 1996), that these hydroxylated monovalent forms of heavy metal cations adsorb on cell surface and significantly decrease their negative charge till to positive value.

The study of (Khassanova, 1996) curried out the comparative analysis of electrophoretical mobility (EPM) and EOE values in the area of electric field with low frequencies for *Escherichia coli* K-12 and *Pseudomonas fluorescence* 71 under effect of Cr(III) in wide pH diapason. It was expected, that in the area of cation existence in monovalent hydroxylated form $Cr(OH_2^+)$ there is the same directed decrease of cell EPM and cell EOE values at electric field frequencies 20-100 Hz. It was conclude that adsorption of hydroxylated form of $Cr(OH_2^+)$ cations on the cell surface significantly decrease negative charge of cells and, correspondingly, DEL of the cell surface. Decrease of DEL relaxation lead to the rise of surface polarization and EOE value in low frequency area of EO spectra. Decrease of EOE value of *Desulfobacterium sp.63* in low frequency area of cell EO-spectrum under the Cr(III) effect at pH 7,0-7,2, observed in our investigation (*fig. 2* (curve - Cr(III)) was similar with data of (Khassanova, 1996). It permits to suggest, that such change of cell EOE value stipulates by adsorption of $Cr(OH_2^+)$ cation forms on cell surface, which lead to decrease of their surface polarization.

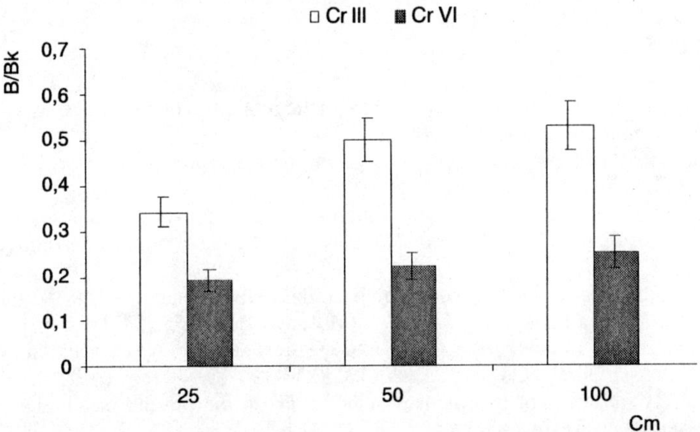

Fig. 3. $\Delta\beta/\beta_\kappa$ (extent of PM damage) of *Desulfobacterium sp.63* cells, incubated with different concentrations of Cr(III) and Cr(VI) (25, 50, 100 μM) for 15 min.

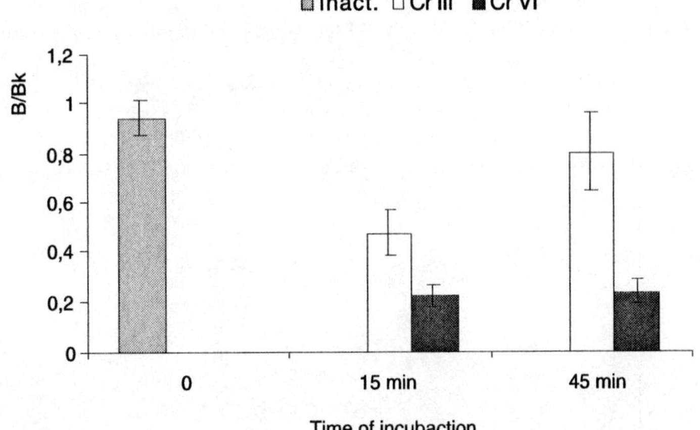

Fig. 4. $\Delta\beta/\beta_\kappa$ (extent of PM damage) of *Desulfobacterium sp.63* cells, heat inactivated, incubated with ions Cr(III) and Cr(VI) (50μM) for 15 and 45 min.

The results of influence of two chromium forms (cation and anion) on the PM barrier properties showed, that the degree of PM damage was significantly higher in case of cation form of chromium. That allows us to suggest different mechanisms of the injuring effect of two chromium forms on cell PM. In the first case, when chromium was in the treatment media in hydroxylated cation form ($Cr(OH_2^+)$) it can be binding with negative groups of PM transport proteins. High toxicity of monovalent hydroxylated cation forms of heavy metals for microbial PM was earlier demonstrated (Khassanova, 1996; Ivanov et al., 1997). Conclusions of these investigations coincide with present results. In case of cell treatment by chromium in anion form ($CrO^{2-}{}_4$), the well known oxidant with strong toxicity for cells (Shi et al., 1999; Fernandes et al., 2000), probably, partial chromium recovery took place with formation of active oxygen forms, which can partly inactivated transport proteins of cell PM.

Thus, present research of the the influence of two chromium forms as a cation and as an anion on electrophysical characteristics of *Desulfobacterium sp.63* showed that the cell treatment by chromium in cation form Cr(III) leads to decrease of cell surface polarization and disturbance of barrier properties of cell PM, whereas chromium presence in $CrO^{2-}{}_4$ form in cell suspension influenced only on cell PM.

REFERENCES

Collins Y.E. Stotzky Y G. Heavy metals alter the electrokinetic properties of bacteria, yeasts and clay minerals. *Applied Environ. Microbiol.* 1992, 58:1592-1600.

De Filippis L.F. The effect of heavy metals compounds on the permeability of *Chlorella* cells. *Z. Pflanzenphysiol.* 1979, 92:33-38.

Fernandes M.A.S. et al. On the mechanism of chromium (VI)-induced toxicity studies in human erythrocyte membrane. *Metal Ions in Biology and Medicine*. V.6 Eds. I. A. Centeno. et al. John Libbey Eurotext, Paris. 2000, 287-289.

Fomchenkov V.M. et al. Electric characteristics of bacterial cells measured when the barrier function of cytoplasmic membrane is disordered. *Microbiologiya* (Moscow). 1986, 55:754-759.

Geier B.M. et al. The effect of mercuric salts on the electrorotation of yeast cells and comparison with theoretical model. *Biochem. et Biophys. acta.* 1987, 900:825-831.

Ivanov A. Yu. et al. Toxic effect of hydroxylated metal ions on the plasma membrane of bacterial cells. *Microbiologiya* (Moscow). 1997, 66:588-594.

Karnachuk O.V. Influence of hexavalent chromium oh hydrogen sulfide formation by sulfate-reducing bacteria. *Microbiologiya* (Moscow). 1995, 64:315-319.

Khassanova L. A. Electrophysical analysis and physiological-biochemical particularities of cell damages by heavy metal ions. Thesis (St. Petersburg). 1996.

Miroshnikov A. I., Fomchenkov V.M., Ivanov A. Yu. Electrophysical analysis and separation. Nauka (Moscow). 1986, 198 p.

Nazarenko V. A. et al. Hydrolysis of metal ions in diluted solutions. Atomizdat (Moscow) 1979, 156 p.

Pfennig N., Widdel F., Truper H.G. The prokaryotes: a handbook on habitats, isolation and indentification of bacteria. Eds. Starr M.P. et al. Berlin: Springer-Verlag, 1981.V.1. P.926.

Shi X. et al. Reduction of chromium (VI) and its relationship to carcinogenesis. *J.Toxicol Environ Health.* 1999, 2:87-107.

Metal Ions in Biology and Medicine: vol. 9. Eds Maria Carmen Alpoim, Paula Vasconcellos Morais, Maria Amélia Santos, Armando J. Cristóvão, José A. Centeno, Philippe Collery.
John Libbey Eurotext, Paris © 2006 pp. 231-1.

Desulfovibrio gigas: toxicity of copper and molybdenum

Lino, A.R.[1,2], Farinha, C.R.[1], Pereira, S.[1], Bursakov, S.A.[3]

[1]*Departamento de Química e Bioquímica, Faculdade de Ciências da Universidade de Lisboa, Campo Grande, 1749-016 Lisboa, Portugal, arlino@fc.ul.pt;*
[2]*Centro de Química e Bioquímica, Faculdade de Ciências da Universidade de Lisboa, Campo Grande, 1749-016 Lisboa, Portugal;*
[3]*REQUIMTE, Departamento de Química, CQFB, Faculdade de Ciências e Tecnologia, Universidade Nova de Lisboa, 2829-516 Caparica, Portugal, sergey@dq.fct.unl.pt*

Sulphate reducing bacteria (SRB) is a group of microorganisms able to carry out the dissimilatory reduction of sulphate to sulphide, a reactive compound that can form insoluble precipitates with heavy metals. SRB require copper and molybdenum at low concentrations as essential micronutrients, however at high concentrations, toxic effect of these elements can be observed.

In this work toxicity of copper and molybdenum was studied by using free and biofilm bound batch cultures of *D. gigas* grown in a semi-defined medium (VMN) with Pipes or phosphate buffer to understand the chemistry and nature of copper, molybdenum and sulphur interactions.

The effect of copper (in the range 0 to 80 μM) was tested at a constant concentration of molybdenum (110 μM) in VMN medium with Pipes buffer. Inhibition effect of 70% was observed in cellular growth at maximal Cu concentration. The presence of Mo in the media increase copper toxicity due to reduction of abiotic copper precipitation and improving copper solubility.

The toxic effects of copper and molybdenum were dependent on concentrations of metals and estimated in terms of inhibition of total cell protein, longer lag times and lower specific growth rates.

The toxic effect of copper was more emphasized in free (80 μM) than in biofilm (150 μM) cultures. Nevertheless biofilm cells were more competent to remove metals from solution.

Keywords: sulfate reducing bacteria; *Desulfovibrio gigas*; toxicity of copper and molybdenum; biofilms

INTRODUCTION

Metal toxicity towards microorganisms is of environmental concern because of possible inhibition of essential microbe-assisted processes, such as the degradation of organic matter and the transfer of accumulated metals to higher organisms in the food chain. Each metal has a particular purpose and each requires specific mechanisms within the cell for uptake, storage and insertion into the protein.

Sulphate reducing bacteria (SRB) carry out dissimilatory reduction of sulphate to sulphide and require copper and molybdenum at low concentrations for growth. However at higher concentrations, toxic effect of these metals can be observed. An interaction of metal ions with nucleic acids, enzyme active sites and an influence on membrane integrity have been reported (1). Metals also undergo biosorption by cell surfaces and extracelular polymeric substances (EPS). EPS comprise a mixture of polysaccharides, proteins, nucleic acids, which varies in composition between species and culture conditions (2).

Free and biofilm bound SRB generate chemically active hidrogen sulphide that interact with metal ions and results in the production of insoluble metal sulfides. Abiotic formation of metal precipitation prevents meaningful quantitative assessment to metal toxicity. Tetrathiomolybdate (MoS_4^{2-}) is able to solubilise freshly precipitated CuS in aqueous medium and enhance the copper bioavailability in presence of H_2S. Confirmation of tetra and trithiomolybdates formation have been accomplished by identification of the characteristic spectral absorption of MoS_4^{2-} in cultural media at certain molybdenum concentrations (4). The ratio between thiomolibdates concentrations depends on the amount of hidrogen sulphide in the medium, varying with time and number of cells in solution.

Reports regarding the toxicity of heavy metals to SRB have generally been qualitative and microbial media have been designed to optimize growth rather than to examine metal tocixity (5). In this study we payed special attention to the composition of culture medium in order to study the bioavailability and toxicity of copper toward *D. gigas* growth. The bacteria were grown in VMN (3) Pipes medium with different concentrations of copper at a constant concentration of molybdenium (110 µM). VMN is a medium where yeast extract is eliminated and a defined vitamin solution is used. In VMN Pipes phosphate buffer is replaced by Pipes buffer to minimize abiotic precipitation.

MATERIALS AND METHODS

Desulfovibrio gigas (ATCC19364) was grown anaerobically at 37 °C, in a semidefined medium VMN with Pipes (piperazine-*NN'*-bis(2-ethanesulfonic acid).

Serum bottles with 100 ml of medium purged with ultra pure nitrogen by 30 min, sealed with butyl rubber septa capped and crimped with an aluminum seals were sterilized for 20 min at 120 °C. In all studies cultures in triplicate were prepared using a 10% (v/v) inoculum in exponential growth phase and incubated at 37 °C. Samples of 0,5 ml were removed to analyze of total cell protein to quantify the growth during 264 hours.

For biofim studies steril mild steel coupons (5 × 1 × 0,1 cm) were transferred to McCartney bottle with 22 ml of medium sterilized at 121 °C during 20 min. Oxygen was purged from bottles with N_2 gas before inoculation by 20 min in order to achieve anaerobic conditions. Experiments were conducted for biofilm growth during 7 days.

Samples of 2 ml from supernatant were removed for metals and protein analysis.

After the described incubation time coupons were transferred to botlles with 15 ml of Tris/HCl buffer 10 mM pH 7,2 with 0,15 M NaCl. Biofilms were removed from coupons by ultrasonic treatment (3 cycles of 5 sec) and sampled for protein analysis and metals determination. Botlles that did not contain inoculum or metals were prepared as control samples.

Molybdenum (Na_2MoO_4) at final concentration of 110 µM and copper ($CuCl_2$) at varied concentrations (0 - 80 µM for free cultures and 0 - 150 µM in biofilms) were added to serum bottles with syringe.

Total cell protein was determined using a quantitative colorimetric Coomassie assay method (6) and metals by atomic absorption spectrophotometry.

Neutral hexoses were quantified by Dubois method (7) and hidrogen sulphide dissolved in the media was determined by methylene blue method.

RESULTS AND DISCUSSION

This study represent assessment of metal toxicity quantified as the inhibition of *D. gigas* growth in VMN Pipes medium for free living and biofilm bound cells for a constant concentration of 110 µM of molybdenum.

The copper toxicity for free living cells was studied by changes in bacterial growth of *D. gigas*, measured based on total cell protein as function of time varying amounts of copper as shown in *figure 1*.

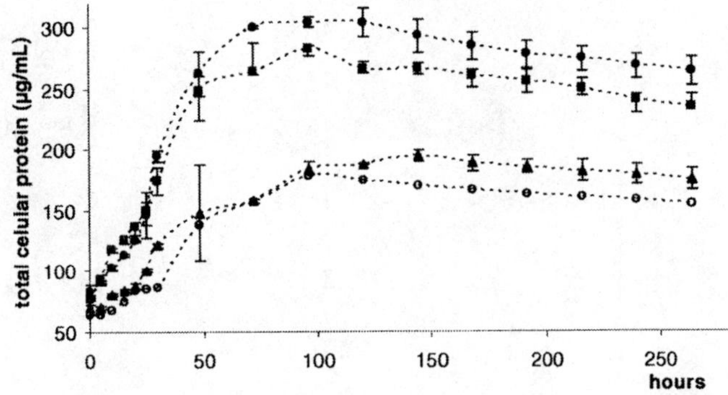

Fig. 1. The growth of *D. gigas* with different concentrations of copper (● 0 µM; ■ 12 µM; ▲ 56 µM; ○ 80 µM) in VMN with Pipes medium. Results present an average of triplicate and error bars indicate standard deviation.

A decrease in final cell protein concentration, longer lag times and lower growth rates were observed for increasing concentrations of copper, indicating the inhibitor effect of this metal in the growth of these bacteria. A reduction of 30% and 70% is observed in specific growth rate of *D. gigas* for copper concentrations of 12 µM and 80 µM, respectively. Lag time of 5 and 10 h are observed to copper concentrations referred.

Specific growth rates, doubling times and percentage of growth inhibition are presented in *table1*.

Table 1. Specific growth rate and doubling time of *D. gigas* in VMN with Pipes medium with different copper concentrations.

[Cu] µM	Doubling time H td	Specific growth rate H^{-1} *µg*	Growth inhibition %
0	7,89±0,07	0,088±0,001	0
12	11,33±0,53	0,061±0,003	30
56	21,98±0,36	0,032±0,002	64
80	27,21±0,78	0,026±0,002	70

The copper concentrations also influence the reduction of sulfate and consequently the production of H_2S. Production of hydrogen sulfide is increased during *D. gigas* growth with time, however increases of metal concentration in solution led to decreases in production of H_2S *(fig. 2)*. The percentage of inhibition of H_2S production at maximum cell protein (96 h of growth) is 52% and 80% for 12 µM and 80 µM copper concentrations *(fig. 3)*.

Copper precipitation in presence of H_2S has been largely discussed and depend of medium and culture conditions (4). Our previous work (3) has shown the toxic effect of molybdenum (110 µM) on the *D. gigas* growth that is demonstrated by the longer lag times and lower growth rates mesuared compared with assay control. However for this particular concentration of Mo, in parallel with increase of the H_2S concentration in solution, an increase of orange coloration was observed due to tri and tetrathiomolybdate production. Spectra with intense absorption peaks at 314 nm and 468 nm are typical of tetratiomolibdates (8) *(fig. 4)*. The formation of tetratiomolibdates inhibite the reaction of H_2S with copper increasing the solubility of this metal in solution.

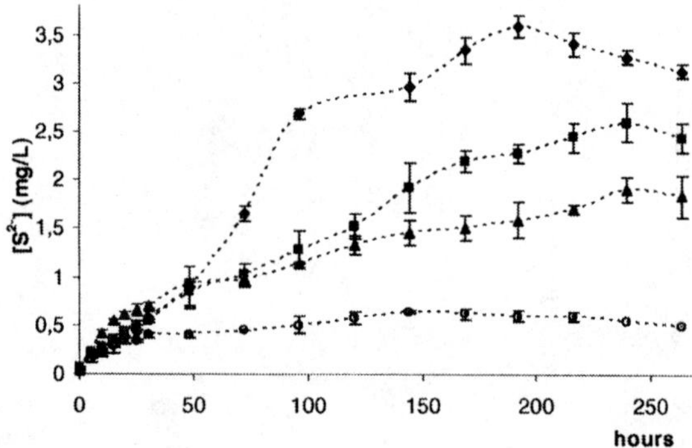

Fig. 2. Hydrogen sulfide production during *D. gigas* growth at different copper concentrations (● 0 μM; ● 12 μM; ● 56 μM; ● 80 μM). The points present an average of triplicate and error bars indicate standard deviation.

The production of tetrathiomolybdates depends of the amount of H_2S soluble in the medium, varying with time and number of cells and copper concentration in cultural media. Tetrathiomolybdates concentration decrease 15% and 43% for copper concentrations of 12 μM and 80 μM at maximum cell protein production (96 h) *(fig. 3)*.

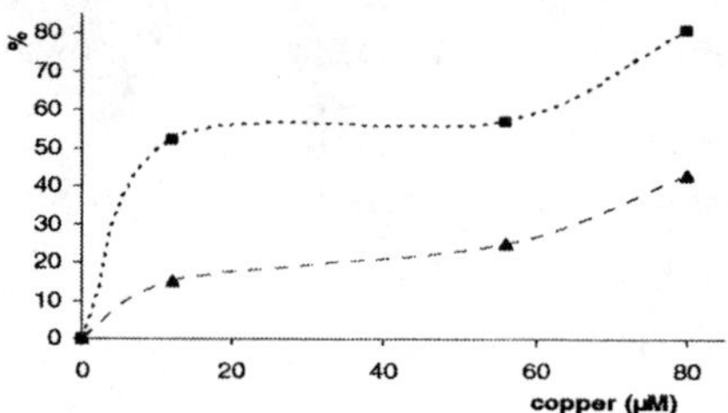

Fig. 3. Inhibition of hydrogen sulfide (●) and tetrathiomolybdate (●) production in presence of different concentrations of copper.

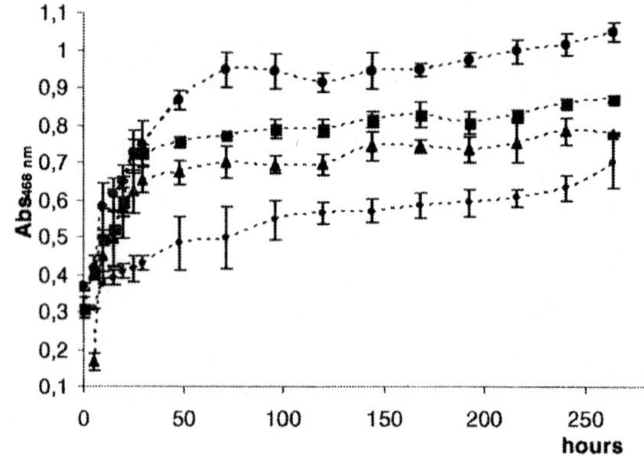

Fig. 4. Absorbance (468 nm) of the cultural media during *D. gigas* growth at different copper concentrations (● 0 μM; ● 12 μM; ● 56 μM; ● 80 μM). The points present an average of triplicate and error bars indicate standard deviation.

Preliminary studies of the inhibitory effect of copper in *D. gigas* biofilm bound growth. Showed that an increase in total cellular protein was observed until seventh day of growth followed by a decline phase for copper concentrations of 0 μM, 80 μM and 150 μM. For copper concentrations of 80 μM and 150 μM a decrease of 35% and 46% in total cellular protein is observed related with control assay for 7 days old biofilms. For free cell of *D. gigas* a decrease of 70% is observed for copper concentration of 80 μM while decrease of 35% is observed in biofilm bound cells showing the protecting effect of the biofilm. Copper determinations by atomic absorption showed than 90% of copper was accumulated by the biofilm. Copper can be accumulated by the biofilm by biosorption on cell surface, bound to EPS or mainly as solid copper sulfides.

Studies concerning EPS composition indicate a higher accumulation of carbohydrates when copper concentrations increase (5% and 24% of neutral hexoses for 80 μM and 150 μM in copper) suggesting that the polysaccharide component of EPS may be responsible for the immobilization of copper in the EPS matrix.

Electron microscopy and EDXA analysis are in course to confirm the nature of copper deposits in the biofilm.

REFERENCES

1. Sani, R.K., Peyton, B.M.; Brown, L.T.; Copper-induced inhibition of growth of *Desulfovibrio desulfuricans* G20: Assessment of its toxicity and correlation with those of zinc and lead; *Applied and Environmental Microbiology* (2001), **67**:4765-4772
2. Beech, I.B. and Cheung, C.W.S. (1995). Interactions of exopolymers produced by sulphate reducing bacteria with metal ions. *Int. Biodet. Biodeg*. **35**, 59-72.
3. Bursakov, S. ; Farinha, C.R. ; Lino, A.R. ; Moura, J.J.G. ; Moura, I., Metal ion influence in sulphate reducing bacteria ; *First International Congress of IMBG*, France, 6-8 September, 2004.
4. Sani, R. K.; Geesey, G.; Peyton, B.M.; assessment of lead toxicity to *Desulfovibrio desufuricans* G20: influence of component of Lactate C medium; *Advances in Environmental Research* (2001), **5**:269-276.
5. Zinkevich, V.; Beech, I. B., Screening of sulphate reducing bacteria, in colonoscopy samples from health and colitic human gut mucosa *FEMS, Microbiology Ecology* (2000), **34**, 147-155.
6. Bradford, M.M.; A rapid and sensitive method for quantification of microgram quantities of protein utilizing the principe of protein dye binding; *Analytical Biochemistry* (1976), **72**:248-254.
7. Dubois, M., Gilles, K.A., Hamilton, J.K., Rebers, P.A., Smith, F. Colorimetric method for determination of sugars and related substances. Analytical Chemistry 1956; 28: 350-56.
8. Quagraine, E.K.; Reid, R.S.; UV/ visible spectrophotometric studies of the interactions of thiomolybdates, copper (II) and other ligands; *Journal of Inorganic Biochemistry* (2001), **85**:53-60.

ACKNOWLEDGMENTS

This work was supported by FCT, POCI/QUI/59119/2004

Metal Ions in Biology and Medicine: vol. 9. Eds Maria Carmen Alpoim, Paula Vasconcellos Morais, Maria Amélia Santos, Armando J. Cristóvão, José A. Centeno, Philippe Collery.
John Libbey Eurotext, Paris © 2006 pp. 236-1.

Cytochromes of *Shewanella* respiratory pathways

Ricardo O. Louro and Carlos A. Salgueiro

Instituto de Tecnologia Química e Biológica da Universidade Nova de Lisboa, Rua da Quinta Grande nº 6, Apt 127, 2780-156 Oeiras, Portugal
REQUIMTE, Departamento de Química, Centro de Química Fina e Biotecnologia, Faculdade de Ciências e Tecnologia da Universidade Nova de Lisboa, 2829-516 Caparica, Portugal

It is in the microbial world that we find the greatest degree of respiratory flexibility with some Bacteria and Archaea being capable of extracting energy for growth from electron-donor/acceptor couples that span more than one volt in the redox scale [1]. Traditional Biochemistry combined with the novel -omics techniques is revealing the wide breadth of respiratory flexibility of some of these organisms and allowing a more in depth exploration of the novel metabolic pathways associated with it.

It has been proposed that the earliest respiratory processes developed by living forms in the primordial Earth relied upon the utilization of Fe(III) or S(0) as electron acceptors. Based on considerations of the environmental conditions in the primordial Earth where photochemically generated Fe(III) should be abundant in the seas, and on the observation of Fe(III) respiration by deep branching Archaea and Bacteria which do not respire S(0) it was proposed that Fe(III) respiration preceded S(0) respiration [2]. Another argument supporting this proposal is the fact the Fe(III) respiration can occur without the recourse to elaborate redox proteins and co-factors. Hydrogen, which was also available in the primordial Earth, can provide the electrons via an externally facing hydrogenase with the resulting protons already available in the correct side of the membrane for electrochemical gradient generation [3].

For many years, work on this and other forms of anaerobic respiratory processes was severely hampered by the difficulty in manipulating the relevant organisms, and the efforts of many talented researchers were required to develop the experimental techniques that nowadays enable the isolation and growth of anaerobic microorganisms in the laboratory (for a review see [4]).

The first fully sequenced genome of an organism capable of growing using metal respiration was that of *Shewanella oneidensis* MR-1[5] and this report was greeted with enthusiasm by the scientific community given the opportunities that it provided for understanding and harnessing the metal respiring capabilities of this organism for bioremediation [6].

Shewanella (S.) species have been isolated from a variety of sources including freshwater and marine sediments, spoiled fish, clinical isolates, and crude oil, and show an impressive respiratory versatility where the metabolism is coupled to the reduction of a variety of electrons acceptors extending from molecular oxygen to S(0) [7]. Furthermore, it was shown that *Shewanella* species can grow using a graphite electrode as electron acceptor therefore opening the possibility for the development of microbial fuel cells [8]. Some species of *Shewanella* display chemotactic behavior in gradients of divalent cations such as Fe(II) and Mn(II) and also towards insoluble Fe(III) and Mn(III) [9], and two broad strategies have been put forward to explain the capability of these organisms to donate electrons to insoluble acceptors, direct contact with the acceptor using cytochromes that are displayed on the outer membrane and the use of soluble electron shuttles excreted into the medium [10, 11].

The great majority of biochemical studies on *Shewanella* focused on proteins purified from *S. frigidimarina* NCIMB400 that was originally isolated from rotting fish [12], and on proteins from *S. oneidensis* MR-1 that was originally isolated from lake Oneida in the USA based on its ability to reduce insoluble Fe(III) and MN(IV) oxides [13].

Prominent in the genome of *S. oneidensis* MR-1 is the presence of a large number of cytochromes and up to 42 have been tentatively identified using pattern matching techniques [14]. Moreover, cytochromes have been implicated in the anaerobic respiration of *Shewanella* in particular that involving the reduction of insoluble metal oxides [10].

Of the multitude of cytochromes in the *Shewanella* genome, six soluble ones exist in significant amounts in the cells of *S. oneidensis* MR-1 *(table 1)* with similar results obtained for *S. frigidimarina* NCIMB400 [14, 15] and PAGE evidence for similar proteins in both species [16].

Table 1. Soluble cytochromes isolated from *Shewanella* sp.

Name	Molecular weight		Redox potential
	S. oneidensis	*S. frigidimarina*	
Cytochrome c_5	9	8.5*	High
Cytochrome c_4	20	20*	High
Bacterial Cytochrome *c* Peroxidase (BCCP)	46	-	High
Cytochrome *c*'	32	11*	High
Small tetraheme cytochrome (STC)	12	12	Low
Favocytochrome c_3 (fcc3)	65	64	Low

* Tentative identification [14]

Of these cytochromes, the most abundant are the cytochrome c_5, the STC, and fcc3 which are present at similar levels of protein concentration [14].

The putative cytochrome c_5 was shown to be more expressed under limited oxygen conditions [14, 15] and its gene together with the gene of cytochrome *c*' is up-regulated in aerobic growth [7]. Analysis of the genome of *S. oneidensis* MR-1 suggests two possible functional roles for the cytochrome c_5. It may function as an electron carrier between the cytochrome bc_1 membrane complex and the terminal cytochrome *c* oxidase, and in addition it may also function as an electron donor to BCCP. The BCCP is a di-heme protein present in larger quantities under low aeration with homology to the *Pseudomonas aeruginosa* ccp and appears to function as a peroxide detoxifying enzyme. The rational for the assignment of cytochrome c_5 as the partner of BCCP relies on the fact that *S. oneidensis* MR-1 lacks a c_8 cytochrome and c_5 is the only high potential soluble cytochrome that is abundant in cell extracts [14].

The soluble low redox potential cytochromes have been implicated in anaerobic respiratory pathways. Using DNA microarrays, 2D PAGE and mass spectrometry the mRNA and protein expression level profiles of *S. oneidensis* MR-1 were investigated under aerobic and anaerobic conditions showing induction of fcc3 [7].

The Flavocytochrome c_3

The genetic context for the flavocytochrome c_3 in the two *Shewanella* species is different for this monocystronic gene which appears to result from the fusion of a tetraheme cytochrome and the flavoprotein subunit of fumarate reductase [14, 17]. The crystallographic structure confirms this showing a N-terminal domain containing four heme binding sites and a C-terminal domain homologous to the membrane bound fumarate reductase flavoprotein [18].

In the bacterium *Wolinella succinogenes* a homologous fumarate reductase is actually encoded by an operon containing three genes, a tetraheme cytochrome, a flavoprotein fumarate reductase and another tetraheme cytochrome homologous to the CymA quinol dehydrogenase from *Shewanella* [19]. In *Shewanella* this tetraheme cytochrome is attached to the periplasmic face of the membrane, is encoded by a monocystronic operon and interacts directly with fcc3 [20, 21].

The flavocytochrome c_3 has unidirectional fumarate reductase activity, with more than 1000 larger Kcat/Km for fumarate reduction reported for the protein from *S. frigidimarina* [22]. The rate limiting step for fumarate reduction is proton delivery to the flavin catalytic site and the intramolecular electron re-equilibration among the four hemes was shown to be faster than the electron delivery by heme IV to the active site [23]. The four hemes have bis-histidine axial coordination which provides a strong ligand field to the central iron that is diamagnetic in the reduced heme and low-spin paramagnetic in the oxidized heme. These conditions are ideally suited for high-resolution paramagnetic NMR studies of the heme domain because the signals of the methyls at the periphery of the heme are shifted outside of the protein envelope towards low field. These shifts assume a pattern that relates to the geometry of the axial histidines therefore facilitating structural determination for novel proteins or assignment to specific hemes for proteins of known structure [24]. NMR spectroscopy studies in the fully oxidized state of the flavocytochrome isolated from *S. frigidimarina* and in a mutant where the axial ligand of heme IV, histidine 61, was replaced by an alanine, allowed the assignment of methyl signals to specific haems in the structure [25]. Dynamic NMR techniques show that for sample concentrations of 0.5 mM the intermolecular electron exchange is slow on the NMR time scale ($<1.51\times10^4$ s^{-1}), whereas the intramolecular exchange is fast ($>9.23\times10^4 s^{-1}$) [25]. Under these conditions NMR experiments performed in partially oxidized samples display a pattern of signals that can be related to the relative redox potentials of the hemes because the paramagnetic shift of each signal is proportional to the degree of oxidation of the respective heme. These data allowed the determination of the order of oxidation of the hemes as II, I, III and IV [25]. The nomenclature of the hemes is based on the order of attachment to the CXXCH motifs in the amino-acid sequence and relates with the distance from the flavin active site. Therefore, the order of oxidation reported above shows that polarization of the electron distribution occurs as the oxidation progresses. The electrons are drained first from the hemes further away from the active site and hemes III and IV are kept reduced until later in the oxidation. This optimizes the availability of electrons to be transferred to the FAD in the active site [25]. This ensures unimpeded transfer to this two electron cofactor and may be at the origin of the observation that proton transfer to the active site is the rate limiting step [23]. The observation that for the H61A mutant the rate limiting step is now electron transfer to the flavin [23], confirms the importance of the correct tuning of the potentials of the hemes to ensure the catalytic performance of this respiratory enzyme, since this mutation necessarily perturbs the redox potential of heme IV to more positive values.

The small tetraheme cytochrome *c*

For the STC the genetic context of its gene is also different between *S. oneidensis* MR-1 and *S. frigidimarina* being upstream to a *b*-type cytochrome in the former and upstream to an assimilatory nitrite reductase in the later [17]. A null mutant for this gene on *S. frigidimarina* gave rise to severe reduction in the ability grow on soluble Fe(III) revealing its participation in Fe(III) respiration [26].

The amino-acid sequence shows 42% identity with the N-terminal domain of fcc3 and a preliminary NMR structure of the STC from *S. frigidimarina* showed that the two are similar in several respects: i) the overall trace of the polypeptide backbone; ii) the location of the heme attaching residues and; iii) overall architecture of the heme core [27]. A semi-empirical model of the electronic structure of the oxidized hemes was utilized to determine the orientation of the axial histidine planes from carbon 13 NMR data measured in un-enriched samples [28]. Hemes I and III have similar orientations of the axial histidine planes which are expected to be parallel and lie in the sector defined by the NA-Fe-ND atoms of the heme. The aromatic planes of the axial histidines of heme IV are expected to have a relatively small angle (34°), whereas for heme II the axial histidines are expected to be close to perpendicular (73°) [28]. These data allowed the disentanglement of the *g* values of the specific hemes therefore allowing the specific assignment of the signals in the EPR spectrum [26]. The order of oxidation of the haems was determined showing that heme IV has the lowest potential followed by heme II, then I, and finally III [27]. Detailed equilibrium thermodynamics studies using dynamic NMR experiments and redox titrations followed by visible spectroscopy showed that the close packing of the hemes allows for heme-heme interactions which are dominated by electrostatic effects [29], with a clear correlation with distance that can be fit to a shielded electrostatic model [30]. Furthermore, the microscopic heme redox potentials are modulated in the physiological pH range by an acid-base group that is predicted to be located in the vicinity of heme III but its nature has not been determined.

The redox potentials of the hemes for the STC from *S. oneidensis* MR-1 were also reported to be pH dependent in the physiological range and the order of oxidation at high pH is I, II, IV and III, which is different to that reported for the STC from *S. frigidimarina* [31]. For this protein, a simple electron harvesting role was proposed based on the easy intermolecular electron transfer allowed by the crystal packing [32].

High resolution crystallographic structures were obtained for the oxidized (0.97Å) and the reduced states (1.02Å) for the STC from *S. oneidensis* MR-1 showing small differences between the two states. The most notorious involves the movement of a lysine side chain (K72) that reduces the solvent exposure of heme III and forms an H-bond to the A-propionate of this heme [32]. This conformational change was proposed to originate a redox-Bohr effect that would be stronger with heme III as was observed for the STC from *S. frigidimarina*. The overall fold is similar to that of the N-terminal domain of the fcc3 with an extended chain of hemes. Despite the extensive sequence identity between these two cytochromes (69%) the order of oxidation of the hemes is different in the two protein with heme III as the highest potential heme in both cases, which forces an endergonic intramolecular electron transfer step if one considers the protein to function as a wire [29]. Furthermore, the order of oxidation in both STC is different to that determined for the heme domain of the fcc3 from *S. frigidimarina*, showing that despite the sequence and structural similarity the tetraheme domain is tuned differently according to function.

Further understanding of the importance of the differences between the two STC and fcc3 will require the study of the other elements of the anaerobic respiratory chains of *Shewanella*.

Anaerobic respiratory chains in *Shewanella*

A central role in the anaerobic respiration of *Shewanella* appears to be played by the membrane bound quinol dehydrogenase cymA which is a tetraheme cytochrome. This protein has homology with the NapC/NirT family of proteins but is monocystronic in the case of *Shewanella* and not incorporated in specific membrane complexes [33]. Iron III respiration involves this protein, the mtrDEF-OmcA-mtrCAB gene cluster that encodes outer membrane decaheme proteins (MtrF, OmcA, MtrC) soluble decaheme cytochromes (MtrD, MtrA) and putative β-barrel proteins (MtrE, MtrB), the STC cytochrome, and the inducible flavocytochrome c_3 (Ifc3) [34]. Vanadate respiration again involves cymA, the outer membrane OmcB(MtrC) and MtrB [35]. CymA also participates in the respiration of fumarate, nitrate, nitrite, manganese and DMSO [36]. From the collected metabolic information a putative organization of the anaerobic respiratory pathways can be proposed *(fig. 1)*.

Despite all this knowledge, the structures of these proteins are for the most part still unknown and the mechanisms by which electron flow is controlled in this multi-branched respiratory chain have not been explored yet. These future steps will be essential to harness the potential for biotechnological applications presented by these organisms.

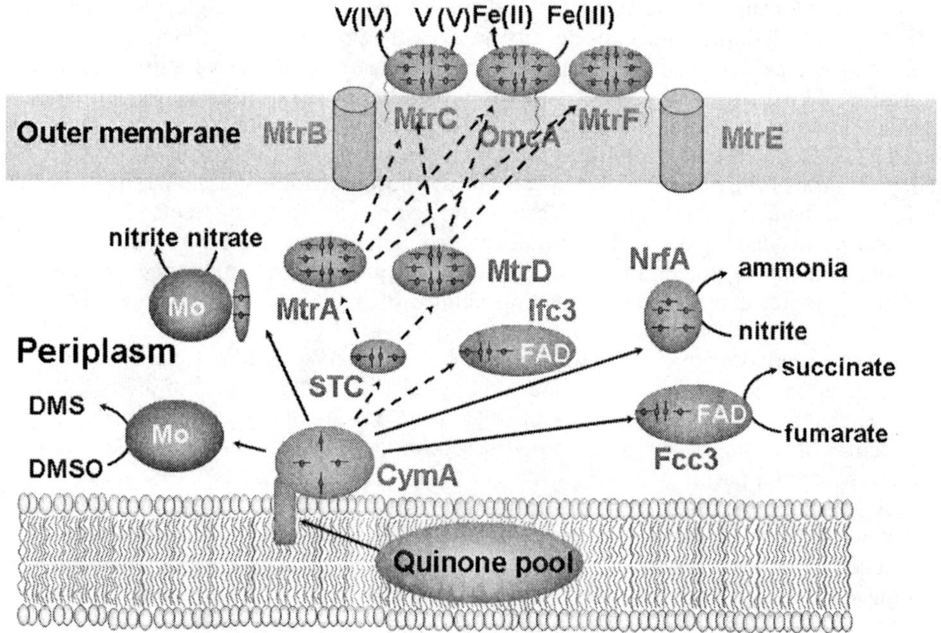

Fig. 1. Schematic Illustration of a few anaerobic respiratory pathways in *Shewanella* sp.
*Putative electron transfer pathways involved in metal respiration are indicated by dashed arrows

REFERENCES

1. Nealson, K.H. and Conrad, P.G. Life: past, present and future. *Phil. Trans. R. Soc. Lond. B* 1999; 354: 1923-1939.
2. Vargas, M. *et al.* Microbiological evidence for Fe(III) reduction on early Earth. *Nature* 1998; 395: 65-67.
3. Richardson, D.J. Bacterial respiration: a flexible process for a changing environment. *Microbiology* 2000; 146: 551-557.
4. Wolf, R.S. Anaerobic life-A centennial view. *J. Bacteriol.* 1999; 181: 3317-3320.
5. Heidelberg, J.F. *et al.* First genome sequence of a dissimilatory iron- and manganese-oxide reducing microbe *Shewanella oneidensis*. *Nat. Biotechnol.* 2002; 20: 1118-1123.
6. Tiedje, J.M. *Shewanella*- the environmentally versatile genome. *Nat. Biotechnol.* 2002; 20: 1093-1094.
7. Beliaev, A.S. *et al.* Gene and protein expression profiles of *Shewanella oneidensis* during anaerobic growth with different electron acceptors. *OMICS* 2002; 6: 39-60.
8. Kim, B. *et al.* Direct electrode reaction of Fe(III) reducing bacterium, *Shewanella putrefaciens*. *J. Microbiol. Biotechnol* 1999; 9: 127-131.
9. Bencharit, S. and Ward, M.J. Chemotactic responses to metals and anaerobic electron acceptors in *Shewanella oneidensis* MR-1. *J. Bacteriol.* 2005; 187: 5049-5053.
10. Meyers, J.M. and Meyers, C.R. Role for outer membrane cytochromes OmcA and OmcB of *Shewanella putrefaciens* MR-1 in reduction of manganese dioxide. *Appl. Environ. Microbiol.* 2001; 67: 260-269.
11. Newman, D.K. and Kolter, R. A role for excreted quinines in extracellular electron transfer. *Nature* 2000; 405: 94-97.
12. Reid, G.A. and Gordon, E.H.J. Phylogeny of marine and freshwater *Shewanella*: reclassification of *Shewanella putrefaciens* NCIMB400 as *Shewanella frigidimarina*. *Int. J. Syst. Bacteriol.* 1999; 49: 189-191.
13. Nealson, K.H. and Saffarini, D. Iron and manganese in anaerobic respiration: environmental significance, physiology and regulation. *Annu. Rev. Microbiol.* 1994; 48: 311-343.
14. Meyer, T.E. *et al.* Identification of 42 possible cytochrome c genes in the *Shewanella oneidensis* genome and characterization of six soluble cytochromes. *OMICS* 2004; 8: 57-77.

15. Morris, C.J. Influence of respiratory substrate on the cytochrome content of *Shewanella putrefaciens. FEMS Microbiol. Lett* 1990; 69: 259-262.
16. Field, S. *et al.* Purification and magneto-optical characterisation of membrane bound multi-heme cytochromes from *Shewanella frigidimarina. J. Biol. Chem.* 2000; 275: 8515-8522.
17. Tsapin, A.I. *et al.* Identification of a small tetraheme cytochrome *c* and a flavocytochrome *c* as two of the principal soluble cytochromes in *Shewanella oneidensis* strain MR-1. *Appl. Environ. Microbiol.* 2001; 67: 3236-3244.
18. Leys, D. *et al.* Structure and mechanism of the flavocytochrome *c* fumarate reductase of *Shewanella putrefaciens* MR-1. *Nat. Struct. Biol.* 1999; 6: 1113-1117.
19. Baar, C. *et al.* Complete genome sequence and analysis of *Wolinella succinogenes. Proc. Natl. Acad. Sci. USA* 2003; 100: 11690-11695.
20. Meyers, C.R. and Meyers, J.M. Cloning and sequence of cyma, a gene encoding a tetraheme cytochrome *c* required for reduction of iron(III), fumarate, and nitrate by *Shewanella putrefaciens* MR-1. *J. Bacteriol.* 1997; 179:1143-1152.
21. Schwalb, C. *et al.* The membrane-bound tetraheme c-type cytochrome CymA interacts directly with the soluble fumarate reductase in *Shewanella. Biochem. Soc. Trans.* 2002; 30: 658-662.
22. Turner, K.L. *et al.* Redox properties of flavocytochrome c_3 from *Shewanella frigidimarina* NCIMB400. *Biochemistry* 1999; 38: 3302-3309.
23. Rothery, E.L. *et al.* Histidine 61: an important heme ligand in the soluble fumarate reductase in *Shewanella frigidimarina. Biochemistry* 2003; 42: 13160-13169.
24. Louro, R.O. *et al.* Electronic structure of low-spin ferric porphyrins: 13C NMR studies of the influence of the axial ligand orientation. *J. Am. Chem. Soc.* 1998; 120: 13240-13247.
25. Pessanha, M. *et al* Redox behaviour of the haem domain of flavocytochrome c3 from *Shewanella frigidimarina* probed by NMR. *FEBS Letts* 2004; 578: 185-190.
26. Gordon, E.H.J. *et al.* Identification and characterisation of a novel cytochrome c_3 from *Shewanella frigidimarina* that is involved in iron(III) respiration. *Biochem. J.* 2000; 349: 153-158.
27. Pessanha, M. *et al.* NMR structure of the haem core of a novel tetrahaem cytochrome isolated from *Shewanella frigidimarina*: identification of the haem specific axial ligands and order of oxidation. *FEBS Letts* 2001; 489: 8-13.
28. Louro, R.O. *et al.* Determination of the orientation of the axial ligands ando f the magnetic properties of the haems in the tetrahaem ferricytochrome from *Shewanella frigidimarina. FEBS Letts* 2002; 531: 520-524.
29. Pessanha, M. *et al.* Thermodynamic characterization of a tetrahaem cytochrome isolated from a facultative aerobic bacterium, *Shewanella frigidimarina*: a putative redox model for flavocytochrome c_3. *Biochem. J.* 2003; 370: 489-495.
30. Louro, R.O. *et al.* Distance dependence of interactions between charged centres in proteins with common structural features. *FEBS Letts* 2004; 576: 77-80.
31. Harada, E. *et al.* A directional electron transfer regulator based on hehe-chain architecture of the small tetraheme cytochrome *c* from *Shewanella oneidensis. FEBS Letts* 2002; 532: 333-337.
32. Leys, D. *et al.* Crystal structures at atomic resolution reveal the novel concept of electron-harvesting as a role for the small tetraheme cytochrome *c. J. Biol. Chem.* 2002; 277: 35703-35711.
33. Groove, J. *et al. Escherichia coli* K-12 genes essential for the synthesis of *c*-type cytochromes and a third nitrate reductase located in the periplasm. *Mol. Microbiol.* 1996; 19: 467-481.
34. Pitts, K.E. *et al.* Characterization of the *Shewanella oneidensis* MR-1 decaheme cytochrome MtrA. *J. Biol. Chem.* 2003; 278: 27758-27765.
35. Carpentier, W. *et al.* Respiration and growth of *Shewanella oneidensis* MR-1 using vanadate as sole the electron acceptor. *Biometals* 2005; 187: 3297-2301.
36. Schwalb, C. *et al.* The tetraheme cytochrome CymA is required for anaerobic respiration with dimethylsulfoxide and nitrite in *Shewanella oneidensis. Biochemistry* 2003; 42: 9491-9497.

Metal Ions in Biology and Medicine: vol. 9. Eds Maria Carmen Alpoim, Paula Vasconcellos Morais, Maria Amélia Santos, Armando J. Cristóvão, José A. Centeno, Philippe Collery.
John Libbey Eurotext, Paris © 2006 pp. 242-1.

Azospirillum brasilense resistance to some heavy metals

Anna V. Tugarova[1]*, Alexander A. Kamnev[1]*, Lyudmila P. Antonyuk[1], Philip H. E. Gardiner[2]

[1]*Laboratory of Plant-Bacterial Symbioses, Institute of Biochemistry and Physiology of Plants and Microorganisms, Russian Academy of Sciences, Saratov, 410049, Russia*
E-mail: molbiol@ibppm.sgu.ru, aakamnev@ibppm.sgu.ru
[2]*Division of Chemistry, School of Science and Mathematics, Sheffield Hallam University, Sheffield, S1 1WB, U.K.*

ABSTRACT

Azospirillum brasilense, a ubiquitous plant-associated rhizobacterium known for its plant-growth-promoting effects, was tested with regard to its resistance to heavy-metal stress. Minimum growth-inhibitory (MIC) and minimum lethal (MLC) concentrations were determined for several HMs; their effects on auxin production by the bacteria under aerobic conditions were also assessed. The results obtained show that strains Sp245 and Sp7 of *Azospirillum brasilense* exhibit a relatively high resistance to cobalt(II), copper(II), zinc(II) and cadmium(II): the MLC values were found to be 0.5 mM (Co^{2+}, Cu^{2+}) and 5 mM (Zn^{2+}, Cd^{2+}) for both the strains. Indole-3-acetic acid concentrations in the culture medium were found to decrease in the presence of 0.2 mM Cu^{2+} or Cd^{2+} under aerobic conditions as a result of HM-induced partial suppression of culture growth.

INTRODUCTION

Plant-growth-promoting rhizobacteria (PGPR) living in associations with roots of higher plants are an essential component of the soil biota. Phytostimulating effects of PGPR have been under investigation for the past decades as a promising field for agrobiotechnology [1, 2]. In contaminated soils, both the partners of such associations are under stress. As heavy metal (HM) pollution of soils is a matter of growing environmental concern (for a recent review see, e.g. [3]), studies on PGPR resistance to HMs can provide valuable information from the "micropartner side" of plant-bacterial interactions under HM stress.

In this study, *Azospirillum brasilense* known as a ubiquitous PGPR [4] was tested with regard to its resistance to HM stress under aerobic conditions. Minimum growth-inhibitory (MIC) and minimum lethal (MLC) concentrations were determined for several HMs; their effects on auxin production by the bacteria were also assessed.

MATERIALS AND METHODS

Azospirillum brasilense strains Sp245 and Sp7 (The Collection of Cultures, IBPPM RAS, Saratov) were used in this study.

Tolerance to HM was estimated visually on a solid agar malate synthetic medium (MSM) [5] supplemented with 3 g l^{-1} NH_4Cl as a nitrogen source. The number of viable cells in the culture was determined by the standard plate method in all cases. The medium was supplemented with one of the HM salts, $CdCl_2$, $CuSO_4$, $ZnSO_4$ or $CoCl_2$ taken at concentrations from 0 (control) to 10 mM. The plates were incubated for 3 days at 31°C.

For IAA analysis, the bacteria were grown for 72 h in the liquid MSM with L-tryptophan (200 mg l^{-1}) as an IAA precursor and 0.5 g l^{-1} NH_4Cl as a nitrogen source, in the absence (control) and in the presence of 2×10^{-4} M $CdCl_2$ or $CuSO_4$ under aerobic conditions. Then the culture liquid was centrifuged (13000*g*; 5 min) to remove the cells, and the supernatant solution was filtered through 0.22 μm filters (Millipore). The IAA content in the culture medium was measured by HPLC with UV spectrophotometric detection using a 150 × 4.6 mm i.d., 5-μm-particle Luna 5u C18(2) analytical column (Phenomenex, USA). The mobile phase used was methanol / distilled water / acetic acid (36 / 64 / 1 volume ratio). The mobile phase flow rate was 0.7 ml min^{-1}. The loop volume was 20 μl; IAA was monitored by UV spectrophotometric detection at 290 nm. The data obtained were statistically treated using MS Excel 97 SR-1.

RESULTS AND DISCUSSION

Minimum lethal concentrations (MLC) of Co^{2+}, Cu^{2+}, Zn^{2+} and Cd^{2+} and minimum growth-inhibitory concentrations (MIC) of Co^{2+} and Cu^{2+} were determined for two strains of *Azospirillum brasilense*: strain Sp245, a facultative endophyte, and strain Sp7, non-endophyte *(table 1)*. The results obtained show that both the strains exhibit a relatively high resistance to the HM toxicants; the MLC values (as well as the MIC values) for any HM were found to be the same for both the strains.

Table 1. Heavy-metal resistance of *Azospirillum brasilense* strains grown on the agar medium

Strain	MIC / MLC values (mM) for different heavy metals			
	Cu	Co	Zn	Cd
A. brasilense Sp7	0.1 / 0.5	0.1 / 0.5	ND / 5	ND / 5
A. brasilense Sp245	0.1 / 0.5	0.1 / 0.5	ND / 5	ND / 5

Note: The minimum growth-inhibitory (MIC) and minimum lethal (MLC) concentrations of heavy metals are shown on the left and on the right of the "/" symbols, respectively (ND - not determined).

It should be noted that the MLC of cadmium(II) found for both the *A. brasilense* strains (5 mM) was much higher than those reported for other associative rhizobacteria. For instance, for some strains of *Azospirillum lipoferum*, *Arthrobacter mysorens* and *Agrobacterium radiobacter* the MLC of cadmium(II) was 0.35 to 0.6 mM, i.e. by an order of magnitude lower, while for *Flavobacterium* sp. L30 the MLC was 0.01 mM [6]. By their cadmium resistance, the following bacteria were closer to *A. brasilense*: *Variovorax paradoxus* (MLC = 0.6 to 3.5 mM), a *Rhodococcus* sp., a *Ralstonia* sp., a *Flavobacterium* sp., a *Pseudomonas* sp. and some other strains (MLC = 2.0 to 4.0 mM) [7].

The *A. brasilense* strains studied were also more resistant to zinc(II): its MLC for strains Sp7 and Sp245 was found to be 5 mM (see *table 1*), which is several times higher than that for *A. lipoferum*, *A. mysorens* and *A. radiobacter*, i.e. 0.8 to 1.5 mM [6]. Nevertheless, for those bacteria the MLC and MIC of Cu^{2+} were in the range of 0.15 to 0.7 and 0.05 to 0.2 mM, respectively. The data on copper(II) MLC obtained in this study for azospirillum (0.5 mM) is within the above-mentioned range (see *table 1*). Therefore, considering the data reported in the literature for other associative rhizobacteria, *A. brasilense* strains Sp7 and Sp245 show a relatively high resistance to copper(II) and a very high resistance to cadmium(II) and zinc(II). As compared to *E. coli*, a well-studied microbiological object [8], *A. brasilense* strains Sp7 and Sp245 were more resistant to cadmium but much more sensitive to cobalt and copper. The resistance of the *A. brasilense* strains studied and of *E. coli* to zinc(II) was similar.

The effects of cadmium(II) and copper(II) at 0.2 mM on IAA production by *A. brasilense* strains Sp245 were also studied under aerobic conditions. Along with IAA analyses, the colony-forming units (CFU) numbers were determined *(table 2)*. It was found that for the culture grown in the presence of 0.2 mM cadmium(II) or copper(II), the IAA concentration was lowered by 38% or 46%, respectively. On the other hand, it was found that the CFU number was also lowered ca. 2-fold and 3.7-fold for Cd^{2+} and Cu^{2+}, respectively (see *table 2*). Thus it may be concluded that the decrease in auxin concentrations in the culture medium found in the presence of 0.2 mM Cd^{2+} or Cu^{2+} under aerobic conditions resulted from HM-induced culture growth suppression but not from a decrease in the average IAA production rate per cell.

Table 2. Growth rate (in terms of colony-forming units, CFU) and indole-3-acetic acid (IAA) production by *Azospirillum brasilense* Sp245 in the presence of heavy metals

Culture medium	CFU, 10^6 cells ml^{-1}	IAA concentration in the medium, 10^{-2} mg ml^{-1}	IAA production rate, 10^{-2} mg per 10^6 cells
Standard (control)	147 ± 12	8.9 ± 0.9	0.6 ± 0.1
With 0.2 mM Cd^{2+}	75 ± 15	5.5 ± 0.6	0.7 ± 0.2
With 0.2 mM Cu^{2+}	40 ± 12	4.8 ± 0.5	1.2 ± 0.4

Note: The data presented were averaged from 5 replicates; confidence intervals are given for confidence probability 95%.

In an earlier work, in order to study the expression of the indole-3-pyruvate decarboxylase gene *(ipdC)*, an *A. brasilense* strain bearing a translational *ipdC-gusA* fusion (pFAJ64) was constructed [9]. Induction of the *ipdC* gene encoding the key enzyme in IAA biosynthesis, indole-3-pyruvate decarboxylase, was found to be inhibited (along with the inhibition of IAA biosynthesis) under aerobic conditions in the logarithmic growth phase [10]. In another recent report [11], IAA biosynthesis by *Azospirillum* strains (including *A. brasilense* Sp7 and Sp245) was shown under aerobic conditions in the presence of tryptophan (0.1 mg ml^{-1}). In the late stationary phase (72 h), *A. brasilense* strains were found to produce 16.5 to 38 μg IAA per mg protein, whereas several *Gluconacetobacter* spp. and *Pseudomonas stutzeri* produced less IAA (1.0 to 2.9 μg IAA per mg protein) [11]. Despite the above-mentioned concusion made by Ona e.a. [10] about IAA biosynthesis inhibition under aerobic conditions in the logarithmic growth phase due to indole-3-pyruvate decarboxylase inhibition, our data and those reported in the literature provide evidence that, in the late stationary phase, aerobically cultivated *A. brasilense* can produce significant amounts of IAA.

In our recent study [12], IAA production by both *A. brasilense* strains Sp7 and Sp245 under *microaerobic* conditions was found to be noticeably decreased in the presence of 0.2 mM Cd^{2+} or Cu^{2+}, while the growth rate (in terms of CFU) was lowered ca. 2-fold for Sp245 only in the case of Cu^{2+}. Thus it may be noted that, with regard to their growth rate, both *A. brasilense* strains Sp7 and Sp245 are more sensitive to HMs under aerobic conditions. As can also be seen from the above data, for both the *A. brasilense* strains studied, cobalt(II) and copper(II) were more toxic (although they are necessary in trace amounts for all living organisms) than cadmium which is known as one of the strongest toxicants for eukaryotes and some prokaryotes.

There are literature data showing that some rhizospheric bacteria can increase plant tolerance to HM stress [6]. Some bacteria of the genus *Azospirillum* were shown to be capable of degrading oil hydrocarbons to a variable extent [13], including strains Sp7 and Sp245 studied here, although these two strains exhibited somewhat lower activity in degrading crude oil.

To conclude, the results obtained and some literature data provide evidence for a high resistance of the bacteria of the genus *Azospirillum* to HMs. This feature, together with their capability of degrading oil hydrocarbons, suggests that their application as PGPR may be advantageous for their host plant to more efficiently counteract the detrimental effects of soil pollution, including their possible role as "micropartners" in soil phytoremediation.

REFERENCES

1. Lucy M., Reed E., Glick B.R. Applications of free living plant growth-promoting rhizobacteria. *Ant. van Leeuwenhoek* 2004; 86: 1-25.
2. Gray E.J., Smith D.L. Intracellular and extracellular PGPR: commonalities and distinctions in the plant-bacterium signaling processes. *Soil Biol. Biochem.* 2005; 37: 395-412.
3. Khan A.G. Role of soil microbes in the rhizospheres of plants growing on trace metal contaminated soils in phytoremediation. *J. Trace Elem. Med. Biol.* 2005; 18: 355-64.
4. Bashan Y., Holguin G., de-Bashan L.E. Azospirillum-plant relationships: physiological, molecular, agricultural, and environmental advances (1997-2003). *Can. J. Microbiol.* 2004; 50: 521-77.
5. Kamnev A.A., Renou-Gonnord M.-F., Antonyuk L.P., Colina M., Chernyshev A.V., Frolov I., Ignatov V.V. Spectroscopic characterization of the uptake of essential and xenobiotic metal cations in cells of the soil bacterium *Azospirillum brasilense. Biochem. Mol. Biol. Int.* 1997; 41: 123-30.
6. Belimov A.A., Kunakova A.M., Safronova V.I., Stepanok V.V., Yudkin L.Yu., Alekseev Yu.V., Kozhemyakov A.P. Employment of associative bacteria for the inoculation of barley plants cultivated in soil contaminated with lead and cadmium. *Microbiology* (Moscow) 2004; 73: 99-106.
7. Belimov A.A., Hontzeas N., Safronova V.I., Demchinskaya S.V., Piluzza G., Bullitta S., Glick B.R. Cadmium-tolerant plant growth-promoting bacteria associated with the roots of Indian mustard (*Brassica juncea* L. Czern.). *Soil Biol. Biochem.* 2004; 37: 241-50.
8. Nies D.H. Microbial heavy-metal resistance. *Appl. Microbiol. Biotechnol.* 1999; 51: 730-50.
9. Vande Broek A., Lambrecht M., Eggermont K., Vanderleyden J. Auxins upregulate expression of the indole-3-pyruvate decarboxylase gene in *Azospirillum brasilense. J. Bacteriol.* 1999; 181: 1338-42.
10. Ona O., Van Impe J., Prinsen E., Vanderleyden J. Growth and indole-3-acetic acid biosynthesis of *Azospirillum brasilense* Sp245 is environmentally controlled. *FEMS Microbiol. Lett.* 2005; 246: 125-32.
11. Pedraza R.O., Ramirez-Mata A., Xiqui M.L., Baca B.E. Aromatic amino acid aminotransferase activity and indole-3-acetic acid production by associative nitrogen-fixing bacteria. *FEMS Microbiol. Lett.* 2004; 233: 15-21.
12. Kamnev A.A., Tugarova A.V., Antonyuk L.P., Tarantilis P.A., Polissiou M.G., Gardiner P.H.E. Effects of heavy metals on plant-associated rhizobacteria: comparison of endophytic and non-endophytic strains of *Azospirillum brasilense. J. Trace Elem. Med. Biol.* 2005; 19: 91-5.
13. Muratova A. Yu., Turkovskaya O.V., Antonyuk L.P., Makarov O.E., Pozdnyakova L.I., Ignatov V.V. Oil-oxidizing potential of associative rhizobacteria of the genus *Azospirillum. Microbiology* (Moscow) 2005; 74(2): 210-15.

ACKNOWLEDGEMENTS

We thank Dr. O.E. Makarov (IBPPM RAS, Saratov) for carrying out IAA analyses. This work was supported in part by NATO (Grants LST.CLG.977664 and LST.NR.CLG.981092), the Russian Academy of Sciences' Commission (Grant No. 205 under the 6th Competition-Expertise of research projects) and the President of the Russian Federation (Grant NSh-1529.2003.4).

VI CELL STUDIES

Metal Ions in Biology and Medicine: vol. 9. Eds Maria Carmen Alpoim, Paula Vasconcellos Morais, Maria Amélia Santos, Armando J. Cristóvão, José A. Centeno, Philippe Collery.
John Libbey Eurotext, Paris © 2006 pp. 249-1.

Random Amplification of Polymorfic DNA Study of Cr(VI)-induced Cancer Cell-like Morphologic and Growth Characteristics on BEAS-2B Cell Line

A.N.D. Costa[1,2], A.M. Urbano[1], V. Moreno[2], P.V. Morais[1] and M.C. Alpoim[1]

1. Departamento de Bioquímica, Universidade de Coimbra, Apartado 3126, 3001-401 Coimbra, Portugal.
2. Department de Química Inorgànica, Universitat de Barcelona, Barcelona, España.

Over the past two decades, several chemical studies have demonstrated the mutagenic and genotoxic capabilities of some of the species formed by the intracellular reduction of Cr(VI) and different active agents were pointed out as candidates to ultimate mutagen. As the vast majority of the *in vivo* surveillance studies, carried out among exposed chromium workers, gave inconclusive results. Whether these apparent conflicting achievements are consequence of the fact that the *in vitro* biological studies, carried out so far, did not completely respect the true conditions observed in the *in vivo* environment, remains to be elucidated, and thus the results obtained have to be taken with extreme caution.

While searching to implement an *in vitro* model that would resemble as much as possible the *in vivo* Cr(VI)-induced lung carcinogenesis, we recently found that sub-lethal chronical doses of Cr(VI) induces, on BEAS-2B cell line, a normal human bronchial epithelial cell line, morphologic and growth characteristics typical of cancer cells. Aiming to evaluate if the acquired characteristics were consequence of genomic mutation both control and modified (exposed) cells were typed by the Random Amplified Polymorphic DNA (RAPD) technique. Nine different primers were used with annealing temperatures ranging from 37ºC to 45ºC. Since each different primer gave a different RAPD pattern, the findings that for each primer used there were no differences on the RAPD patterns between the control and Cr(VI)-modified cells, seems to suggest that those cancer like characteristics, acquired upon continuous Cr(VI) exposure, were not a consequence of Cr(VI)-induced DNA damage but probably a Cr(VI)-disruption of the epigenetic control of the genome. It's thus possible that the epigenetic control may trigger of the carcinogenic process as it favors genomic instability.

INTRODUCTION

Action-reaction principle let us to think that a carcinogen should be a mutagen as cancer depends on mutation. This is true but should not be taken strictly as the carcinogen may act over non genetic material that plays a role in the genetic control and stability. This less conventional route is highlighted in several types of cancers where anomalous epigenetic control allow the genetic instability necessary for cancer development [1]; so we should be open minded to this possibility. The research work on Cr(VI)-induced carcinogenesis, stated in epidemiological studies over chromium workers, have been conditioned by the visibility given by the *in vitro* chemical studies to the mutagenic potential of the Cr(VI) species when they meet the intracellular reductive environment. Binary and ternary Cr-DNA adducts, protein-Cr-DNA cross-links, bi-functional DNA-Cr-DNA inter-strand cross-links and even Cr(VI)-reduction by products like reactive oxygen species have been pointed as ultimate carcinogens. These mutagens may damage DNA but can they exist in sufficient amount in a living cell to play their roles? So far, *in vivo* surveillance studies carried out among chromium workers gave inconclusive results while biological *in vitro* studies that detected some of these mutagens and their DNA injuries did not respect the essential condition that carcinogenesis is a process of viable living cells. The use of cellular systems as biological models is a powerful tool if the system does represent the modelized environment (biotic and abiotic). The epidemiological studies show us that Cr(VI)-induced lung cancers is a slow process originated by chronic exposures [2]. A mimetic cellular system should emphasise these characteristics.

Based on those concepts while attempting to implemented an *in vitro* cellular model that would resemble as much as possible the *in vivo* Cr(VI)-induced lung carcinogenesis by chronic expure of a normal human bronchial epithelial cell line to sub-lethal doses of Cr(VI). Upon several passages we observated the acquisition of morphologic and growth characteristics typical of cancer cells. This achievement promt us to search if these Cr(VI)-induced characteristics resulted from DNA damage.

MATERIALS AND METHODS

Biotic component

As a model of bronchial epithelial cells we used adherent cultures of the non tumorigenic cell line BEAS-2B (European Collection of Cell Cultures, n.95102433), cultured with a LHC-9 serum-free media (BEGM from Clonetics Corporation) and additivated with insulin, bovine pituitary extract, epidermal growth factor, transferrin, hydrocortisone, epinefrin, triiodothyronine, retinoic acid and gentamicin/anphotericin-B (BEGM Bullet Kit from Clonetics Corporation).

Abiotic component

The source of Cr(VI) ions was provided to the system adding to the culture media appropriate amounts of potassium dichromate solutions.

Tuning of the carcinogenic cellular system

Despite the representativity of both biotic and abiotic components the exposure regimen assumes a central role in the reliability of the all system. Taking this to consideration we performed an exhaustive toxicological study to know the tolerance and the response of the system to the presence of Cr(VI). As the cancer development depends on important exposures that do not compromise life we picked up those "growth-arrest-almost-apoptotic" conditions that allowed us to keep the cells in culture. After some weeks at these conditions the cultures acquired morphological and growth characteristics typical of the carcinogenic development (data not published).

RAPD-PCR typing of DNA

The RAPD-PCR technique is widely used to compare genomic variances between similar genomes and the variances appear like differences in the random amplification patterns of the compared genomes [3].

Cells of a 70 days exposed culture to 1 μM or 2 μM Cr(VI) and of a 70 days non exposed culture (control) were harvested and the DNA extracted. The DNA from the exposed and the control cultures was then randomly amplified using 9 distinct 10-mer sequence primers and different annealing temperature accordingly to Welsh *et al.* [3]. The randomly amplified DNA fragments were separated by electrophoresis and stained with ethidium bromide for visualization.

RESULTS

We report here preliminary results of a comparative study over the DNA of non exposed-normal cells and Cr(VI) exposed-modified cells presenting cancer cell characteristics.

Figure 1 illustrates the amplification patterns obtained with 9 different RAPD-PCRs. As shown each different primer gave a different RAPD pattern, however for each primer used there were no differences on the RAPD patterns between the control non exposed population and two modified populations by 70 days exposure to 1 and 2 μM Cr(VI). These data shows that under the experimental conditions used the altered phenotype acquired during chronic exposure to Cr(VI) is not addressable to any detectable Cr(VI)-induced genomic mutation.

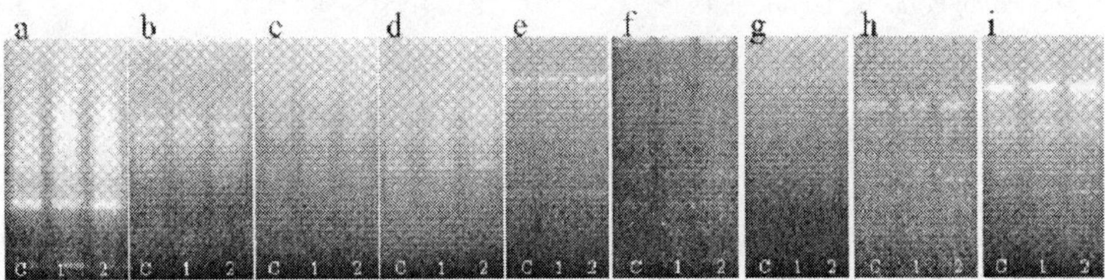

Figure 1. Comparative RAPD-PCR patterns of exposed-modified cultures, lanes 1 and 2 (1 and 2 μM Cr(VI) exposure respectively), and a non exposed control, lane C. Each group a, b, c, d, e, f, g, h, i refers to a distinct random amplification reaction.

CONCLUSION

The results obtained do not prove that the Cr(VI)-induced morphologic and growth characteristics like - cancer cells on BEAS-2B cell line is independent of its mutagenic potential but they suggest the possible role of epigenetic events as the first step contributors to the carcinogenic process.

REFERENCES

1. Robin Holliday. DNA methylation and Epigenotypes. *Biochemistry* 2005; 70: 500-504.
2. Chromium, nickel and welding. *IARC Monographs on the Evaluation of Carcinogenic Risk of Chemicals to Humans* 1990; 49: 463-474.
3. Welsh J, McClelland M. Fingerprinting genomes using PCR with arbitrary. *Nucleic Acids Research* 1990; 18: 7213-7218.

Metal Ions in Biology and Medicine: vol. 9. Eds Maria Carmen Alpoim, Paula Vasconcellos Morais, Maria Amélia Santos, Armando J. Cristóvão, José A. Centeno, Philippe Collery.
John Libbey Eurotext, Paris © 2006 pp. 252-1.

Removal of mercury by inflammatory cells: a study by SEM coupled with X-ray microanalysis

Elisabete M. Cunha, and Artur P. Águas

Department of Anatomy, ICBAS (Abel Salazar Institute for Biomedical Sciences), and UMIB (Unit for Multidisciplinary Investigation in Biomedicine), University of Porto, Lg. Prof. Abel Salazar, 2, 4099-003 Porto, Portugal, European Union.

E-mail: mcunha@icbas.up.pt

SUMMARY

Phagocytes remove and store mercury (Hg) that enters the body. Macrophages and granulocytes respond in opposite ways to Hg: macrophages loose cell viability, neutrophils become protected from apoptosis. A number of studies have been devoted to the investigation of the effect of mercury (Hg) *in vivo* on the physiology of phagocytes, namely with regards to ingestion and killing of microbes. We have investigated here a different view of the interaction between Hg and phagocytes: how the two major cell types of phagocytes, i.e., macrophages and neutrophilic granulocytes, take up and store microparticles of Hg. For that, Hg was injected in two inflamed body cavities of mice (peritoneal and subcutaneous pouches). Because we have used a large amount of Hg ($HgCl_2$, 25 mg in 500 μL of PBS) it is plausible to consider that virtually all of the inflammatory cells of mice were exposed to Hg particles. The mice died 2-4 min later and the cell exudates were harvested and studied by scanning electron microscopy coupled with X-ray elemental microanalysis (SEM-XRM). More than half of the phagocytes showed ingested Hg; a higher percentage of macrophages (around 70%) than neutrophils (around 50%) were positive for the metal. This investigation document that Hg is fastly ingested as small particles by phagocytes, and also that endocytosis of Hg increases with the degree of cell activation and that Hg is internalising by pinocytosis.

INTRODUCTION

Mercury (Hg) has been widely used as a constituent of commercial products and some ointments used in traditional medicine. For instance, Hg is a component of thermometers, blood pressure cuffs, batteries, switches and fluorescent light bulbs. Large quantities of metallic mercury are employed as electrodes in the electronic production of chlorine and sodium hydroxide from saline. The increasing uses of Hg may cause accidental and occupational exposures to the metal (1). At the moment, fish consumption, dental amalgams and vaccines are major sources of concern of Hg causing harmful effects on humans (2). The toxic effects of mercury depend on the chemical form, the dose, the duration of exposure and the route of entry into the body. Methylmercury (CH3HgCl) is more toxic to living organisms than the inorganic forms of Hg (3). Hg can diffuse across the alveolar membrane into the erythrocytes of blood circulation and is rapidly oxidized to ionic mercury (Hg^{2+}) after inhaled Hg (4). In contrast, mercuric chloride (HgCl2) can not readily traverse the blood-brain barrier. Less than 10% of HgCl2 is directly absorbed to mammals via gastrointestinal tract (5). One of the main target organs of mercuric chloride is the kidney where Hg^{2+} ions are accumulated and produce tissue damage (6, 7). Hg entering the body is known to impair macrophage function (8). We have investigated how Hg is ingested by inflammatory phagocytes (macrophages and neutrophils) using a high-resolution method (scanning electron microscopy) coupled with X-ray microanalysis (SEM-XRM).

METHODS

Forty-eight female 6-8 weeks old BALB/c mice, weighing 25 g, were used in this study. They were obtained from a Spanish breeder (Charles River Laboratories SA, Spain). The animals were kept under standard animal house conditions, in accordance with the European Union law on animal protection (directive 86/609/EC). In half of the mice, inflammation was induced in a subcutaneous air pouch; the other half of the mice were submitted to peritoneal inflammation experimental group was made up of 6 mice, for that, the mice were injected with a phlogistic solution of 500 µL of 3% bovine serum albumin (BSA) in PBS. A lethal dose of mercuric chloride ($HgCl_2$, 25 mg in 500 µL of PBS) was injected in the peritoneal or air-pouch cavities of the mice 6, 24, 48 and 72 hours after the phlogistic inoculation of BSA. The animals died 2-4 minutes after the $HgCl_2$ injection. Cytological slides of the exudates were obtained in a cytocentrifuge. These preparations were used for quantification of cell types by light microscopy (Giemsa staining) or for scanning electron microscopy (SEM). The preparations were processed and mounted on metal stubs and coated by carbon under vacuum and examined in a JEOL JSM-6301F scanning electron microscope (SEM) that was coupled to a Noran Voyager X-ray elemental microanalyser (XRM) with a EDS (Energy Dispersive Spectrometry) detection system. SEM-XRM allows the *in situ* identification of Hg upon the detection of the characteristic elemental spectra of this metal. SEM micrographs of the samples were derived from secondary and backscattered electron imaging modes.

RESULTS

Studies of leukocyte kinetics of cells harvested from the two inflammation models, subcutaneous air pouch and the peritoneal cavity, showed that 72 hours after BSA injection, macrophages were the predominant cell type in the peritoneal cavity and neutrophils were the most numerous cell types in the subcutaneous air pouch. A significant difference between the two cavities was found with regards to the distribution of Hg dots per phagocyte: after 24 hours of inflammation, the phagocytes from the peritoneal cavity ingested 3 times more Hg than the inflammatory cells from the subcutaneous air pouch. We also observed that as the inflammation progressed a higher percentage of Hg-positive phagocytes were observed. The most significant difference in the Hg intake between the two cell types of inflammatory phagocytes was observed in mice that had been submitted to BSA-induced inflammation for 72 hours.

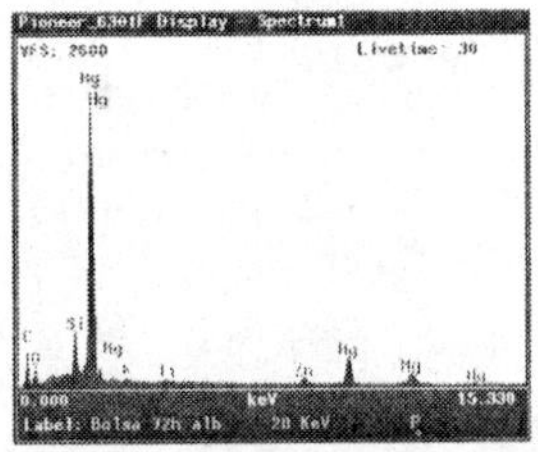

Figure 1. X-ray elemental microanalysis spectrum of cellular inclusion observed by SEM and containing Hg as revealed by the peaks of the Hg element.

DISCUSSION

This study shows that Hg particles can be detected inside the cytoplasm of inflammatory macrophages and granulocytes by using XRM-SEM technique. We found that the main inflammatory leukocytes in peritoneal cavity and subcutaneous air pouch were neutrophils after *in situ* injection of BSA 24 hrs before, and mononuclear cells after injection of BSA 72 hrs before. The percentage of Hg-positive cells at 72 hrs of inflammation was higher for macrophages (70%) than for neutrophils (50%).

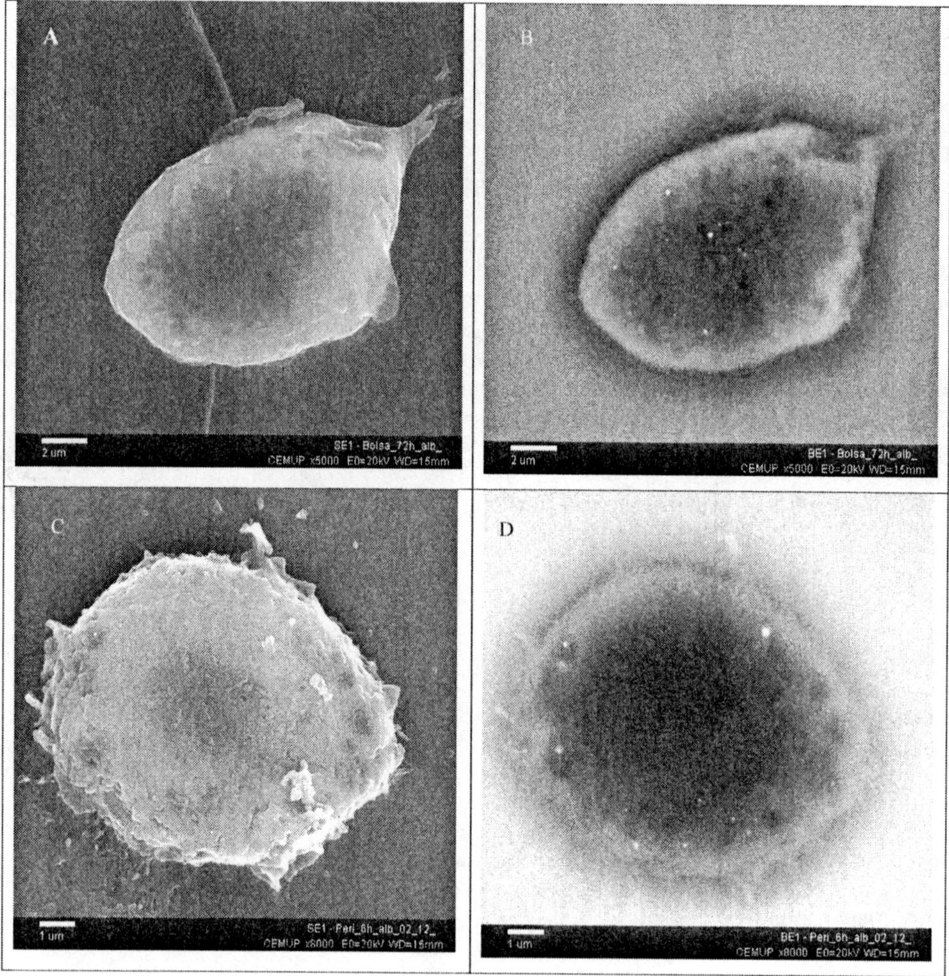

Figure 2. SEM micrographs of a neutrophil (A and B) from a subcutaneous air pouch of mouse that was injected 72 hours before with BSA and of a macrophage (C and D). The surface morphology of the cells is shown on the left images by secondary electron imaging mode of SEM. The use of back secondary electrons imaging mode of SEM reveals intracellular Hg as expressed by the white spots. Black bars at the bottom of the images indicate magnification.

Hg ingesting by inflammatory cells has been reported by some investigators. Christensen and others (1988) concluded that the uptake of Hg by macrophages is depended on the concentration of Hg reaching phagocytes. They also found that mercury chloride stimulated the release of H_2O_2 from peritoneal neutrophils of Lewis but not from BN rats, both *in vivo* and *in vitro*. They also showed the ultrastructure of Hg intake: Hg was located mainly inside lysosome and also in nucleus and cytoplasm of macrophages.

Contrino et al. (1992) postulate that no structural or functional changes are observed in neutrophils treated with low concentrations of Hg.

We show here that phagocyte affinity for Hg depends on the timing of the inflammatory reaction. This work was focused on the "immediate" interaction between inflammatory cells and Hg, rather than on the long-term intracellular handling of Hg by the cells. The herein data suggest the following conclusions: (i) Hg is fastly ingested as small particles by phagocytes; (ii) endocytosis of Hg increases with the degree of activation of the phagocytes, and (iii) phagocytes ingest Hg by pinocytosis.

REFERENCES

1. Toxicology profile for mercury. Atlanta: Agency for toxic Substances Disease Registry, 1999.
2. FDA. Action level for mercury on fish, shellfish, crustaceans, and other aquatic animals. Federal Register 1999; 44: 3990-3993.
3. Clarkson TW. The three modern faces of mercury. Environmental Health Perspectives 2002; 110: 11-23.
4. Berlin M, Ullberg S. Accumulation and retention of mercury in the mouse. An autoradiographic study after a single intravenous injection of mercuric chloride. Arch Environ health 1963; 6: 589-601.
5. WHO. Environmental health criteria 118. Inorganic mercury. World health Organization, Geneva, 1991.
6. Cunha EM, Silva DP, Águas AP. High-resolution identification of mercury in particles in mouse kidney after acute lethal exposure. A study by scanning electron microscopy coupled with X-ray microanalysis. BioMetals 2003; 16: 583-590.
7. Cunha EM, Cherdwongcharoensuk D, Águas AP. Quantification of particles of lethal mercury in mouse víscera: high-resolution study of mercury in cells and tissues. Toxicology and Industrial Health 2003; 19: 55-61.
8. Soltys J, Boroska Z, Dvoroznakova E. Effects of concurrently administered copper and mercury on phagocytic cell activity and antibody levels in guinea pigs with experimental ascariasis. Journal of Helminthology1997; 71: 339-344.
9. Christensen M, Mogensen SC, Rungby J. Toxicity and ultrastructural localization of mercuric choride in cultured murine macrophages. Archives of Toxicology 1988; 62: 440-446.
10. Christensen MM. Histochemical localization of autometallographically detectable mercury in tissue of the immune system from mice exposed to mercuric chloride. The Histochemical Journal 1996; 28: 217-225.
11. Contrino J, Kosuda LL, Marucha P, Kreutzer DL, Bigazzi PE. The in vitro effects of mercury on peritoneal leukocytes (PMN and macrophages) from inbred Brown-Norway and Lewis rats. International Journal Immunopharmacology 1992; 14: 1051-1059.

ACKNOWLEDGEMENTS

The authors are grateful to Professor Carlos M. Sá, director of CEMUP, and to Dr. Daniela Silva for expert help with SEM-XRM. We thank Dr. Madalena Costa for technical assistance. This work was funded by grants from FCT (POCTI/BSE/36188/2000 and UMIB (Unit for Multidisciplinary Investigation in Biomedicine), Portugal.

Metal Ions in Biology and Medicine: vol. 9. Eds Maria Carmen Alpoim, Paula Vasconcellos Morais, Maria Amélia Santos, Armando J. Cristóvão, José A. Centeno, Philippe Collery.
John Libbey Eurotext, Paris © 2006 pp. 256-1.

Cr(VI) effect on *Ochrobactrum tritici* strain 5bvl1 respiration capacity

Romeu Francisco[1], António Moreno[2], Maria Carmen Alpoim[3] and Paula V. Morais[1,3]*

[1]*Instituto do Ambiente e Vida, 3004-517 Coimbra, Portugal.*
[2]*Departamento Zoologia, Faculdade de Ciências e Tecnologia da Universidade de Coimbra, 3004-517 Coimbra, Portugal.*
[3]*Departamento Bioquímica, Faculdade de Ciências e Tecnologia da Universidade de Coimbra, Apartado 3126, 3001-401 Coimbra, Portugal.*

The present work focuses on the effect of Cr(VI) on cell respiration of strain *Ochrobactrum tritici* 5bvl1, previously isolated from a contaminated wastewater treatment plant and considered both resistant and able to reduce this metal with a cytosolic NADH-dependent enzyme. Cr(VI) decreased O_2 consumption in this strain, especially for concentrations above 4 mM Cr(VI). KCN stopped cell respiration and CCCP worked as an uncoupler, increasing cell respiration rate. The effect of CCCP was dependent on Cr(VI) concentration. When in presence of 8 mM Cr(VI), the oxygen consumption was very low, and no stimulation of respiration was noticed when adding the proton motive force uncoupler CCCP. These results lead us to conclude that there was a toxic effect affecting the normal cell metabolism and/or the electron flow at the membrane level. However, experiments realized with the type strain of *O. tritici* LMG 18957, a strain sensible to Cr(VI), showed no Cr(VI) respiration inhibition, pointing to the possibility that an inhibition of respiration in strain 5bvl1 could be linked in some extent to mechanisms of resistance.

INTRODUCTION

Chromium is a widespread industrial waste. The soluble hexavalent chromium (Cr(VI)) is an environmental contaminant, widely recognized to act as a carcinogen, mutagen and teratogen towards humans, animals and plants (13). The fate of chromium in the environment is dependent on its oxidation state. While Cr(VI) is readily bioavailable due to its high solubility, Cr(III) compounds are much less toxic because they are extremely insoluble under pH near neutral conditions and cannot penetrate cells due to their large size, which makes reduction of Cr(VI) to Cr(III) a good method in detoxification of contaminated soils and waters.

Several bacteria belonging to a variety of genera have been reported to possess chromate reductase activity, converting Cr(VI) compounds to the less toxic Cr(III). There is evidence for both aerobic (10, 7) and anaerobic (3, 2) reduction pathways with different microbes. While anaerobic reduction seems to be associated to the cell membrane, a few enzymes have been described as cytosolic or periplasmic (11, 8). The anaerobic strategies could involve cytochromes, nitrite reductase [Fe] or [NiFe] hidrogenase (12, 2). The aerobic strategies described until now were related to soluble enzymes dependent on NAD(P)H (10, 7). In order to begin an efficient bioremediation strategy, it is necessary to gather information on the physiological effects caused by the presence of Cr(VI).

The present work focuses on the effect of Cr(VI) on respiration of strain *Ochrobactrum tritici* 5bvl1 recently isolated and identified in our laboratory (5, 1). We therefore evaluated the oxygen consumption of resting cells in the presence of Cr(VI), the effect of glucose and the effects of CCCP and KCN on respiration.

MATERIAL AND METHODS

Bacteria and growth conditions

O. tritici strain 5bvl1 was previously isolated from activated sludge in a chromium-contaminated area (5), is resistant up to 10 mM Cr(VI) (growth rates between 0.175 h^{-1} and 0.025 h^{-1}) and able to reduce Cr(VI) up to 1.7 mmol l^{-1} (1). The type strain of *O. tritici* LMG 18957^T,obtained from LMG Culture Collection (Laboratorium voor Microbiologie, Universiteit Gent), is a Cr(VI)-sensible strain able to reduce Cr(VI) when inoculated at high-density cell suspension, although at lower amounts then strain 5bvl1. The strains were maintained at -80° C in Nutrient Broth (NB, Difco) containing 15% (w/v) glycerol. The strains were cultured in buffered mineral medium (MMH) as described in Branco *et al.* (2004). In all experiments with chromium, chromium was used as sodium dichromate ($Na_2Cr_2O_7$).

Cell respiration assays

Strain 5bvl1 was grown in MMH medium with different concentrations of glucose. A volume of 20 ml of culture (OD 1.0) was centrifuged at 15 000 × g and the pellet cells were ressuspended in 200 µl Tris-HCl 100 mM, pH 7.0. Oxygen consumption by bacteria cells was measured in Tris-HCl 100 mM, pH 7.0, at 30°C, in a 1 ml chamber, using a Clark-type electrode (Yellow Springs Instruments Co., Inc.) connected to a Linear 1200 register. The respiratory rates are expressed in nmol O_2.min^{-1}.cell^{-1}, considering the oxygen solubility in water at 28°C and 1 atm as 233 µM (4). A variety of respiratory substrates were tested, including glucose (0.5% (w/v)). CCCP (11.7 µM) was used as an uncoupling agent, and potassium cyanide (1.5 mM) as an inhibitor of the respiratory chain. The effect of different concentrations of Cr(VI) on respiration stimulated by 0.5% (w/v) glucose was tested in cells grown both in the presence of 0.1% or 0.5% (w/v) glucose. An identical experiment was made with a resting cells suspension of *O. tritici* type strain (LMG 18957^T) previously grown in 0.1% (w/v) glucose, to serve as control. The number of cells used in each assay was of 2.8×10^{10} as estimated by plating samples in Nutrient Agar (Difco) and counting the colony forming units (CFU) after incubation at 30°C during 48 h.

RESULTS

Effects of Cr (VI) on cells respiration

Glucose was the only carbon source tested that stimulated respiration in the assays *(fig. 1)*. The oxygen consumption of *O. tritici* strain 5bvl1 cells was inhibited by Cr(VI), and a decrease of 82% was observed in the presence of 8 mM Cr(VI) (from 7.5×10^{-10} to 1.3×10^{-10} nmol O_2. min^{-1}. cell^{-1}). In contrast, cells of *O. tritici* type strain (LMG 18957^T) never showed a respiration inhibition caused by Cr(VI) exceeding 20% and stabilized above 4mM Cr(VI). In fact, only a decrease of 14.7% was observed in the presence of 8 mM Cr(VI) (from 8.8×10^{-10} to 7.5×10^{-10} nmol O_2. min^{-1}.cell^{-1}). Oxygen consumption of strain 5bvl1 cells was increased by CCCP, but when 6 mM Cr(VI) were present in the buffer, the stimulation was weak. When 8 mM Cr(VI) were present, no respiratory stimulation was visible in strain 5bvl1. Potassium cyanide stopped the oxygen consumption on both strains.

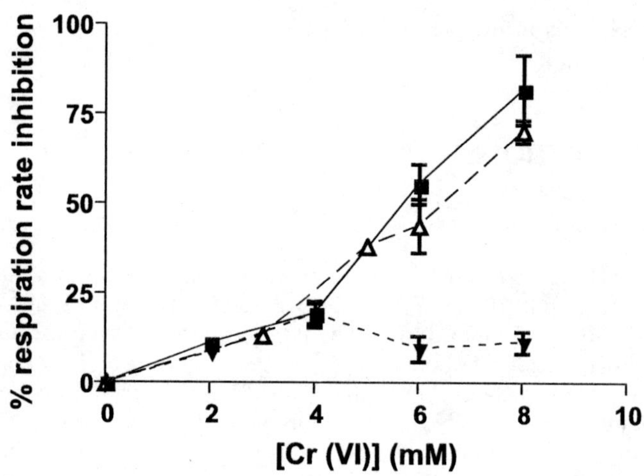

Figure 1. Respiration rate inhibition by various Cr(VI) concentrations on cells of *O. tritici* strain 5bvl1 previously grown on 0.1% glucose (■) or 0.5% glucose (△) and on cells of *O. tritici* type strain (LMG 18957) previously grown in 0.1% glucose (▼).

DISCUSSION

O. tritici strain 5bvl1 was described as a strain Cr(VI)-resistant, Cr(VI)-reducing, halotolerant and alkilotolerant although unable to grow in anaerobiose in the presence of Cr(VI) (1). We also noticed that strain 5bvl1 used a cytosolic NADH-dependent enzyme to reduce Cr(VI) (data not shown).

Cr(VI) inhibited respiration of strain 5bvl1 but a higher resilience was observed in the presence of higher glucose concentrations. The results obtained were expected when active mechanisms of resistance and reduction are present. Interestingly, the internal electron donors present in cells deprived of glucose were sufficient to maintain Cr(VI) reduction for at least 24 hours.

The respiration of type strain of *O. tritici*, which is a Cr(VI) sensible strain able to reduce Cr(VI) at low levels (1), is not inhibited by Cr(VI). In contrast, *O. tritici* strain 5bvl1 is resistant up to 10 mM Cr(VI) and able to reduce high Cr(VI) amounts (1) but the respiration rate is strongly decreased in the presence of Cr(VI) specially for concentrations above 4 mM. The decrease of respiration seems to indicate a toxic effect even in this Cr(VI)-resistant strain, since a loss on cell viability may contribute in some extent to a decrease in the number of active breading cells (6). However, we cannot exclude the possibility of an effect caused in some extent by mechanisms of resistance, since the type strain, supposedly deprived of mechanisms of resistance, showed no inhibition of respiration by Cr(VI).

The results obtained with CCCP in strain 5bvl1 confirm the respiration inhibition caused by Cr(VI). The addition of CCCP to cells in the presence of 8 mM Cr(VI) (consuming oxygen at a very slow rate and near to the strain maximum Cr(VI) tolerance) did not increase the respiration rate, probably due to the lack of a proton gradient, and not to a failure in uncoupling the respiratory chain. If Cr(VI) resistance in strain 5bvl1 is due to a proton motive force-dependent resistance protein responsible for the extrusion of Cr(VI) like ChrA (9), the absence of such a gradient, caused by the presence of high Cr(VI) concentrations, which inhibits cell respiration, would compromise the effectiveness of resistance towards Cr(VI) and further contribute to the dissipation of the proton gradient. It is possible that CCCP will also cause the same effect leading to the accumulation of Cr(VI) inside the cell.

In conclusion, our work demonstrated evidences suggesting a relation between Cr(VI) and the elements associated to the respiratory chain especially for Cr(VI) concentrations of 4 mM or higher.

Further studies for elucidation of the relation between respiratory chain and the Cr(VI) reduction ability of *O. tritici* strain 5bvl1 is needed in order to evaluate the potential of the strain for the bioremediation of Cr(VI)-contaminated sites or industrial effluents.

REFERENCES

1. Branco R., Alpoim M.C. & Morais P.V. *Ochrobatrum tritici* strain 5bvl1 - characterization of a Cr(VI)-resistant and Cr(VI)-reducing strain. *Can J Microbiol* 2004. 50: 697-703.
2. Chardin B., Giudici-Orticoni MT, De Luca G., Guigliarelli B. & Bruschi M. Hydrogenases in sulfate-reducing bacteria function as chromium reductase. *Appl Microbiol Biotechnol* 2003. 63: 315-321.
3. Daulton T.L., Little B.J., Lowe K. & Jones-Meehan J. *In situ* environmental cell-transmission electron microscopy study of microbial reduction of chromium(VI) using electron energy loss spectroscopy. *Microsc Microanal* 2001; 7: 470-485.
4. Estabrook R.W. Mitochondrial respiratory control and the polarography measurement of ADP/O ratios. *Methods Enzymol* 1967; 10: 41-47.
5. Francisco R., Alpoim M.C. & Morais P.V. Diversity of Chromium-resistant and - reducing bacteria in a chromium-contaminated activated sludge. *J Appl Microbiol* 2002; 92: 837-843.
6. Konopka A. & Zakharova T. Quantification of bacterial lead resistance via activity assays. *J Microbiol Methods* 1999; 37: 17-22.
7. Kwak Y.H., Lee D.S. & Kim H.B. *Vibrio harveyi* nitroreductase is also a chromate reductase. *Appl Environ Microbiol* 2003; 69: 4390-4395.
8. McLean J. & Beveridge T.J. Chromate reduction by a Pseudomonad isolated from a site contaminated with chromated copper arsenate. *Appl Environ Microbiol* 2001; 67: 1076-1084.
9. Nies D.H., Koch S., Wachi S., Peitzsch N. & Saier M.H. Jr. CHR, a novel family of prokaryotic proton motive force-driven transporters probably containing chromate/sulfate antiporters. *J Bacteriol* 1998; 180: 5799-5802.
10. Park C.H., Keyhan M., Wielinga B., Fendorf S. & Matin A. Purification to the homogenity and characterization of a novel *Pseudomonas putida* chromate reductase. *Appl Environ Microbiol* 2000; 66: 1788-1795.
11. Shen H. & Wang YT. Characterization of enzymatic reduction of hexavalent chromium by *Escherichia coli* ATCC 33456. *Appl Environ Microbiol* 1993; 59: 3771-3777.
12. Viamajala S., Peyton B.M., Apel W.A. & Petersen J.N. Chromate/nitrite interactions in *Shewanella oneidensis* MR-1: evidence for multiple hexavalent chromium [Cr(VI)] reduction mechanisms dependent on physiological growth conditions. *Biotechnol Bioengin* 2002; 78: 770-778.
13. World Health Organization. Chromium. *Environ Health Criter* 1988; 61: 11-144.

ACKNOWLEDGEMENTS

This research was funded by Fundação para a Ciência e Tecnologia (FCT), Portugal, under POCTI and FEDER programs, contract POCTI/BSE/42414/2001. R. Francisco was supported by a Ph.D. scholarship from FCT (SFRH/BD/10742/2002). We thank A. P. Chung for technical support in cell respiration experiments.

Metal Ions in Biology and Medicine: vol. 9. Eds Maria Carmen Alpoim, Paula Vasconcellos Morais, Maria Amélia Santos, Armando J. Cristóvão, José A. Centeno, Philippe Collery.
John Libbey Eurotext, Paris © 2006 pp. 260-1.

Anticancer activity of the lanthanum drug KP772 (FFC24): impact of the cellular P53 status

Heffeter P.[1], Jakupec M.A.[2], Dornetshuber R.[3], Elbling L.[1], Sutterlüty H.[1], Micksche M.[1], Keppler B.K.[2], Berger W.[1]

[1]*Institute of Cancer Research, Department of Medicine I, Medical University Vienna, Borschkegasse 8a, 1090 Vienna;*
[2]*Institute of Inorganic Chemistry, University of Vienna;*
[3]*Institute for Pharmacology, University of Vienna, 1090 Vienna, Austria.*

[Tris(1,10-phenanthroline) lanthanum(III)] trithiocyanate (KP772; FFC24) is a new compound, in which lanthanum centers a complex built by three 1,10-phenathroline molecules. Recently, we have demonstrated that KP772 is a promising new anticancer agent exerting potent activity against a wide range of tumor cell lines in vitro and a colon carcinoma xenograft model in vivo. Moreover, it was demonstrated that KP772 exerts antiproliferative effects by distinct induction of cell cycle arrest in G_0/G_1 followed by induction of apoptosis which is not mediated by DNA damage and radical formation [1].

MATERIAL AND METHODS

Drugs

[Tris(1,10-phenanthroline)lanthanum(III)] trithiocyanate (KP772; FFC24; *fig. 1*) was prepared at the Institute of Inorganic Chemistry-Bioinorganic, Environmental and Radiochemistry, University of Vienna (Vienna, Austria) according to the procedure described by Hart and Laming [2]. The compound was dissolved in water and diluted into culture media at the concentrations indicated.

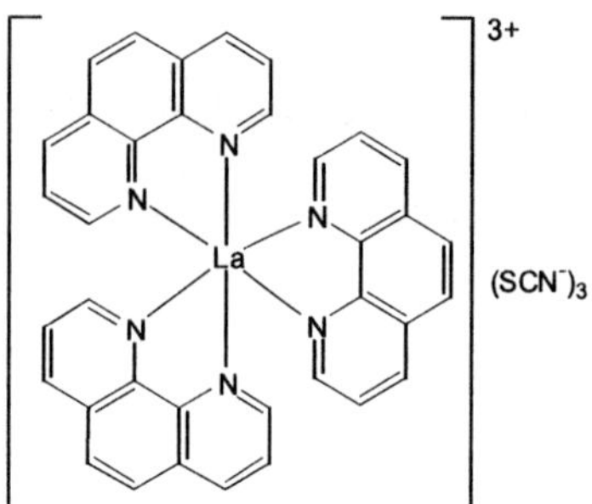

Figure 1. [Tris(1,10-phenanthroline)lanthanum(III)] trithiocyanate (KP772; FFC24)

Cell Culture

The following human cell lines were derived from American Type Culture Collection (Manassas, VA): the promyelocytic leukaemia cell line HL60, the non-small cell lung cancer cell lines A549, and the hepatocellular carcinoma cell line Hep3B. The colon carcinoma cell line HCT116 and respective sublines with deleted p53, p21, or bax genes were generously donated by Bert Vogelstein, John Hopkins University, Baltimore. HCT116 cell lines were grown in McCoy's culture medium, all other cells in RMPI 1640 both supplemented with 10% fetal bovine serum. Cultures were regularly checked for *Mycoplasma* contamination.

Cytotoxicity Assays

Cells were plated (2×10^4 cells/ml) in 100 µl per well in 96-well plates and allowed to recover for 24 h. Drugs were added in another 100 µl growth medium and cells exposed for 72 h. The proportion of viable cells was determined by an MTT-based vitality assay following the manufacturer's recommendations (EZ4U, Biomedica, Vienna, Austria). Cytotoxicity was expressed as IC_{50} values calculated from full dose-response curves (drug concentrations including a 50% reduction of cell survival in comparison to the control cultured in parallel without drugs).

Western Blot Analysis

Cell fractionation, protein separation and western blotting were performed as described [3]. The following antibodies were used: anti-p53 monoclonal mouse DO-7 (NeoMarkers, CA, USA), dilution: 1:500; anti-p21^{Waf1} polyclonal rabbit C-19 (Santa Cruz Biotechnology, CA, USA), dilution: 1:1000. All secondary, peroxidase-labelled antibodies from Pierce were used at working dilutions of 1:10000.

Cell Cycle Analysis

10^5 HCT116 cells were seeded into 6-well plates, allowed to recover for 24 h, and then treated with 1 and 2.5 µM KP772. To analyse cell cycle distribution, cells were collected, washed with PBS, in 70% ethanol and stored at 4 °C. For analysis, cells were transferred into PBS, incubated with RNAse (10 µg/ml) for 30 min at 37 °C, treated with 5 µg/ml propidium iodide for 30 min and then analyzed by flow cytometry using FACS Calibur (Becton Dickinson, Palo Alto, CA). The resulting DNA histograms were quantified using the Cell Quest Pro software (Becton Dickinson and Company, New York, USA).

^{3}H-Thymidine Incorporation Assay

A549 cells (3×10^3 cells/well) were seeded into 96-well plates, and treated 24 h later with the drug for another 24 h. Culture medium was replaced by a 2 nM ^{3}H-thymidine solution (diluted in full culture medium; radioactivity: 25 ci/mM). After 4 h incubation at 37 °C, cells were washed 3 times with PBS. Cell lysates were prepared and the radioactivity determined as described [4].

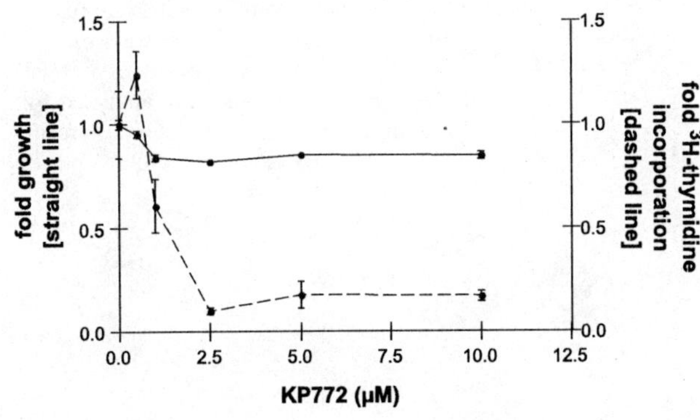

Figure 2. DNA synthesis and cell viability of A549 cells were determined by ^{3}H-thymidine incorporation and MTT assay, respectively, after 24 h treatment with KP772 at the indicated concentrations [1].

P53 Transfection

P53-positive cell clones were obtained from the p53 (-/-) Hep3B cell line by transfection with the temperature-sensitive p53val143 vector as described [1]. For analysis of drug sensitivity, Hep3B/p53 and Hep3B/c (vector control) cells were plated on 96-well microstate plates at a density of 4×10^3/100 µl RPMI/well. After incubation for 24 h, cells were starved for another 24 h to reduce cell proliferation. On the next day two test groups were defined: group 1 was transferred to 32 °C (wt p53) for 24 h, group 2 remained at 37 °C (mutated p53). Subsequently, drugs were added in 100 µl culture medium with 10% serum and after 1 h incubation the first group was transferred from 32 to 37 °C. Exposure was continued for another 72 h and cell viability was measured by EZ4U kit.

RESULTS

Impact of KP772 on DNA synthesis and cell cycle distribution

The effects of KP772 on DNA synthesis were determined by ^{3}H-thymidine incorporation assays. KP772 treatment dramatically inhibited ^{3}H-thymidine incorporation in A549 lung cells *(fig. 2)* within 24h, indicating a complete inhibition of DNA synthesis. To further characterise the effects of KP772 on cell proliferation, cell cycle distribution of KB-3-1 and HL60 cells was analysed *(fig. 3)*. A significant reduction of cells in G_2/M and S phases was detectable in both cell lines following a 24 h treatment. In addition to the G_0/G_1 arrest, a significant proportion of cells had entered apoptosis in HL-60 cells indicated by the appearance of a subG_0/G_1 peak.

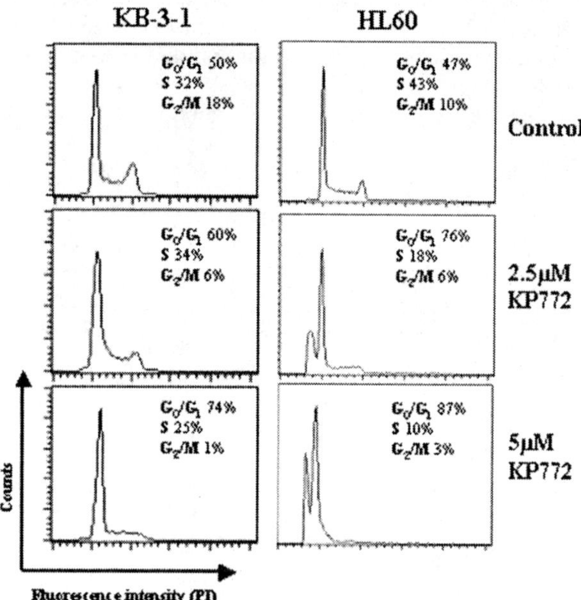

Figure 3. Changes in the cell cycle distribution of KB-3-1 and HL60 cells treated with increased concentrations of KP772 for the indicated times were analysed by PI staining and flow cytometry. Percentages of cells in G_0/G_1, S and G_2/M phase are indicated.

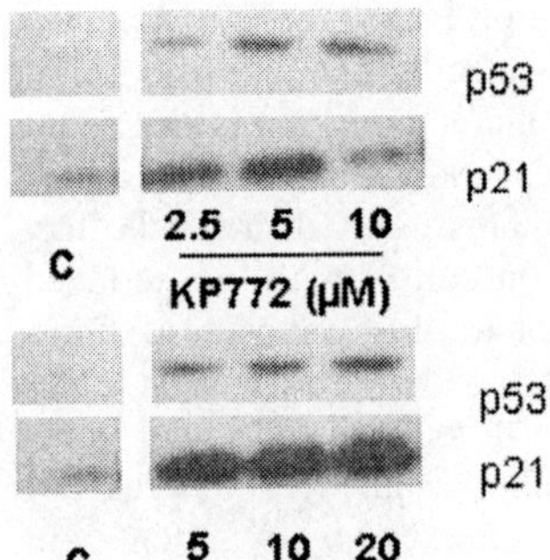

Figure 4. Induction of wild-type p53 and p21[Waf1] in A549 cells by treatment for 6 h and 24 h, respectively, with KP772 or bleomycin at the indicated concentrations was analysed via Western blotting [1].

Table 1. Cytotoxic activity of KP772 against tumor cell models (72 h treatment) as compared to the cellular p53 status.

		IC_{50} (µM)[a]	
Cell line	P53	mean	± SD
A459	wt	1.5	0.1
Hep3B	(-/-)	2.2	0.8
HL60	(-/-)	1.2	0.9
KB-3-1	mut	2.6	0.7
HTC116	wt	1.4	0.3

[a]Means and SD of at least two independent experiments in triplicates.

Impact of the p53 status on KP772-induced cytotoxicity

Various types of stress lead to activation of wild-type p53 and consequently arrest cell cycle predominantly in G_0/G_1 phase via induction of the cyclin-dependent kinase inhibitor p21[Waf1] [6]. Generally, the anticancer activity of KP772 did not correlate with the cellular p53 status *(table 1)* and for example p53 (-/-) HL-60 cells were especially sensitive against KP772-induced apoptosis *(fig. 3)*. Next we analysed whether treatment with KP772 induces p53 and p21[Waf1] in A549 cells containing wild type p53 [7]. After 6 h treatment, dose-dependent p53 induction could be observed in the KP772-treated cells *(fig. 4)*. P21[Waf1] upregulation became detectable only after 24 h treatment. Induction of p53/ p21[Waf1] by bleomycin followed the same pattern but was distinctly stronger as compared to KP772.

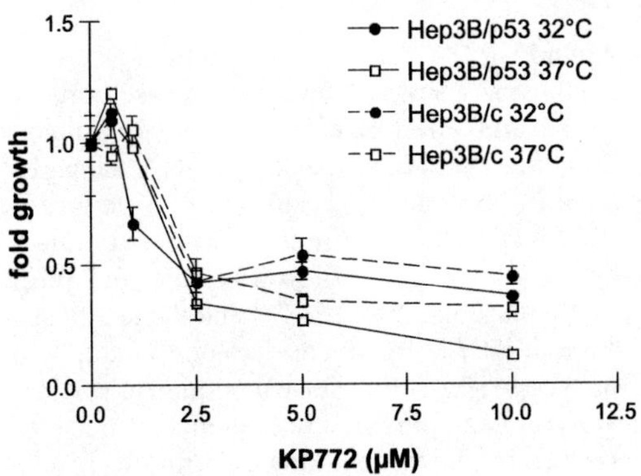

Figure 5. Hep3B celles (p53-/-) were stably transfected with a vector containing a temperature-sensitive p53 gene (wild-type at 32 °C, mutated at 37 °C) (Hep3B/p53) or the control vector (Hep3B/c). Growth arrested cells were treated with KP772 as described in Material and Methods. Dose-response curves derived from two independent experiments in triplicates are shown [1].

Based on the upregulation of wild type p53 by KP772 we used p53-null Hep3B-cells transfected with a temperature-sensitive p53 variant (Hep3B/p53) [1] to further determine the contribution of wild-type p53 to the anticancer activity of KP772. In this cell model the ectopic p53 is in mutant conformation at 37 °C and has wild-type conformation at 32 °C. Independent of the p53 status, Hep3B cell proliferation was significantly reduced at 32 °C leading to a distinctly decreased effect of KP772 (data not shown). To avoid the influence of temperature on cell growth, we reduced proliferation in all experimental groups by serum starvation 24 h prior to drug exposure. After a one hour drug exposure, cells were returned to 37 °C to allow now unimpeded proliferation. Only at 1 µM KP772, a significantly enhanced cytotoxicity of KP772 against cells treated under wild-type p53 conditions was detectable *(fig. 5)*. At higher drug concentrations, however, a weak opposite effect got obvious. This indicates that, although p53 expression is induced by treatment with KP772, it only weakly contributes to its anticancer activity.

To further analyse the impact of apoptosis- and cell cycle-regulating proteins, we used HCT116 colon carcinoma cells and subclones with selective deletion of p53, p21 or bax. IC_{50} values for these cell models are given in *table 2*. Overall, the sensitivity of the tested HCT116 cells was very similar (~ 1.4µM), without any significant differences. Nevertheless, in p21 (-/-) cells a constant tendency towards hypersensitivity against KP772 was observed, while p53 (-/-) tend to slight resistance against KP772.

Additionally, p53(-/-) cells were found to arrest preferentially in early S instead of G_0/G_1-phase of the cell cycle *(fig. 6)*.

Table 2. Cytotoxic activity of KP772 against HCT116 cell models at 72 h treatment.

	IC_{50} (µM)[a]	
Cell line	mean	± SD
HCT116 p53 (+/+)	1.1	0.3
HCT116 p53 (-/-)	1.3	0.8
HCT116 p21 (+/+)	1.7	0.2
HCT116 p21 (-/-)	1.2	0.4
HCT116 bax (+/+)	1.5	0.4
HCT116 bas (-/-)	1.4	0.7

Means and SD of at least two independent experiments in triplicates.

DISCUSSION

The anticancer activity of the new lanthanum compound KP772 has recently been demonstrated to be based on profound blockade of DNA synthesis, cell cycle arrest at the G_0/G_1-S-phase border, and induction of apoptosis [1]. During chemotherapy, accumulation of cells in G_0/G_1 is usually the result of the respective cell cycle check point activation as a consequence of DNA damage. Molecularly this process is often mediated by activation of p53 causing besides cell cycle arrest predominantly at G_1 phase also induction of apoptosis. Most of these 53 functions involve transcription factor activity resulting in enhanced expression of several anti-proliferative and pro-apoptotic proteins like for, example, the cyclin-dependent kinase inhibitor $p21^{Waf1}$ and the apoptosis inducing bax [6]. Despite the lack of DNA damage through KP772 treatment, we found induction of p53 and the downstream gene $p21^{Waf1}$ in p53-wild type A549 cells. Correspondingly, several examples of DNA damage-independent induction of p53 for example as a consequence of nucleotide depletion, hypoxia and block of transcription have been reported [8]. However, in our hands p53-dependent signalling had only a minor influence on the cytotoxic activity of KP772, again suggesting that DNA damage is not the major reason for the activity of the lanthanum drug. Also disruption of the p53 target genes bax and p21 exerted no significant influences on KP772-induced effects. Additionally, HL60 and Hep3B cells, which both are p53 (-/-) [9], are highly sensitive to apoptosis induction by KP772. Moreover, we found no induction of $p21^{Waf1}$ in KP772-treated p53 (-/-) HL-60 cells (data not shown). As also the p53 (-/-) cells exhibited a distinct cell cycle arrest at G_1/S border, the upregulation of $p21^{Waf1}$ via p53 does not seem to be essential for the KP772-induced cell cycle arrest. Summarizing, the profound cell cycle arrest of KP772-treated cells does not primarily depend on the activation of the cell cycle checkpoints activated by the $p53/p21^{Waf1}$ axis but on yet unknown mechanism. The elucidation of the precise interplay of the underlying molecular mechanisms is currently subject of ongoing experiments.

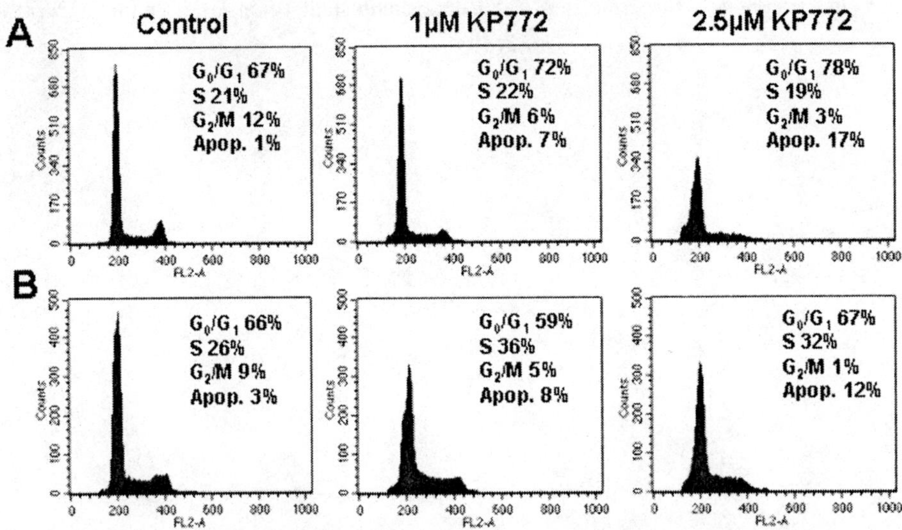

Figure 6. Changes in the cell cycle distribution of (A) HCT116 p53 (+/+) an (B) HCT116 p53 (-/-) cells treated with 1 or 2.5 µM of KP772 for 24 h were analysed by PI staining and flow cytometry. Percentages of cells in G_0/G_1, S, G_2/M phase and apoptosis are indicated.

REFERENCES

1. Heffeter P, Jakupec MA, Korner W, Wild S, von Keyserlingk NG, Elbling L, Zorbas H, Korynevska A, Knasmuller S, Sutterluty H, Micksche M, Keppler BK, and Berger W. Anticancer activity of the lanthanum compound. *Biochem Pharmacol* 2006; 71: 426-40.
2. Hart FA and Laming FP. Complexes of 1,10-phenanthroline with lanthanid chlorides and thiocyanates. *J Inorg Nucl Chem* 1964; 26: 579-585.
3. Berger W, Elbling L, and Micksche M. Expression of the major vault protein LRP in human non-small-cell lung cancer cells: activation by short-term exposure to antineoplastic drugs. *Int J Cancer* 2000; 88: 293-300.
4. Berger W, Elbling L, Minai-Pour M, Vetterlein M, Pirker R, Kokoschka EM, and Micksche M. Intrinsic MDR-1 gene and P-glycoprotein expression in human melanoma cell lines. *Int J Cancer* 1994; 59: 717-23.
5. Heffeter P, Pongratz M, Steiner E, Chiba P, Jakupec MA, Elbling L, Marian B, Korner W, Sevelda F, Micksche M, Keppler BK, and Berger W. Intrinsic and acquired forms of resistance against the anticancer ruthenium compound KP1019. *J Pharmacol Exp Ther* 2005; 312: 281-9.
6. Oren M. Decision making by p53: life, death and cancer. Cell Death Differ 2003; 10: 431-42.
7. Bai F, Matsui T, Ohtani-Fujita N, Matsukawa Y, Ding Y, and Sakai T. Promoter activation and following

induction of the p21/WAF1 gene by flavone is involved in G1 phase arrest in A549 lung adenocarcinoma cells. *FEBS Lett* 1998; 437: 61-4.

8. Blagosklonny MV, Demidenko ZN, and Fojo T. Inhibition of transcription results in accumulation of Wt p53 followed by delayed outburst of p53-inducible proteins: p53 as a sensor of transcriptional integrity. *Cell Cycle* 2002; 1: 67-74.
9. Banerjee D, Lenz HJ, Schnieders B, Manno DJ, Ju JF, Spears CP, Hochhauser D, Danenberg K, Danenberg P, and Bertino JR. Transfection of wild-type but not mutant p53 induces early monocytic differentiation in HL60 cells and increases their sensitivity to stress. *Cell Growth Differ* 1995; 6: 1405-13.

AKNOWLEGEMENTS

This work was supported by the Faustus Forschung Austria AG and by Medizinischer-Wissenschaftlicher Fonds des Bürgermeisters der Bundeshauptstadt Wien, grand number 2460.

Metal Ions in Biology and Medicine: vol. 9. Eds Maria Carmen Alpoim, Paula Vasconcellos Morais, Maria Amélia Santos, Armando J. Cristóvão, José A. Centeno, Philippe Collery.
John Libbey Eurotext, Paris © 2006 pp. 267-1.

Organic and aqueous extracts from particulate matter ($PM_{2.5}$) and their effects on the immunological response of beas cells

*Jimenez-Velez B. D., Gioda A., Fuentes-Mattei E.

Center for Environmental and Toxicological Research, Department of Biochemistry, School of Medicine, Medical Sciences Campus, University of Puerto Rico, P.O. Box 365067, San Juan, Puerto Rico 009, 36-5067, Tel-FAX 787-758-8784, bjimenez@rcm.upr.edu

ABSTRACT

The immunological response of organic and aqueous extracts in particulate matter ($PM_{2.5}$) from an urban industrialized area (Guaynabo) and a reference site (Fajardo), in Puerto Rico was assessed using a human respiratory tract cell line. Organic (hexane, acetone) and aqueous extracts were analyzed for trace metal content and evaluated for the immune response on human bronchiotracheal cell (BEAS-2B) line measuring 17 human cytokines (Bio-Plex/Luminex Cytokine Array System). Results from these experiments revealed that both organic extracts from Guaynabo and Fajardo exert a significant increase on the release of Il-6 and IL-1b while significantly inhibiting the secretion of IL-8. Conversely, only the aqueous extracts from the industrialized site induced IL-6, IL-8 and IL-1b. C-CSF and MCP-1 were significantly inhibited by organic extracts and aqueous extracts. Metal concentrations are directly related to cytokine induction. High levels of V and Ni concentrations were measured in these extracts. Some of metals found originate from anthropogenic sources, however there is also a significant influence due to natural Sahara dust events. Sahara storm events (with high metal content) are common during certain seasons in the Caribbean and have been identified as possible sources responsible for adverse effects on the respiratory system. High incidence of asthma has been reported in the Guaynabo area and could be related to the abundance of high metal content in particulate matter. This research provides the tools for studying the effects of specific metal species in particulate air matter and evaluating their role on the development of respiratory diseases such as Asthma.

INTRODUCTION

Epidemiological studies have demonstrated a high association between particulate air pollution ($PM_{2.5}$) and several health problems related with respiratory illnesses, cardiovascular disease mortality, acute bronchitis, and asthma attacks (1-3). Ultra fine particle constituents, organic components, the presence of biological material, and the transition metal components in particulate matter are some of the factors suggested of causing these adverse cardiopulmonary health effects (3). Fine particles less than $PM_{2.5}$ have been reported to be dominated by anthropogenic emissions (4-5). The absorption of the fine fraction of the atmospheric particulate matter is the main event initiating a signal cascade of molecular immune responses in the respiratory tract and can also play an indirect role on metabolic and immune responses in the digestive system. Experiments with rodents have indicated that particles and metal content especially transition metals, cause inflammation and interfere with host defense function of lung macrophages (6-8). Furthermore, in vitro experiments with human macrophages exposed to urban particles showed cytotoxicity, production of oxygen radicals, and release of various cytokines, suggesting that these cells are important targets of particulate pollution leading to the release of mediators of lung injury and inflammatory responses (9-10). Consequently, cytokines can influence the airway inflammatory response and contribute to respiratory airway lesions in asthma and Chronic Obstructive Pulmonary Disease (11).

In addition, many studies have shown that organic particles such as diesel can enhance or stimulate the secretion of a number of cytokines in airway epithelial cells. However, very little research has been performed using the organic extracts from $PM_{2.5}$. The purpose of this study was to evaluate the immune response of airway epithelial cells to organic compounds and soluble metals from fine particles $PM_{2.5}$ obtained at two locations in Puerto Rico.

METHODOLOGY

Sampling and analysis Procedures (PM2.5)

Particulate matter ($PM_{2.5}$) was sampled in an urban/industrialized area (Guaynabo) and in a reference site (Fajardo) in Puerto Rico. Samples were collected for 72-hour on Teflon filters using a Fine Particle Chemical Speciation Air Sampler (RAAS 2.5-400 - Andersen Instruments Inc.). Teflon filters were weighed and conditioned at temperatures of 20-23 ± 2°C and a humidity of 40 ± 5%. Particulate matter collected on the filters, were Soxhlet extracted using organic solvents (Acetone and Hexane) and highly purified water. Metals (As, Cd, Fe, Pb, Ni and V) were analyzed means of Atomic Absorption (Perkin Elmer AAnalyst 800) following EPA standard methods.

Treatment and Quantification of cytokines

BEAS-2B human bronchial epithelial cells were plated at densities of 70,000 per well in a 24-wells plate and maintained growing for 48 hours until 80%-90% confluence was achieved using supplemented KGM bullet kit media (Cambrex). We tested the effect of organic extracts (1μg/mL or 100μg/mL) obtained from composite samples (7-8 month Sept/2000-Sept/2001) on BEAS-2B cell line. The aqueous extracts were tested at three different concentrations 0.6%, 20% and 50%. Three different concentrations of aqueous extract were evaluated (0.6%, 20% and 50%) in media. Every treatment was made in triplicates. Cytokine concentrations released to the supernatant media were determined using the Bio-Plex/Luminex Human Cytokine 17-plex panel Assay (Bio-Rad Lab. Inc.) for seventeen different human cytokines (IL-2, IL-4, IL-6, IL-8, IL-10, IL-5, IL-7, IL-12, IL-13, IL-17, GM-CSF, IFN-γ, TNF-α, IL-1β, G-CSF, MCP-1 (MCAF) and MIP-1β) after 24 hrs of exposure.

RESULTS

The average levels of $PM_{2.5}$ at the industrialized site (Guaynabo) was 11.6 $\mu g/m^3$ as compared to 8.5 $\mu g/m^3$ collected at the reference site (Fajardo). The amount of $PM_{2.5}$ was always greater throughout the year (± 30%) at the urban/industrialized site. However, the amount of organic extracts obtained from $PM_{2.5}$ collected at the reference site during the summer was greater than at the urban site. This data agrees with higher $PM_{2.5}$ concentrations detected during the summer months when coincides with Sahara dust storms arriving from Africa (12).

The average annual trace metal determined in airborne particulate matter at both stations is presented in *table 1*. The average concentrations were always higher at the urban/industrialized site for all metals except Fe. Average concentrations as low as 0.055 ng/m^3 for Cd and as high as 103 ng/m^3 for Fe were obtained (12). In this case high metal concentrations were also detected during Sahara events.

Table 1. Annual average trace metal concentrations (ng/m^3) in $PM_{2.5}$, obtained at Guaynabo and Fajardo, Puerto Rico (n = ± Standard error of the mean).

Site	As	Cd	Fe	Ni	Pb	V
Guaynabo	0.39	0.055	93	17	3.0	40
Fajardo	0.09	0.015	103	1.9	0.57	1.4

Aqueous extracts

Analyses of 17 human cytokines revealed effects on three of these, IL8, IL6 and MCP-1. The average concentrations of these three cytokine released by BEAS cells after 24 hrs of exposure to aqueous extracts of $PM_{2.5}$ are summarized in *table 2*. The effect of aqueous extracts at three different concentrations exerted different responses on cytokine release dependent on the concentration tested. The greatest immune response was on IL-6 and IL-8 for aqueous extracts of $PM_{2.5}$ (leachate fraction) exposure at 20% concentration. This response was detected on the leachate extract obtained from $PM_{2.5}$ at the urban/industrialized site (Guaynabo) while not detected at the reference site at this concentration. At 50% of $PM_{2.5}$ aqueous extract from Guaynabo resulted in cytokine inhibition of IL-6 and MCP-1. While examining the aqueous metal concentration *(table 3)* and correlating it with cytokine response the main effect appears to be associated with concentrations of As, Ni with IL-8 while Fe, V, Cd and Pb were not as strong. These analyses were perform just to provide a vague idea of possible associations and therefore need to be evaluated further with a thorough analyses. Significant concentrations of metals were detected in $PM_{2.5}$ from Guaynabo. This is a site where metals are present due to common activities of industries and fuel combustion. Otherwise in Fajardo, a reference site, was measured lower metal concentrations *(table 1)* since less anthropogenic of metal influence is expected. The marked effect of the Guaynabo aqueous extract on immune response on human bronchial epithelial cells seems to be associated with the higher metal content in $PM_{2.5}$. Guaynabo, characteristics of high concentrations of V and Ni were abnormal to those found in other areas. A detailed study on dose response and speciation of these metals needs to be conducted in order to validate and confirm our results.

Table 2. Cytokine concentrations (pg/mL) (and standard error) produced by BEAS cells treated with aqueous extract of particulate matter ($PM_{2.5}$) from two different sites (Guaynabo and Fajardo) in Puerto Rico (n = 3).

	Cytokines - 0.6% aqueous extract		
	IL-8	**IL-6**	**MCP-1**
Fajardo	124.4 (±7.4)	59.7 (±2.03)	69.3 (±0.5)
Guaynabo	na	na	na
CNT	108.6 (±7.9)	73 (±8.17)	55.2 (6±.31)
	20% aqueous extract		
	IL-8	IL-6	MCP-1
Fajardo	226.7 (±3.6)	143.0 (±19.8)	39.9 (±1.7)
Guaynabo	575.6 (±20)	388.2 (±6.34)	42.1 (±3.0)
CNT	306.9 (±8.8)	129.2 (±1.66)	49.7 (±1.2)
	50% aqueous extract		
	IL-8	IL-6	MCP-1
Fajardo	na	na	na
Guaynabo	409 (±53.5)	61.05 (±1.02)	31.25 (±1.8)
CNT	446.5 (±25)	165.7 (±25)	68.9 (±12.1)

na: not analyzed; CNT: negative control

Table 3. Average metal concentrations in the aqueous extracts obtained from $PM_{2.5}$ of Guaynabo and Fajardo and tested for immunological response.

0.6%	As	Cd	Fe	Ni	Pb	V
Fajardo	0.02	0.011	1.60	0.58	0.23	0.21
Guaynabo	0.10	0.082	26.77	2.96	0.48	15.18
20%	As	Cd	Fe	Ni	Pb	V
Fajardo	0.7	0.4	53.4	19.3	7.6	7.1
Guaynabo	3.4	2.7	892.2	98.8	16.1	505.9
50%	As	Cd	Fe	Ni	Pb	V
Fajardo	1.8	1.0	133.5	48.3	18.9	17.7
Guaynabo	8.6	6.8	2230.5	247.1	40.2	1264.7

Organic extract

The effect of organic extracts on the release of human cytokines from the airway epithelial cells (BEAS) was similar to those obtained with aqueous extracts. Three major cytokines released by these cells after 24 hrs of exposure with the organic extracts were, IL-8, IL-6 and MCP-1. The average concentrations of these three cytokine released by BEAS cells are summarized in *table 4*. In our aqueous extracts exposure experiments at 20% we found the highest induction for IL-6 (3 fold) followed by a 1.9 fold induction in IL-8 *(table 2)*. This cytokine (IL-6) was also found to respond highly (5 fold increase) to acetone extracts at 100 ug/mL *(fig. 1)*, however, the response was not site specific (induction at both sites Guaynabo and Fajardo) as found in the aqueous extract.

Table 4. Summary of Cytokines concentrations (pg/mL; and standard error, SE) released by BEAS cells after 24 hours treatment with organic extracts (hexane or acetone) from particulate matter ($PM_{2.5}$) collected at two different sites (Guaynabo and Fajardo) in Puerto Rico (n = 3).

BEAS-B2 cells 24hr Treatment	Hul IL-6 pg/ml	Hu IL-8 pg/ml	Hu MCP-1 pg/ml
0.1% DMSO (carrier)	807 (+/-) (+/- 196.64)	1486.7 (+/- 165.76)	804.33 (+/- 124.59)
1ug/ml PM2.5 Guaynabo (acetone extract)	686 (+/- 129.48)	1363.3 (+/- 81.718)	792.33 (+/- 59.795)
100ug/ml PM2.5 Guaynabo (acetone extract)	4290 (+/- 412.59)	578.67 (+/- 37.777)	9.633 (+/- 9.633)
100ug/ml PM2.5 Fajardo (acetone extract)	4543.3 (+/- 118.37)	(+/- 18.774)	0
100ug/ml PM2.5 Guyanabo (hexane extract)	1273.3 (+/- 106.51)	1313.3 (+/- 95.975)	433.67 (+/- 81.11)
100ug/ml PM2.5 Fajardo (hexane extract)	911.67 (+/- 41.571)	903.67 (+/- 103.72)	288.17 (+/- 98.023)

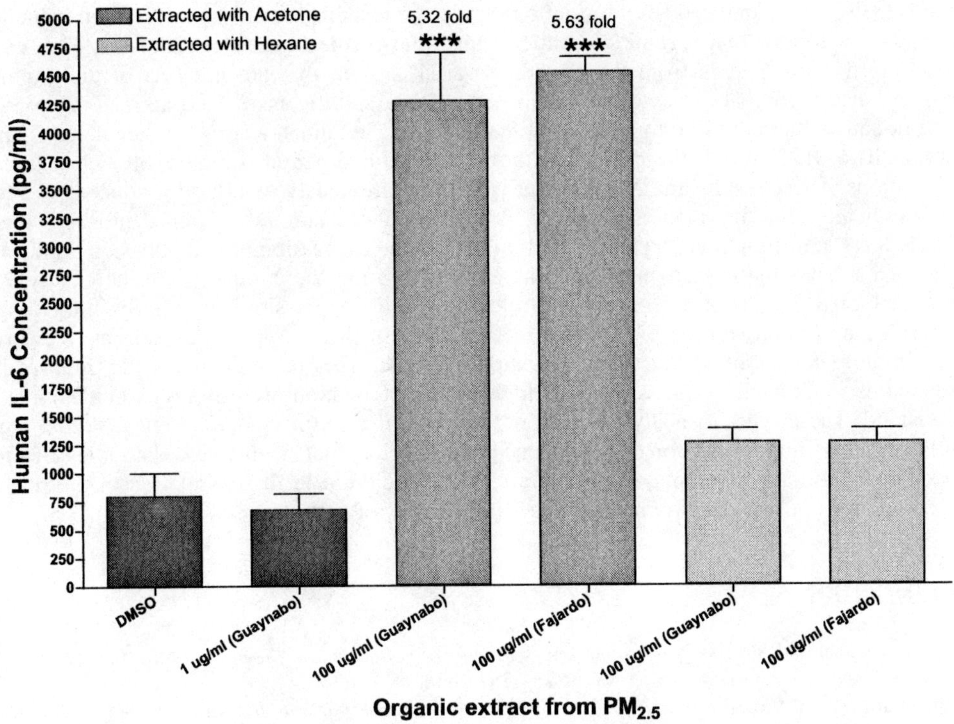

Figure 1. Effects of different organic extract (hexane or acetone) concentrations from $PM_{2.5}$ on IL-6 induction by BEAS cells after 24 hours exposure. Extracts obtained from particulate matter collected at two different sites (Guaynabo and Fajardo) in Puerto Rico. The DMSO bar represents the control and each bar is the mean of three experiments (n = 3). Error lines illustrates the SE of the mean.

This finding suggests that there is an intrinsic polar component in $PM_{2.5}$ acetone extract that induces the synthesis and release of IL-6 from BEAS cells. This component is not present in the non-polar extract fraction (hexane) of $PM_{2.5}$. Whether this component is a metal or an organic compound is yet to be determined. Metal analyses of PM_{10} organic extracts have shown that the mayor metal extracted in the acetone fraction is Cu while Fe constitute the main component in the hexane extract. In addition, acetone $PM_{2.5}$ organic extracts from both Guaynabo and Fajardo have components that inhibit the secretion of IL-8 and MPC-1 cytokines. This cytokine has been previously reported to be induced in airway epithelial cell by PM_{10} aqueous extracts (13). MPC-1 is a chemotactic protein similar to GM-CSF which plays a key role in monocytes recruitment. Both aqueous and organic extracts inhibit this cytokine in BEAS cells at high concentration. This effect seems to be associated with polar and non-polar extract components. Nevertheless, the polar components seem to contain a stronger inhibitor. The presence of these type of compounds in $PM_{2.5}$ could compromise and delay the response of the immune system to events of high particulate matter insults.

CONCLUSION

Much research has been done showing the importance of soluble metals and their role on generating reactive oxygen species (ROS). It has also been demonstrated that many of these ROS are generated in neutrophils and other cells from the immune system such as primary macrophages after exposure to air particulate matter are responsible for cytokine release. However, other mechanisms than particle induced ROS formation seem to be responsible for the differential induction of IL-8 (14). We show that organic constituents may play a role in such mechanisms. This study demonstrate that other cells from the respiratory track system that are not part of the immune system can also participate in cytokine release and play a significant role inflammatory process. This work shows that exposure to aqueous extract of $PM_{2.5}$ in human airway epithelial cells cause effects on IL-6, IL-8, which are proinflamatory cytokines and can also inhibit MCP-1 at higher concentrations. These results are in agreement with those previously reported for aqueous extracts of PM_{10} indicating that the inducing component of particulate matter are retained in $PM_{2.5}$. Interleukin IL-6 is a multifunctional cytokine that influences the expression of cell adhesion molecules which can mediates the movement of inflammatory cells from the circulation to the airway epithelium or lumen. Metals play an important role on cytokine expression particularly in the lungs. There are several main sources of airborne metals in Puerto Rico, Sahara dust storms, industrial and automobile emissions are just some example of these. This research states the grounds for future studies to directed towards the toxicological characterization of airborne particulate matter on the island. These types of analyses could provide useful data for epidemiological studies were it could serve as fingerprints for the prevalence and development of diseases. The identification of specific organic air pollutants on immune response could aid in the elucidation of the role of these compounds on the development of specific diseases.

REFERENCES

1. Dockery, D.W. et al (1993). *An Association Between Air Pollution and Mortality in Six U.S. Cities*. The New England Journal of Medicine. 329 (24): 1753-1808.
2. Reichhardt, T. (1995). *Weighting the Health Risks of Airborne Particulates*. Environ. Sci. Technol. 29 (8): 360-364.
3. Darwin et al. (2000) Evaluation of organic extracts from airborne particulate matter in Puerto Rico. Evironmental Health Perspective, 108:635-640.
4. Walls et al. 1988. Measurements of aerosol size distributions for nitrate and major ionic species, Atmos. Environ. 22, 1649-1656.
5. Ohlström, M.et al. (2000). *Fine-particle emissions of energy production in Finland*. Atmospheric Environment 34: 3701-3711. 6
6. Chen, L. et al. (1992). Effects of fine and ultrafine sulfuric acid aerosols in guinea pigs: Alterations in alveolar macrophage function and intracellular pH. Toxicol. Appl. Pharmacol. 113, 109-117.
7. Dreher, K., et al. (1996). Soluble transition metals mediate the acute pulmonary injury and airway hyperreactivity induced by residual oil fly ash articles. Chest. 109, 33S-34S.
8. Kodavanti, U P. et al. (1997). Genetic variability in combustion particle-induced chronic lung injury. Am. J. Physiol. 272, L521-l532.
9. Becker, S. et al. (1996). Stimulation of human and rat alveolar macrophages by urban air particulates: Effects on oxidant radical generation and cytokine production. Toxicol. Appl. Pharmacol. 141, 637-648.
10. Pritchard R, J. et al. (1996). Oxidant generation and lung injury after particulate air pollutants exposure increase with the concentration of associate metals. Inhal. Toxicol. 8, 457-477.
11. Fujii Takeshi et al. (2001) Particulate matter induces cytokine expression in human bronchial epithelial cells. American Journal of Respiratory Cell and Molecular Biology. Vol. 25, pp. 265-271. 7.
12. Acevedo Figueroa, D.A., Rodríguez-Sierra, C.J. and Jiménez-Velez, B.D. (2006). "Concentrations of heavy metals, arsenic and elemental and organic carbon in atmospheric fine particles (PM2.5) from Puerto Rico" Ind. Health Environ. In press March.
13. Frampton, M. W., A. J. Ghio, et al. (1999). "Effects of aqueous extracts of PM(10) filters from the Utah valley on human airway epithelial cells." Am J Physiol 277 (5 Pt 1): L960-7.
14. Hetland R.B et al. (2001) Importance of soluble metals and reactive oxygen species for cytokine release induced by mineral particles. Toxicology 165: 133-14.

Metal Ions in Biology and Medicine: vol. 9. Eds Maria Carmen Alpoim, Paula Vasconcellos Morais, Maria Amélia Santos, Armando J. Cristóvão, José A. Centeno, Philippe Collery.
John Libbey Eurotext, Paris © 2006 pp. 273-1.

Study of DNA strand breaks and apoptosis in spleen cells of mice continuously exposed to non-radioactive cesium chloride

Andreyan N. Osipov

Moscow Scientific and Industrial Association "Radon", 2/14, 7th Rostovsky lane, 119121 Moscow, Russia; E-mail: aosipov@radon.ru

ABSTRACT

The aim of the present work was to study the DNA strand breaks level and apoptotic cells rate changes in spleen cells of mice continuously exposed to non-radioactive cesium chloride. CBA/lac male-mice 4-5 weeks old were exposed to cesium chloride (70 mg Cs+/l) given instead drinking water for different time (40-270 days) and compared with control mice. The level of DNA strand breaks in spleen cells was determined by the alkaline single cell gel electrophoresis (comet) assay. The percent of apoptotic cells was counted using by the DNA diffusion assay. The results of our studies showed that long-term exposure of mice to cesium chloride induces a significant increase in the DNA strand breaks level, starting from 120 day of the experiment. The effect recorded was 40-50% higher the control level. Further prolongation of exposure time leads to further increase in the DNA strand breaks level. Thus, the level of DNA strand breaks at 270 day of cesium chloride exposure was (3-4 fold higher the control level. The high percent of apoptotic spleen cells (~ 10%) was simultaneously detected in the same animals. The results of this study showed high genotoxic and cytotoxic effects in mouse spleen cells after continuous (270 day) cesium chloride uptake in mice. It is possible that the strong increase of the DNA strand breaks level in spleen cells at 270 day of cesium chloride exposure is reflected of the DNA fragmentation process during apoptosis induced by cesium ions.

INTRODUCTION

Non-radioactive cesium chloride has widely been used for cancer therapy [1] and in experimental models to produce various ventricular arrhythmias [2]. However, the data about genotoxicity and cytotoxicity of non-radioactive cesium chloride are very scarcity and fragmented. The first reports about clastogenic effects of cesium chloride on mouse bone marrow cells *in vivo* have been appeared in the beginning 1990 years [3, 4].

The aim of this work was to study the DNA strand breaks level and apoptotic cells rate in spleen cells of CBA/lac male-mice exposed to non-radioactive cesium chloride (70 mg Cs+/l) given instead drinking water during 40, 120 and 270 days.

MATERIALS AND METHODS

4-5 week old CBA/lac male mice weighting 12-14 g (purchased from "pitomnik-Stolbovaya") were used in experiments. The mice were placed in plastic cages 7 days prior to cesium chloride exposure. Distribution of animals into control and experimental groups was random. Mice were given standard dry feed and water *ad libitum*. Two independent experiments with identical conditions were performed, utilizing totally 120 mice.

Cesium chloride was dissolved in drinking water up to a final concentration of 70 mg/l cesium chloride. The solution was given to animals instead drinking water for different time (40-270 days). According to our calculations, one mouse drank 3 to 5 ml of the solution a day.

Suspension of spleen cells in phosphate buffered saline (pH 7.4) containing 0.14 M NaCl, 2.7 mM KCl, 3 mM NaN_3, was filtered through nylon mesh at 4°C. Cell concentrations were counted using hemocytometer.

Alkali single cell gel electrophoresis (comet assay) was carried out as described by Singh et al. [5]. According to the assay, a number of alkali labile sites and single-strand breaks is proportional to a number of DNA fragments and to distance DNA migrated from the nucleus after alkali electrophoresis of agarose-immobilized single cells. Fluorescent dye Hoechst 33258 (Sigma Chemical Co, St. Louis, MO, USA) was used to visualize DNA. Analysis was performed using the "Lumam I-2" fluorescent microscope (LOMO, Russia). 100 comets were counted from each slide. Comets were divided into classes 0-4 (0 corresponded to no visible tail, 4 - total migration of DNA from the nucleus into the tail) depending on the shape (diameter, tail length, etc.). This method of visual damage is considered as a valid way for DNA damage analysis [6]. The results of the visual classification were subsequently confirmed using the analytic package image analysis software (Kinetic Imaging, Liverpool, UK).

A number of comets in each class was recorded and the average comet index (ACI) was calculated as: ACI = $(1{\cdot}n1 + 2{\cdot}n2 + 3{\cdot}n3 + 4{\cdot}n4)/\Sigma$ n1 - n4 - a number of comets in classes 1-4, HΣ - the sum of counted comets, including comets in class 0.

Percentage of apoptotic cells was determined by the DNA diffusion assay described elsewhere [7].

Statistical analysis of experimental results was performed using the Student t-test. Results are presented as averages for a group of animals ± standard errors.

RESULTS AND DISCUSSION

Fig. 1 shows the results of the ACI determination in spleen cells from mice chronically exposed to cesium chloride and control animal.

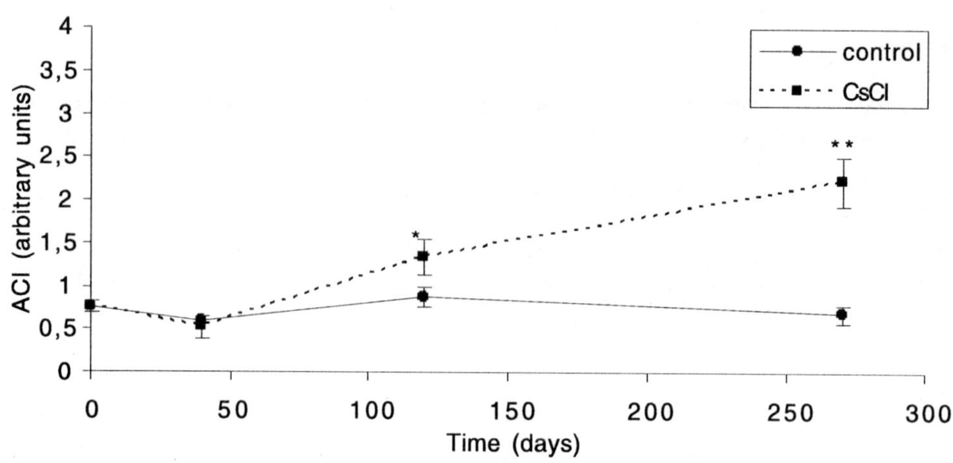

Figure 1. Response - exposure time curve of the average comet index (ACI) of DNA comets of spleen cells in mice chronically exposed to cesium chloride (70 mg Cs+/l).

It was found that the ACI of spleen cells in control animals is slight varied during experiment time within 0.4-0.9 *(fig. 1)*. This can be associated with age depending changes in proliferative and metabolic activity of cells. Long-term exposure of mice to cesium chloride induces a significant increase in the DNA strand breaks level, starting from 120 day of the experiment. The effect recorded was 40-50% higher the control level. Further prolongation of exposure time leads to further increase in the DNA strand breaks level. Thus, the level of DNA strand breaks at 270 day of cesium chloride exposure was ~ 3-4 fold higher the control level.

Mathematical analysis of the data have shown that a response - exposure time curve for cesium chloride exposure is perfectly fitted by a linear regression ACI = 0.55 + 0.006*T as well as a exponential function ACI = 0.62*exp(0.005*T), where T is exposure time in days. It is need more experiential points to choice the best mathematical model correctly described the changes in the DNA strand breaks level induced by long-term exposure of mice to cesium chloride. Establishing of the optimal model (threshold or no-threshold models) is very important for understanding of cesium chloride biological action mechanism.

The comet assay has a strong advantage versus standard biochemical methods of DNA damage determination. This is a possibility of differentiation of cells on DNA damage level that gives additional information about the biological processes caused an increase in the level of DNA damage. *Fig. 2* presents the DNA comet distribution of spleen cells into the different DNA strand breaks level comet classes in mice chronically exposed to cesium chloride during 270 days and control mice.

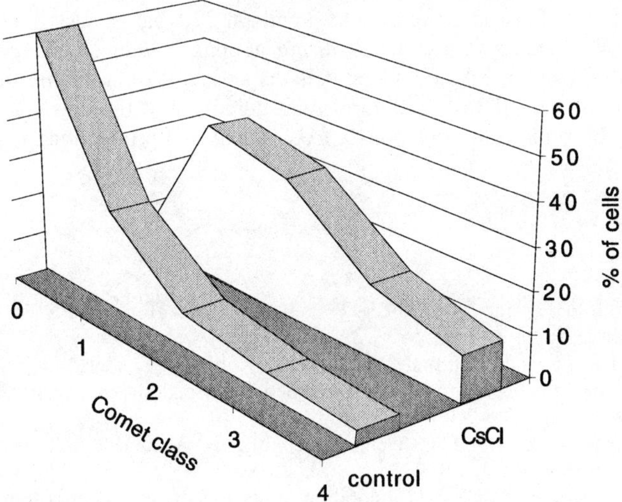

Figure 2. DNA comet distribution of spleen cells in mice chronically exposed to cesium chloride during 270 days and control mice.

As shown in *fig. 2*, at 270 days of cesium chloride exposure a significant shift in the distribution of spleen cells to an increase in the percent of cells with high DNA strand breaks level is observed in exposed mice.

It was reported that cesium ions enter the cell, modify plasma membrane integrity and alter some specific cytoplasmic components, e.g. the cytoskeleton [8]. Strong increase in the percent of spleen cells with high DNA strand breaks level in long-term cesium chloride exposed mice can reflect apoptosis activation by cesium chloride, supposedly through a mitochondrial way. Really, in mice received the cesium chloride solution during 270 days a statistically significant increase in the percent of apoptotic spleen cells is found *(fig. 3)*. It is interestingly; that the total number of spleen cells in mice drank the cesium chloride solution significantly did not changed during all experimental time. This fact can be explained by development of compensatory proliferation of cells in response to cell death.

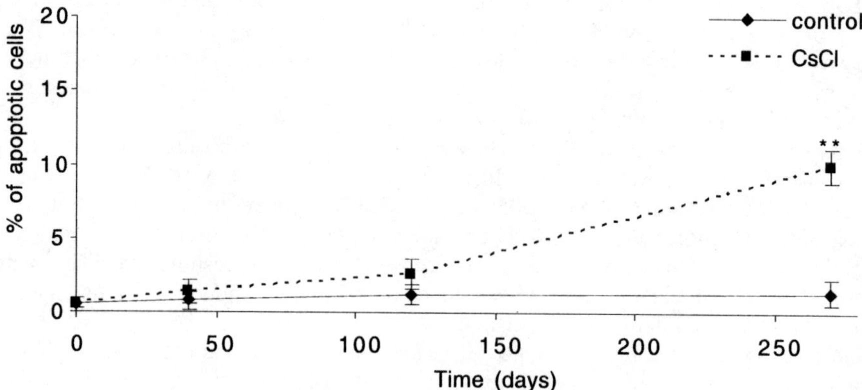

Fig. 3. Exposure time depending changes in the percent of apoptotic spleen cells in mice chronically exposed to cesium chloride (70 mg Cs+/l).

In concussion, the results of this study showed high genotoxic and cytotoxic effects in mouse spleen cells after continuous (270 day) cesium chloride uptake in mice. It is possible that the strong increase of the DNA strand breaks level in spleen cells at 270 day of cesium chloride exposure is reflected of the DNA fragmentation process during apoptosis induced by cesium ions. Overall increase in the level of DNA breaks in spleen cells as a result of chronic cesium chloride uptake can be also partially associated with structural rearrangement of the chromatin during gene expression activation, cell proliferation response, free radical overproduction, and DNA repair activation.

REFERENCES

1. Brewer K. The High pH Therapy for Cancer, Tests on Mice and Humans. *Pharmacology Biochemistry & Behaviour* 1984; 21 Suppl. 1: 1-5.
2. Senges JC, Sterns LD, Freigang KD, Bauer A, Becker R, Kubler W, Schoels W. Cesium chloride induced ventricular arrhythmias in dogs: three-dimensional activation patterns and their relation to the cesium dose applied. *Basic Res Cardiol* 2000; 95(2): 152-62.
3. Ghosh A, Sharma A, Talukder G. Clastogenic effects of cesium chloride on mouse bone marrow cells in vivo. *Mutat Res* 1990; 244(4): 295-98.
4. Ghosh A, Sen S, Sharma A, Talukder G. Inhibition of clastogenic effects of cesium chloride in mice in vivo by chlorophyllin. *Toxicol Lett* 1991; 57(1): 11-17.
5. Singh NP, McCoy MT, Tice RR, Schneider EL. A simple technique for quantification of low levels of DNA damage in individual cells. *Exp Cell Res* 1988; 175: 184-91.
6. Kobayashi H, Sugiyama C, Morikawa Y, Hayashi M and Sofuni T. A comparison between manual microscopic analysis and computerized image analysis in the single cell gel electrophoresis assay. *MMS Commun* 1995; 3: 103-15.
7. Singh NP. A simple method for accurate estimation of apoptotic cells. *Exp Cell Res* 2000; 256(1): 328-37.
8. Santini MT, Paradisi S, Straface E, Malorni W. Cesium ions influence cultured cell behavior by modifying specific subcellular components: the role of membranes and of the cytoskeleton. *Cell Biol Toxicol* 1993; 9(3): 295-06.

Metal Ions in Biology and Medicine: vol. 9. Eds Maria Carmen Alpoim, Paula Vasconcellos Morais, Maria Amélia Santos, Armando J. Cristóvão, José A. Centeno, Philippe Collery.
John Libbey Eurotext, Paris © 2006 pp. 277-1.

Mercury induces cytotoxicity and the externalization of phosphatidylserine HK-2 human renal proximal tubule cells

Dwayne J. Sutton[1] and Paul B. Tchounwou[1]

[1]*Molecular Toxicology Research laboratory, NIH-Center for Environmental Health, College of Science, Engineering and Technology, Jackson State University, 1400 Lynch Street, Box 18540 Jackson, Mississippi 39217; Email: paul.b.tchounwou@jsums.edu*

ABSTRACT

Mercury is one of the most environmentally abundant toxic metals, and is known to produce cellular injury in the kidneys. The kidneys serve as a target organ for toxins due to its extremely high blood flow (20 - 25%) of the cardiac output. Hence, heavy metals such as mercury that enter the blood stream will travel to the kidneys. The primary function of the kidneys is to concentrate waste products, including heavy metals such as mercury. Transport and binding sites in the kidneys are present in the proximal tubules, and mercury may alter the structure and function of the proteins and membranes in these cells. These changes may result in long term residual effects. Heavy metals such as mercury elicit adverse effects in the proximal tubule and it is the epithelial cells of the proximal tubule that reabsorbs the mercury that is filtered out of the glomerulus. This research was therefore designed to evaluate the dose response relationship in human renal proximal tubule cells following exposure to mercury. Cytotoxicity was evaluated using the MTT-assay for cell viability. The Annexin-V assay was performed by flow cytometry to determine the extent of phosphatidylserine externalization in HK-2 cells exposed to mercury. Cells were exposed to mercury for 24 hours at doses of 0, 1, 2, 3, 4, 5, and 6 µg/mL. Cytotoxicity experiments yielded a LD_{50} value of 4.65 ± 0.6 µg/mL upon 24 hours of exposure, indicating that mercury is highly toxic. The percentage of cells undergoing early apoptosis were $0.70 \pm 0.03\%$, $10.0 \pm 0.02\%$, $11.70 \pm 0.03\%$, $15.20 \pm 0.02\%$, $16.70 \pm 0.03\%$, $24.20 \pm 0.02\%$, and $25.60 \pm 0.04\%$ for 0, 1, 2, 3, 4, 5, and 6 µg/mL of mercury respectively, indicating a dose response relationship with regards to mercury induced cytotoxicity, and early apoptosis in HK-2 cells.

INTRODUCTION

All forms of mercury are toxic and exert their effects in a number of organs, tissues, and cell systems. The kidneys are the primary target organ where inorganic mercury is taken up, accumulated, and induces toxicity [1, 2, 3]. In humans and other mammals, the kidneys are the primary target where inorganic mercuric ions accumulate after exposures [4]. In vivo, inorganic mercury has been shown to be a potent and specific nephrotoxicant that accumulates predominantly in the kidneys and selectively in the proximal tubule cells [5, 6]. The intrarenal content of mercury has been shown to correlate with the severity of mercury induced nephropathy and cellular injury, but only up to the point where injury occurs [7, 8, and 9]. A variety of renal systems have shown an extremely steep dose response relationship for inorganic mercury. These systems include the in vivo treatment of rats and rabbits [10, 11, 12, and 13], renal cortical slices [14], isolated segments of proximal tubules from rabbits [15, 16], freshly isolated proximal tubular cells from rats [17], and primary cultures of renal cortical cells from rats [18, 19]. In some of these systems, a threshold effect was generally observed in that no cellular death was observed up to a certain dose. However, above that dose cell death progressed rapidly, and in some but not all of these systems, an all or none response was observed. This suggests that subtoxic doses of mercury are having biochemical and physiological effects, but not to an extent where they can be measured.

It is known that endogenous ligands such as glutathione bind to mercury, and may act as a buffer to prevent functional changes from occurring [20]. Accordingly, above a certain dose or concentration of mercury, the buffer is depleted. Then the mercuric ions can bind readily to critical nucleophilic groups in the cell causing functional impairment. It is likely that intracellular sulfhydryl-containing proteins such as metallothionein or low-molecular weight thiols such as glutathione function in the capacity of buffers.

Physiological and pathological alterations in cellular function in the kidney may have many diverse roles that modify the susceptibility to mercury induced renal injury. We must understand the biochemical and molecular actions of mercury in the kidney and also the intracellular buffering capacity of the kidney itself. Knowledge of the molecular and cellular mechanisms of mercury induced toxicity in the target organ the kidney and the target cells, namely the epithelial cells lining the proximal tubule is essential for early diagnosis and treatment regimens.

MATERIALS AND METHODS

Chemical and growth medium

Reference solution of mercury (10,000 μg/mL). CAS No. 7439-97-6, Lot No. B0095024 was purchased from EM Science (Gibbstown, New Jersey). Gibco Keratinocyte-SFM Medium Cat. No. 10724-011, Lot No. 1261258 was purchased from Invitrogen Corporation, Carlsbad Corporation. Supplements for Keratinocyte-SFM Medium (Recombinant Epidermal Growth Factor 5 ng/mL and Bovine Pituitary Extract 0.05 mg/mL) Lot No. 1277572 were purchased from Invitrogen Corporation, Carlsbad, California. Penicillin-Streptomycin Lot No. 3000342 and fetal bovine serum Lot no.3863047 were purchased from American Type Culture Collection, Manassas, VA. Hanks Balanced Salt Solution Lot. No. 2000257 was also purchased from American Type Culture Collection, Manassas, VA. Trypsin - EDTA without calcium and magnesium Lot No. 3000396 was also purchased from American Type Culture Collection, Manassas, VA. Dulbecco's Phosphate Buffered Saline Solution without Calcium Chloride and without magnesium chloride Lot. No. 1270494 was purchased from the Invitrogen Corporation, Carlsbad. California.

Cell Culture

Human renal proximal tubule cells (HK-2, ATCC No. 2190) were purchased from American type Culture Collection (Manassas, VA). In the laboratory, cells were stored in liquid nitrogen until use. They were next thawed by gently agitation of their containers (vials) for 2 minutes in a water bath at 37°C. After thawing, the content of each vial was transferred to a 75 cm^2 diluted with Keratinocyte-Serum Free Medium with 10% fetal bovine serum (FBS), 1% streptomycin and penicillin, 5 ng/mL recombinant epidermal growth factor, 0.05 mg/ml of bovine pituitary extract, and incubated and allowed to grow to eighty percent confluency as recommended by the manufacturer. Cells were then washed with Hanks Balance Salt Solution twice. Flasks were then treated with 1, 2, 3, 4, 5, and 6 ug/mL for 24 hours, and a control that received no treatment.

MTT Cell Viability Assay

The MTT [3-(4, 5-dimethylthiazol-2-yl)-2, 5-diphenyltetrazolium bromide] assay was determined using a commercially available kit (MTT Cell Proliferation Assay Catalog No. 30-1010K obtained from ATCC Manassas, VA). HK-2 cells were exposed to serial doses (0, 1, 2, 3, 4, 5, and 6 μg/mL) of mercury in 1% dimethyl sulfoxide (DMSO) and incubated at 37° C for 24 hours. The MTT assay for cell viability was performed using a microplate reader at 550mn to determine the cell viability of HK-2 cells to mercury and the lethal dose (LD_{50}).

Flow cytometric analysis of phosphatidylserine externalization

Annexin V binding to cells was determined using a commercially available staining kit (Annexin V-FITC Apoptosis Detection Kit - BD Biosciences Catalog No. 556570; obtained from BD Pharmingen (San Diego, CA). After exposure, mercury stimulated cells were washed twice with Hanks Balanced Salt Solution and collected through trypsinization/centrifugation. For Annexin V staining collected cells were washed twice with cold PBS and resuspended in 1x binding buffer at a concentration of 1×10^6 cells/ml. One hundred microliters of the solution was transferred to a 5 ml culture tube. Five microliters of Annexin V-FITC and propidium iodide was added. The cells were gently vortexed and incubated in the dark at room temperature for 15 minutes. Four hundred microliters of the binding buffer was added to each tube (one per concentration). The cells were then analyzed by flow cytometry within one hour as recommended by the manufacturer of the kit.

RESULTS AND DISCUSSION

Figure 1 shows the effects of mercury on the viability of HK-2 cells. The data presented in this figure indicates a strong dose response relationship with respect to the cytotoxicity of mercury. As the dose increases, the number of viable cells decreases in a dose dependent manner. The LD_{50} value for mercury was computed to be 4.65 μg/mL upon 24 hours of exposure, indicating that mercury is highly toxic to the cells. In previous cytotoxicity studies in our laboratory for $HepG_2$ cells exposed to mercury, the LD_{50} was computed to be 3.5 ± 0.6 indicating that liver cells are more sensitive to mercury exposure with regards to cytotoxicity [21].

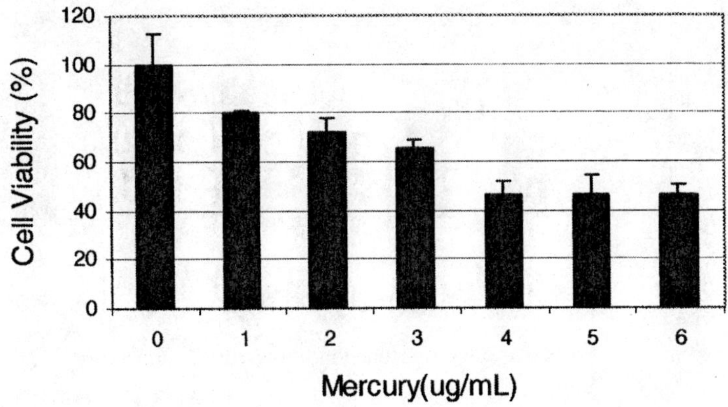

Fig. 1. Cytotoxicity of mercury to HK-2 cells

Figure 2 show the histogram analysis in which the annexin positive cells are show in M2 and the annexin negative cells are show in M1 for the control and 6 μg/mL.

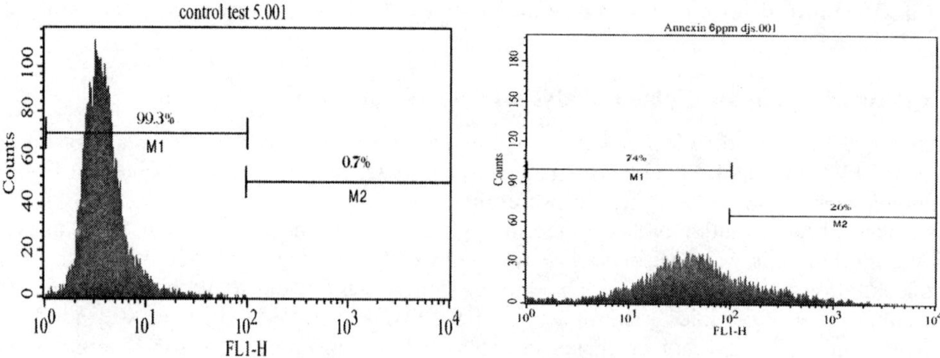

Fig. 2. Flow cytometry analysis of annexin-5 in control cells, and mercury-treated HK-2 cells at 6 μg/ml

Figure 3 shows the annexin positive HK-2 cells in response to mercury exposure. The percentage of Annexin V positive cells were 0.7 ± 0.3%, 10.0 ± 0.02%, 11.70 ± 0.03%, 15.20 ± 0.02%, 16.70 ± 0.03%, 24.20 ± 0.02%, and 25.60 ± 0.04% for 0, 1, 2, 3, 4, 5, and 6 μg/mL of mercury respectively. Previous Annexin V analysis in our laboratory with HepG2 cells exposed to mercury showed the percentage of annexin positive cells in response to mercury exposure were 0.03 ± 0.3%, 5.19 ± 0.04%, 6.36 ± 0.04%, and 8.84 ± 0.02% indicating that the kidney cells are entering early apoptosis at a faster rate than the liver cells [22].

Our findings clearly establish a strong dose response relationship between mercury exposure, cytotoxicity, and early apoptosis in HK-2 cells exposed to mercury.

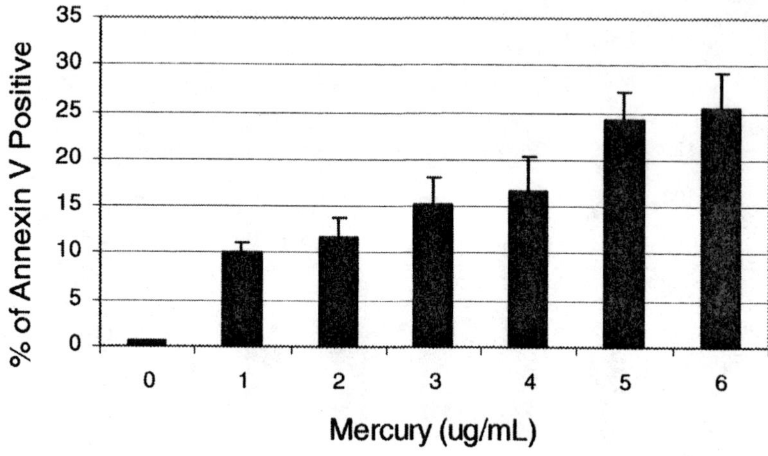

Fig. 3. Percentages of annexin-5 positive cells as a function of mercury treatment

REFERENCES

1. Zalups, R.K., and Barfus, D.W. (1996). Nephrotoxicity of inorganic mercury co -administered with L-cysteine. *Toxicology* ***109****:15-29.*
2. Cannon, V.T., Zalups, R.K., and Barfuss, D.W. (2001). Amino acid transporters involved in luminal transport of mercuric conjugates of cysteine in rabbit proximal tubule. *J Pharmacol Exp Ther* ***298****:780-789.*

3. Lash, L.H., Putt, D.A., and Zalups, R.K. (1998). Role of extracellular thiols in accumulation and distribution of inorganic mercury in rat renal proximal and distal tubular cells. *J Pharmacol Exp Ther* ***285**:1039-1050.*
4. Cannon, V.T., Barfuss, D.W., and Zalups, R.K. (2000). Molecular homology and luminal transport of Hg^{2+} in the renal proximal tubule. *Journal of the American Society of Nephrology* ***11**:394-402.*
5. Zalups, R.K. (1991a). Autometallographic localization of inorganic mercury in the kidney of rats: Effect of unilateral nephrectomy and compensatory renal growth. *Exp. Mol. Pathol.* ***54**:10-21.*
6. Zalups, R.K. (1991b). Method for studying the in vivo accumulation of inorganic mercury in segments of the nephron in the kidney of rats treated with mercuric chloride. *J. Pharmacol Methods* ***26**:89-104.*
7. Bohets, H.H., Van Thielen, M.N., Van Der Biest, I., Van landeghem, G.F., D'Haese, P.C., Nouwen, E.J., De Broe, M.E. and Dierlickx, P.J. (1995). Cytotoxicity of mercury compounds in LLC-PK1, MDCK and human proximal tubular cells. *Kidney Int.* ***47**:395-403.*
8. Burton, C.A., Hatlelid, K., Divine, K., Carter, D.E., Fernando, Q., Brendel, K., and Gandolfi, A.J. (1995). Glutathionine effects on toxicity and uptake of mercuric chloride and sodium arsenite in rabbit renal cortical slices. *Environ Healt Perspec* ***103**(Suppl. 1):81-84.*
9. Girardi, G., and Elias, M.M. (1991). Effectiveness of N-acetylcysteins in protecting against mercuric chloride-induced nephrotoxicity. *Toxicology* ***67**:155-164.*
10. Zalups, R.K., and Diamond, G.L. (1987). Mercuric chloride induced nephrotoxicity in the rat after unilateral nephrectomy and compensatory renal growth. *Virchows Arch B* ***53**:336-346.*
11. Zalups, R.K., Parks, L., Cannon, V.T., and Barfuss, D.W. (1998). Mechanisms of action of 2,3,-dimercaptopropane-1sulfonate and the transport, disposition, and toxicity of inorganic mercury in isolated perfused segments of rabbit proximal tubules. *Mol Pharmacol* ***54**:353-363.*
12. *Zalups, R.K., and Lash, L.H. (1990). Effects of uninephrectomy and mercuric chloride on renal glutathionine homeostasis. J Pharmacol Exp Ther* ***254**:962-970.*
13. Zalups, R.K. (1991c). Renal accumulation and intrarenal distribution of inorganic mercury in the rabbit: Effects of unilateral nephrectomy and dose of mercuric chloride. *J Toxicol Environ Health* ***33**:213-228.*
14. Reugg, C.E., Gandolfi, A.J., Nagle, R.B., and Brendel, K. (1987). Differential patterns of injury to the proximal tubule of renal cortical slices following in vitro exposure to mercuric chloride, potassium dichromate, or hypoxic conditions. *Toxicol Appl Pharmacol* ***90**:261-273.*
15. Barfus, D.W., Robinson, M.K., and Zalups, R.K. (1990). Inorganic mercury transport in the proximal tubule of the rabbit. *Journal of the American Society of Nephrology* ***1**:910-917.*
16. Zalups, R.K. (1993a). Early aspects of the intrarenal distribution of mercury after the intravenous administration of mercuric chloride. *Toxicology* ***79**:215-228.*
17. Lash, L.H., and Zalups, R.K. (1992). Mercuric chloride-induced cytotoxicity and compensatory hypertrophy in rat kidney proximal tubular cells. *J Pharmacol Exp Ther* ***261**:819-829.*
18. Smith, M.A., Acosta, D., and Bruckner, J.V. (1986). Development of a primary culture system of rat kidney cortical cells to evaluate the nephrotoxicity of xenobiotics. *Food Chem Toxicol* ***24**:551-556.*
19. Lash, L.H., Putt, D.A., and Zalups, R.K. (1999). Influence of exogenous thiols on inorganic mercury-induced injury in renal proximal and distal tubular cells from normal and uninephrectomized rats. *J Pharmacol Exp Ther* ***291**:492-502.*
20. Zalups, R.K., and Lash, L.J. (1997). Depletion of glutathionine in the kidney and the renal disposition of administered inorganic mercury. *Drug Metab Dispos* ***25**:516-523.*
21. Sutton, D.J., Tchounwou, P.B., Ninashvilli, N., Shen, E. (2002). Mercury induces cytotoxicity and transcriptionally activates stress genes in human liver carcinoma ($HepG_2$) cells. *Int. J. Mol. Sci* ***3**:965-984.*
22. Sutton, D.J., and Tchounwou, P.B. (2004). Mercury induced externalization of phosphatidylserine in human liver carcinoma (HepG2) cells. *Metal Ions in Biology and Medicine 8:123-126.*

ACKNOWLEDGEMENT

This research was financially supported in part by a grant from the National Institutes of Health (Grant No. 1G12RR13459) through the center for Environmental Health, and in part by a grant from the U.S. Department of Army (Grant No. DACA-42-02-C-0057) through the MACERAC Program. We thank Dr. Abdul Mohamed and Dr. Richard Price for their support in this work.

Metal Ions in Biology and Medicine: vol. 9. Eds Maria Carmen Alpoim, Paula Vasconcellos Morais, Maria Amélia Santos, Armando J. Cristóvão, José A. Centeno, Philippe Collery.
John Libbey Eurotext, Paris © 2006 pp. 282-1.

Tris(8-quinolinolato)gallium(III) exerts strong antiproliferative effects in melanoma cells

Valiahdi S.M.[1], Jakupec M.A.[1], Marculescu R.[2], Keppler B.K.[1]

[1] *Institute of Inorganic Chemistry, University of Vienna, Waehringer Strasse 42, 1090 Vienna, Austria*
[2] *Clinical Institute of Medical and Chemical Laboratory Diagnostics, Medical University of Vienna, Waehringer Guertel 18-20, 1090 Vienna, Austria*
E-mails: seied.valiahdi@univie.ac.at; michael.jakupec@univie.ac.at; rodrig.marculescu@meduniwien.ac.at; bernhard.keppler@univie.ac.at

BACKGROUND

Malignant melanoma is a very aggressive tumor with a rapidly increasing global incidence and a high rate of primary resistance to chemotherapy. Prognosis of disseminated disease is poor, and the response rates and median survival achieved with the established chemotherapeutic drug dacarbazine (DTIC) do not exceed 20% and 9 months, respectively [1]. The increasing demand for treatment options contrasts with the failure of most investigational drugs.

Among many other compounds with antineoplastic properties, gallium nitrate has been explored for its clinical efficacy as an antimelanoma drug. In a phase I dose-escalation study, 3 of 19 patients with advanced melanoma treated with gallium nitrate given by continuous infusion over 7 consecutive days had experienced disease stabilization [2], prompting the initiation of a phase II study in this setting. However, this trial yielded a disappointing overall response rate of only 3% (1 partial response with nearly complete resolution of metastases for seven months and two disease stabilizations for 3+ months in a total of 31 evaluable patients), forcing the investigators to conclude that further evaluation of gallium nitrate in patients with malignant melanoma is not justified [3].

Nevertheless, attempts to utilize gallium-67 scintigraphy for the detection and surveillance of occult metastatic disease in melanoma patients showed that these tumors can regularly be visualized by gallium tracers [4]. An overall sensitivity of 82% and specificity of 99% has been reported [5]. Even though the clinical utility remained controversial ever since, it is without doubt that melanomas avidly accumulate gallium, thus providing a rationale for the development of gallium drugs with emphasis on this malignancy.

With the aim of overcoming the limitations experienced with the clinical use of gallium salts, in particular the severe dose-limiting toxicities associated with the high plasma gallium levels observed after intravenous infusion, the inconvenience of continuous infusion over several days and the unsatisfactory oral bioavailability, the lipophilic gallium complex tris(8-quinolinolato)gallium(III) (KP46, FFC11) *(fig. 1)* has been explored in preclinical tumor models [6] and recently been evaluated in an orally administered formulation in a phase I trial in solid tumors patients with promising results [7]. This compound is expected to allow the accumulation of gallium in tumors from comparatively low steady-state plasma concentrations, thereby expanding the pharmacological capacity of this metal. In order to provide a basis for further preclinical and clinical studies, we investigated KP46 for its antimelanoma potency *in vitro* in a variety of human melanoma cell lines.

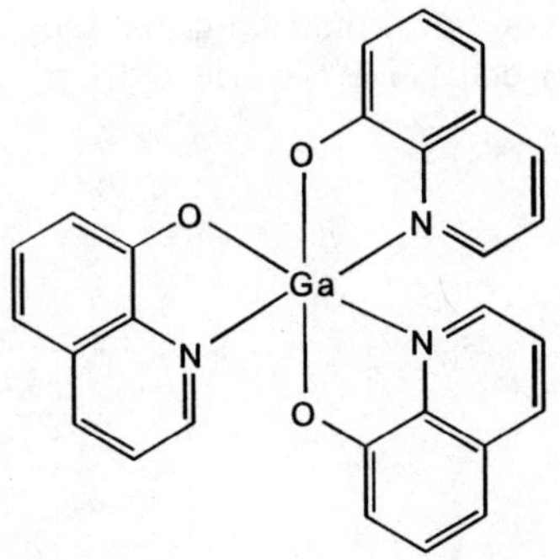

Fig. 1. Structural formula of tris(8-quinolinolato)gallium(III) (KP46, FFC11).

MATERIALS AND METHODS

518A2, 607B, A375, MEL-JUSO, SK-MEL-28 (all melanoma), 41M, CH1 (both ovarian carcinoma), SK-BR-3 (mammary carcinoma), HT29 and SW480 (both colon carcinoma) cells were propagated as adherent monolayer cultures in Minimal Essential Medium (MEM) supplemented with 10% heat-inactivated fetal bovine serum, 1 mM sodium pyruvate, 2 mM *L*-glutamine and 1% non-essential amino acids (100×). Cultures were maintained at 37 °C in a humidified atmosphere containing 5% CO_2.

Cytotoxicity of KP46 was determined in comparison to dacarbazine and cisplatin by means of a colorimetric microculture assay (MTT assay). Briefly, cells were harvested from subconfluent cultures by trypsinization and seeded into 96-well microculture plates in appropriate cell densities ensuring exponential growth throughout drug exposure. After a 24 h pre-incubation, cells were exposed to serial dilutions of the test compounds in complete MEM (as described above). Because of the limited aqueous solubility of KP46, stock solutions had to be prepared in DMSO and diluted such that the effective DMSO content in the medium did not exceed 1%, whereas dacarbazine and cisplatin were dissolved directly in the medium. After 96 h exposure, drug solutions were replaced by 7.5 : 1 mixtures of RPMI1640 medium (supplemented with 10% heat-inactivated fetal bovine serum and 2 mM *L*-glutamine) and MTT solution (5 mg/ml PBS). After incubation for 4 hours, the medium/MTT mixtures were removed, and the formazan crystals developed by vital cells were dissolved in DMSO. Optical densities at 550 nm were measured with a microplate reader. The quantity of vital cells was expressed in terms of T/C values by comparison to untreated control microcultures, and 50% inhibitory concentrations (IC_{50}) were calculated from concentration-effect curves by interpolation.

RESULTS

The IC_{50} values of KP46 obtained by the MTT assay in the five melanoma cell lines are in a relatively narrow range of low micromolar concentrations (0.8-2.5 μM). When compared to a small cell panel representing other solid tumors (ovarian, mammary and colon carcinoma), most melanoma cell lines (with the exception of SK-MEL-28) clearly rank among the KP46-sensitive cell lines *(figs. 1, 2A)*.

The cytotoxic potency of KP46 is higher than that of the established antimelanoma drug dacarbazine in all five melanoma lines. In the least dacarbazine-sensitive cell line (SK-MEL-28), KP46 is even 26 times more potent (based on comparison of IC_{50} values). Furthermore, the cytotoxicity of KP46 is only slightly (1.1-2.0-fold) lower than that of cisplatin. The concentration-effect curves depicted in *figure 2B-F* reveal that KP46 yields consistently steeper curves than the two reference drugs under the same conditions, indicating that only a comparatively low increase of KP46 concentration is required for enhancing the effects from cytostatic to cytocidal.

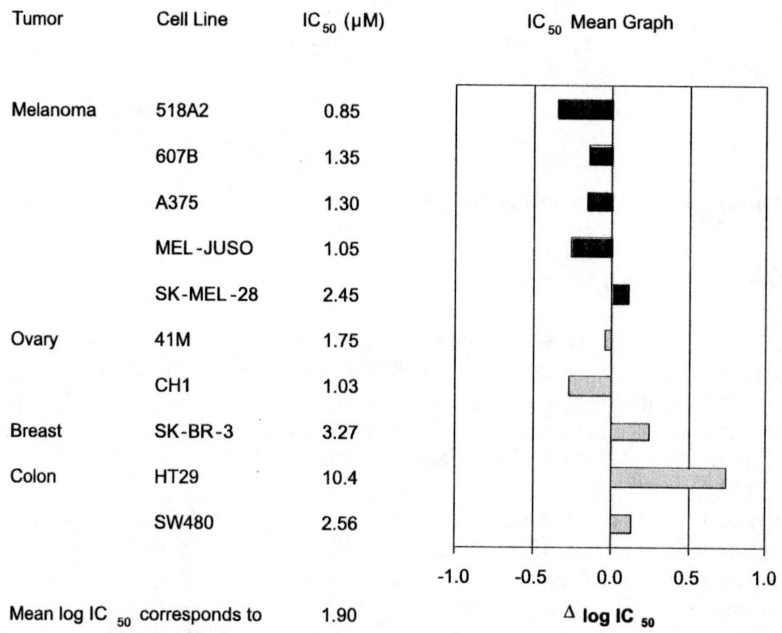

Fig. 1. IC_{50} mean graph of KP46 in five melanoma cell lines (black) and five other human tumor cell lines (grey), representing the deviations from the mean log IC_{50} (averaged over all cell lines). Bars oriented to the left indicate a higher sensitivity, bars oriented to the right a lower sensitivity than the average. Values were obtained by the MTT assay (96 h exposure) and are the means of three independent experiments.

DISCUSSION

Based on the clinical activity spectrum of gallium nitrate, lymphoma [8] and bladder cancer [9] have constantly been among the malignancies aimed at by the development of new antineoplastic gallium compounds. Preliminary signs of efficacy with 1 partial response and 2 disease stabilizations in a total of 4 patients with renal cell carcinoma observed in a phase I trial of tris(8-quinolinolato)gallium(III) (KP46, FFC11) have moved renal cell carcinoma into the center of interest for further studies [7].

The organ affinity patterns of gallium (compare ref. [10]) might also justify attempts to utilize this metal for the treatment of osteosarcomas and hepatocellular carcinomas. Furthermore, clinical experience with low-dosed gallium nitrate suggests potential benefits in multiple myeloma because of the attenuating effects on bone resorption rather than its cytostatic activity [11]. The well-known osteotropic and antiosteolytic properties also provide a rationale for the treatment of patients with secondary bone involvement from solid tumors such breast cancer [12].

Despite the modest clinical effectiveness of gallium nitrate in malignant melanoma, the avidity of this tumor for gallium, the improved pharmacological properties of the gallium complex KP46 and the *in vitro* data presented here indicate that, in addition to the spectrum of tumors delineated above, further studies exploring the therapeutic potential of this compound in preclinical melanoma models are warranted.

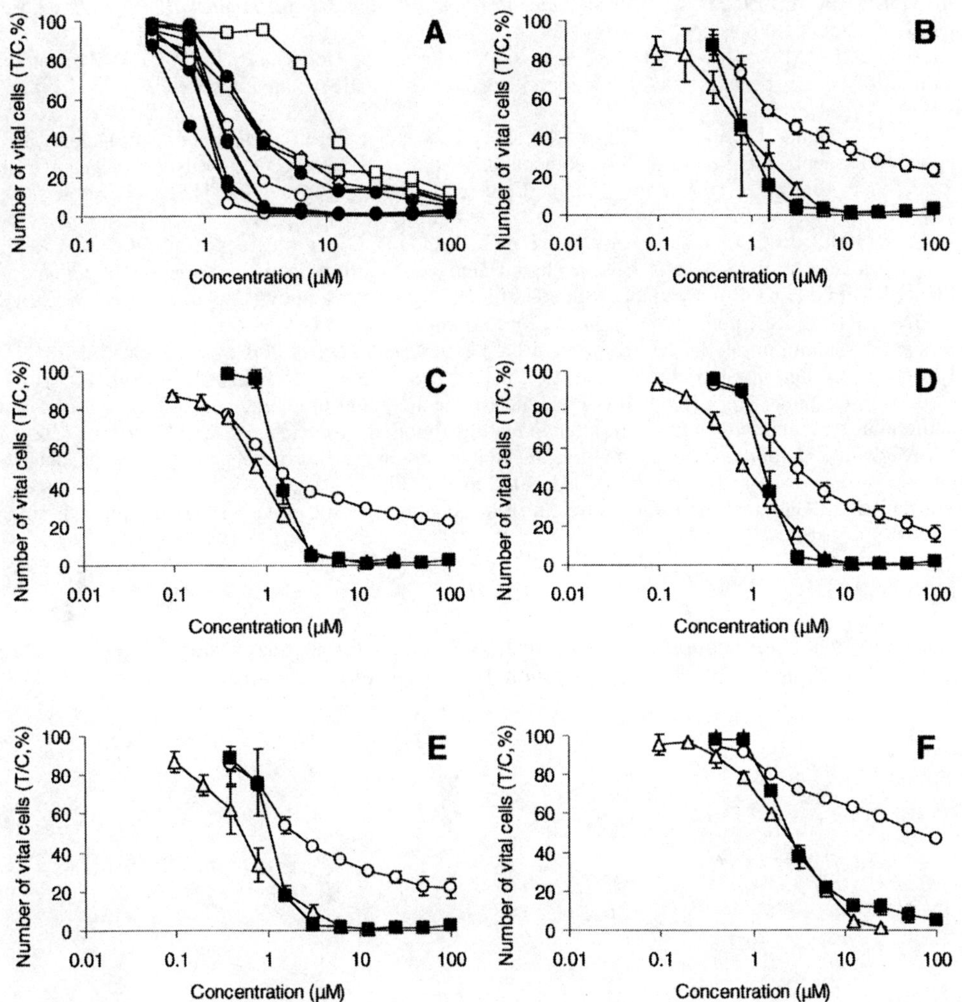

Fig. 2. Concentration-effect curves of KP46 in five human melanoma cell lines (black symbols) and five other human tumor cell lines representing ovarian, mammary and colon carcinoma (white symbols) (A); and comparison of concentration-effect curves of KP46 (- ■ -), dacarbazine (- ○ -) and cisplatin (- △ -) in 518A2 (B), 607B (C), A375 (D), MEL-JUSO (E) and SK-MEL-28 cells (F), obtained by the MTT assay (96 h exposure).

REFERENCES

1. Eigentler TK, Caroli UM, Radny P, Garbe C. Palliative therapy of disseminated malignant melanoma: a systematic review of 41 randomised clinical trials. *Lancet Oncol* 2003; 4: 748-59.
2. Bedikian AY, Valdivieso M, Bodey GP, Burgess MA, Benjamin RS, Hall S, Freireich EJ. Phase I clinical studies with gallium nitrate. *Cancer Treat Rep* 1978; 62: 1449-53.
3. Casper ES, Stanton GF, Sordillo PP, Parente R, Michaelson RA, Vinceguerra V. Phase II trial of gallium nitrate in patients with advanced malignant melanoma. *Cancer Treat Rep* 1985; 69: 1019-20.
4. Van der Wall H, McLaughlin AF, Southee AE. Gallium scintigraphy in tumor diagnosis and management.

In: Murray IPC, Ell PJ, eds. *Nuclear Medicine in Clinical Diagnosis and Treatment*, Vol 2, 2nd ed. Edinburgh: Churchill Livingstone, 1998: 813-29.

5. Kirkwood JM, Myers JE, Vlock DR, Neumann R, Ariyan S, Gottschalk A, Hoffer P. Tomographic gallium-67 citrate scanning: useful new surveillance for metastatic melanoma. *Ann Intern Med* 1982; 97: 694-9.
6. Thiel M, Schilling T, Gey DC, Ziegler R, Collery P, Keppler BK. Tris(8-quinolinolato)gallium(III), a novel orally applied antitumor gallium compound. In: Fiebig HH, Burger AM, eds. *Relevance of Tumor Models for Anticancer Drug Development. Contributions to Oncology*, Vol 54. Basel: Karger, 1999: 439-43.
7. Hofheinz RD, Dittrich C, Jakupec MA, Drescher A, Jaehde U, Gneist M, Keyserlingk N Graf v, Keppler BK, Hochhaus A. Early results from a phase I study on orally administered tris(8-quinolinolato)gallium(III) (FFC11, KP46) in patients with solid tumors - a CESAR study (Central European Society for Anticancer Drug Research - EWIV). *Int J Clin Pharmacol Ther* 2005; 43: 590-1.
8. Straus DJ. Galium nitrate in the treatment of lymphoma. *Semin Oncol* 2003; 30, Suppl 5: 25-33.
9. Einhorn L. Galium nitrate in the treatment of bladder cancer. *Semin Oncol* 2003; 30, Suppl 5: 34-41.
10. Collery P, Domingo JL, Keppler BK. Preclinical toxicology and tissue gallium distribution of a novel antitumour gallium compound: tris(8-quinolinolato)gallium(III). *Anticancer Res* 1996; 16: 687-92.
11. Niesvitzky R. Gallium nitrate in multiple myeloma: prolonged survival in a cohort of patients with advanced-stage disease. *Semin Oncol* 2003; 30, Suppl 5: 20-4.
12. Warrell RP Jr. Gallium nitrate for the treatment of bone metastases. *Cancer* 1997; 80, Suppl 8: 1680-5.

ACKNOWLEDGMENT

This work has been supported by the Austrian Council for Research and Technology Development and by Faustus Forschung Translational Drug Development AG.

Metal Ions in Biology and Medicine: vol. 9. Eds Maria Carmen Alpoim, Paula Vasconcellos Morais, Maria Amélia Santos, Armando J. Cristóvão, José A. Centeno, Philippe Collery.
John Libbey Eurotext, Paris © 2006 pp. 287-1.

Arsenic trioxide mediated cytotoxicity and oxidative stress, in breast and lung carcinoma cell lines

Alice M. Walker, Jacqueline J. Stevens and Paul B. Tchounwou

Molecular Toxicology Research Laboratory, Molecular and Cellular Biology Research Laboratory, NIH-Center for Environmental Health, College of Science, Engineering and Technology, Jackson State University, 1400 JR Lynch Street, Box 18540, Jackson, Mississippi, USA; email: paul.b.tchounwou@jsums.edu

ABSTRACT

Arsenic is a metalloid that is commonly found in soil, water and air. It is an element that has no known physiological function but is present in the body as a result of environmental exposure. The primary source of human exposure is through drinking water and food. Arsenic acts on cells through a variety of mechanisms influencing numerous signal transduction pathways resulting in cellular effects such as apoptosis induction, growth inhibition and angiogenesis inhibition. Although arsenic has been reported to induce reactive oxygen species formation and oxidative stress in liver cells and hematopoetic cells, its effects on breast and lung cells are not well elucidated. The primary objective of this research is to evaluate the effects of arsenic cytotoxcity and to determine whether arsenic induces oxidative stress in breast and lung carcinoma cell lines.

To achieve this goal, breast cancer (MCF-7) and lung cancer (A549) cells were cultured following standard protocols, and exposed to various doses of arsenic trioxide for 48 h. The 3-(4, 5 dimethyl-thiazoyl-2-yl) 2,5diphenyl-tetrazolium bromide (MTT) assay was performed to determine the cytotoxicity, and the thiobarbituric acid test was performed to evaluate the degree of lipid peroxidation and oxidative stress. Data obtained from the MTT assay indicated that arsenic significantly reduced the viability of MCF-7 and A549 cells. Upon 48 hr of exposure, the LD_{50} values from arsenic trioxide treatment were 11.5 and 14.1 µg/ml for A549 cells and MCF-7 cells, respectively. The result of the thiobarbituric acid test demonstrated that arsenic trioxide treatment resulted in a significant increase ($p < 0.05$) of malondialdehyde-MDA, indicating that oxidative stress may play a key role in arsenic-induced toxicity in the breast and lung cells.

INTRODUCTION

Arsenic is a metalloid that is ubiquitous in the environment. People may be exposed to arsenic in three ways; by ingestion of contaminated food and water, by inhalation of contaminated air, aerosols or particulates, and by dermal or skin contact. The toxicity of arsenic depends upon its chemical form; the organic forms being usually less harmful than the inorganic ones (1). Acute exposure, whether from ingested or inhaled arsenic, can damage many tissues and organ systems including the nervous system, respiratory system, cardiovascular system, gastrointestinal tract, and skin. Intense acute arsenic exposure can be fatal (2). Chronic exposure to arsenic has been associated with several adverse health effects including vascular, peripheral neuropathy, exacerbation of the complications of diabetes, cardiac arrhythmias, liver and kidney toxicity, anemia, and leukopenia, and several types of cancers (2).

The major mechanism by which arsenic exerts its toxic effect is through impairment of cellular respiration by inhibition of various mitochrondrial enzymes, and phosphorylation. Most toxicity of arsenic results from its ability to interact with sulfhydryl groups of proteins and enzymes, and to substitute phosphorus in a variety of biochemical reactions (3, 4). Arsenic *in vitro* reacts with protein sulfhydryl groups to inactivate enzymes, such as dihydrolipoyl dehydrogenase and thiolase, thereby producing inhibited oxidation of pyruvate and betaoxidation of fatty acids (5). Arsenical compounds have shown to induce oxidative stress in mammalians cells (3, 6). The objective of this study is to determine the cytotoxic effects of arsenic trioxide in breast and lung carcinoma cell lines and to assess whether arsenic toxicity is mediated via oxidative stress in these cell lines. To accomplish this objective, lipid peroxidation is used as an indicator of oxidative stress, and as a biomarker to ascertain cellular injury. It has been reported that the peroxidation of lipids in cell membranes can damage these biologic structures by disrupting fluidity and permeability. Lipid peroxidation can also adversely affect the function of membrane bound proteins such as enzymes and receptors (7).

MATERIALS AND METHODS

Cell Lines and Chemicals

The breast cancer cell line (MCF-7) was generously provided by Dr Ernest Izevbigie, Department of Biology, Jackson State University; Jackson, MS. The human lung carcinoma cell line (A549), the F-12 K medium and trypan blue were purchased from American Type Culture collection (ATCC) (Manassa, VA). The RPMI 1640 medium, fetal bovine serum (FBS), penicillin/streptomycin/fungizone, phosphate buffered saline (PBS) and trypsin versene were purchased from Invitrogen (Grand Island, NY). BCA protein assay kit was obtained from Pierce (Rockford, IL). Arsenic trioxide (As_2O_3) was purchased from Fisher Scientific (Houston, TX) and the MTT [3-(4, 5-dimethylthiazol-2-yl)-2, 5-diphenyltetrazolium bromide] reagent was obtained from Sigma Chemical Company (St. Louis, MO). The lipid peroxidation assay kit was purchased from EMD Bioscience (San Diego, CA).

Cell Culture

MCF-7 cells were maintained in RPMI 1640 supplemented with 10% FBS, and 1% penicillin (10,000 units/ml), streptomycin (10,000 μg/ml) and fungizone mixture. A549 cells were maintained in F12-K medium supplemented in 10% FBS and 1% penicillin, streptomycin and fungizone mixture, as adherent cells. The cells were grown in a humidified incubator under an atmosphere of 95% air and 5% CO_2 at 37°C to sub-confluence (80-95%). The culture medium for each cell line was replaced every 48 hours. After growing to 80-95% confluence, the medium was aspirated off and the cell monolayer was washed three times with sterile phosphate buffered saline (PBS). The cell monolayer was treated with 1 mL trypsin versene per plate and incubated briefly at 37°C. The cells were then viewed microscopically to ensure a complete cell detachment. Cells were re-suspended in RPMI 1640 complete medium for MCF-7 and F-12K complete medium for A549, stained with 4% trypan blue (1 to 2 minutes), and counted with a hemocytometer. The cells were seeded at a density of 5×10^5 cells in 13×100 mm tissue culture plates, prior to arsenic trioxide treatment.

Cytotoxicity Assay

MCF-7 and A549 cells were seeded in a 96-well plates with 5000 cells per well for a period of 24 hours at 37°C in a 5% CO_2 humidified incubator. The medium was removed and replaced with various doses of arsenic trioxide using deionized water as solvent. The plates were treated with arsenic trioxide at 0.78, 1.58, 3.125, 6.25, 12.5, 25, 50 μg/ml doses for 18, 24, and 48 hrs. The MTT assay was performed as previously described, and optical densities were read on a microtiter plate reader (Bio-Tek Instruments Inc) at a wavelength of 550 nm (8). A data analysis was performed to determine the chemical doses required to reduce cell viability by 50% (LD_{50}s).

Lipid Peroxidation Assay

MCF-7 and A549 cell lines were seeded at a density of 3×10^5 cells in 13×100 mm tissue culture plates. The cells were then grown in a humidified incubator under an atmosphere of 95% and 5% CO_2 at 37°C, to 75% confluence. The medium was aspirated from the cell monolayer and treated with 4 ml of various doses of arsenic trioxide (0, 4, 6, 8, 10 µg/ml). The experiment was carried out in triplicates. The control was grown in the absence of As_2O_3. After 48 hr exposure time, the treatments were removed and the cells were removed from the plate by scraping. The cells were collected and resuspended in 1 ml of PBS, and were washed three times with PBS pH 7.4. The cell lysis was by homogenization (Omni GLH homogenizer) and sonication (Branson sonifier). The lipid peroxidation assay was performed according to the manufacture protocol (Calbiochem-EMD Biosciences, Inc.). Optical densities were read at 586 nm on a Varian Cary 300 Bio UV-Visible spectrophotometer.

Statistical Analysis

The absorbance values obtained per treatment were converted to percentages of cell viability. Regression analysis was performed on cell viability data and the resulting equation was used to compute the lethal dose required to produce a 50% reduction (LD_{50}) in cell viability. Statistical analysis for differences in mean levels of MDA was done using student's t-test for comparing two sample sets, and ANOVA for multiple sample sets. P-values less than 0.05 were considered statistically significant.

RESULTS

Data obtained from the bioassay with MCF-7 cells revealed a strong dose response with the cytotoxicity of arsenic trioxide. The mean percentages of cell viability were 100% ± 0.8, 85% ± 5%, 72% ± 7%, 72% ± 3%, 5.4 ± 0.2%, 5.5% ± 0.3% and 6.3% ± 0.7% (18 hr); 100% ± 6%, 97% ± %5, 93% ± 0.3%, 110% ± 1%, 40% ± 2%, 6% ± .03% and 6% ± 0.2% (24 hr); and 100% ± 1%, 85% ± 6%, 72% ± 13%, 72% ± 4%, 5.4% ± 4%, 5.5% ± 7% and 6.2% ± 11% (48 hr) for 0, 1.56, 3.125, 6.25, 12.5, 25 and 50 µg/ml of arsenic trioxide, respectively *(fig. 1)*. A time-dependent response was also observed. Arsenic trioxide doses required to reduce cell viability by 50% were computed to be 21.5, 18.4 and 15.3 µg/ml for 18, 24 and 48 hrs of exposure, respectively.

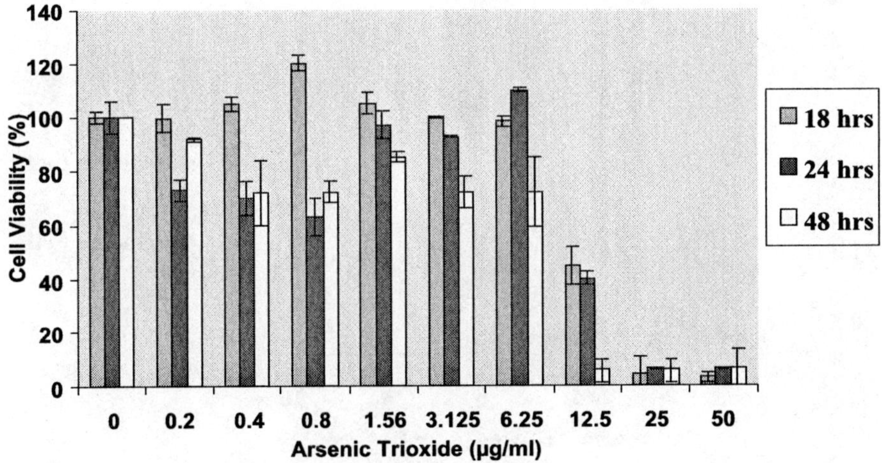

Fig. 1. Cytotoxic effect of arsenic trioxide on MCF-7 cells

Tests with A549 cells also revealed a strong dose response with cytotoxicity of arsenic trioxide. The mean percentages of cell viability were 100% ± 6%, 122% ± 8%, 131% ± 1, 146% ± 6%, 80% ± 2%, 27% ± 5% and 27% ± 5% (18 hr); 100% ± 5%, 136% ± 13%, 149% ± 8%, 115% ± 3%, 49% ± 9%, 4% ± 5% and 4% ± 3% (24 hr); and 100% ± 6%, 95% ± 8%, 90% ± 5%, 71% ± 12%, 27% ± 4%, 2% ± 4%, and 2% ± 1% for 0, 1.56, 3.125, 6.25, 12.5, 25 and 50 µg/ml of arsenic trioxide. Computed LD_{50} values of 32.24, 25.76 and 11.5 µg/ml were obtained for 18, 24, and 48 hrs of exposure, respectively.

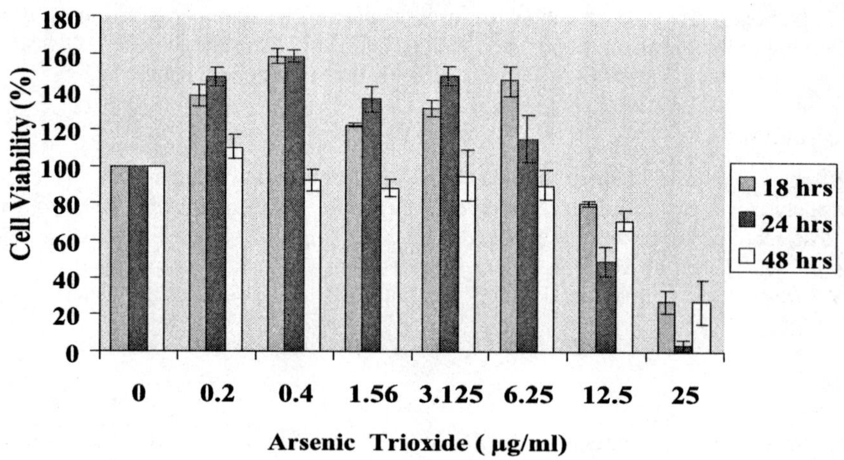

Fig. 2. Cytotoxic effect of arsenic trioxide on A549 cells

Lipid Peroxidation

Figure 3 shows the results from the lipid peroxidation assay of arsenic trioxide toxicity to MCF-7 and A549 cells. The MDA levels in MCF-7 cells were 0.50±0.0, 0.75±0.35, 0.50±0.71, 1.50±0.71, 1.25±0.35 and 1.25±0.35 uM in 0, 2, 4, 6, 8, and 10µg/ml arsenic trioxide, respectively. The MDA levels in A549 cells were 0.25±0.35, 0.25±0.35, 2.50±0.71, 4.0±0.0, 2.5±0.0 and 2.5±0.0 in 0, 2, 4, 6, 8, and 10µg/ml arsenic trioxide, respectively.

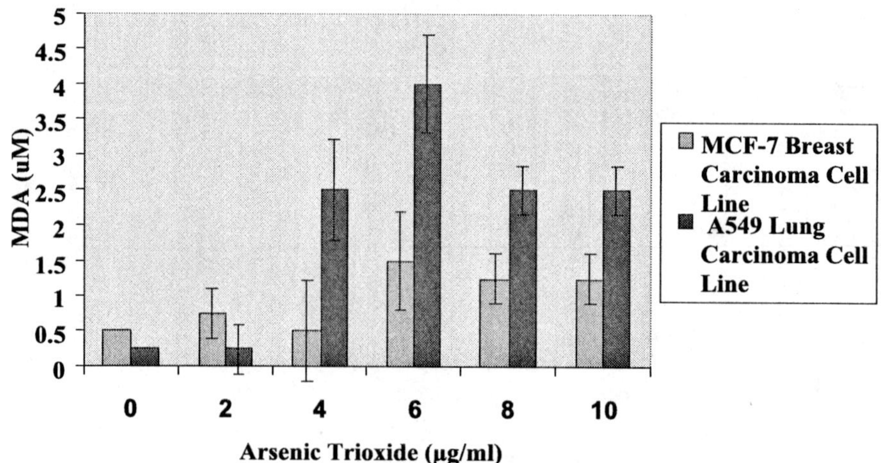

Fig. 3. MDA levels in MCF-7 and A549 cells exposed to arsenic trioxide.

DISCUSSION

Cytotoxicity is a tool for ascertaining the negative effect of a chemical compounds such as arsenic trioxide in biological systems. Toxicity is dependent upon the chemical species, the route of exposure, and other factors (9). In this study, it was demonstrated that arsenic trioxide is acutely toxic to both breast carcinoma cells (MCF-7) and lung carcinoma cells (A549). There was a time and dose-dependent response with regard to arsenic trioxide toxicity to the two cell lines. A biphasic response was obtained showing a slight increase in cell viability within the dose range of 0-0.8 μg/ml in MCF-7 and dose range of 0-0.4 μg/ml in A549, followed by a gradual decline. The median lethal doses (LD_{50}s) of arsenic trioxide for MCF-7 cells were 21.5, 18.4, 15.3 μg/ml upon 18, 24, and 48 hr treatment, respectively. LD_{50} values for A549 cells were 32.24, 25.79 and 11.5 μg/ml upon 18, 24, 48 hr treatment, respectively. This study demonstrated that cytotoxicity differs in human cell lines, indicating that some cell types are more sensitive than others (9, 10). The cytotoxicity occurred at higher levels of exposure whereas proliferation occurred at lower doses.

Chow *et al.* reported that the arsenic trioxide exhibited inhibitory effects on the proliferation of MCF-7 cells in a dose and time dependent manner, and found the LD_{50} to be 8, 1.8 and 1.2 μM upon 1-, 2-, and 3- day treatments respectively (11). Chow *et al.* also pointed out that arsenic was capable of reducing cell survival in MCF-7 cells via the suppression of the estrogen induced growth stimulatory effects in MCF-7 cells (11). Studies in our laboratory have revealed that arsenic trioxide is acutely toxic to human carcinoma cells ($HepG_2$). Upon 48 hr exposure, the LD_{50} value was 8.55±0.58 μg/mL (4). This study indicated that arsenic trioxide is less toxic in breast and lung carcinoma compared to the liver carcinoma cells. Graham-Evans *et. al* (10) studied the cytotoxicity effect of arsenic trioxide on several established human cell lines such as keratinocytes (HaCat), dermal fibroblast (CRL 1904), monocytes (THP-1/A23187), and melanocytes (1675). These authors reported that arsenic was toxic at high doses to keratinocytes (6 μg/ml), fibroblasts (1.5 μg/ml), monocytes (0.19 μg/ml) and toxic at lower doses in melanocytes (0.19 μg/ml) (10).

Malondialdehyde (MDA) has been used to evaluate lipid peroxidation and DNA damage caused by exogenous free radicals or endogenous reactive oxygen species. In this study, we investigated the effect of oxidative stress in breast and lung cancer cell lines treated with arsenic trioxide by evaluating MDA production. We found a dose-dependent increase in MDA production in both cell lines, with increasing doses of arsenic trioxide. In the MCF-7 cell line, there was an increase of MDA production from 0 to 6 μg/ml (2.5 μM), followed by a decrease in production that reaches 1.5μM at both 8 and 10 μg/ml. We believe that this decrease is related to the decrease in the number of viable cells at higher levels of arsenic trioxide exposure. In the A549 cell line, our findings revealed a gradual increase of MDA production to 4 μM at the 6 μg/ml dose, and a 50% reduction (2 μM) at both 8 and 10 μg/ml doses. The lung carcinoma cell line (A549) showed a higher level of MDA production (4 μM at 6 μg/ml) compared to the breast carcinoma cell line at the same dose (2 μM at 6 μg/ml). This is indicative that the lung cells appear to be more sensitive to arsenic-induced oxidative stress than the breast cells. It has been reported that because of hormonal activity, the breast is a constant target for oxidative stress, a process that occurs in the breast ductal system where it is surrounded by adipose tissues (12).

REFERENCES

1. Miller, W.H, Schipper, H.M., Lee, J.S., Waxman, S., Mechanisms of action of arsenic trioxide. Cancer Research 2002, 62, 3893-3903.
2. Frumkin, H., Thun, M.J., Arsenic. CA J. Clin., 2001, 51, 254-262.
3. Tchounwou, P.B., Yedjou, C.G., Dorsey, W.C., Arsenic trioxide induced transcriptional activation of

stress genes and expression of related proteins in human liver carcinoma cells (HepG2). Cell. Mol. Biol., 2003, 49 (7), 1071-1079.
4. Li, J.H., Rossman, T.C., Inhibition of DNA ligase activity by arsenite: A possible mechanism of its comutagenesis. Mol. Toxicol. 1989, 2, 1-9.
5. Belton, J.C., Benson, N.C., Hanna, M.L., Taylor, R.T., Growth inhibition and cytotoxic effects of three arsenic compounds on cultured Chinese hamster ovary cells. J. Environ. Sci. Health 1985, 20A, 37-72.
6. Jingbo, P.I., Hiroshi, Y., Yoshito, K., Guifan, S., Takahiko, Y., Hiroyuki, A., Claudia, H.R., Nobuhiro, S., Evidence for oxidative stress caused by chronic exposure of Chinese residents to arsenic contained in drinking water. Environ. Health Perspect. 2002, 110(4), 331-336.
7. Bergamini, C.M., Gambetti, S., Dondi, A., Cervellati C., Oxygen, reactive oxygen species and tissue damage. Curr Pharm Des 2004, 10(14), 1611-1626.
8. Mosman, T., Rapid colorimetric assay for cellular growth and survival: applications to proliferation and cytotoxicity assays. J. Immunol. Methods 1988, 65, 55-63.
9. Tchounwou, P.B., Wilson, B.A., Abdelghani, A.A, Ishaque, A.B, Patlolla, A.K., Differential cytotoxicity and gene expression in human liver carcinoma ($HepG_2$) cells exposed to arsenic trioxide, and monosodium acid methanearsonate (MSMA). Int. J. Mol. Sci., 2002, 3, 1117-1132.
10. Graham-Evans, B., Tchounwou, P.B., Cohly, H.H.P., Cytotoxicity and proliferation studies with arsenic in established human cell lines: Keratinocytes, melanocytes, dendritic cells, dermal fibroblasts, micro-vascular endothethial cells, monocytes and T-cells. Int. J. Mol. Sci., 2003, 4, 13-21.
11. Cho, S.K.Y., Chan, J.Y.W., Fung, K.P., Inhibition of cell proliferation and the action mechanisms of arsenic trioxide As_2O_3 on human breast cancer cells. J. Cell. Biochem., 2004, 93(1), 173-187.
12. Brown, N.S., Bicknell, R., Hypoxia and oxidative stress in breast. Oxidative stress: its effect on the growth, metastatic potential and reponse to therapy of breast cancer. Breast Cancer Res. 2001, 3, 323-327.

ACKNOWLEDGEMENTS

This research supported by a grant from the National Institutes of Health (Grant NO.1G2RR13459), through the NCRR-RCMI Center for Environmental Health at Jackson State University (JSU). We thank Dr. Abdul K. Mohamed, Dean of the College of Science, Engineering and Technology at JSU for his support of this research.

Metal Ions in Biology and Medicine: vol. 9. Eds Maria Carmen Alpoim, Paula Vasconcellos Morais, Maria Amélia Santos, Armando J. Cristóvão, José A. Centeno, Philippe Collery.
John Libbey Eurotext, Paris © 2006 pp. 293-1.

Lead nitrate-induced oxidative stress in human liver carcinoma ($HepG_2$) cells

Clement Yedjou, Matthew Steverson and Paul Tchounwou

Molecular Toxicology Research Laboratory, NIH-Center for Environmental Health, College of Science, Engineering and Technology, Jackson State University, 1400 Lynch Street, P.O. Box 18540, Jackson, Mississippi, USA.

ABSTRACT

Most research on lead has focused on its effects on organ systems such as the nervous system, the red blood cells, and the kidneys which are considered to be the primary targets of lead toxicity. However, its molecular mechanisms of toxicity are still largely unknown. In this research, we used $HepG_2$ cells as a model to study the cytotoxicity and oxidative stress associated with exposure to lead nitrate. We hypothesized that oxidative stress plays a key role in lead nitrate induced cytotoxicity. To test this hypothesis, we performed the MTT [3-(4, 5-dimethylthiazol-2-yl)-2, 5-diphenyltetrazolium bromide] assay for cell viability and the thiobarbituric acid test for lipid peroxidation. Data obtained from the MTT assay indicated that lead nitrate significantly reduced the viability of $HepG_2$ cells. Data generated from the thiobarbituric acid test showed a significant increase ($p \leq 0.05$) in MDA levels in lead nitrate-treated $HepG_2$ cells compared to control cells. Lead nitrate treatment significantly increased cellular content of reactive oxygen species (ROS), as evidenced by the increase in MDA, a lipid peroxidation by-product.

INTRODUCTION

Lead is a ubiquitous metal that has been used by humans for more than 3 millennia. Exposure to lead occurs mainly via inhalation of lead-contaminated dust particles or aerosols, and ingestion of lead-contaminated food, water, and paints (1). There are many published studies that have documented the adverse effects of lead in children and the adult population. In the United States, at least three million children suffer the neurotoxic effects (memory impairement) of lead exposure. In addition to effects on the nervous system, low-level lead exposure may result in increased blood pressure, diminished male fertility, and nephrotoxicity (2). Epidemiological studies have reported an association between exposure to lead compounds and increased risk of adverse developmental effects such as congenital malformations, low birth weight, spontaneous abortion, decreased sperm count in men, and neurodevelopmental abnormalities in offsprings (3, 4).

Lead toxicity on different biological systems and functions is well documented (5, 6). Recent studies in our laboratory have demonstrated that lead nitrate is cytotoxic to human liver carcinoma ($HepG_2$) cells (6). Although intensive investigations have focused on the toxicology of lead, its molecular mechanisms are not well elucidated. The objective of the present study was to use $HepG_2$ cells as a model to evaluate the role of oxidative stress in lead-induced cytotoxicity.

MATERIAL AND METHODS

Chemicals and media

Reference solution (1000 ± 10 ppm) of lead nitrate (CAS No. 10099-74-8, Lot No. 981735-24) with a purity of 100% was purchased from Fisher Scientific in Fair Lawn, New Jersey. Dulbecco's Modified Eagle's Minimal Essential Medium (DMEM, Lot. 1016511) was purchased from Life Technologies in Grand Island, New York.

Cytotoxicity assay

In the laboratory, parental $HepG_2$ cells stored in liquid nitrogen were thawed by gentle agitation of their containers (vials) for 2 minutes in a water bath at 37°C. Cell culture and lead nitrate exposure were performed as previous described in one of our recent publications (6). Cytotoxicity assay was performed using the MTT {3-(4, 5-dimethylthiazol-2-yl)-2, 5-diphenyltetrazolium bromide} method. The absorbance was read at a wavelength of 550 nm using microtiter plate reader (Bio-Tek Instruments Inc) (7, 8).

Assay of Lipid Peroxidation

Aldehydes such as MDA and HAE are formed during lipid peroxidation. The concentration of MDA was measured by using a lipid peroxidation assay kit Calbiochem Novabiochem, San Diego, CA). Briefly, 2×10^6 $HepG_2$ cells/mL untreated as a control and treated with different lead nitrate doses were cultured in a total volume of 10 ml growth medium for 48 hrs. After the incubation period, cells were collected in 15 mL tube, followed by low-speed centrifugation. The cell pellets were re-suspended in 0.5 ml of Tris-HCl, pH 7.4, and lysed using a sonicator (W-220; Ultrasonic, Farmingdale, NY) under the conditions of duty cycle 25% and output control 40% for 5 sec on ice. The protein concentration of the cell suspension was determined using a protein assay kit (BioRad, Hercules, C.A.). A 200µl aliquot of the culture medium or 2 mg of cell lysate protein was assayed for MDA according to the lipid peroxidation assay kit protocol (Calbiochem-Novabiochem, San Diego, CA). The absorbance of the sample was monitored at 586 nm, and the concentration of MDA was determined from a standard curve.

Statistical Analysis

Results were presented as means ± SDs. Statistical analysis was done using one way analysis of variance (ANOVA) for multiple samples and Student's t-test for comparing paired sample sets. *P*-values less than 0.05 were considered statistically significant. The percentages of cell viability and MDA levels were presented graphically in the form of histograms, using Microsoft Excel computer program.

RESULTS

Cytotoxicity assay

The MTT result of the cytotoxic effect of lead nitrate on human liver carcinoma ($HepG_2$) cells following 48 hrs of exposure is shown in *(fig. 1)*. As indicated in this figure, there was a gradual decrease in the viability of $HepG_2$ cells, with increasing doses of lead nitrate. This figure indicates a strong dose-response relationship with regard to lead toxicity. Although the assay involved six different doses of lead nitrate (control - 0 µg/mL, 3.12 µg/mL, 6.2 µg/mL, 12.25 µg/mL, 25 µg/mL and 50 µg/mL), only four doses (control - 0 µg/mL, 3.12 µg/mL, 12.25 µg/mL, and 50 µg/mL) are depicted in *fig. 1*, for clarity (of presentation) purposes. After 48 hrs of exposure, the percentages of cell viability were 100.0 ± 0.0%, 82.0 ± 12.0%, 55.0 ± 5.8%, and 40.0 ± 12.0% for the control,

3.12 μg/mL, 12.25 μg/mL, and 50 μg/mL of lead nitrate, respectively, indicating a dose-dependent response with regard to the cytotoxic effect of lead nitrate. The dose of lead nitrate required to produce 50% reduction in the viability of $HepG_2$ cells (LD_{50}) was computed to be 37.5 ± 9.2 μg/mL, upon 48 hrs of exposure.

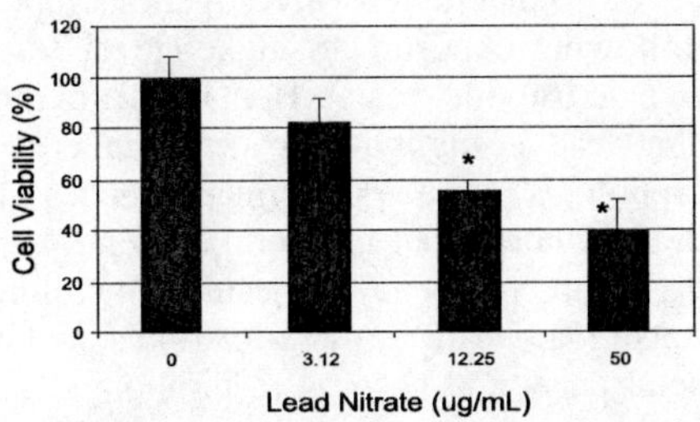

Fig. 1. Cytotoxicity of lead nitrate to $HepG_2$ cells. Each point represents a mean ± SD of eight individual measurements. *Significantly different from the control by ANOVA; $p < 0.05$.

Lipid peroxidation Assay

The standard curve generated from this assay is shown in *(fig. 2)*, and the effect of lead nitrate on MDA production in $HepG_2$ cells is represented in *(fig. 3)*. The data presented demonstrate that lead nitrate treatment resulted in a significant increase in malondialdehyde (MDA) formation, a major indicator of lipid peroxidation. Upon 48 hrs of exposure, the MDA levels were computed to be 1 ± 0, 2.25 ± 0.35, 3.75 ± 0.35, 8.25 ± 0.35, and 11.75 ± 1.05 μM in 0, 10, 20, 30, and 40 μg/mL of lead nitrate, respectively.

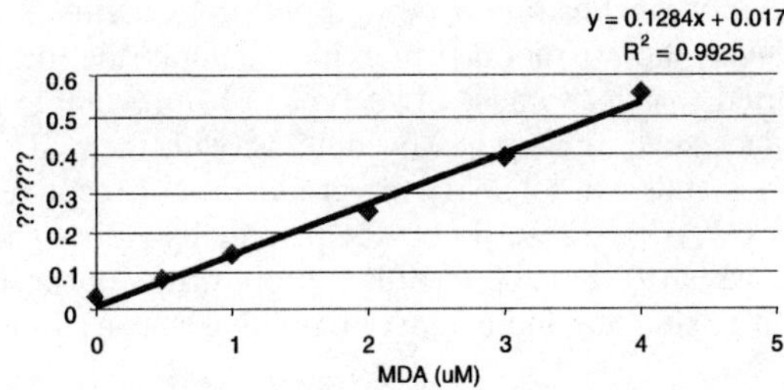

Fig. 2. MDA standard curve showing the net absorbance at 586 nm as a function of MDA concentration.

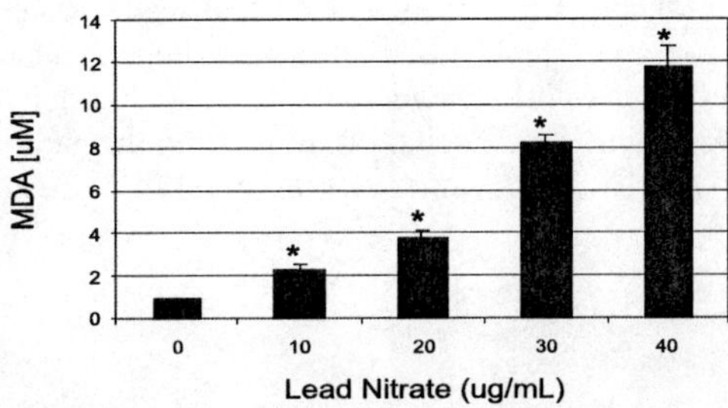

Fig. 3. Effects of lead nitrate on MDA production in $HepG_2$ cells. Each point represents a mean ± SD of three measurements. *Significantly different from the control by ANOVA; $p < 0.05$.

DISCUSSION

Cytotoxicity of lead

Data obtained from the present study clearly indicate that lead nitrate is highly cytotoxic to human liver carcinoma cells. The LD_{50} was computed to be 37.5 ± 9.2 μg/mL upon 48 hrs of exposure. These results support those of previous investigations reporting a marked reduction in the viability of $HepG_2$ cells following exposure to higher levels of lead (6, 9). We previously reported a similar trend with arsenic trioxide-treated $HepG_2$ cells in our laboratory (10). Data from a recent study also indicate that lead is highly toxic to immune cells; inhibiting cell adhesion property, and altering cell morphology in the splenic macrophages of mice (11). Although fatal, lead poisoning occurs rarely in the United States, several epidemiological have pointed out that it represents a medical and public health emergency, especially in children consuming high amounts of lead-contaminated flake paints (12). Death in these lead-poisoned children has been associated with extreme lethargy with facial palsy and gasping respirations consistent with lead encephalopathy, and severe hematologic abnormalities (12).

Lipid peroxidation Assay

Lipid peroxidation is a well-established mechanism of cellular injury in both plants and animals, and is used as an indicator of oxidative stress in cells and tissues (13). In the present study, we assessed the degree of lipid peroxidation by estimating the levels of malondialdehyde (MDA) in lead nitrate-treated $HepG_2$ cells. Our results clearly showed that the treatment of $HepG_2$ cells with lead nitrate resulted in a significant increase of malondialdehyde levels, a major indicator of lipid peroxidation. Upon 48 hrs of exposure, the MDA level value was computed to be 11.75 ± 1.05 μM at highest dose tested. A series of recent studies showed that rats exposed to lead had an elevation of blood pressure accompanied by a marked increase of lipid peroxidation product (MDA) in the plasma and tissue; and a substantial reduction in urinary excretion of stable NO metabolites (NOx) (14, 15). Metal-induced lipid peroxidation is mostly attributed to increased production of free radicals (16). Damage to cell organelles produced by lipid peroxidation has been demonstrated by many investigations. However, there is not a firm evidence about the mechanism of lipid peroxidation. Studies have reported that lead causes two types of unfavorable processes in biological systems. Firstly, it inactivates several enzymes by binding with their SH-groups. Secondly, lead ions, similar to other heavy metals can intensify the production of reactive oxygen species (ROS) leading to oxidative stress (17, 18). These processes potentially affect and destroy cell structure through the metabolic pathway (19). In support of this proposition, our results indicate that excess lead nitrate increases lipid peroxidation, indicative of oxidative stress, a biomaker of cellular injury.

CONCLUSIONS

Results from this study indicate at the cellular level that lead nitrate significantly reduced the viability of human liver carcinoma ($HepG_2$) cells in a dose-dependent manner. At the molecular level, lead treatment resulted in a significant increase in malondialdehyde (MDA) formation, an end product of lipid peroxidation in $HepG_2$ cells. Findings from this study indicate that lead nitrate is highly cytotoxic to $HepG_2$ cells. This cytotoxicity is found to be mediated by oxidative stress, a biomarker of cellular injury.

REFERENCES

1. Agency for Toxic Substances and Disease Registry (ATSDR): Toxicological Profile for Lead. Public Health Service, U.S. Department of Health and Human Services, Atlanta, GA, 1999.

2. Fishbein, A.: Occupational and environmental exposure to lead. In Environmental Occupational Medicine (W. M. Rom, Ed.), 1998, pp. 973-996, Lippincott-Raven Publishers, Philadelphia.
3. Wadi SA, Ahmad G: Effects of lead on the male reproductive system in mice. J Toxicol Environ Health, 1999, 56: 513-521.
4. Apostoli P, Kiss P, Stefano P, Bonde JP, Vanhoorne M: Male reproduction toxicity of lead in animals and humans. Occup Environ Med, 1998 55: 364-374.
5. Todd, A. C.; Wetmur, J. G.; Moline, J. M.; Godbold J. H.; Levin, S. M.; Landrigan, P. J.: Unraveling the chronic toxicity of lead: an essential priority for environmental health. Environ Health Perspect, 1996. 104, 141-146.
6. Tchounwou, P. B.; Yedjou, C.G.; Foxx, D.; Ishaque, A.; and Shen, E.: Lead induced cytotoxicity and transcriptional activation of stress genes in human liver carcinoma cells. Mol. Cell. Biochem, 2004, 255, 161-170.
7. Mosmann, T.: Rapid colorimetric assay for cellular growth and survival: applications to proliferation and cytotoxicity assays. J Immunol Methods, 1983, 65 (1-2): 55-63.
8. Bradford MM. A rapid and sensitive method for the quantification of microgram quantities of protein utilizing the principle of protein-dye binding. Anal Biochem, 1976, 72: 248-254.
9. Tchounwou, P.B.; Wilson, B.; Schneider, J. and Ishaque, A.: Cytogenic assessment of arsenic trioxide toxicity in the Mutatox, Ames II and CAT-Tox assays. Metal Ions Biol. Med, 2000, 6, 89-91.
10. Tully, D. B.; Collins, B. J.; Overstreet, J. D.; Smith, C.S.; Dinse, G. E.; Mumtaz, M. M.; Chapin, R. E.: Effects of arsenic, cadmium, chromium and lead on gene expression regulated by a battery of 13 different promoters in recombinant $HepG_2$ cells. Toxicol Appl Pharmacol, 2000, 168, 79-90.
11. Tchounwou, P.B.; Yedjou, C. G. and Dorsey, W. C.: arsenic trioxide induced transcriptional activation and expression of stress genes in human liver carcinoma cells (hepg2). Cellular and Molecular Biology™. 2003, 49 (7), 1071-1079.
12. Sengupta, M.; Bishayi, B.: Effect of lead and arsenic on murine macrophage response. Drug Chem Toxicol, 2002, 25, 459-472.
13. Centers for Disease control (CDC). Fatal pediatric lead poisoning, New Hampshire, 2000. Morb Mort Weekly Rep, 2001, 50(22), 457-459.
14. Esterbaur H., Schaur r. j., and Zoller H.: Chemistry and Biochemistry of 4-Hydroxynonenal, Malonaldehyde and related Aldehydes; Free Rad. Biol. Med. 1991, 11: 81-128.
15. Mazhoudi, S.; Chaoui, A.; Ghorbal, M.H.; and El Ferjani, E.: Response of antioxidative enzymes to excess copper in tomato (*Lycopersicm esculentum*, Mill). Plant Sci, 1997, 127, 129-137.
16. Gonick, H. C.; Ding, Y.; Bondy, S. C.; Ni, Z.; Vaziri, N. D.: Lead-induced hypertension: interplay of nitric oxide and reactive oxygen species. Hypertension, 1997, 30, 1487-1492.
17. Ding, Y.; Vaziri, N. D.; Gonick HC.: Lead-induced hypertension, II: response to sequential infusions of L-arginine, superoxide dismutase, and nitroprusside. Environ Res, 1998, 76, 107-113.
18. Prasad, K.V.S.K.; Paradha Saradhi, P. & Sharmila, P.: Concerted action of antioxidant enzymes and curtailed growth under zinc toxicity in *Brassica juncea*. Environ. Exp. Botany, 1999, 42, 1-10.
19. Clijsters, A.; Cuypers, A.; and Vangronsveld, J.: Physiological responses to heavy metals in higher plants. Defence against oxidative stress. Z. Naturforsch, 1999, 54c, 730-734.
20. Stroinski, A.; and Kozlowska, M.: Cadmium-induced oxidative stress in potato tuber. Acta Soc. Bot. Po, 1997, 66, 189-195.

ACKNOWLEDGEMENTS

This research was financially supported by a grant from the National Institutes of Health (Grant No. 1G12RR13459), through the RCMI-Center for Environmental Health at Jackson State University. The authors thank Dr. Abdul Mohamed, dean of College of Science, Engineering and Technology, for his technical support of this research.

Metal Ions in Biology and Medicine: vol. 9. Eds Maria Carmen Alpoim, Paula Vasconcellos Morais, Maria Amélia Santos, Armando J. Cristóvão, José A. Centeno, Philippe Collery.
John Libbey Eurotext, Paris © 2006 pp. 298-1.

Oxidative stress in human leukemia (HL-60), human liver carcinoma ($HepG_2$), and human (Jurkat-T) cells exposed to arsenic trioxide

Clement G. Yedjou and Paul B. Tchounwou

Molecular Toxicology Research Laboratory, NIH-Center for Environmental Health, College of Science, Engineering and Technology, Jackson State University, 1400 Lynch Street, P.O. Box 18540, Jackson, Mississippi, USA.

ABSTRACT

Recent studies have shown that arsenic trioxide (ATO) can induce a clinical remission in patients with acute promyelocytic leukemia. However, the molecular mechanisms of action remain to be elucidated. In this research, we performed the MTT assay to evaluate the cytotoxic effects of ATO to HL-60 cells and to compare their relative sensitivity to that of $HepG_2$, and Jurkat T cells. We also performed the thiobarbituric acid test to determine the levels of malondialdehyde (MDA) plus 4-hydroxy-2 (E)-nonenal (4-HAE) production in these three cell lines following exposure to ATO. The result of MTT assay clearly demonstrated that ATO has a significant cytotoxic effect on HL-60, Jurkat, and $HepG_2$ cells; showing 24 hrs LD_{50} values of 6.4 ± 0.6 µg/mL, 15 ± 3.84 µg/mL, and 23.2 ± 6.03 µg/mL, respectively. These data indicated that HL-60 cells are about twice as sensitive to arsenic toxicity compared to Jurkat T cells and about 3 times more sensitive to arsenic trioxide compared to $HepG_2$ cells. The result of the thiobarbituric acid test demonstrated that arsenic trioxide treatment resulted in a significant increase ($p < 0.05$) of MDA and HAE production, indicating that oxidative stress plays a key role in arsenic induced toxicity and cell injury. MDA and HAE levels were significantly higher in ATO-treated HL-60 cells, indicating that these cells appear to be more sensitive to oxidative stress than $HepG_2$ and Jurkat-T cells. In summary, these results indicate that the pharmacology of ATO as an effective anti-cancer drug is associated with its cytotoxic effects in human promyelocytic leukemic cells. This cytotoxicity is found to be mediated by oxidative stress, a biomarker of cellular injury.

INTRODUCTION

Arsenic trixiode has been shown to inhibit both proliferation and viability when tested against a panel of lymphoma cell lines (1), and arsenicals have activity *in vitro* against myeloma cell lines and primary myeloma cells (2). Recently, arsenic trioxide (Trisenox) has been used as an anticancer agent in the treatment of acute promyelocytic leukemia. One of the major mechanisms by which arsenic exerts its toxic effect is through impairment of cellular respiration by the inhibition of various mitochondrial enzymes, and the uncoupling of oxidative phosphorylation. In addition, arsenic toxicity results from its ability to interact with sulphydryl groups of proteins and enzymes, and to substitute phosphorous group in a variety of biochemical reactions (3).

Although arsenic trioxide (ATO) has cytotoxic effects on several cancer cells, its molecular mechanisms of action remain to be elucidated. Hence, the aim of the present study was to assess the relative sensitivity of HL-60, Jurkat, and $HepG_2$ cells to ATO toxicity and to assess the role of oxidative stress in ATO-induced cytotoxicity.

MATERIALS AND METHODS

Chemicals and Test Media

Arsenic trioxide (As_2O_3), CASRN 1327-53-3, MW 197.84, with an active ingredient of 100% (w/v) arsenic in 10% nitric acid was purchased from Fisher Scientific in Houston, Texas. Growth medium RMPI 1640 containing 1 mmol/L L-glutamine was purchased from Gibco BRL products (Grand Island, NY). Ninety six- well plates were purchased from Costar (Cambridge, MA). Fetal bovine serum (FBS), antibiotics (penicillin G and streptomycin), phosphate buffered saline (PBS), and MTT assay kit were obtained from Sigma Chemical Company (St. Louis, MO).

Tissue Culture

In the laboratory, cells were stored in the liquid nitrogen until use. They were thawed by gentle agitation of their containers (vials) for 2 minutes in a bath at 37°C. After thawing, the content of each vial of cell was transferred to a 25 cm^2 tissue culture flask, diluted with up to 10 mL of RMPI 1640 (HL-60 and Jurkat T-cells) or DMEM ($HepG_2$ cells) containing 1 mmol/L L-glutamine (GIBCO/BRL, Gaithersburg, MD) and supplemented with 10% (v/v) fetal bovine serum (FBS), 1% (w/v) penicillin/streptomycin. The 25 cm^2 culture flasks (2×10^6 viable cells) were observed under the microscope, following by incubation in a humidified 5% CO_2 incubator at 37°C. Three times a week, they were diluted to maintain under the same conditions at a density of 5×10^5/mL and harvested in the exponential phase of growth. The cell viability was assessed by the trypan blue exclusion test (Life Technologies) and manually counted using a hemocytometer.

Cytotoxicity/MTT Assay

Human leukemia HL-60 cells and human Jurkat-T cells were maintained in RMPI 1640. Human liver carcinoma ($HepG_2$) cells were maintained in DMEM. Both RPMI 1640 and DMEM containing 1 mmol/L L-glutamine were supplemented with 10% (v/v) fetal bovine serum (FBS), 1% (w/v) penicillin/streptomycin, and incubated at 37°C in humidified 5% CO_2 incubator. To 180 µL aliquots in six replicates of the cell suspension (5×10^5/mL) seeded to 96 well polystyrene tissue culture plates, 20 µL aliquots of ATO solutions (1.25, 2.5, 5, 10, 20, and 40µg/mL) were added to each well using distilled water as solvent. Cells incubated in culture medium alone served as a control for cell viability (untreated wells). All chemical exposures were carried out in 96 well tissue culture plates for the purpose of chemical dilutions. Cells were placed in the humidified 5% CO_2 incubator for 24 hrs at 37°C. After incubation, 20 µL aliquots of MTT solution (5 mg/mL in PBS) were added to each well and re-incubated for 4 hours at 37°C following by low centrifugation at 800 rpm for 5 min for HL-60 and Jurkat-T cells. Then, the 200 µL of supernatant culture medium were carefully aspirated and 200 µL aliquots of dimethylsulfoxide (DMSO) were added to each well to dissolve the formazan crystals, following by incubation for 10 minutes to dissolve air bubbles. The culture plate was placed on a Biotex Model micro-plate reader and the absorbance was measured at 550 nm. The amount of color produced is directly proportional to the number of viable cell. All assays were performed in six replicates for each dose. Cell viability rate was calculated as the percentage of MTT absorption as follows: *% survival = (mean experimental absorbance/mean control absorbance×100).*

Assay of Lipid Peroxidation

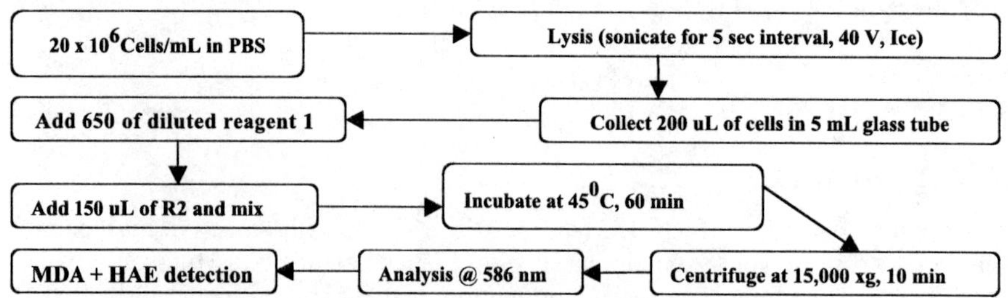

Fig. 1. Schematic representation of the steps in Lipid Peroxidation assay

Statistical Analysis

Data were presented as means ± SDs. Statistical analysis was done using one way analysis of variance (ANOVA) for multiple samples and Student's t-test for comparing paired sample sets. *P*-values less than 0.05 were considered statistically significant. The percentages of cell viability, and MDA plus HAE levels were presented graphically in the form of histograms, using Microsoft Excel computer program.

RESULTS

Cytotoxicity/MTT Assay

Data presented in *(fig. 2)* clearly demonstrate that arsenic trioxide has a significant cytotoxic effect on HL-60, Jurkat, and $HepG_2$ cells. LD_{50} values of 6.4 ± 0.57 μg/mL, 15 ± 3.84 μg/mL, and 23.2 ± 6.03 μg/mL were computed for HL-60, Jurkat, and $HepG_2$ cells, respectively. These data indicate that HL-60 cells are about twice as sensitive to ATO compared to Jurkat T-cells and about 3 times more sensitive to ATO compared to $HepG_2$ cells *(fig. 2, 3)*. Taken together, our results demonstrated a strong dose-response relationship with regard to ATO cytotoxicity. At low doses of exposure, arsenic trioxide produces a slight increase in cell viability. On the other hand, it produces a non-linear gradual decrease in cell viability at higher doses.

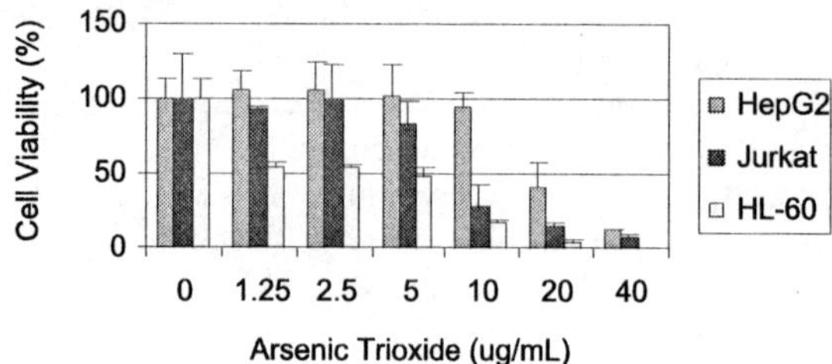

Fig. 2. Cytotoxicity of ATO to $HepG_2$, Jurkat, and HL-60 cells.

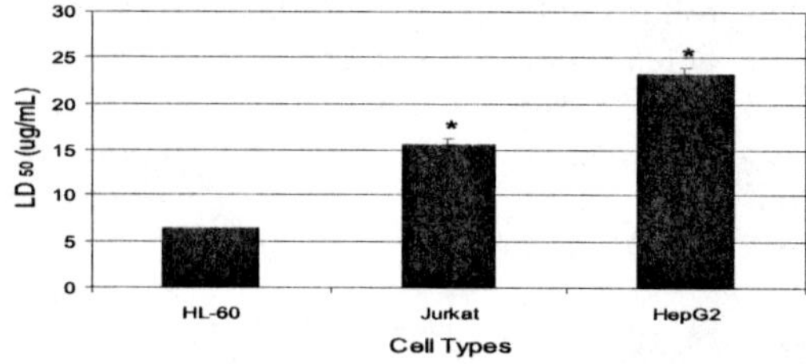

Fig. 3. Mean values of 24 h-LD_{50} of ATO to HL-60, Jurkat, and HepG2 cells.

Lipid Peroxidation Assay

The standard curve generated from lipid peroxidation assay is presented in *(fig. 4)*, and the effect of arsenic trioxide on lipid peroxidation is presented in *(fig. 5)*. Results of this assay indicated an elevated production of MDA plus HAE in ATO-treated cells compared to the control cells. At low doses of exposure, the release of MDA plus HAE was higher in HL-60 cells compared to Jurkat and HepG2 cells, indicating that HL-60 cells are more sensitive to ATO than other cell lines.

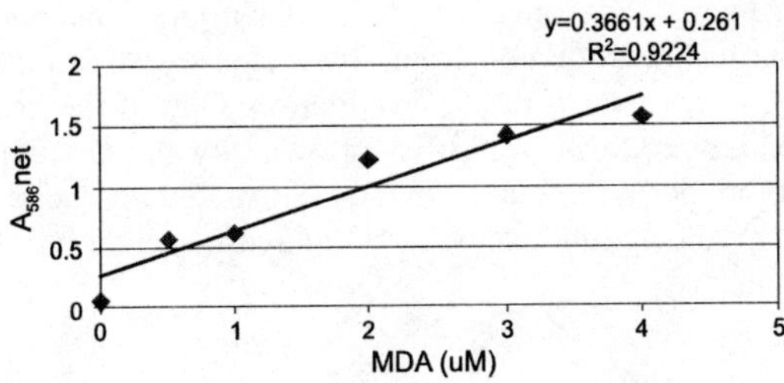

Fig. 4. MDA standard curve showing the net absorbance at 586 nm as a function of MDA concentration.

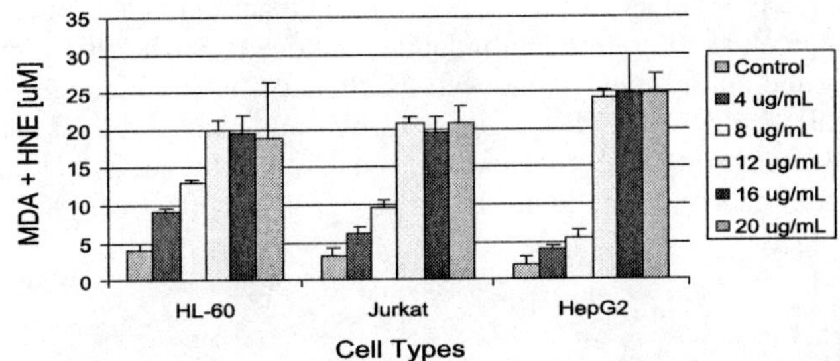

Fig. 5. Effects of different concentrations of ATO on MDA plus HAE production in HL-60, Jurkat, and $HepG_2$ cells.

DISCUSSION

Cytotoxicity/MTT Assay

Cytotoxicity can be defined as the cell killing property of a chemical compound independent from the mechanism of death. We examined the cytotoxic effect of arsenic trioxide (ATO) on the HL-60, Jurkat, and $HepG_2$ cells. Findings from our study clearly showed that ATO is highly cytotoxic to these three cell lines. Several studies have addressed the cytotoxicity of arsenic to various cells. A study has shown that when using 0.5 to 1 μM/L of ATO, apoptosis was induced in the monocytic cells line NB_4 (4). Cytotoxicity studies of two multiple myeloma (MM) derived cell lines, RPMI 8226 and U266, found that 1.0 μM/L ATO inhibited cell proliferation resulting in a weak degree of apoptosis induction, and 2.0 μM/L ATO- induced cell apoptosis. These results showed that ATO exerts apoptosis inducing and growth-inhibiting effects on MM derived cells (5). Recently, we reported that ATO is cytotoxic to human liver carcinoma ($HepG_2$) cells, showing a LD_{50} of 8.55 ± 0.58 μg/mL after 48 hrs of exposure (6, 7). Findings from other studies suggest that low doses of arsenic are effective in APL and show considerable promise in preclinical models of other tumor types (8). Taken together, these results indicated that HL-60 cells are more sensitive to ATO than $HepG_2$ cells and many other cell lines.

Lipid Peroxidation Assay

Because heavy metals such as arsenic are powerful catalysts of lipid peroxidation processes (9), the induction of lipid peroxidation in arsenic trioxide -treated cells was determined by estimating the levels of malondialdehyde (MDA) plus 4-hydroxy-2 (E)-nonenal (4-HAE). Our results demonstrated that ATO treatment resulted in a significant increase ($p < 0.05$) of MDA plus HAE, indicating that oxidative stress plays an important role in arsenic induced toxicity and cell injury.

These studies suggest that the pharmacology of ATO as an effective anti-cancer drug is associated with its cytotoxic effects in human promyelocytic leukemic cells, which is found to be mediated through oxidative stress, a biomarker of cellular injury. Damage to cell organelles produced by lipid peroxidation has been demonstrated by many investigations. However, there is not a firm evidence about the mechanism of lipid peroxidation. One of the primary effects of ATO in the cell is induction of oxidative stress, which is followed by the development of apoptosis (10, 11). The metal-induced lipid peroxidation is mostly attributed to increased production of free radicals (9, 12). Our results indicate that excess ATO increased oxidative stress, as is evident from increased lipid peroxidation.

CONCLUSIONS

Arsenic trioxide exerts a potent cytotoxic effect on human leukemia (HL-60) cells and other cell lines by inhibiting cell proliferation and inducing cell death. Such effects have been observed in cultured cell lines and animal models, as well as clinical studies. Findings from these studies indicate that the pharmacology of ATO as an effective anti-cancer drug is associated with its cytotoxic effects in human promyelocytic leukemic cells. This cytotoxicity is found to be mediated by oxidative stress, a biomarker of cellular injury.

REFERENCES

1. Zhang K, Ohnishi K, Shigeno K, Fujisawa S, Naito K, Nakamura S, Takeshita K, Takeshita A, Ohno R.: The induction of apoptosis and cell cycle arrest by arsenic trioxide in lymphoid neoplasms. Leukemia (Baltimore), 1998, 12: 1383-1391.
2. Rousselot P, Labaume S, Marolleau J. P., Larghero J, Noguera M. K., Brouet J. C., Fermand J. P.: Arsenic trioxide and melarsoprol induce apoptosis in plasma cell lines and in plasma cells from myeloma patients. Cancer Res. 1999, 59: 1041-1048.
3. Li J. H. and Rossman T.C.: Inhibition of DNA ligase activity by arsenite: A possible mechanism of its comutagenesis. Mol. Toxicol., 1989, 2: 1-9.
4. Chen C-S., and Siegel D. M.: Arsenical keratosis. eMedicine J. 2001, 2 (6).
5. Jai P., Chen G., Huang X., Cai X., Yang J., Wang L., Zhou Y., Shen Y., Zhou L., Yu Y., Chen S., Zhang X., Wang Z.: Arsenic trioxide induces multiple myeloma cell apoptosis via disruption of mitochondrial transmembrane potentials and activation of caspace-3. Chin. Med. J. (Engl), 1999 (114), 19-24.
6. Tchounwou P. B., Wilson B. A., Abdelgnani A. A., Ishaque A. B., Patlolla A. K.: Differential cytotoxicity and gene expression in human liver carcinoma (HepG2) cells exposed to arsenic trioxide and monosodium acid methanearsonate (MSMA). Int J Mol Sci. 2002, 3: 1117-1132.
7. Tchounwou P. B., Yedjou C. G., and Dorsey W. C.: Arsenic trioxide induced transcriptional activation and expression of stress genes in human liver carcinoma cells (HepG2). Cellular and Molecular Biology™ 2003, 49 (7), 1071-1079.
8. Soignet S. L., Frankel S. R., Douer D., Tallman M. S., Kantarjian H., Calleja E., Stone R. M., Kalaycio M., Scheinberg D. A., Steinherz P., Sievers E. L., Coutré S., Dahlberg S., Ellison R., Warrell R. P. Jr.: United States multicenter study of arsenic trioxide in relapsed acute promyelocytic leukemia, J. Clin. Oncol. 2001, 19: 3852-3860.
9. Halliwell, B. and Gutteridge, J.M.C.: Oxygen toxicity, oxygen radicals, transition metals and disease. Biochem. J, 1984, 219: 1-14.

10. Smith K. R., Klei L.R., and Barchowsky A.: Arsenite stimulates plasma membrane NADPH oxidase in vascular endothelial cells. Am J Physiol Lung Cell Mol Physiol 2001, 280: L442-9.
11. Martindale JL and Holbrook NJ.: Cellular response to oxidative stress: signaling for suicide and survival. J Cell Physiol, 2002, 192:1-15.
12. Aust S.D., Marehouse L.A., and Thomas C. E.: Role of metals in oxygen radical reactions. J. Free Radic. Biol. Med, 1985, 1: 3-25.

ACKNOWLEDGEMENTS

This research was financially supported by a grant from the National Institutes of Health (Grant No. 1G12RR13459), through the RCMI-Center for Environmental Health at Jackson State University. The authors thank Dr. Abdul Mohamed; Dean of College of Science, Engineering and Technology, for his technical support in this research.

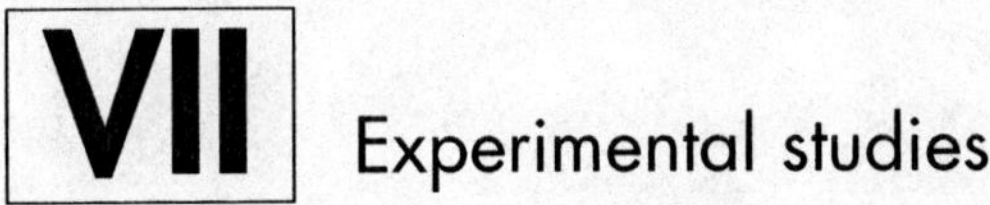

VII Experimental studies

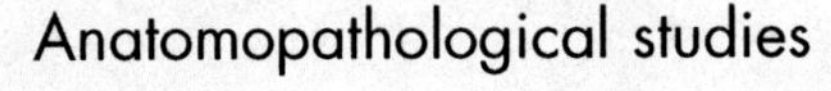

Anatomopathological studies

Metal Ions in Biology and Medicine: vol. 9. Eds Maria Carmen Alpoim, Paula Vasconcellos Morais, Maria Amélia Santos, Armando J. Cristóvão, José A. Centeno, Philippe Collery.
John Libbey Eurotext, Paris © 2006 pp. 309-1.

The effect of iron-gluconate on the carp liver: histological and morphometrical studies

Gordana Gregorović, Nada Kralj-Klobučar, Mirjana Kalafatić, Gordana Lacković

University of Zagreb, Faculty of Sciences, Department of Zoology, Rooseveltov trg 6, 10000 Zagreb, Croatia

The aim of this study was to monitor iron accumulation in carp (*Cyprinus carpio* L.) liver under conditions of chronic exposure to low waterborne iron concentrations. Carp were held for 70 days in aquaria with constant iron concentration (1 mg/L) in the form of iron-gluconate. Perl's reaction was used to detect iron in the liver tissue. Iron depositions were analyzed by light microscope and thereafter also by image analyser (LUCIA G 4.81) by which the surface of iron depositions were measured. Iron started to accumulate in the liver tissue on the 14th day of treatment and was located in the sinusoidal endothelium as mildly diffuse reaction. Much less was found in the cytoplasm of hepatocytes in the form of grain and diffuse reaction. Following the 35th day of treatment iron was also accumulated in macrophages. Continued treatment increased the quantity of iron depositions in liver tissue. The results indicate that long-term exposure of carp to low iron concentrations of iron-gluconate causes significant accumulation ($p<0,05$) of this metal in the carp liver.

INTRODUCTION

Iron is a metal of vital importance for many organisms because it is involved in a plethora of metabolic processes. It is an integral part of proteins, in the first place of haemoglobin and myoglobin, where it participates in oxygen binding and transport. It is also a part of cytochromes which enable the processes of cell respiration, enzymes which participates in the synthesis of DNA, RNA and catalases, peroxidases and dehydrogenases (succinate dehydrogenase, mitochondrial NADH dehydrogenase).

Although iron is an essential element, its metabolism in fish is poorly described. The latest researches [1] have shown that iron metabolism in fish is similar to the metabolism in other vertebrates, although fish are unique among the other vertebrates because of having two routes of metal acquisition, from the diet and from the water. In the water at neutral pH iron is in ferric (Fe^{3+}) form [2]. Prior to import into the gut or branchial epithelia of fish, ferric iron is reduced to ferrous iron (Fe^{2+}) via ferric reductase [3]. Ferrous iron than enters the epithelial cell by protein, divalent metal transporter (DMT). The export of Fe^{2+} form the epithelial cell to the blood is mediated by another protein, iron regulator transporter, termed ferroportin [4]. Ferroportin is located on the basolateral membrane of the epithelial cell [5]. The export of iron from the cell by that transporter depends on the presence of a hephaestin; a membrane bound copper containing oxidase [6]. Hephaestin oxidases Fe^{2+} to Fe^{3+} which bind to transferrin in the blood [7]. In this form iron is transported to liver and other tissues. The liver is the major iron storage where it can be stored in hepatocytes and/or reticuloendothelial cells.

Although essential for life, increased accumulation of tissue iron has been associated with toxicity. The mechanisms by which excess iron exerts its toxic effects include formation of free radicals that damage DNA, RNA, proteins, sugars, organelle and cell membrane lipids [8] that can result in cell injury or death. The extent of toxicity will be dictated by the terms of exposure, metal concentration, its biochemical form and by the localisation of the iron in the tissue.

Iron distribution in the liver can be demonstrated by the histochemical and morphometrical methods. The aim of this study was to monitor iron accumulation in liver tissue under conditions of long term exposure of fish to maximum allowed waterborne iron in the form of iron-gluconate and to determine whether that long term exposure influences histological changes of liver tissue. To evaluate this changes computerised image analysis was applied.

MATERIAL AND METHODS

Experimental animals were carp approximately 15 cm long, kept in aquaria with aerated waterworks water at room temperature. They were divided into two groups: a control group of 16 carp and experimental group of 108 carp treated with iron in the concentration of 1 mg l^{-1} added in the form of iron-gluconate. The water was changed daily (with addition of a certain quantity of iron-gluconate). Liver tissue samples of the control and treated animals were taken immediately after sacrifice, every day during first four days of treatment, and after that in intervals of two, three, four or seven days until the final 70th day of treatment. Immediately after dissection, the tissue was fixed in 10% formaldehyde, dehydrated and embedded in paraplast. Tissue blocks were cut by microtome into 6 µm thick sections. The sections were used for histochemical proof of iron by Perls' reaction [9]. The method includes incubation of deparaffined sections in a mixture of 4% potassium ferrocyanide and 4% hydrochloric acid for 90 min (3×30 min) at room temperature. After the Perls' reaction the accumulated iron appears as blue depositions. Some sections were counterstained with nuclear fast red. Iron depositions in the liver tissue were analyzed by light microscope Nikon Eclipse E600, and thereafter also by image analyser (LUCIA G 4.81) by which the surface of iron depositions were measured. Statistical elaboration of the results was made by computer programme STATISTICA 5.0. Variation analysis and Duncan test were used to assess statistical significance. Differences were considered significant at $p = 0.05$.

RESULTS

In the carp liver of the control group, Perls' reaction showed no iron deposits. In the experimental group the first visible reaction indicating presence of iron in the tissue was found on the 14th day of treatment and was located in the sinusoidal endothelium as weak diffuse reaction *(fig. 1)*. Much less iron was also found in the cytoplasm of the hepatocytes in the form of grain and diffuse reaction. On the 14th day of treatment, the measured surface of Perls' positive depositions, which mark the accumulated iron, were 69, 9 µm^2 *(fig. 5)*. One week later (21st day) all samples were negative. On the 28th day of the treatment half of the samples were also negative, while the other half had more iron in the tissue in comparison to the 14th day. On the 28th day the surface of Perls' positive structures were almost eleven times larger in relation to the value measured two weeks earlier *(table 1, fig. 5)*. Following the 35th day of treatment iron was also accumulated in macrophages *(fig. 3)*. Diffuse reaction in the sinusoidal endothelium was stronger compared to the previous days of treatment. On the 35th day iron was found in all of the samples. Therefore, the measured area was larger compared to the day 28 *(table 1, fig. 5)*. Further treatment, up to the 56th day, led to the continuous enlargement of the Pearl-positive deposits *(table 1, fig. 5)*. After the 56th day, the level of iron in the tissue rapidly increased. On the 61st day of treatment the amount of iron deposits was double compared to the day 56th *(table 1, fig. 5)*. A strong diffuse reaction was present in the sinusoidal endothelium *(fig. 2)* as well as in gall capillaries. A stronger reaction was also found in hepatocytes. Grains were larger in number and size and more intensive in colour. The reaction in macrophages was also significantly stronger compared to the previous days of testing *(fig. 4)*. High value of the measured areas remain after the 61st day, and continue to increase very slowly until the last day of treatment (day 70) *(table 1, fig. 5)*. The results showed that after the treatment with iron-gluconate the surface of Pearl-positive depositions has increased almost 10,000 times compared to the control one.

The statistical significance of differences between control and experimental group was made with the test of variation analysis. The test showed that the value p is significantly lower from 0.05 (p = 8, 41526E-09) which indicates that the differences in surfaces of iron depositions between particular days of sampling are statistically important. In order to determine which days during the treatment particularly differ in relation to one another, a "post-hock" testing was done.

The results of the Duncan test show that the surfaces of iron depositions measured in samples analyzed on the 56th, 61st, 66th and 70th day are significantly larger than the surfaces measured on 14th and 21st day of treatment.

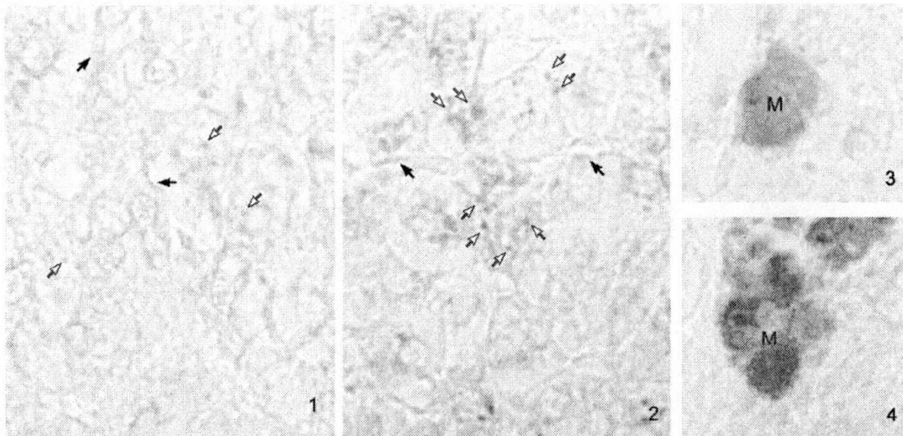

Fig. 1-4. Carp liver sections stained with Perl's reaction. × 1000. Fig. 1. On the 14th day of treatment iron was located in the sinusoidal endothelium as weak diffuse reaction (black arrows) and much less in the cytoplasm of hepatocytes in the form of grains (white arrows). Fig. 2. On the 61st day of treatment there is more iron depositions in the liver tissue. Diffuse reaction in the sinusoidal endothelium is stronger (black arrows) in comparison to the 14th day. In the hepatocytes cytoplasm there are more grain depositions (white arrows) which are bigger and more intensively coloured. Fig. 3. Diffuse reaction in the macrophage (M) on the 35th day of treatment. Fig. 4. On the 61st day of treatment diffuse reaction in the macrophage (M) is much stronger compared to the previous days.

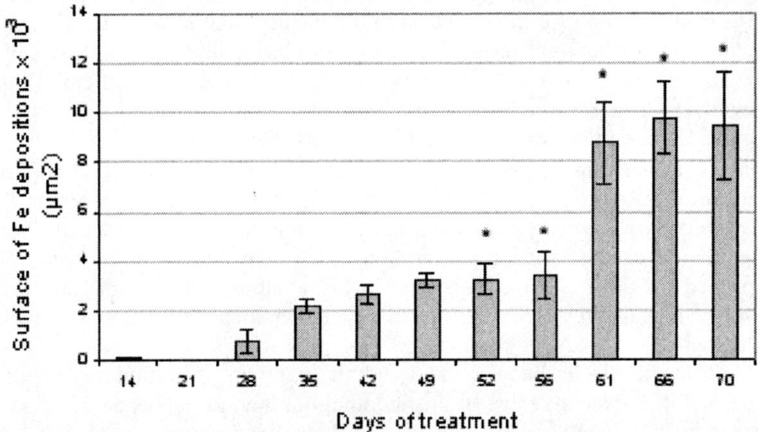

Fig. 5. Average values of Perls' positive surfaces during exposure to iron-gluconate. Four samples per day were analysed. Asterisks indicated statistically significant differences ($p<0.05$; analysis of variance, post-hoc Duncan test). Error bars are also showed.

Table 1. Mean value of the measured areas of iron deposited in liver tissue in iron-gluconate treatment.

Days of treatment	Surface of Fe depositions/μm^2
Control	0
1-14	0
14	69,8929
21	0
28	762,0411
35	2190,7099
42	2671,5474
49	3238,5130
52	3247,1919
56	3415,8339
61	8763,9370
66	9762,8655
70	9490,1313

DISCUSSION

Many researches showed that iron accumulation in the liver tissue depends on iron concentration, exposure period, its source, sort of salt and animal species.

Accumulated iron can be distributed in two basic histologic patterns that differ in their pathogenic implications and pathologic consequences.

Younes and associates [10] showed that repeated treatment of rats with i.p. injections with iron-dextran led to an accumulation of iron in Kupffer cells while no iron could be detected in hepatocytes, endothelium or macrophages. Their results also showed that in animals fed on diet containing 3, 5% iron-fumarate for three weeks, iron deposits were located mainly in hepatocytes, Kupffer cells and to a lesser extent in macrophages. Similar results were archived by Wang and associates [11]. They found iron deposits in hepatocytes and occasional Kupffer cells after feeding rats on a diet with 2%-2, 5% carbonyl iron for 23 weeks. The same results described Stal et al. [12] in rats received diets with 2, 5% carbonyl iron for 6-9 weeks.

Observations of iron exposure on fish liver are rare. There are very few studies that have assessed the accumulation of iron by fish from the water. Our research assesses the effect of waterborne iron-gluconate exposure on liver iron accumulation in carp during extended contamination. Our histological analysis of the preparation has shown that at the moment, when iron in tissue can be proved for the first time, it is located in the sinusoidal endothelium and much less in the cytoplasm of hepatocytes. The same results were obtained by histological examination of Schwartz and associates [13]. After the treatment of pigs with a low level of iron (0,5 g Fe/kg b. w.), it was found primarily in the sinusoidal endothelium, and in minimum quantities in hepatocytes. The fact that iron deposits more in the endothelium than in the hepatocytes was confirmed by the research done by Caperna and associates [14]. In their research, a day old piglets were injected intramusculary with iron-dextran (50 mg Fe/kg b. w.). After their 2nd, 6th and 11th day iron deposits in hepatocytes and sinusoidal cells (Kupffer and endothelial) were measured. The results showed an increase in the concentration of iron in hepatocytes, endothelial cells and Kupffer cells by 5, 62 and 54 times more than in the control group. Higher concentration of iron in endothelial cells and Kupffer cells were also found on the 6th and 11th day.

Our results showed that the further treatment increased the value of iron in sinusoid endothelium. Ultrastructural changes of sinusoid endothelium which can result from the direct toxic effect of the deposited iron or increased production of free radicals were studied by Basset and associates [16]. Their research showed that the acute exposure to colloidal iron caused changes in the endothelial cells, Kupffer cells and stellate cells, which were not visible under a light microscope. Transmission electron microscope showed activated Kupffer and stellate cells, while endothelial cells were defenestrated and thinned.

All these findings suggest that iron may be taken up by liver endothelium first and than transported to parenchymal cells. In addition to these findings, researches by Kishimoto and Tavassoli [15] can be quoted. They show that iron-transferrin complex first binds to the luminal surface of sinusoidal endothelium but not to Kupffer cells or hepatocytes.

Our results also showed that apart from hepatocytes, iron was significantly accumulated in macrophages and that the amount of iron in the tissue was increased with the length of treatment. The increase of iron quantity in tissues corresponding to the length of treatment is confirmed by morphometric measuring, which have shown that the surfaces of iron deposition increase until the end of treatment (70th day), when an increase of almost 10 000 times was recorded in comparison to the control. Similar results were obtained by Rodriques and Pereira [17]. After intraperitoneal injection with iron-dextran (10 mg/ml) in sea bass, values of iron concentration in liver were 15-fold higher than control values. Rainbow trouth on high-Fe diet (175 mg Fe/kg food) also increased iron accumulation in the liver. Conversely, these fish on low-Fe diet for 8 weeks did not show tissue iron depletion [18].

Conclusively, our results indicate that long-term exposure of carp to even low waterborne iron concentrations of iron-gluconate causes significant accumulation of this metal in the carp liver.

REFERENCES

1. Bury NR, Walker PA, Glover CN. Nutritive metal uptake in teleost fish. *J. Exp. Biol.* 2003; 206: 11-23.
2. Asien P, Enns C, Wessling-Resnick M. (2001). Chemistry and biology of eukaryotic iron metabolism. *Int. J. Biochem. Cell Biol.* 2001; 33: 940-959.
3. Bury N, Grosell M. Iron acquisition by teleost fish. *Comp. Biochem. Physiol.* 2003; 135**C**: 97-105.
4. Donovan A, Brownlie A, Zhou Y, Shepard J, Pratt SJ, Moynihan J, Paw BH, Drejer A, Barut B, Zapata A, Law TC, Brugnara C, Kingsley PD, Palis J, Fleming MD, Andrews NC, Zon LI. Positional cloning of zebrafish ferroportin1 identifies a conserved vertebrate iron exporter. *Nature* 2000; 403: 776-781.
5. McKie AT, Marciani P, Rolfs A, Brennan K, Wehr K, Barrow D, Miret S, Bomford A, Peters TJ, Farzaneh F, Hediger MA, Hentze MW, Simpson RJ. A novel duodenal iron-regulated transporter, IREG1, impicated in basolateral transfer of iron to the circulation. *Mol. Cell* 2000; 5: 299-309.
6. Vulpe CD, Kuo YM, Murphy TL, Cowley L, Askwith C, Libina N, Gitschier J, Anderson GJ. Hephaestin, a ceruloplasmin homologue implicated in intestinal iron transport, is defective in the sla mouse. *Nature Genet.* 1999; 21: 195-199.
7. Ford MJ. (2001). Molecular evolution of transferrin: Evidence for positive selection in salmonids. *Mol. Biolol. Evol.* 2001; 18: 639-647.
8. Stal P. Iron as a hepatotoxin. *Dig. Dis.* 1995; 13: 205-222.
9. Pearse AGE. Histochemistry: Theoretical and Applied. Edinburgh and London: Churchill Livingstone, 1972, 1518.
10. Younes M, Eberhardt I, Lemoine R. Effect of iron overload on spontaneous and xenobiotic-induced lipid peroxidation *in vivo.* J. Appl. Toxicol. 1989; 9: 103-108.
11. Wang GS, Eriksson LC, Xia L, Olsson J, Stal P. Dietary iron overload inhibits carbon tetrachloride-induced promotion in chemical hepatocarcinogenesis: effects on cell proliferation, apoptosis, and antioxidation. *J. Hepatol.* 1999; 30: 689-698.
12. Stal P, Johansson I, Ingelman-Sundberg M, Hagen K, Hultcrantz R. Hepatotoxicity induced by iron overload and alcohol. *J. Hepatol* 1996; 25: 538-546.

13. Schwartz KA, Fisher J, Adams ET. Morphologic investigations of the Guinea pig model of iron overload. Toxicol. Pathol. 1993; 21: 311-320.
14. Caperna TJ, Failla ML, Steele NC, Richards MP. Accumulation and metabolism of iron-dextran by hepatocytes, Kupffer cells and endothelial cells in the neonatal pig liver. Journal of Nutrition 1987; 117: 312-320.
15. Kishimoto T, Tavassoli M (1987) Transendothelial transport (transcytosis) of iron-transferrin complex in the rat liver. Am. J. Anat. 1987; 178: 241-249.
16. Bassett ML, Dahlstorm JE, Taylor MC, Koina ME, Maxwell L, Francais D, Jain S, McLean AJ. Ultrastructural changes in hepatic sinusoidal cells acutely exposed to colloidal iron. Exp. Toxicol. Pathol. 2003; 55: 11-16.
17. Rodriques PNS, Pereira FA. A model for acute iron overload in sea bass (*Dicentrarchus labrax* L.). *Lab. Animal.* 2004; 38: 418-424.
18. Carriquiriborde P, Handy RD, Davies SJ. Physiological modulation of iron metabolism in rainbow trout *(Oncorhynchus mykiss)* fed low and high iron diets. *J. Exp. Biol.* 2004; 207: 75-86.

Metal Ions in Biology and Medicine: vol. 9. Eds Maria Carmen Alpoim, Paula Vasconcellos Morais, Maria Amélia Santos, Armando J. Cristóvão, José A. Centeno, Philippe Collery.
John Libbey Eurotext, Paris © 2006 pp. 315-1.

An *in vivo* Study on the Effects of Hexavalent Chromium Contaminated Drinking Water on Rat Livers

A.I. Rafael[1], A. Almeida[2], I. Parreira[3], P. Santos[2], A.M. Cabrita[1], and M.C. Alpoim[3]

[1]*Faculdade de Medicina da Universidade de Coimbra, Portugal*
[2]*Centro de Histocompatibilidade do Centro HUC, Coimbra, Portugal*
[3]*Departamento de Bioquímica da FCTUniversidade de Coimbra, Portugal*

SUMMARY

In industrial areas chromium compounds are widespread in soil, sediments and ground-water, mostly as result of hazardous disposal practices. In the case of aquatic systems the contamination with chromium is chiefly resulting from chromium contaminated industrial and domestic waste-water effluents. It is known that the valence state of chromium depends on the pH and the redox potential and, thus, in an aquifer under high oxidative conditions and neutral pH the hexavalent chromium [Cr(VI)] species predominates.

Epidemiological animal studies have established that Cr(VI) compounds are toxic, and carcinogenic and, in spite of the protective mechanisms, long term exposures to particulate Cr(VI) compounds if often related to an increased risk of respiratory tract cancer in humans.

Although some authors claim that Cr(VI) compounds also injure the gastrointestinal system this issue is object of debate. The controversy around the theme incited us to carried out a study on which human exposure to highly Cr(VI)-contaminated drinking water was mimicked by exposing along 8 weeks male Wistar rats (6) to Cr(VI)-contaminated water (Cr(VI) concentration 20 ppm). The purpose of this study was to evaluate the possible health effects resulting from ingestion of an highly Cr(VI)-contaminated drinking water. To this end the liver of Cr(VI)-exposed rats and control rats was subject to a careful microscopic and histological examination, and the expression of genes related to apoptosis (caspases 3 and 8, and Tp53) as well as of Tgf-β was assessed by RT-PCR on the liver of both control rats and Cr(VI)-exposed rats. The increased expression of all the genes related to apoptosis and of Tgf-β and the concomitant observed alterations on cell and tissue morphology, decreased cell size, inflammatory infiltration, and fibrosis following Cr(VI) ingestion do, in fact, suggest that ingestion of water contaminated with high levels of Cr(VI) caused liver injury, and that there is an ongoing growth/repair process mediated by the growth factor Tgf-β

INTRODUCTION

Some Cr(VI) compounds are recognized occupational human lung carcinogens through chronic inhalation (1). Some studies also revealed that 4 out of 5 chrome plating workers exposed to chromium trioxide exhibited severe liver damage, and Cr(VI) exposure has been strongly associated with several other adverse health effects (2). However, there are also numerous other studies revealing the inconsistency of the widespread toxic and carcinogenic effects of hexavalent chromium compounds towards humans occupationally exposed (3).

Orally ingested Cr(VI) is considered not genotoxic, at doses that overwhelm the drinking water standards for chromium, thus supporting the lack of carcinogenicity of Cr(VI) by the oral route observed in some studies. In a study with adult volunteers given a 10 mg single dose of Cr(VI) in water, demonstrated that 99.7% of the ingested Cr(VI) was reduced to Cr(III) within the upper intestinal tract. No adverse health effects were also observed in rats fed 25 ppm Cr(VI) for 1 year (4) or 134 ppm Cr(VI) for 6 months (5). However, this data is not supported by other data available using both animal and human volunteers and thus the intense debate around the theme (2).

The findings that in some industrial areas the Cr(VI) concentration in the aquifers greatly overwhelms the maximum recommended by EPA (the current US EPA maximum chromium water level is 50 µg $Cr.dm^{-3}$), and the controversy of thresholds in carcinogenesis, particularly in the case of genotoxic carcinogens like Cr(VI) (3), lead us to carried out a study on which human exposure to highly Cr(VI)-contaminated drinking water was mimicked by exposing along 8 weeks male Wistar rats (6) to highly Cr(VI)- contaminated water (Cr(VI) concentration 20 ppm). The purpose of this study was to evaluate the possible hepatotoxicity resulting from a continuous ingestion of a highly Cr(VI)-contaminated water. To this end the liver of Cr(VI)-exposed rats and control rats was subject to a careful microscopic and histological examination, and the expression of genes related to apoptosis (caspases 3 and 8, and Tp53) and Tgf-β was assessed by RT-PCR on the liver of both control rats and Cr(VI)-exposed rats.

MATERIAL AND METHODS

12 male Wistar rats, 4 months old at the beginning of the experimental study, and weighing around 500 g each were used. The animals were separated in 2 groups, one group was exposed to 20 ppm Cr(VI)-contaminated drinking water for 8 weeks, while the other group, control, was given Cr(VI)-uncontaminated drinking water along the same period of time. All the procedures were in accordance with the Guiding Principles in the Use of Animals in Toxicology expressed in Portuguese and EEC law.

Animals were weighed before the sacrifice. Livers were removed after the sacrifice, weighed, and samples were taken for microscopic and histological examination. The remaining liver was stored in RNA later for the gene expression studies.

The histological study of livers was carried out using several dying techniques, H&E, PAS, Masson trichromium, and the biomarker caspase 3.

RT-PCR was used to evaluate gene expression. To this end total liver lysates were processed according to the protocol from *RNeasy® Mini Kit* for Isolation of Total RNA extraction from animal tissues (Qiagen). 1 µg total RNA was reverse transcribed to cDNA using 1.25 U/µl of MuLV RT - TaqMan® Gold RT-PCR kit (Applied Biosytems) and were stored at -20°C. Relative quantification of gene expression by real-time PCR was performed using Assays-on-Demand™ Gene Expression (Applied Biosystems, Foster City, USA): 20X Mixture of primers and probes TaqMan® MGB (FAM) for caspase 3 (Casp3), caspase 8 (Casp8), Tp53 and Tgf-β were used together with TaqMan® Universal PCR Master Mix, No Amperase UNG (Applied Biosystems) and Pre-Developed TaqMan Assay Reagent 20X 18SrRNA (Applied Biosystems) as endogenous control.

RESULTS

Macroscopic evaluation of the livers of Cr(VI)-exposed animals showed no significant alteration with exception of increased weight relative to the weight of the control group. The histological study of the livers revealed alterations on cell and tissue morphology, decreased cell size, inflammatory infiltration, and fibrosis, carbohydrates were not present.

Relative quantification of gene expression in liver tissue from rats exposed to Cr(VI) was performed using the $\mathbf{2^{-\Delta\Delta Ct}}$ **method**, where $\Delta\Delta Ct = (C_{T,target} - C_{T,reference})$ sample - $(C_{T,target} - C_{T,reference})$

control group; the target represents the target gene of interest (Casp3, Casp8, Tp53 or Tgf-β) and the reference represents a housekeeping gene (18SrRNA), The sample represents the liver tissue from rats exposed to Cr(VI) and the control represents the tissue from control group rats.

Quantification of gene expression by real-time PCR revealed moderate upregulation of Casp3, Casp8 and Tp53 in liver tissue from Cr(VI) treated animals; whereas Tgf-β exhibited a large variation comparatively to the control group *(fig. 1)*.

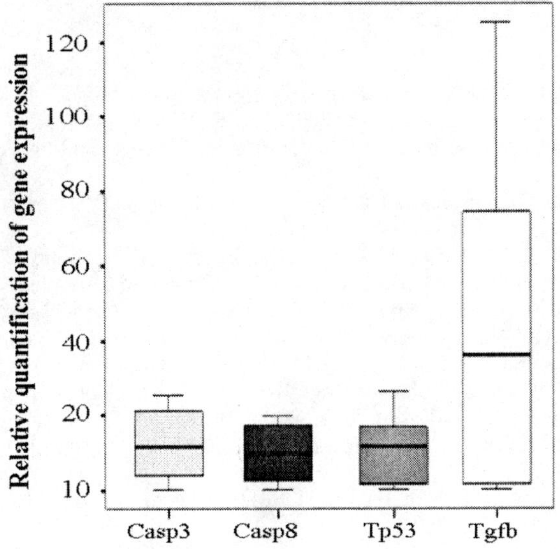

Fig. 1. Relative quantification of Casp3, Casp8, Tp53 and Tgf-β cDNA in liver tissue from rats exposed to Cr(VI), using $2^{-\Delta\Delta Ct}$ method on real-time PCR.

DISCUSSION

The activation of Casp3 and Casp8, over expressed 16 times more in rats exposed to Cr(VI) than in the control ones, suggest that following exposure to high doses of Cr(VI) there is an ongoing apoptotic process in the liver of Cr(VI)-exposed animals. Moreover, the large over expression observed for Tgf-β, a growth factor whose active transcripts are normally absent in a normal liver, might be a strong indicator of apoptosis/growth undergoing process in response to hepatotoxic injury caused by Cr(VI). In fact, it is known that in a healthy liver hepatocytes rarely divide. However, following chemical or physical injury hepatocytes progress from the G0 phase to the G1 phase of the cell cycle. Growth factors regulate this process through both stimulatory and inhibitory signaling. Tgf-β controls hepatocyte growth presumably through an autocrine feedback mechanism (6). After partial hepatectomy the active Tgf-β controls hepatocyte growth either by cell cycle arrest or apoptosis. Previous studies have demonstrated that active Tgf-β induces cell cycle arrest (7) in the G1 phase or alternatively, controls epithelial cell growth, specifically hepatocytes, by inducing apoptosis (6), while the latent Tgf-β is a potent stimulus for hepatic fibrogenesis (8). Data obtained with recent studies carried out with rats also confirmed that following liver injury Tgf-β regulates hepatocytes proliferation mostly by apoptosis mediated by Casp3 and 8 (6). The increased expression of all the genes related to apoptosis and of Tgf-β, and the concomitant observed alterations on cell and tissue morphology, decreased cell size, inflammatory infiltration, and fibrosis following Cr(VI) ingestion do, in fact, suggest that ingestion of water contaminated with high levels of Cr(VI) caused liver damage and that there is an ongoing growth/repair process involving the growth factor Tgf-β.

CONCLUSION

This study suggests that Tgf-β may have important hepatic growth regulatory functions following a Cr(VI)-induced hepatic injury. Apoptosis, via caspase activation, appears to be the mechanism of hepatocyte growth/repair control, and activation of Tgf-β may be an important regulatory step in hepatocyte growth/repair control.

REFERENCES

1. O'Brien T, Ceryak S, Patierno SR Complexities of chromium carcinogenesis: role of cellular response, repair and recovery mechanisms. *Mutat Res* 2003; 533: 3-36.
2. Costa M. Toxicity and carcinogenicity of Cr(VI) in animal models and humans. *Critical Rev Toxicol* 1997; 27: 431-442.
3. De Flora, S. Threshold Mechanisms and site specificity in chromium(VI) carcinogenesis. *Carcinogenesis* 2000; 21: 533-541.
4. MacKenzie RD, Byernum RU, Decker C, Hoppert CA, Langham FF. Chronic toxicity studies: Hexavalent and trivalent chromium administered in drinking water. *Am Med Assoc Arch Ind Health* 1958; 18: 232-234.
5. Borneff J, Engelhardt K, Grien W, Kunte H, Reichert J. Kanzerogene substanzen in wasser und boden. Mausetrankwersach mit 3,4-benzpyren unt kaliumchromat. *Arch Hygiene Bakteriol* 1968; 152: 45-53.
6. Schrum LW, Bird MA, Salcher O, Burchardt E-R, Grisham JW, Brenner DA, Rippe RA, Behrns KE. Autocrine expression of activated transforming growth factor-b 1 induces apoptosis in normal rat liver. *Am J Physiol Gastrointest Liver Physiol* 2001; 280: 139-148.
7. Alexandrow M, Moses H. Transforming growth factor Band cell cycle regulation. *Cancer Res* 1995; 55: 1452-1457.
8. Brenner D, Rippe R, Rhodes K, Trotter T, Breindl M. Fibrogenesis and type I collagen gene regulation. *J Lab Clin Med* 1994; 124: 755-760.

Distribution

Metal Ions in Biology and Medicine: vol. 9. Eds Maria Carmen Alpoim, Paula Vasconcellos Morais, Maria Amélia Santos, Armando J. Cristóvão, José A. Centeno, Philippe Collery.
John Libbey Eurotext, Paris © 2006 pp. 321-1.

Concentrations of As, Cd, Hg and Pb in fish and shellfish: intake by the population of Catalonia, Spain

Falcó G[1], Bocio A[2], Llobet JM[1,2], Domingo JL[2],*

[1]*Toxicology Unit, School of Pharmacy, University of Barcelona, Barcelona, Spain*
[2]*Laboratory of Toxicology and Environmental Health, School of Medicine, "Rovira i Virgili" University, Reus, Spain. *joseluis.domingo@urv.net*

INTRODUCTION

For most people, diet is the main route of exposure to metals. Fish and seafood is one of the food groups with a highest contribution to dietary intake of metals. Recently, in a study performed in Catalonia (Spain) we found that among 11 analyzed food groups, fish and seafood showed the highest concentrations of arsenic (As), cadmium (Cd), mercury (Hg) and lead (Pb) [1]. These results were in accordance with previously reported data from a number of investigations carried out in various regions and countries [2-7]. With respect to the dietary intake of pollutants, it is important to remark that the European Union has recommended some restrictions for fish and seafood intake, especially for children, pregnant women, and breastfeeding mothers [8], which is mainly based on the potential methylmercury content of this food group.

In Spain, although there are some limits for metal contents in commercial fish and shellfish, the number of species included is rather reduced. Since a preventive point of view, it is important to perform periodic surveys focused on metal contents in fish and seafood. These programs allow to detect health risks for different groups of population and to establish dietary recommendations. The aim of the present study was to determine the levels of As, Cd, Hg and Pb in edible samples of 14 fish and seafood species, which constitute the most consumed by the population of Catalonia. The contribution to the daily intake of these metals through the consumption of fish and seafood was also estimated.

MATERIALS AND METHODS

Sampling

Between March and April 2005, edible fish and seafood was randomly acquired in local fish markets and supermarkets from six cities (Barcelona, Tarragona, Lleida, Hospitalet de Llobregat, Terrassa and Girona) of Catalonia, Spain, which all have an important number of inhabitants (70,000-2,000,000). According to data from the last consume survey published by the Spanish Ministry of Agriculture, Fishery and Nutrition [9], the 14 most consumed species of fish and seafood were included in the study. Samples included six species of blue fish: sardine *(Sardine pilchardus)*, tuna *(Thunnus thynnus)*, anchovy *(Engraulis encrasicholus)*, mackerel *(Scomber scombrus L.)*, swordfish *(Xiphias gladius)* and salmon *(Salmo salar L.)*; three species of white fish: hake *(Merluccius merluccius L.)*, red mullet *(Mullus surmuletus)* and sole *(Solea vulgari)*, and five species of cephalopods and shellfish: cuttlefish *(Sepia esculenta)*, squid *(Loligo vulgaris)*, clam *(Tapes decussatus)*, mussel *(Mytilus galloprovincialis L.)* and shrimp *(Parapenaeus longirostris)*. For analytical purposes, composites were made up by 20 individual samples of each species. A total of 42 samples were analysed for As, Cd, Hg and Pb concentrations.

Analytical methods and instrumentation

About 0.5 g of homogenized samples were pre-digested under pressure with 5 ml of 65% nitric acid (Suprapur, E. Merck, Darmstadt, Germany) in Teflon vessels for 8 h at room temperature. Subsequently, solutions were heated at 85°C for 8 additional hours. On completion of the digestion and after adequate cooling, solutions were filtered and made up to 25 ml with deionised water. Concentrations of As, Cd, Hg and Pb, were determined by inductively coupled plasma-mass spectrometry (ICP-MS, Perkin Elmer Exlan 6000). Rhodium was used as internal standard. The accuracy of the instrumental methods and the analytical procedures was checked by duplication of samples.

Dietary exposure and health risk assessment

The daily intake of As, Cd, Hg and Pb through fish and seafood consumption was calculated by multiplying the respective metal concentration in each species by the weight of that species consumed by an average individual from Catalonia [10]. For calculations, when the metal levels were under their respective detection limits (LOD), the concentration was assumed to be one-half to the detection limits (ND = 1/2 LOD). LOD were the following: As and Hg, 0.05 µg/g, and Cd and Pb, 0.02 µg/g. Calculations for health risk assessment were mainly based on the comparison of As, Cd, Hg and Pb daily intakes by each group of population with the respective provisional tolerable weekly intakes (PTWI).

RESULTS AND DISCUSSION

Table 1 shows the concentrations of As, Cd, Hg and Pb in the 14 species of fish and seafood included in this study. The highest As concentration was found in red mullet, 16.6 µg/g fresh weight. Shrimp and sole showed also remarkable As concentrations, 6.3 and 6.1 µg/g, respectively. Tuna and salmon were the species with the lowest As concentration. The As levels found in sardine and mussel were similar to those found in our previous survey [1], while the current As concentration of hake doubled that previously [1]. For Cd, the highest concentration was found in clam and mussel: 0.14 and 0.13 µg/g fresh weight, respectively. The concentration found in mussels was similar to that previously found, while sardine and hake showed higher Cd levels [1]. The highest concentration of Hg corresponded to swordfish with 1.93 µg/g fresh weight. Hg concentration in mussel did not change in comparison to the previous survey [1]. However, the current levels of sardine and hake increased in relation to that survey [1]. Finally, the highest Pb concentrations were noted in mussel and salmon: 0.15 and 0.10 µg/g fresh weight, respectively. For mussel, Pb concentration did not change in comparison with the previous level [1], while Pb levels in sardine and hake increased significantly.

The average daily intake of As, Cd, Hg and Pb by children (boys and girls), male and female adolescents, male and female adults, and male and female seniors are depicted in *figures 1-4*. The highest As intake corresponded to male seniors, 218 µg/day, whereas the lowest intake of this element corresponded to girls, 111 µg/day. For all groups, the main contributor to As intake was hake, which represented between 23.6% and 60.1% of total As intake through fish consumption. The As intake through sole and shrimp was also notable. For Cd, male seniors were the group with the highest intake, 1.34 µg/day. In contrast, boys showed the lowest Cd intake (0.48 µg/day). For all groups, cuttlefish was the main species responsible for Cd intake, ranking between 4.2% and 35.7% for boys and girls, respectively. Male adults was the group with the highest Hg intake (9.89 µg/day), whereas girls and female seniors, with 5.60 and 5.99 µg/day, were the groups with the lowest Hg intake through fish consumption. The main contributor to these intakes corresponded (in all groups) to tuna, which represented contributions ranking between 25.6% for female seniors to 59.8% for female adolescents. Hake showed also a remarkable contribution to Hg intakes. In turn, male seniors were the group with the highest Pb daily intake through fish consumption (2.48 μg), while the group of girls showed the lowest Pb intake (1.27 μg/day). For all age/sex groups, hake was the species with the highest contribution to the daily intake of Pb, which ranked between 29% for male adolescents and 69.4% for girls.

Table 1. Mean concentrations of As, Cd, Hg and Pb (μg/g wet weight) in fish and seafood.

	As	Cd	Hg	Pb
sardine	3.67	0.01	0.08	0.04
tuna	1.13	0.01	0.48	0.02
anchovy	4.63	0.01	0.08	0.01
mackerel	4.19	0.01	0.09	0.02
swordfish	2.10	0.05	1.93	0.02
salmon	1.90	0.01	0.05	0.10
hake	4.10	0.01	0.19	0.05
red mullet	16.6	0.01	0.23	0.03
sole	6.09	0.01	0.08	0.03
cuttlefish	2.99	0.07	0.02	0.01
squid	4.26	0.05	0.06	0.05
clam	2.23	0.14	0.02	0.06
mussel	2.23	0.13	0.02	0.15
shrimp	6.31	0.02	0.12	0.01

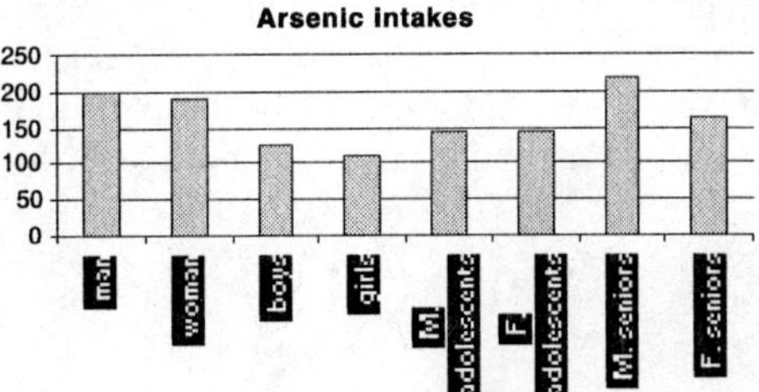

Fig. 1. As intake (μg/day) though fish and seafood for different groups.

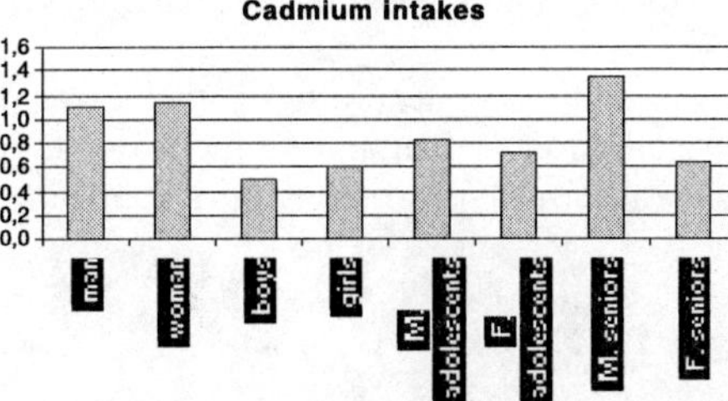

Fig. 2. Cd intake (μg/day) through fish and seafood for different groups.

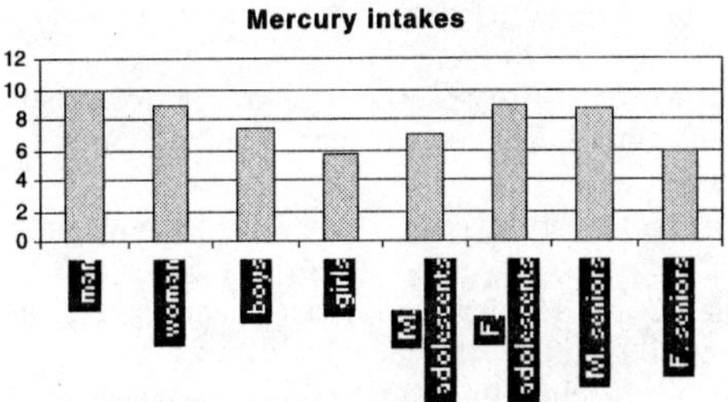

Fig. 3. Hg intake (μg/day) through fish and seafood for different groups.

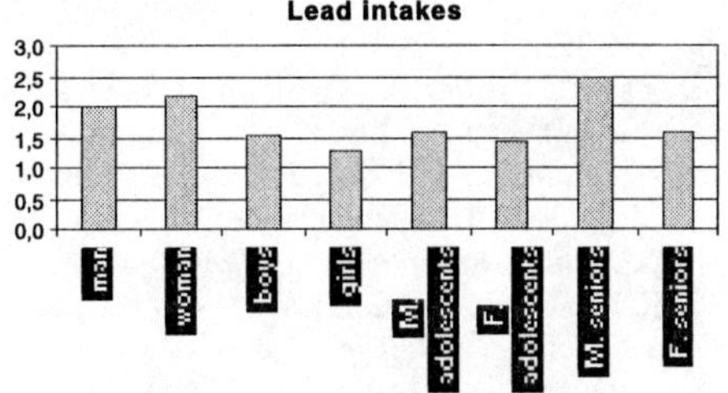

Fig. 4. Pb intake (μg/day) through fish and seafood for different groups.

For the assessment of health risks due the above metal intakes, these have been compared with the current provisional tolerable weekly intakes (PTWI) for As, Cd, Hg and Pb [11]. For inorganic As, the PTWI is 15 μg/kg of body weight/week (or 129 μg/day for a subject of 60 kg). In the present study, all analyses were carried out for total (organic and inorganic) As. However, it is well-known that most As found in fish and shellfish is organic As, which is the less toxic form.

According to the literature, the percentage of inorganic As in fish and shellfish ranked between 0.02 and 11% [6], whereas the maximum acceptable daily intake for As set by the WHO is 3000 µg for a subject of 60 kg. Taking this into account, the intake of inorganic As here estimated would not be of concern for any studied age/sex group. Carcinogenic risk assessment was done according to the slope factor established for As: 1.5 $(mg/kg/day)^{-1}$ [12]. The carcinogenic risk for a male adult during an estimated life of 70 years would be 1.8×10^{-4}. The As intake is similar to that found in our previous survey in Catalonia, 203.3 µg/day [1], and higher than that reported for Chile, 44.7 µg/day [13].

For Cd, the PTWI is 7 µg/kg/week. The intake of Cd represented around 2% of this value in all age/sex groups. The current estimated Cd intake through fish and seafood is lower than that found in our previous survey in Catalonia, 3.33 µg/day [1], and in a recent study in Chile, 9.2 µg/day [13], whereas it is comparable to that reported in Greece, 0.7-1.1 µg/day [14]. For Hg, all intakes were under the PTWI, 5 µg/kg/week. Boys presented the maximum intake, 2.2 µg/kg/week. Assuming the estimation that 90% of Hg in fish and shellfish is as methylmercury [15], intakes for all groups of population would be under the safety limit of 1.6 µg/kg/week (excepting boys, 1.96 µg/kg/week). The current intake of Hg through fish and seafood by the population of Catalonia has no changed since our previous survey, 8.9 µg/day [1]. However, it means a high intake comparing to that recently reported for countries such as Chile, 1.6 µg/day [13]. Finally, the estimated Pb intake was, in all age/sex groups, lower than the PTWI value, 25 µg/kg/week. The maximum intake was found in boys with 0.45 µg/kg/week. The current intake is lower than that of our recent survey, 4.7 µg/day [1], and comparable with that found in Chile, 1.7 µg/day [13]. In a recent survey carried out in Canary Islands (Spain), region with an estimated consumption of fish and seafood comparable to Catalonia, the mean intake of Pb was notably higher (16.8 µg/day) [5], than the current one.

In summary, according to the above, the current intakes of As, Cd, Hg and Pb through the consumption of fish and seafood by the general population of Catalonia, Spain, do not mean, in general terms, specific health risks for the consumers.

REFERENCES

1. Llobet JM, Falcó G, Casas C, Teixidó A, Domingo JL. Concentrations of arsenic, cadmium, mercury, and lead in common foods and estimated daily intake by children, adolescents, adults and seniors of Catalonia, Spain. *J Agric Food Chem* 2003; 51: 838-42.
2. Leblanc JC, Malmauret L, Guérin T, Bordet F, Boursier B, Verger P. Estimation of the dietary intake of pesticide residues, lead, cadmium, arsenic and radionuclides in France. *Food Addit Contam* 2000; 17: 925-32.
3. Ysart G, Millar P, Croasdale M, Crews H, Robb P, Baxter M, de L'Argy C, Harrison N. UK total diet study. Dietary exposures to aluminium, arsenic, cadmium, chromium, copper, lead, mercury, nickel, selenium, tin and zinc. *Food Addit Contam* 2000; 17: 775-86.
4. McIntosh DL, Spenglet JD, Özkaynak H, Tsai LH, Ryan PB. Dietary exposure to selected metals and pesticides. *Environ Health Perspect* 1996; 104: 202-9.
5. Rubio C, González-Iglesias T, Revert C, Reguera JI, Gutiérrez AJ, Hardisson A. Lead dietary intake in a Spanish population (Canary Islands). J Agric Food Chem 2005; 53: 6543-49.
6. Muñoz O, Devesa V, Suñer MA, Velez D, Montoro R, Urieta I, Macho ML, Jalón M. Total and inorganic arsenic in fresh and processed fish products. *J Agric Food Chem* 2000; 48: 4369-76.
7. Bordajandi L, Gomez G, Abad E, Rivera J, Fernández-Bastón M, Blasco J, González M. Survey of persistent organochlorine contaminants (PCBs, PCDD/Fs, and PAHs), and heavy metals (Cu, Cd, Zn, Pb and Hg), and arsenic in food samples from Huelva (Spain): levels and health implications. *J Agric Food Chem* 2004; 52: 992-1001.
8. European Comission Health and Consumer Protection Directorate General. Information note. Methyl mercury in fish and fishery products. Brussels, 2004.
9. Ministerio de Agricultura, Pesca y Alimentación. Secretaria General de Agricultura y Alimentación. Dirección General de Alimentación. La Alimentación en España. Madrid, 2004.

10. Serra Majem L, Ribas L, Salvador G, Castells C, Serra J, Jover L, Treserras R, Farran A, Román B, Raidó B, Taberner JL, Salleras L, Ngo J (2003) Avaluació de l'estat nutricional de la població catalana 2002-2003. Evolució dels hàbits alimentaris i del consum d'aliments i nutrients a Catalunya (1992-2003).
11. FAO/WHO. Evaluation of Certain Food Additives and Contaminants; Technical Report Series 837, World Health Organization: Geneva, Switzerland, 1993.
12. US EPA. Risk based concentration table, January-June 1996. US Environmental Protection Agency Region 3, Philadelphia, PA, USA.
13. Muñoz O, Bastias JM, Araya M, Morales A, Orellana C, Rebolledo R, Velez D. Estimation of the dietary intake of cadmium, lead, mercury and arsenic by the population of Santiago (Chile) using a total diet study. *Food Chem Toxicol* 2005; 43: 1647-55.
14. Karavoltsos S, Sakellari A, Scoullos M. Cadmium exposure of the Greek population. *Bull Environ Contam Toxicol* 2003; 71: 1108-15.
15. Storelli M, Storelli A, Giacominelli-Stuffler R, Marcotrigiano G. Mercury speciation in the muscle of two commercially important fish, hake *(Merluccius merluccius)* and striped mullet *(Mullus barbatus)* from the Mediterranean Sea: estimated weekly intake. *Food Chem* 2005; 89: 295-300.

Metal Ions in Biology and Medicine: vol. 9. Eds Maria Carmen Alpoim, Paula Vasconcellos Morais, Maria Amélia Santos, Armando J. Cristóvão, José A. Centeno, Philippe Collery.
John Libbey Eurotext, Paris © 2006 pp. 326-1.

Measuring lead in bone by non-invasive K-shell X-ray fluorescence and atomic absorption spectrometry: lead distribution, homogeneity, and validation issues

Patrick J. Parsons[1], Katherine M. Hetter[1], Yan Yan Zong[1], David Bellis[1], Frank S. Blaisdell[1], Neeta R. Ginde[2] and Andrew C. Todd[2]

[1]*Wadsworth Center, New York State Department of Health, PO Box 509, Albany, NY, 12201-0509 USA,*
[2]*Department of Community and Preventive Medicine, Mount Sinai School of Medicine, One Gustave L. Levy Place, Box 1057, New York NY, 10029-6574 USA.*

SUMMARY

K-shell X-ray fluorescence (KXRF) has been used for many years for non-invasive *in vivo* measurements of bone lead (Pb) levels in human-subject studies. Typically, the tibia is the most commonly selected bone site for human measurements, but calcaneus and patella have also been measured. In this study, a number of long bones from Pb-dosed animals were analyzed for Pb, using both KXRF and electrothermal atomic absorption spectrometry. The principal aims were to examine the distribution of Pb in various bones types, and to assess the validity of KXRF measurements by comparing them to ETAAS measurements that are traceable to certified reference materials. Caprine (goat) bones were removed from Pb-dosed animals *post mortem*, cleaned, defatted, and analyzed for Pb content by ETAAS, using the validated method. Results indicated considerable accumulation of Pb at the epiphyses (joint ends) of the tibia and femur, and enriched levels of Pb in trabecular (spongy) bones such as the patella and calcaneus, when compared to cortical (dense, compact) tibia bone. Considerable Pb heterogeneity was evident from ETAAS analysis of triplicate samples of bone fragments. In follow-up work on Pb-dosed caprine tibiae, Pb was enriched at the tibia surface relative to the tibia core. A comparison between KXRF measurements of bone Pb in the bare tibiae (no overlying tissue) and ETAAS measurements of surface and core materials showed KXRF to be in closer agreement with ETAAS surface bone measurements than with core bone measurements. The ETAAS results are consistent with our previous study of human tibiae; tibia surface lead is greater than tibia core lead. The change in tibia Pb concentration along the bone shaft, as detected by ETAAS, is also reflected in the corresponding KXRF-measured Pb concentrations. These data underline the significance of developing certified bone lead standards for KXRF measurements.

INTRODUCTION

K-shell X-ray fluorescence (KXRF) has been used for many years for *in vivo* measurements of bone lead levels in human-subject studies. The most commonly used KXRF instrumental configuration consists of a ^{109}Cd radioactive spot source coupled with a liquid nitrogen-cooled high-purity germanium detector, arranged with the source in a backscatter geometry. Lead-doped plaster-of-Paris phantoms are typically used to calibrate the KXRF system, and analytical results are typically reported in units of micrograms of Pb *per* gram of bone mineral. Such systems have been used in population-based studies of lead exposure and adverse health effects. Currently, there are around 15 systems located worldwide.

The measurement of lead in bone is attractive because, unlike blood lead, it represents cumulative exposure, thereby including exposures that occurred decades previously. The residence time of lead in bone has been estimated to be on the order of decades, and more recent work has established that residence times differ for differing bone compartments. For example, whereas lead stored in cortical (compact) bone has a residence time of approximately 25 years, lead stored in trabecular (spongy) bone has a residence time that is closer to 15 years. In contrast, blood lead levels reflect exposure only over the past 4-6 weeks. When *in vivo* measurements of bone lead are taken *via* KXRF, the most common bone sites analyzed are the mid-shaft of the tibia, the patella, and the calcaneus. The mass of bone typically sampled using a ^{109}Cd arrangement is approximately 25 - 30 g in the tibia.

The questions of how uniformly Pb is distributed in various long bones and, in particular, how that distribution might affect KXRF bone lead measurements, have been a subject of interest to us recently [1-3].

METHODS AND INSTRUMENTATION

Electrothermal Atomic Absorption Spectrometry (ETAAS)

Bone lead measurements were made using a Perkin-Elmer Model Z5100 atomic absorption spectrometer equipped with an HGA 60 electrothermal atomization unit (*i.e.*, graphite furnace) and a transverse Zeeman background correction system (hereafter this system will be referred to simply as AAS). Animal bone samples (0.2 - 2.0 g) were scraped clean of adhering tissue, washed and defatted, and then digested in ultrapure concentrated nitric acid using microwave-assisted heating in a CEM Model 2100 microwave digestion system (CEM, Matthews NC). The furnace AAS method has been fully validated [4] and has been used in previous studies of lead in human and animal bones [2, 3].

K-Shell X-Ray Fluorescence Spectrometry (KXRF)

Details of the "spot source" KXRF bone lead measurement system [5] used in our studies have been described elsewhere [6]. Briefly, a ^{109}Cd source of approximate activity 960 MBq (26 mCi) was used; detector output pulses were passed to a digital signal processor (Model 2060; Canberra Industries, Meriden, CT) that was operated with a rise time of 2.4 μs; spectra were acquired for 30 min (true time); and the KXRF system was calibrated using lead-doped plaster-of-Paris phantoms that ranged in lead concentration from a nominal blank to 106 μg Pb *per* g plaster (equivalent to 155 μg Pb *per* g bone mineral [7]). The detector/source combination was mounted on a platform that could be moved with millimeter precision in all three spatial dimensions.

Bone samples

In this study, we had access to a number of bone samples of caprine (goat) and bovine (cow) origin. The animals had been previously dosed over many years with lead, administered as lead acetate, as part of another program to produce blood lead pools. These blood lead pools are routinely prepared for distribution to clinical laboratories that participate in the New York State Department of Health's proficiency testing program. As the animals reach the end of their useful working lives, the facility veterinarian recommends euthanasia. Dissection is performed *post mortem,* and the long bones are removed and transported to the Trace Elements Laboratory for ETAAS analysis. Once the overlying tissue has been removed, the bones are cleaned, defatted, and freeze-dried to constant weight. In addition to caprine and bovine bones, we have analyzed a number of human bones that were made available to us through the Mt. Sinai School of Medicine. These bones were the subject of another KXRF study that has been reported previously [2].

In our initial studies of caprine bones, we analyzed selected locations from the femur, tibia, patella, and calcaneus from the left limb. Each bone segment sampled was analyzed for lead in triplicate, by sub-dividing the section into three, smaller samples. In more detailed work, the individual tibia was systematically analyzed for lead using two analytical techniques: (a) non-destructive KXRF analysis of the intact bare bones at 2-cm intervals along the bone shaft, and (b) AAS analysis of the 2-cm tibia cross-sections that were previously analyzed by KXRF. Each 2-cm cross section was removed and then further separated into (i) 1-2 mm thick sections of the tibia surface and (ii) the bone core, using a diamond-disc saw. The proximal epiphyses were sub-divided into three distinct sections: epiphyses, tibia tuberosity, and the condyle region. The distal epiphyses were also sub-divided into three distinct sections: epiphyses, medial malleolus, and the lateral malleolus. No attempt was made to separate the epiphyseal surface from the deeper bone structure. The surface and core fragments, and the epiphyseal segments, were sub-divided into approximately equal portions and were analyzed for Pb in duplicate by AAS.

For validation and quality-control purposes, we analyzed Standard Reference Material (SRM) 1486 Lead in Bone Meal and SRM 1400 Bone Ash, from the National Institute of Standards and Technology (NIST, Gaithersburg, MD).

RESULTS AND DISCUSSION

The analysis of various caprine long bones by AAS showed that Pb is not uniformly distributed along the proximal-distal shaft of bones that comprise the pelvic limb *(fig. 1)*. There appears to be some enrichment of Pb evident at one or more epiphyses, certainly in most animals studied. The data in *figure 1* indicate that for trabecular (spongy) bones, such as the patella and calcaneus, there is a relative enrichment of lead. The large variation in lead concentrations found between sub-samples is reflected by the error bars that indicate the maximum and the minimum values found for each bone segment sampled.

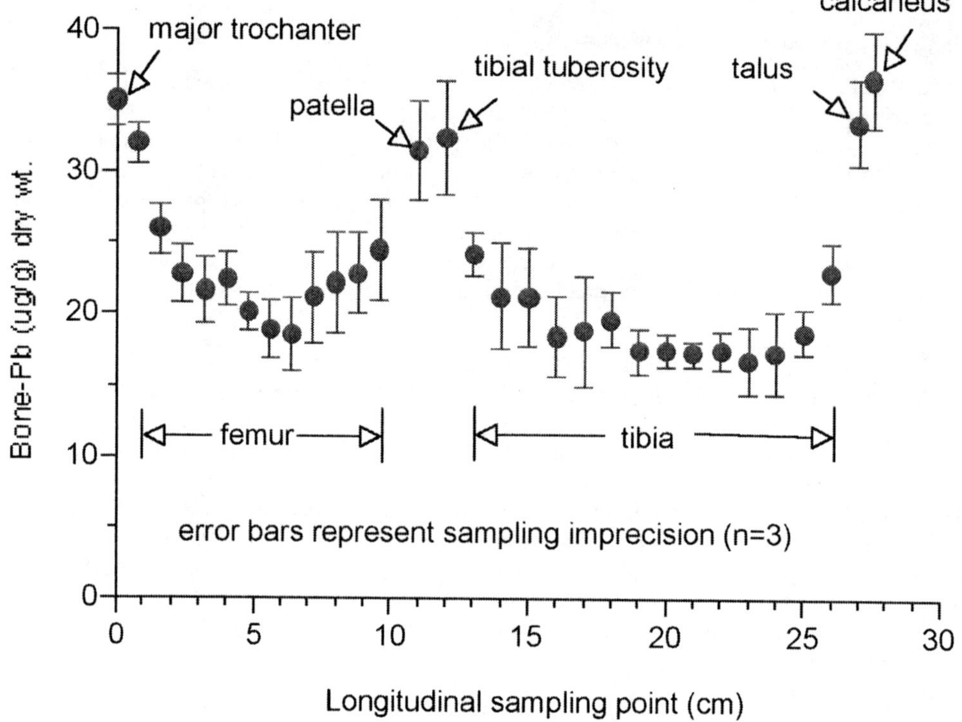

Fig. 1. Distribution of lead as measured by AAS (µg/g, dry weight) along the left pelvic limb of a lead-dosed goat (82-11).

Lead concentrations (AAS) from the duplicates were averaged, and core-surface values were plotted separately as a function of tibia location *(fig. 2)*. The error bars shown for AAS measurements indicate the maximum and minimum found at each site sampled. For the KXRF measurements of bare bones, the error bars denote the standard deviation of the mean Pb value calculated from 5 replicate measurements, in units of µg/g dry weight bone.

It is evident that lead is enriched at the surface of caprine tibia relative to the bone core. Moreover, KXRF measurements more closely match the AAS-measured Pb concentrations of the bone surface than those of the bone core. This is entirely consistent with our findings in human bones reported previously [2]. Variations in AAS-measured lead concentrations within the cross-sectional area of the tibia, as well as along the bone shaft, are evidence of the non-uniform distribution of lead in this bone compartment. The trend along the bone is also reflected in the KXRF-measured Pb data.

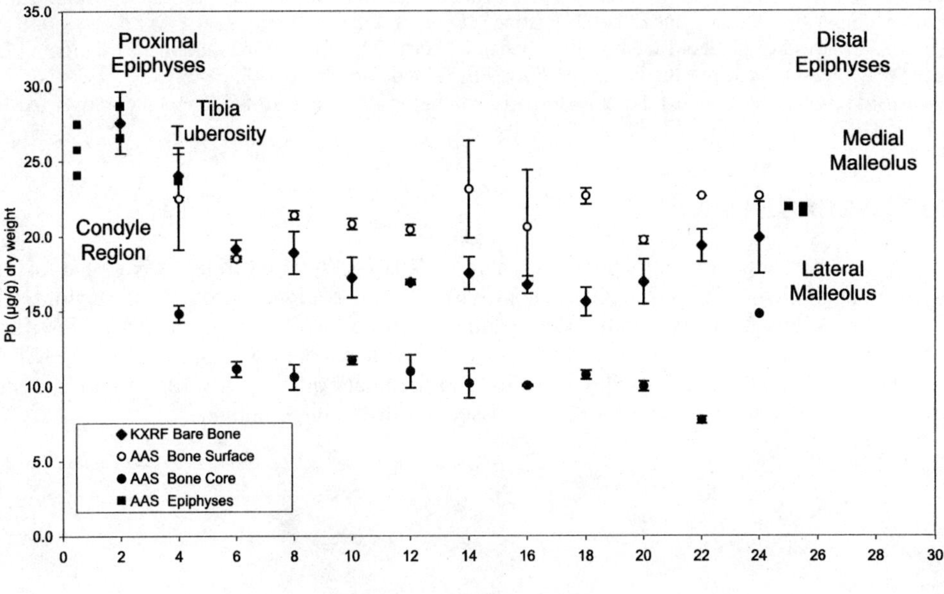

Fig. 2. Distribution of lead within the tibia of a lead-dosed goat (93-12) as measured by (a) AAS (● core and ○ surface) and (b) KXRF (◆ bare-bone) methodologies.

CONCLUSION

Thus far, non-destructive KXRF data obtained from caprine bones, prior to destructive AAS analysis, seem to reflect an enrichment of lead at the epiphyses and an elevated level of lead in the calcaneus. Moreover, KXRF tibia lead concentrations (in µg/g dry wt.) more closely match the AAS concentrations (in µg/g dry wt.) found at the tibia surface than the AAS concentrations in the bone core. Further investigation of the effect of both proximal-distal and surface-core bone lead inhomogeneities on bone lead XRF measurements would be valuable.

REFERENCES

1. Parsons PJ, Zong YY, Matthews MR (1995) Development of bone-lead reference materials for validating in vivo XRF measurements. In: Predecki PK, Bowen DK, Gilfrich JV, Goldsmith CC, Huang TC, Jenkins R, Noyan IC, Smith DK (eds). Advances in X-Ray Analysis. Plenum Press, New York, p. 625-632.
2. Todd AC, Parsons PJ, Tang S, Moshier EL (2001) Individual Variability in Human Tibia Lead Concentration. Environmental Health Perspectives 109:1139-1143.
3. Todd AC, Parsons PJ, Carroll S, Geraghty C, Khan FA, Tang S, Moshier EL (2002) Measurements of lead in human tibiae. A comparison between K-shell x-ray fluorescence and electrothermal atomic absorption spectrometry. Physics In Medicine & Biology 47:673-687.
4. Zong YY, Parsons PJ, Slavin W (1996) Accurate and precise measurements of lead in bone using graphite furnace atomic absorption spectrometry with Zeeman-effect background correction. J Anal At Spectrom 11:25-30.
5. Todd AC, McNeill FE (1993) In vivo measurements of lead in bone using a ^{109}Cd "spot" source Human Body Composition Studies. In: Ellis KJ, Eastman JD (eds). Plenum Press, New York, p. 299-302.
6. Todd AC, Carroll S, Godbold J, Moshier E, Khan F (2001) The effect of measurement location on tibia lead XRF measurement results and uncertainty. Phys. Med Biol. 46:29-40.
7. Todd AC (2000) Coherent scattering and matrix correction in bone-lead measurements. Phys Med Biol 45:1953-1963.

ACKNOWLEDGEMENTS

This project was supported in part by grant number R01 ES12424-02 from the National Institute of Environmental Health Sciences (NIEHS), a division of the National Institutes of Health (NIH). Its contents are solely the responsibility of the authors and do not necessarily represent the official views of the NIEHS, NIH. We thank William Schoonmacher and Kevin Jarvis of the Griffin Laboratory, and Ciaran Geraghty, Steven Smith and members of the Trace Elements Laboratory at the Wadsworth Center for help with gross dissection of the large animals.

Metal Ions in Biology and Medicine: vol. 9. Eds Maria Carmen Alpoim, Paula Vasconcellos Morais, Maria Amélia Santos, Armando J. Cristóvão, José A. Centeno, Philippe Collery.
John Libbey Eurotext, Paris © 2006 pp. 331-1.

Primary Data about accumulation of Rhenium in tumor tissue

Zhabitskaya Elena[1], Tykhomyrov Artem[1], Musichenko Maria[1], Shitelman Zoya[2], Glushkova Lidia[2], Shevtsov Nickolay[2], Blank Avraam[2], Shtemenko Natalia[1], Shtemenko Alexander[3]

[1]*Dnepropetrovsk National University, 13, Naukoviy by-street, 49050, Dnepropetrovsk;*
[2]*Institute for Single Crystals of National Academy of Science of Ukraine; 60, Lenin ave., Kharkov, Ukraine;*
[3]*Ukrainian State Chemical-Technological University, 8, Gagarin avenue, 49005 Dnepropetrovsk, Ukraine*

ABSTRACT

It was previously shown that radioactive isotopes $^{183,\,184}$Re did not accumulate in any body parts of healthy rats and were excreted completely in 24 hours being introduced as potassium perrhenate. In our works cluster Rhenium compounds with organic ligands in liposome forms are investigated as antitumor substances. The main purpose of this paper was to analyze whether Rhenium accumulates in any organ of tumor-bearing rats.The most quantity of Re was found in urine collected during 21 days (100ppm), in tumor (0.5ppm - 2ppm) and in liver (1ppm). Other organs are not characterized by sufficient Re levels compared to control animals. Such a large quantity of Re in malignant tissue may contribute to antitumor activity of cluster Rhenium compounds in the process of chemoprevention.

INTRODUCTION

Early experiments devoted to distribution of Re in animals, discussed in [1-2], showed low toxicity and significant efflux of the investigated substance such as potassium perrhenate. Introduction of the rhenium salt independently from the mode of injection (peritoneally, intravenously) in different doses led to quickly excretion of the injected dose, for example, to urinary excretion of 92% of injected $^{183,\,184}$Re in 24 hours; by 16 days excretion was essentially complete - urine 94% and feces 5%. Later investigation of distribution of ^{188}Re(V)-DMSA in mice [3] supported earlier conclusions about essential excretion of rhenium substances during 1-2 hours after introductions. Some investigations, based on radiotherapeutic properties of rhenium isotopes, used different radioactive rhenium substances with intratumoral injections [4, 5] as accumulation of an antitumor agent in tumor cells is one of the most important property of the drug shown both in preclinical and clinical settings [6]. In these and other works biodistribution of Re depends on structure of used substances, mode of injections, conditions of the experiments, kind of animals and diseases, etc. As we work with cluster rhenium compounds with organic ligands and explore the idea of their own anticancer activity not connected with radioactivity [7], the main purpose of this paper is to analyze whether Rhenium accumulates in any organ of tumor-bearing rats in conditions and during experiments, elaborated by us.

MATERIALS AND METHODS

Cluster rhenium compound with organic ligand with formula:

$[Re_2(i\text{-}C_3H_7CO_2)_4Cl_2]$, where $i\text{-}C_3H_7CO_2R$ = isobutiric, - (Re1), synthesized according to procedure described in [8], have been tested.

Wistar rats weighting 100-120g were experimental animals. Two types of experiments were accomplished: A - acute doze of Re1 (14,4 mg/kg) in liposome form [9] was introduced peritoneally to healthy animals; after 24 hours (A1) and after 48 hours (A2) animals were sacrified under chlorophormium anesthesia. Liver, spleen, kidneys, urine (collected 21 days), erythrocytes, plasma, brain, bones, skin, heart, lungs and thyroid gland were taken for weighting and analysis. B - animals were inoculated by tumor carcinoma Guerin (T8) cells. The cells were taken in the Institute of Oncology and Experimental Pathology by R.E. Kavetskiy (Kiev). The intraperitoneal administration of the Re1 at the dose of 7μM/kg according to the scheme of antioxidant therapy [10] in liposome forms began on the 3 day after the inoculation of the tumor cells and was repeated every 2 days until day 21. On the day all organs described in experiment A and tumors were isolated and weighted. Rhenium content was determined by means of atomic emission spectrometry (spectrograph DFS-8, generator IVS-28) after mineralization of investigated materials.

RESULTS AND DISCUSSION

In all described experiments no observed-adverse-effect (NOAEL) [11] was established. Weight of isolated organs was the same as in control group of animals. That confirms low toxicity of Re1. Data about content of rhenium in different isolated biological material, where Re was detected, are presented in the *table*.

Table. Content of Re (ppm) in biological material.

Biological material	Experiment A1	Experiment A2	Experiment B
liver	1-2	1-2	1-2
spleen	-	-	10
kidneys	10-20	20-30	20
urine	90-100	10-50	10-20
erythrocytes	≤0,5	≤0,5	0,5-1
plasma	-	-	0,5-1
brain	-	-	≤0,5
thyroid glands	-	-	0,5-1
tumor	-	-	0,5-2

It is difficult to discuss or to compare the data obtained as there is no any data about distribution of rhenium carboxylates or rhenium cluster compounds in living organism at all. Accumulation of Re in spleen, kidneys, liver and excretion in essential quantities is not surprising facts as was previously described for a range of metal-organic substances. Accumulation of elements of the VII Periodic group by thyroid glands is described in [12]. Primary results, presented here, show in fact a very important thing - accumulation of Re1 in tumor in detectable amounts. Accumulation of a certain agent, such as cisplatin, for example, depends on two factors: drug uptake and drug efflux. There are some reagents, that enhance cisplatin accumulation (dipyridamole, amphotericine B, cyclosporine), decrease cisplatin efflux and increase cytotoxic activity of cisplatine. The mechanism, by which these substances decrease cisplatin efflux is not fully understood, but may be explained by their ability to increase cell membrane permeability through different ways. The clinical use of cisplatin faces a number of serious problems. Due to its reactive nature, most of the drug is rapidly inactivated by bonding to proteins upon entry in the blood by intravenous administration and never reaches the tumor in an active form [13]. Binding to proteins is considered a major cause of the many dose-limiting toxicities exhibited by cisplatin such as nephro-, oto-, and neurotoxicity [14-15]. One approach to try and circumvent these drawbacks of cisplatin is to encapsulate the drug in liposomes [16]. Preclinical studies showed that compared with the free drug, liposomal formula improved stability, prolonged circulation time, increased antitumor effect, and reduced toxicity [17]. In our experiments: 1. we used Re1 - a substance, which have symmetric structure *(fig.)*.- four hydrophobic isobutiric ligands around cluster fragment - that may enhance transport through membranes analogically to dipyridamole, for example; 2. we used liposomes of Re1, that helped to avoid binding to proteins and to reach tumor.

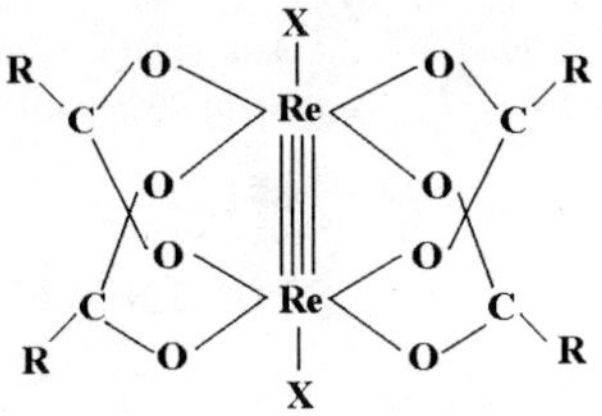

Fig. Structure of Re1. R=tetraisobutiric, X=CL

CONCLUSIONS

Cluster rhénium compound with isobutiric ligands being introduced to tumor-bearing animals in liposomes accumulated in tumor in detectable quantities. Elaborated experimental procedure is promising, requires further investigations and may be effective in anticancer research.

REFERENCES

1. W., Scott K.G., Hamilton J.G. The distribution of radioisotopes of same heavy metals in the rat. *Univ. Calif. Publs Pharmacol.* 1957; 3, N1: 1-34.
2. Oliynik S.A., Shtemenko N.I., Gorchakova N.O., Shtemenko, A.V, et al. *Toxicology of Rhenium substances. Problems of Toxicilogy (Ukrainian).* 2001; N1: 11-15.
3. Dadachova E., Chapman J. ^{188}Re(V)-DMSA revitized. Preparation and biodistribution of a potential radiotherapeutic agent with low kidney uptake. *Nuclear Medicine Communications*, 1998: 19: 173-181.
4. Wang S., Lin W., Chen M., et al. Biodistribution of rhenium-188 Lipiodol infused via the hepatic artery of rats with hepatic tumors. *European Journal of Nuclear Medicine*, 1196: 23: N1: 13-17.
5. Wang S., Lin W., Chen M., et al. Intratumoral Injection of Rhenium-188 Microspheres into an Animal Model of Hepatoma. *The Journal of Niclear Medicine*, 1998: 39: N10: 1752-1757.
6. Fuertes M.A., Alonso C., Perez J.M. Biochemical Modulation of Cisplatin Machanism of Action: Enhancement of Antitumor Activity and Circumvention of Drug Resistance. *Chemical Reviews*: 2002.
7. Collery P., Shtemenko N., Shtemenko A., Bourleaud M., Etienne J.C., Maymard I., Loriquet P. Supplementation by rhenium compounds instead of iron compounds during the treatment by erythropoeitin of anemia in cancer patients. *In: Metal Ions in Biology and Medicine John Libbey Eurotext Paris* 2004; 8: 534-7.
8. Shtemenko A.V., Golichenko A.A., Domasevitch K.V. Synthesis of Novel Tetracarboxylato Dirhenium(III) Compounds and Crystal Structure of them. Z. *Naturforsch* 2002; 56b: 381-5.

9. Shtemenko AV, Shtemenko N.I, Oliynik SA, Zelenuk MA. Lyposome forms of rhenium cluster compounds in models of Haemolytic anemia. *In Metal Ions in Biology and Medicine. Eds. Khassanova LK, Collery P, Maymard I, Khassanova Z, Etienne JC. John Libbey Eurotext, Paris* 2002; 7: 558-61.
10. Meerson F.Z., Evstigneeva M.E., Ustinova E.E. Effect of chronic haemolytic anemia on heart contractile function and increase of its resistance to hipoxia. *Pat. Physiol. and Exp. Therap.(Rus)* 1983; N5: 25-9.
11. Collery P., Domingo J.L., Keppler B.K. Preclinical Toxicology and Tissue Gallium Distribution of a Novel Antitumor Gallium Compound: Tris (8-Quinolinolato) Gallium III. *Anticancer Research*, 1996: 16: 687-692.
12. Baumann E.J., Searle N.Z., Yalow A.A. et al. Behavior of the Thyroid Toward Elements of the Seventh Periodic Group *Amer. J. Physiol.* 1956; 185, N1: 71-76.
13. Howe-Grant M. E., and Lippard S. J. Aqueous platinum(II) chemistry; binding to biological molecules.1980. *In "Metal Ions in Biological Systems"*. 1999; XI: 63-125.
14. Calvet H., Judson I., and van der Vijgh W. J. Platinum complexes in cancer medicine. *Cancer Surv.* 1993; 17: 189-217.
15. Hacker M.P. In "Toxicity of Anticancer Drug". 1991; 82.
16. Newman M.S., Colbern G.T., Working P.K., et al. Comparative pharmacokinetics, tissue distribution, and therapeutic effectiveness of cisplatin encapsulated in long-circulating, pegylated liposomes (SPI-077) in tumor-bearing mice. *Anticancer Research.* 1999; 43: 1-7.
17. Vaage J., Donovan D., Wipff E., et al. Therapy of a xenografted human colonic carcinoma using cisplatine or doxorubicin encapsulated in long-circulating pegylated stealth liposomes. *Int. J. Cancer.* 1999; 80: 134-7.

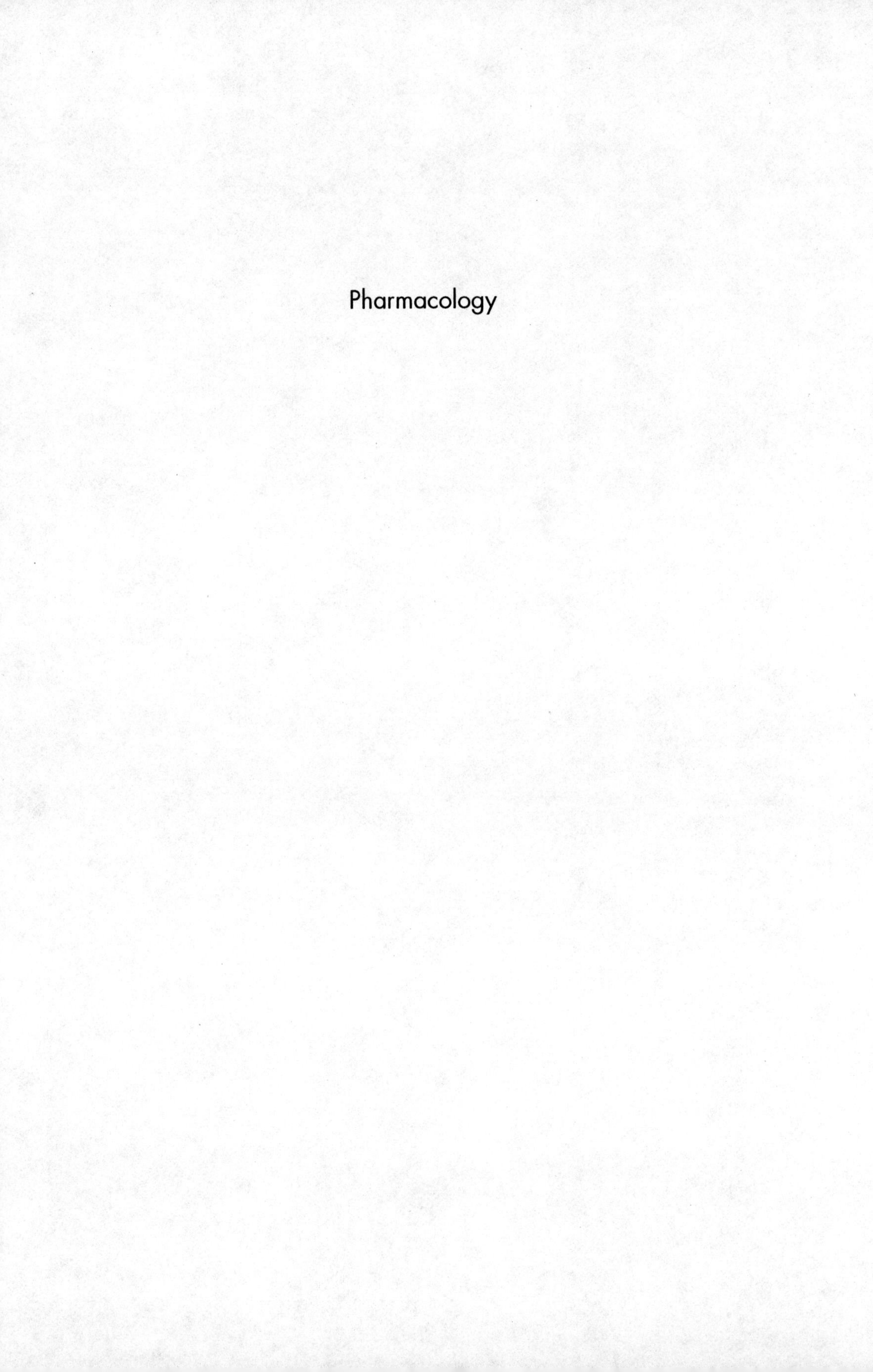

Pharmacology

Metal Ions in Biology and Medicine: vol. 9. Eds Maria Carmen Alpoim, Paula Vasconcellos Morais, Maria Amélia Santos, Armando J. Cristóvão, José A. Centeno, Philippe Collery.
John Libbey Eurotext, Paris © 2006 pp. 337-1.

Zinc concentrations in supplemented mice during perinatal stages

Aguilar AE, Lastra MD, Munguía N, Soriano A, Saldivar L

School of Chemistry, National University of Mexico
Cd Universitaria, Fac Química, UNAM, México DF, México 04510
lastraa@servidor.unam.mx

INTRODUCTION

Growth retardation, immune dysfunctions and cognitive impairment are major effects of zinc deficiency. The effects caused by the lack of zinc during pregnancy are disastrous.

These effects are reversible with zinc supplementation. The biochemical pathways in immune cells that involve zinc as a major actor are not well known, as well as the intracellular zinc concentrations in the immune cells and in various stages and sites of the immune system.

MATERIAL AND METHODS

Experimental Design

BALB/c mice (mice strain in which every member is genetically identical, normally utilized for immunological studies) were divided into groups according to Zn oral supplementation (+Zn, -Zn) (500 mg/L Zn acetate, reagent grade (Zn $(C_2H_3O_2) \bullet 2H_2O$), Mallinckrodt, Mexico) and periods of administration during gestation (1, 2, 3 weeks).

Collection of samples

Maternal venous blood samples and embryos were collected after 1, 2 and 3 weeks of gestation. The splenocytes were deposited into styrene containers and the erythrocytes were eliminated by lysis. Spleen cells were adjusted to 10^9 cells/mL. All samples were transferred to sterile polystyrene tubes. All collection tubes had been checked for possible trace elements contamination in advance of the experiments. Samples were freezed at -70 °C.

Trace element analysis

Suprapur nitric acid 65% (HNO_3, Merck, Darmstadt Germany), hydrogen peroxide 30% (H_2O_2, Merck, Darmstadt Germany), were used. Deionized distilled water (ddw, 18MΩcm) was prepared by Barnstead deionization. Primary standards (1000 mg/L PE PURE, Perkin Elmer) were used to prepare working standard mixtures (in 2% HNO_3).

Samples digestion was performed in a constant temperature equipment (Thermolyne, USA) at 100 °C for 24 h and registered as dry weight. Nitric acid (1 mL) and hydrogen peroxide (2 mL) were added to the samples and filtered 24 h later. Completely clear, colorless, homogenous digests were obtained, and subsequently diluted. Reagent blanks were also prepared. The Zn concentration was obtained by Atomic Absorption Spectrometry. The detection and quantification limits were quantified [1, 2]. In order to validated the method and results we utilized the NIST (Standard Reference Material, 1577b, bovine liver).

Statistical analysis

ANOVA test was performed for statistical analysis. A *p*-value less than 0.05 was considered significant.

RESULTS AND DISCUSSION

Results showed that zinc serum concentrations in treated mice (+Zn) increase throughout gestation with a particularly important elevation in the last gestational week (from 668 µg/L to 1100 µg/L) as compared with the non treated mice (-Zn) *(fig. 1 a, b)*. The increase of zinc in circulation is proportional to the intracellular zinc concentration in splenocytes *(fig. 2 a, b)*. The intracellular zinc concentrations (12 µg/10^9 cells, 28 µg/10^9 cells and 35 µg/10^9 cells, in the weeks 1, 2, and 3 respectively) showed a tendency to gradual increase in +Zn mice while in the -Zn mice, this tendency is towards descent. The splenocytes zinc concentrations became extremely low in the 3rd week of gestation in -Zn dams (7 µg/10^9 cells) which may open an opportunity to infections.

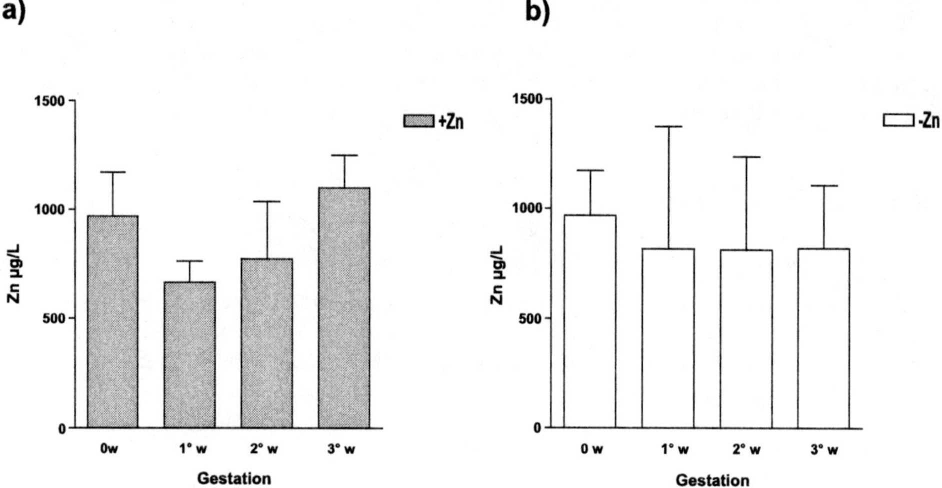

Fig. 1. Zinc serum concentrations

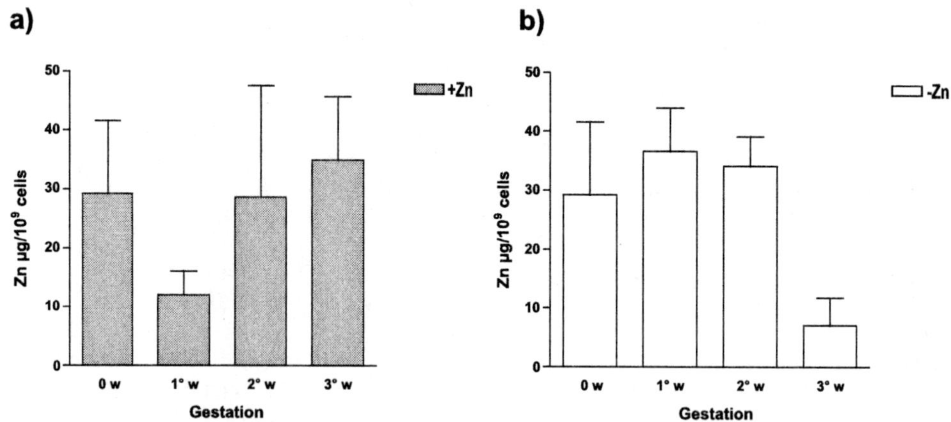

Fig. 2. The intracellular zinc concentration in splenocytes. (b) p<0.05)

The parallel increase of Zn in serum and intracellular Zn, in +Zn dams may result in an elevation of the functional capacities of the immune cells as previously shown by the action of zinc over the production of pro inflammatory cytokines [4].

Murine pregnancy is characterized by transient splenomegaly, whereby immunological changes are not well characterized. The weight of the spleen reaches a peak on day-10 in mice. Thereafter, on day-15 of pregnancy, lymphocyte apoptosis is seen in the spleen indicating the deletion of peripheral sensitized cells. This results in decrease in spleen weight to that of non-pregnant mice [3].

We observed increase in the splenic index (SI) (indicative of cellular immune response *status*) both in +Zn and -Zn pregnant dams in the 1st week of gestation (day-8). The SI became normal in the 2nd week of pregnancy (day-15) with a drop to almost half on the third week of gestation (where the weight augmentation of pregnant dams, has a negative effect on the SI, in addition to the spleen returning to normal weight) *(fig. 3a, b)*.

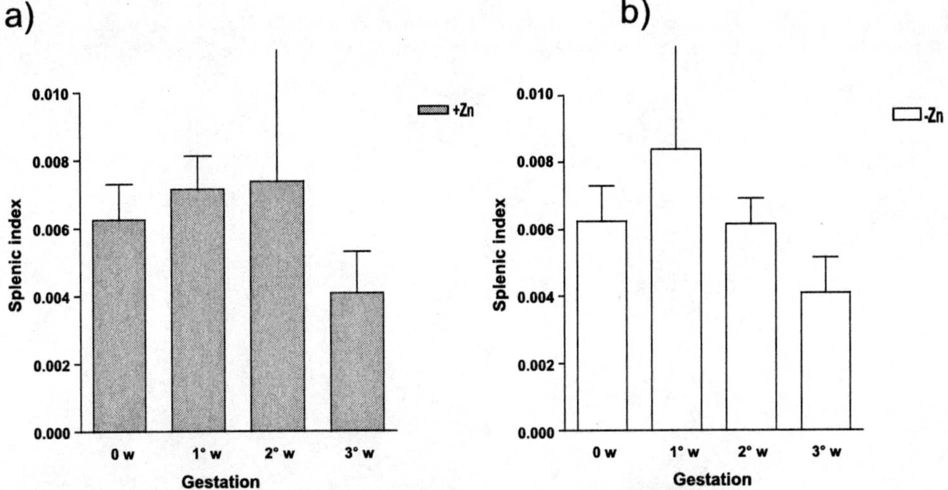

Fig. 3. Splenic index gestation in treated and not treated mice. (a), b) $p<0.05$)

Embryos zinc show a significant increase the 1st week (day-8) in +Zn pregnant dams, with a dramatic drop in the 2nd and 3rd week, probably due to the gestational physiology and the homeostatic characteristics of the placenta *(fig. 4)*.

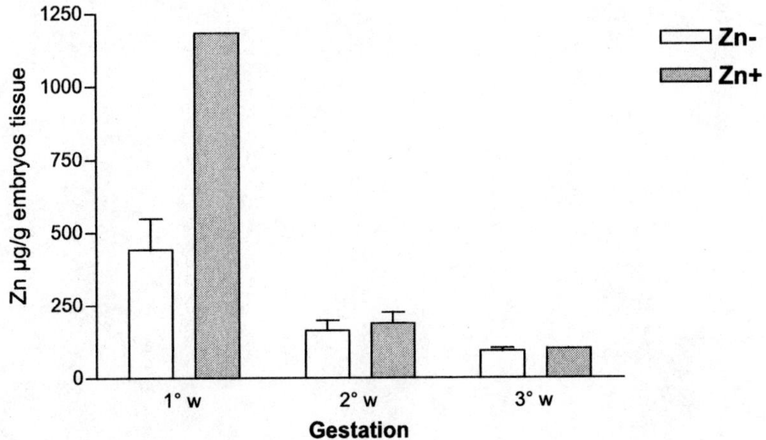

Fig. 4. Embryos tissue concentrations ($p<0.05$)

We conclude that the zinc concentrations in serum as well as in the splenocytes were significantly increased in +Zn pregnant dams which particularly, in the case of zinc deficiencies, might be favorable to the immune response during these periods.

REFERENCES

1. Miller JC y Miller JN. Métodos de calibración en análisis instrumental: regresión y correlación. In: Pearson Educación, ed. *Estadística y Quimiometría para Química Analítica*, 4ª Edición. España: Prentice Hall, 2002: 111-152.
2. Osada H, Watanabe Y, Nishimura Y, Yukawa M, Seki K, Sekiya S. Profile of trace element concentrations in the feto-placental unit in relation to fetal growth. *Acta Obstet Gynecol Scand* 2002; 81: 931-937.
3. Hegde UC, Ranpura S, D'Souza S, Raghavan VP. Immunoregulatory pathways in pregnancy. *Indian J Biochem Biophys* 2001; 38: 207-19.
4. Lastra MD, Aguilar AE, Cabañas M, Hernández R, Humanez K, Pastelín R. IL-1, TNF-alpha and IL-12 secreted by zinc induced murine macrophages in vivo and in vitro. *J Trace Elem Exp Med* 2004; 17: 123-35.

Metal Ions in Biology and Medicine: vol. 9. Eds Maria Carmen Alpoim, Paula Vasconcellos Morais, Maria Amélia Santos, Armando J. Cristóvão, José A. Centeno, Philippe Collery.
John Libbey Eurotext, Paris © 2006 pp. 341-1.

Effect of Depleted Uranium Exposure on Mouse Midbrain Catecholamine Levels

Wayne Briner

Department of Psychology, University of Nebraska at Kearney, Kearney, NE 68849 USA

BACKGROUND: Depleted uranium (DU) has been shown to have a variety of neurocognitive and hormonal effects. Humans demonstrate differences in cognitive testing and serum prolactin levels. Animals demonstrate differences in development, activity levels and responses to novel stimuli. Central nervous system (CNS) lipid oxidation has also been demonstrated. **Aims:** Determine if DU affects the catecholamine synthetic pathway in mice. **Methods:** Mice were exposed to DU acetate at 0, 38, or 75mg/L in drinking water for 2 weeks. At the end of two weeks the animals were tested in an open-field apparatus for 5 minutes, line crossing and rearing behavior were measured. Two days after the initial open-field trial animals were again tested in the open-field. The brains were then quickly removed and the midbrain prepared and the concentrations of tyrosine, norepinephrine, and epinephrine were determined by ion pairing HPLC with UV detection. Lipid oxidation was assayed using the thiobarbituric acid method. **Results:** Behavioral and lipid oxidation of mice reflected previous findings. Significant relationships were found between DU dose and midbrain tyrosine and epinephrine levels. **Conclusion:** These preliminary findings indicate that DU exposure alters the metabolism of catecholamines in the mouse midbrain.

INTRODUCTION

Depleted uranium (DU) is a heavy metal by-product of enriching uranium for nuclear energy or nuclear weapons production. DU is chemically identical to native uranium but is 40% less radioactive than the parent element. The vast majority of DU is used by the military where, because of its pyrophoric properties and high density, it is used in armor and armor penetrating munitions. When used as a penetrator, DU combusts creating a mixture of DU compounds, primarily oxides, which are then deposited around the impact area.

Exposure to DU may occur when handling the weapons or armor, if struck by DU containing shrapnel, inhalation of DU dust, exposure of the skin to DU dust, or by oral ingestion of DU containing soil or dust. DU is primarily an alpha and beta particle emitter, and because of its low radioactivity, skin exposure of external regions of the body is of little concern. However, inhalation or ingestion of DU would allow direct exposure to DU's low-level radioactivity as well as direct chemical activity in the body. DU exposure by inhalation is probably the greatest route of exposure. Direct chemical activity of DU may be more of a concern than DU's radioactivity. When DU is used as a kinetic energy penetrator the explosive impact and combustion of DU produces a cloud of fine DU containing particulates that can remain in the air for several hours. Roughly 50% of the particles in the cloud are respirable and lodge in the alveoli and solublize, with DU entering the bloodstream for an extended period. Once DU has entered the alveoli it may have a pulmonary half-life of nearly 4 years. Exposure to DU may continue after the end of combat operations because DU has little mobility in the soil. This allows it to continue to be an exposure risk via inhaled or ingested dust [1].

There is considerable interest in the potential chemical and radiologic toxicity of DU. DU munitions were used in the Persian Gulf War, the Kosovo police action, and the conflicts in Afghanistan and Iraq. It has been estimated that 320 tons of DU were deposited in Iraq soils during Desert Storm and an estimated 13 tons deposited in Kosovo. There are estimates that 176 tons of DU were used in the 2003 Iraq War. A great deal of public concern about DU toxicity has been generated in the United States and even more so in Europe and the Middle East. Much of the debate about the effects, or lack of effects, of DU is rhetorical because of the lack of empirical data on DU exposure. Human studies that focus on DU are lacking, most focus on "Gulf War Syndrome" making the effects of DU difficult to discern. Few human studies have focused on DU only.

Human studies focusing on DU exposure have primarily been conducted on Gulf War veterans. Elevated DU levels were found in spot sampled urine of Gulf War veterans with retained DU fragments. Another study found that lowered performance on computerized neuropsychological tests was related to urinary DU levels, as were elevated prolactin levels. A study of an enlarged Gulf War cohort seemed to indicate urinary DU levels were not elevated in veterans that were simply present in the theater of war, unless DU fragments were embedded [2].

Studies indicate that DU does cross the blood brain barrier and accumulates in the central nervous system, including the hippocampus, where electrophysiologic changes have been demonstrated. Preliminary studies in our laboratory have found that DU exposure in drinking water alters the development and behavior of mice and the open-field behavior of rats. These early studies also found evidence of oxidation of brain lipids in exposed mice [3, 4].

In light of the evidence presented above we set out to determine if DU exposure would produce changes in catecholamine levels in the mouse midbrain. Catecholamines are linked to a variety of beahviors and several catecholamine containing nuclei are found in the midbrain. We also examined the behavior and CNS lipid oxidation of mice exposed to DU.

METHODS

Male and female Swiss-Webster mice 30 days of age and housed under standard laboratory conditions were exposed to depleted uranium acetate dihydrate at concentrations of 0, 38, or 75mg/L in drinking water for 2 weeks. At the end of two weeks the animals were tested in an open-field apparatus for 5 minutes. While in the open-field line crossing and rearing behavior were measured. Two days after initial testing the measures of open-field behavior were repeated.

After the final open-field test the mice were anesthetized with chloroform, heads removed, brain quickly dissected onto a cold plate and the midbrain and cerebral cortex dissected and frozen at -20 °C for chemical analysis.

Frozen midbrains were dissected in half, along the saggital midline and each half was homogenized in a solution of 0.1N perchloric acid. The homogenate was centrifuged for 5 minutes. Concentration of tyrosine, norephinephrine, and epinephrine were determined by injection of 20microL of the supernant into an HPLC. The column consisted of a Zorbax SB C-18 4.6×250mm with 5 micron particles. The mobile phase consisted of 5% acetylnitrile with 50mM KH_2PO4, 100mg/L EDTA, 200mg/L 1-octane-sulfonic acid, pH 3.0 in water. Substances were detected with a UV detector at 240nm. Concentrations of unknowns were calculated from known standards.

Lipid oxidation was assayed using the thiobarbituric acid (TBA) assay. Briefly, a weighed sample of frontal pole was homogenized and incubated with a solution of 3% TBA, 0.4% SDS and 7.7% acetic acid, pH 3.5, at room temperature, overnight. After incubation a mixture of butanol and pyridine (15:1) was introduced. The organic layer was removed and absorbance read at 532nm. Concentrations were calculated against known concentrations of the standard MDA.

RESULTS

In general, the animals suffered no obvious ill effects from the DU exposure. Open-field testing demonstrated increases in activity consistent with findings reported previously (data not presented). Brain lipid oxidation was increased in a dose dependent fashion, consistent with previous reports (data not shown).

Analysis of midbrain tyrosine levels demonstrated a trend toward a dose dependent increase (p=.13; *fig. 1*). Norepinephrine levels demonstrated a nonsignificant decrease in the experimental groups *(fig. 2)*. Midbrain epinephrine levels demonstrated a dose dependent increase similar to the trend seen for tyrosine (p=.13; *fig. 3*).

Midbrain epinephrine levels demonstrated a significant relationship with the change (session 1-session 2) in open-field rearing activity (r(27)=-.34; p<.05, one tail; *fig. 4*).

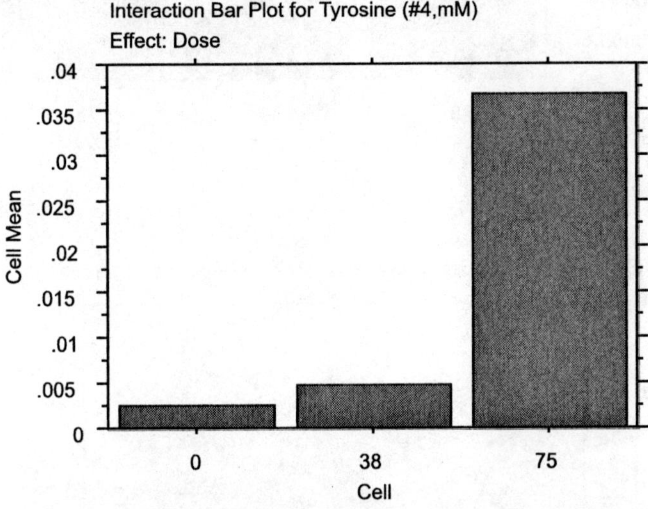

Fig. 1. Effect of DU exposure on midbrain tyrosine levels. X axis is dose of DU. Y axis is tyrosine levels in mM. Tyrosine levels are increased in the 75mg/L groups, p=.06, compared to control.

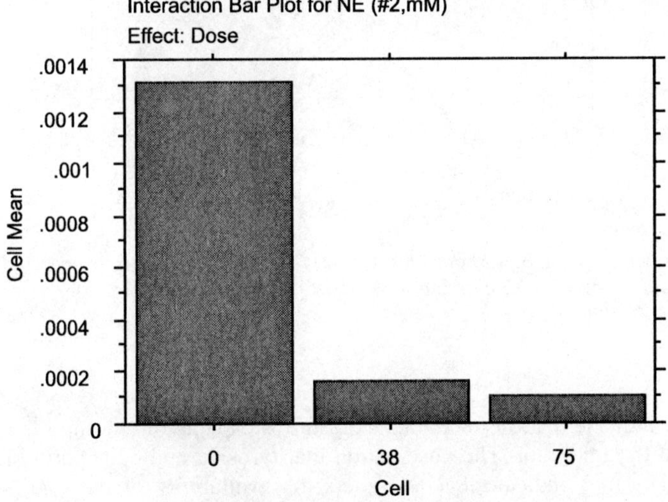

Fig. 2. Effect of DU exposure on midbrain norepinephrine levels. X axis is dose of DU. Y axis is norepinephrine levels in mM. There are no statistically significant differences.

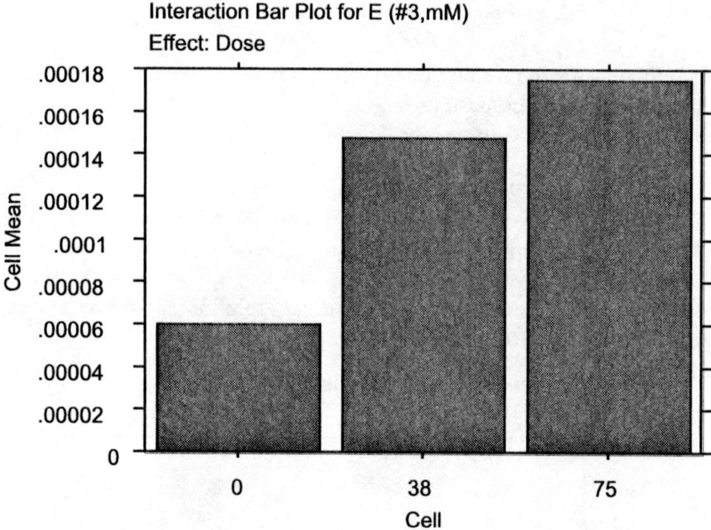

Fig. 3. Effect of DU exposure on midbrain epinephrine levels. X-axis is dose of DU. Y-axis is midbrain epinephrine levels in mM. Control and 75mg/L groups are significantly different at p<.05.

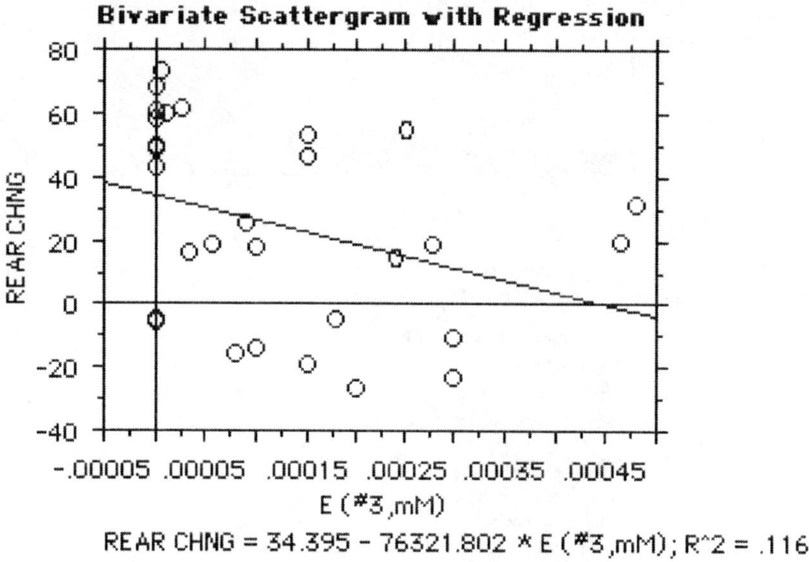

Fig. 4. Relationship between midbrain epinephrine levels (mM) and change in open-field rearing activity between session 1 and session 2. The correlation is statistically significant (p<.05).

DISCUSSION

These findings indicate that, in mice, DU exposure is capable of altering the levels of tyrosine and epinephrine in the midbrain. The observation that tyrosine and epinephrine levels are altered in very similar ways may indicate that DU alters the availability of tyrosine, the precursor for epinephrine. It is puzzling however, that norepinephrine levels are altered in a manner nearly opposite that of epinephrine and tyrosine, suggesting that tyrosine may be shunted to norepinephrine production, depleting the availability of tyrosine for epinephrine synthesis. The finding that epinephrine levels are related to open-field activity is consistent with our understanding of the role of epinephrine in behaviour. The findings suggest that the behavioural effects of DU are at least partly mediated by altering the activity of epinephrine in the midbrain.

REFERENCES

1. Durakovic, A, Horan P, Dietz L, Zimmerman I. Estimate of the time zero lung burden of depleted uranium in Persian Gulf War veterans by the 24-hour urinary excretion and exponential decay analysis, *Mil Med* 2003; 168: 600-5.
2. McDiarmid M, Keogh J, Hooper F, McPhaul K, Squibb K, Kane R, DiPino R, Kabat M, Kaup B, Anderson L, Hoover D, Brown L, Hamilton M, Jacobson-Kram D, Burrows B, Walsh M. Health effects of depleted uranium on exposed Gulf War veterans, *Environ Res* 2000; 82: 168-80.
3. Briner W, Murray, J. Effects of short-term and long-term depleted uranium exposure on open-field behavior and lipid oxidation in rats. *Neurotox Teratol* 2005; 27: 135-44.
4. Pellmar T, Keyser D, Emery C, Hogan J. Electrophysiological changes in hippocampal slices isolated from rats embedded with depleted uranium fragments. *Neurotox* 1999; 20: 785-92.

Metal Ions in Biology and Medicine: vol. 9. Eds Maria Carmen Alpoim, Paula Vasconcellos Morais, Maria Amélia Santos, Armando J. Cristóvão, José A. Centeno, Philippe Collery.
John Libbey Eurotext, Paris © 2006 pp. 346-1.

Dietary Vitamin E, But Not Coenzyme Q10, Reduces Labile Iron In Rat Tissues

Chow, C. K. and Ibrahim, W.

Graduate Center for Nutritional Sciences, University of Kentucky, Lexington, KY 40506-0054, U.S.A. (e-mail: ckchow@uky.edu)

FREE RADICAL-INDUCED OXIDATIVE DAMAGE

Mitochondrion is the principal supplier of the energy required for sustaining life. Mitochondrial electron transport system consumes over 85% of all the oxygen utilized by the cells, and up to 5% of the oxygen consumed by the mitochondrial respiratory chain undergoes one electron reduction, typically by the semiquinone form of coenzyme Q, to generate superoxide (1, 2). The superoxide formed may be converted to other reactive oxygen species under normal physiological conditions. The conversion of superoxide to hydrogen peroxide is catalyzed by superoxide dismutase. Hydrogen peroxide formed can be reduced to water by the activity of glutathione peroxidase or catalase. Also, in the presence of transition metal ions, superoxide and hydrogen peroxide may serve as precursors of hydroxyl radicals. Additionally, superoxide can react readily with nitric oxide to form peroxynitrite. Hydroxyl radicals and peroxynitrite are the two most oxidizing radicals that are likely to arise in biological systems (3).

Reactive oxygen/nitrogen species may react with cellular components with resultant degradation and/or inactivation of essential cellular constituents. Consequent to its generation of superoxide and related reactive oxygen species, mitochondrion plays a critical role in the pathway leading to cell injury and death. Due to its high reactivity, hydroxyl radical is regarded as the initiator of DNA damage after ionizing radiation and oxidative stress. In addition to irreversible damage of mitochondrial DNA, reactive oxygen/nitrogen species can cause oxidative damage to membrane lipids and proteins, and result in mitochondrial dysfunction and ultimately cell death. Proximal to the influx of reactive oxygen species, mitochondrion, particularly its DNA, is susceptible to oxidative damage and mutation because mitochondrion lacks protective histones and effective repair systems (4). Increased oxidative lesions, deletions, point mutations, and aberrant forms are associated with mitochondrial DNA of postmitotic tissues upon aging (5). Mitochondrial defects encompassing complexes I-IV of the electron transport chain characterize a relatively large number of neurodegenerative diseases. Free radical-induced oxidative damage is increasingly implicated as an important contributor in the pathogenesis of cancer, cardiovascular disease, aging and other degenerative diseases (6, 7).

ROLE OF VITAMIN E AND COENZYME Q10 IN ANTIOXIDANT DEFENSE

Vitamin E is the major lipid-soluble chain-breaking antioxidant that prevents free radical-initiated peroxidative tissue damage, and plays a central role in the overall antioxidant defense (8, 9). The antioxidant property of vitamin E is attributable to its more rapidly reaction with peroxy radicals several orders of magnitude faster than with acyl lipids. The free radical scavenging reaction of vitamin E reduces the available superoxide and related reactive oxygen/nitrogen species. However, the mechanism by which vitamin E exerts its protective effect against oxidative tissue damage has yet to be delineated.

As stated above, mitochondrion is the major source of reactive oxygen/nitrogen species, which are generated continuously by its respiratory chain (1, 2). The mitochondrial inner membrane has the highest concentration of vitamin E, and disruption of mitochondial ultrastructure is one of the earliest pathologic events observed in the skeletal muscle of vitamin E-deficient animals. Also, *de novo* synthesis of xanthine oxidase, which catalyzes the formation of superoxide, is markedly increased in the skeletal muscle of vitamin E-deficient rabbits, and its activity is significantly higher in the liver of vitamin E-deficient rats. These reports suggest an increased mitochondrial superoxide production during vitamin E deficiency and an important role of superoxide in the pathogenesis of vitamin E-deficiency (9).

Coenzyme Q is a lipid-soluble compound composed of a redox active quinoid moiety and a hydrophobic tail. The compound is an essential cofactor in the mitochondrial electron transport chain and plays important roles in energy production (10). The reduced form of coenzyme Q (ubiquinol) may act as an antioxidant by scavenging reactive oxygen/nitrogen species and forms ubisemiquinone in biological systems (11). Coenzyme Q is considered an important antioxidant because it can be regenerated by intracellular reducing mechanisms, and is present in relatively high concentrations (12). Protection against oxidative damage by coenzyme Q has been demonstrated in liposomes, low density lipoproteins, biological membranes, proteins and DNA.

Sufficient coenzyme Q is synthesized by enzymes in the endoplasmic reticulum and Golgi membranes, and then transported to other cellular organelles under normal conditions. A unique feature of coenzyme Q10, not shared by most endogenously synthesized bioactive compounds, is that its content can be greatly augmented by exogenous administration, and that dietary coenzyme Q10 does not seem to interfere with the metabolism of endogenous coenzyme Q. Experimental data available suggest that dietary coenzyme Q10 is taken up into circulation at a variable degree, and significant uptake occurs mainly in such organs as liver and spleen (13, 14).

Both vitamin E and coenzyme Q are essential for maintaining functions and integrity of mitochondria, and high concentrations of these compounds are found in its inner membrane of mitochondria. There is an interaction between exogenously administered vitamin E and coenzyme Q10 in terms of uptake and tissue retention. Moderate levels of vitamin E enhance tissue uptake and/or retention of dietary coenzyme Q10, while high levels of vitamin E may compete with coenzyme Q10 and thus suppressing its absorption and/or uptake (14). This is probably because both vitamin E and coenzyme Q10 have a similar absorption/transport mechanism.

ROLE OF LABILE IRON IN FREE RADICAL-INDUCED OXIDATIVE DAMAGE

Labile iron or free iron associated with low molecule mass has the potential to participate in redox cycling and catalyze the formation of hydroxyl radical from superoxide/hydrogen peroxide (15, 16). The state and levels of labile iron or available form of iron can be modified by oxidants or reductants acting on cell iron sources. In addition to damaging some biological molecules directly, superoxide and hydrogen peroxide may be converted to the more reactive hydroxyl radicals in the presence of transition metal ions. Also, transitional metal ions may catalyze the decomposition of lipid hydroperoxides to form alkoxyl, peroxyl and other radicals, which in turn may initiate or accelerate oxidation reactions.

While transition metal ions play a key role in catalyzing the formation of hydroxyl radicals and initiating oxidative cell damage, the vast majority of transition metals are transported and bound to proteins, and are not available to catalyze the formation of hydroxyl radicals under normal conditions. However, results obtained from *in vitro* and cell culture studies suggest that several compounds, including superoxide and hydrogen peroxide, may release iron from such protein complexes as mitochondrial iron-sulfur clusters, transferrin and ferritin. Therefore, the conditions that favor superoxide generation may also lead to an increased iron release, and initiate oxidative damage. On the other hand, factors that reduce mitochondrial superoxide generation are expected to attenuate iron release and oxidative damage.

EFFECT OF DIETARY VITAMIN E ON LABILE IRON

Vitamin E has long been recognized as the major lipid-soluble antioxidant preventing against oxidative tissue damage (8, 9). However, the mechanism by which vitamin E delays or protects against oxidative tissue degeneration remains to be delineated. Information available suggests that an increased mitochondrial superoxide production is associated with vitamin E deficiency, and vitamin E status may alter tissue levels of labile iron (9).

Iron overload is associated with increased oxidative damage and dietary vitamin E may alter iron metabolism and attenuate its toxicity. Also, dietary vitamin E has been shown to dose-dependently reduce the generation/levels of superoxide and/or hydrogen peroxide in rodent tissues (17, 18). Superoxide and/or hydrogen peroxide has potential to release labile or available form of iron from its protein complexes. Since labile or available form of iron is capable of catalyzing the formation of hydroxyl radicals as well as the decomposition of lipid hydroperoxides to form more free radicals (15, 16), an increase in labile iron is expected to cause an increase in the levels of oxidation products. Thus, vitamin E may exert its antioxidant function by attenuating iron release by reducing available superoxide. Indeed, dietary vitamin E has also been shown to reduce the levels of labile iron or loosely bound iron, as well as lipid peroxidation products in rats (19). These data supports the notion that labile or available form of iron plays an important role in initiating peroxidative damage to membrane lipids.

While the nature or chemical identity of the labile iron or loosely bound iron pool detected is not yet clear, the findings suggest that vitamin E may attenuate the release of iron from its protein complexes by mediating the level and/or generation of superoxide. However, it is possible that increased oxidative stress caused by inadequate vitamin E may damage cellular components that contain iron and resulting in its release.

EFFECT OF DIETARY COENZYME Q10 ON SUPEROXIDE GENERATION AND LABILE IRON

In order to determine if the influence of dietary vitamin E to attenuate mitochondrial superoxide generation and labile iron levels is a unique property of the compound, the effect of dietary coenzyme Q10, in the presence or absence of vitamin E, on mitochondrial superoxide generation and labile iron was studied in rats. Twenty-four twelve-month-old male Sprague-Dawley rats were fed a basal low vitamin E diet (10 IU vitamin E/kg) supplemented with 500 mg coenzyme Q10/kg diet and either 0, 100, or 1300 IU vitamin E/kg diet for 28 days. Another animal group received no supplementation. Feed and water were provided *ad libitum*. At the end of the feeding period, rats were killed following blood withdrawal via heart puncture, and portions of liver and spleen were analyzed for the rates of mitochondrial hydrogen peroxide generation, as well as the levels of labile iron and lipid peroxidation products.

Mitochontrial generation of hydrogen peroxide was measured by monitoring the oxidation of p-hydroxyphenylacetate (PHPA) coupled to the enzymatic reduction of hydrogen peroxide by horseraddish peroxidase according to the modified procedure of Hyslop and Sklar (20). The rate of hydrogen peroxide released was determined fluorometrically at an excitation of 318 nm and emission of 405 nm. Due to the presence of superoxide dismutase in mitochondria, measurement of hydrogen peroxide is same as measuring superoxide. The level of labile iron was measured according to the modified procedure of Kime et al. (21). Freshly prepared tissue homogenate was mixed with nitrilotriacetic acid, pH 7.0, and then diluted with 5 mM Mops buffer, pH 7.0. The filtrate of 10 kDa ultracentrifuge filter was mixed with 1 M thioglycolic acid, 0.25% bathophenanthroline in isopropyl alcohol, and saturated potassium acetate. The ferrous-bathophenanthroline colored complex was then extracted with ethanol-chloroform (1:4), and the absorbance measured at 533 nm. The levels of lipid peroxidation products, mainly malondialdehyde, were measured by the modified procedure of Li and Chow (22) fluorometrically with excitation at 515 nm and emission at 550 nm following isobutanol extraction. Data obtained were analyzed using analysis of variance followed by Tukey's multiple comparison test and correlation analysis.

As expected, dietary vitamin E dose-dependently decreased the rates of mitochondrial hydrogen peroxide generation, and the levels of labile iron and lipid peroxidation products in the liver, and to a lesser degree in the spleen. Dietary coenzyme Q10 partially reduced rates of mitochondrial hydrogen peroxide generation, and the levels of labile iron and lipid peroxidation products, while the levels of vitamin E were increased in the liver of animals receiving low vitamin E in the diet. Dietary coenzyme Q10 had relatively little effects on the spleen. The results obtained suggest that dietary vitamin E, but not coenzyme Q10, exerts its protective effect against oxidative damage by reducing the generation and/or levels of superoxide, which in turn attenuates iron release from its protein complex. The results also support the view that coenzyme Q10 spares vitamin E when dietary vitamin E is low.

POSSIBLE SIGNIFICANCE

Among the biological functions proposed for vitamin E, protection against free radical-initiated peroxidative damage is the most widely accepted one (8, 9). It has long been recognized that dietary vitamin E alters iron metabolism and protects against oxidative damage resulting from iron overload. The findings that dietary vitamin E dose-dependently reduced the rate of mitochondrial superoxide generation, as well as levels of labile iron and lipid peroxidation products observed suggest that vitamin E may exert its antioxidant function by limiting the generation and/or level of superoxide. By reducing the generation and/or levels of superoxide, dietary vitamin E not only reduces levels of harmful free radicals, but also limits the release of iron from its protein complex. Thus, vitamin E may protect against oxidative damage or exert its antioxidant function by directly scavenging oxidants/free radicals, and/or reducing mitochondrial superoxide generation. By reducing superoxide and available labile iron, the possibility of hydroxyl radical formation is also reduced.

In addition to its antioxidant property, vitamin E may also function as a biological response modifier independent of its antioxidant function (9, 23). By reducing the generation and/or levels of superoxide and other reactive oxygen/nitrogen species, dietary vitamin E may modulate the activation and/or expression redox-sensitive biological response modifiers, and thereby attenuates the cellular events leading to subsequent cell death/apoptosis and onset of cardiovascular, cancer, aging and other degenerative diseases (9). However, since only dietary vitamin E, but not coenzyme Q10, reduces the rates of mitochondrial superoxide generation, and the levels of labile iron and lipid peroxidation products, this property of vitamin E may or may not be attributable to its antioxidant function. More study is needed to clarify this view.

In summary, the results obtained showed that dietary vitamin E, but not coenzyme Q10, dose-dependently reduced the rates of mitochondrial superoxide generation, and levels of labile iron and lipid peroxidation products in the liver and spleen of rats. As superoxide has potential to release iron from its protein complexes and be converted to hydroxyl radicals in the presence of labile or available form of iron, dietary vitamin E may protect against peroxidative tissue damage by attenuating the generation and/or levels of superoxide.

REFERENCES

1. Shigenaga MK, Hagen TM, Ames BN. Oxidative damage and mitochondrial decay in aging. *Proc Nat Acad Sci USA* 1994; 91: 10771-10778.
2. Lenaz G. Role of mitochondria in oxidative stress and aging. *Biochim Biophys Acta* 1998; 1366: 53-67.
3. Squadrito GL, Pryor WA. Oxidative chemistry on nitric oxide: The roles of superoxide, peroxynitrite, and carbon dioxide. *Free Rad Biol Med* 1998; 25: 392-403.
4. Wallace DC, Brown MD, Melov S, Graham B, Lott M. Mitochondrial biology, degenerative disease and aging. *Biofactors* 1998; 7: 187-190.
5. Ames BN, Shigenaga MK, Hagen M. Oxidants, antioxidants, and the degenerative diseases of aging. *Proc Nat Acad Sci USA* 1993; 90: 7915-7922.
6. Chow CK. Nutritional influence in cellular antioxidant defense systems. *Am J Clin Nutr* 1979; 32: 1066-1081.
7. Yu BP. Cellular defense against damage from reactive oxygen species. *Physiol Rev* 1994; 74: 139-162.
8. Chow CK. Vitamin E and oxidative stress. *Free Rad Biol Med* 1991; 11: 215-232.
9. Chow CK. Biological functions and metabolic fate of vitamin E revisited. *J Biomed Sci* 2004; 1: 295-302.
10. Ernster L, Dallner G. Biochemical, physiological and medical aspects of ubiquinone function. *Biochem Biophys Acta* 1995; 1271: 195-204.
11. Forsmark-Andree P, Lee CP, Dallner G, Ernster, L. Lipid peroxidation and changes in the ubiquinone content and the respiratory chain enzymes of submitochondrial particles. *Free Rad Biol Med* 1997; 22: 391-400.
12. Kagan V, Serbinova E, Packer L. Antioxidant effects of ubiquinones in microsomes and mitochondria are mediated by tocopherol recycling. *Biochem Biophys Res Commun* 1990; 169: 851-857.
13. Zhang Y, Aberg F, Appelkvist EL, Dallner G, Ernster L. Uptake of dietary coenzyme Q supplement is limited in rats. *J Nutr* 1995; 125: 446-453.
14. Ibrahim W, Bhagavan H, Chopra R, Chow CK. Dietary coenzyme Q10 and vitamin E alters concentrations of coenzyme Q and vitamin E in rat tissues and mitochondria. *J Nutr* 2000; 130: 2343-2348.
15. Minotti G, Aust SD. Redox cycling of iron and lipid peroxidation. *Lipids* 1992; 27: 219-226.
16. Keyer K, Imlay JA. Superoxde accelerates DNA damage by elevating free iron levels. *Proc Natl Acad Sci USA* 1996; 93: 13635-13640.
17. Chow CK, Ibrahim W, Wei ZH, Chan AC. Vitamin E regulates mitochondrial hydrogen peroxide generation. *Free Rad Biol Med* 1999; 27; 580-587.
18. Lass A, Sohal RS. Effect of coenzyme Q10 and alpha-tocopherol content of mitochondria on the production of superoxide anion radicals. *FASEB J.* 2000; 14: 87-94.
19. Ibrahim W, Chow CK. Dietary vitamin E reduces tissue labile iron. *J Biochem Mol Toxicol* 2005; 19: 298-303, 2005.
20. Hyslop PA, Sklar LA. A quantitative fluorometric assay for the determination of oxidant production by polymorphonuclear leukocytes: Its use in the simultaneous fluorometric assay of cellular activation processes. *Anal Biochem* 1984; 141: 280-286.
21. Kime R, Gibson A, Yong W, Hider R, Powers H. Chromatographic method for the determination of non-transferrin-bound iron suitable for use on the plasma and bronchoalveolar lavage fluid of preterm babies. *Clin Sci* 1996; 91: 633-638.
22. Li XY, Chow CK. An improved method for measuring malondialdehyde in biological samples. *Lipids* 1994; 29: 73-75.
23. Traber MG, Packer L. Vitamin E: beyond antioxidant function. *Am J Clin Nutr* 1995; 62: 1501S-1509S.

Metal Ions in Biology and Medicine: vol. 9. Eds Maria Carmen Alpoim, Paula Vasconcellos Morais, Maria Amélia Santos, Armando J. Cristóvão, José A. Centeno, Philippe Collery.
John Libbey Eurotext, Paris © 2006 pp. 351-1.

Inheritance of susceptibility: mercury kinetics in two mouse strains (A.SW and B10.S) and their F1 generation

Nielsen J.B.[1], Ekstrand J.[2], Zalups R.K.[3], Söderkvist P.[4], Hultman P.[2]

[1]*Environmental Medicine, Institute of Public health, University of Southern Denmark, Denmark*
(e-mail: jbnielsen@health.sdu.dk)
[2]*Molecular and Immunological Pathology, Department of Molecular Medicine, Linköping University, Sweden*
(e-mail: perhu@imk.liu.se)
[3]*Division of Basic Medical Sciences, Mercer University School of Medicine, Macon, USA*
(e-mail: zalups_rk@mercer.edu)
[4]*Cell Biology, Department of Biomedicine and Surgery, Linköping University Sweden*
(e-mail: petso@ibk.liu.se).

ABSTRACT

The whole-body retention (WBR) and organ deposition of inorganic mercury depend on strain as well as gender. These genetic traits have previously been demonstrated to affect the susceptibility towards various adverse effects of inorganic mercury, e.g. induction of renal damage and different systemic autoimmune responses. This susceptibility is linked to certain inbred strains, but few studies have addressed the inheritance of various aspects of this susceptibility. The purpose of the present study was to compare the toxicokinetics of inorganic mercury in two mouse strains with known differences in mercury kinetics (A.SW and B10.S) with their F1 generation (A.SW male × B10.S female). All mice were exposed to radiolabelled $HgCl_2$ (^{203}Hg; 2 mg/L) in the drinking water for six weeks. WBR of mercury was measured in a whole-body counter at regular intervals throughout the experimental period, followed by measurements of deposition in liver, kidneys, spleen, and heart at the end of the experiment. After six weeks, WBR in A.SW males was significantly higher than in any other group of both genders. The gender-related difference in WBR observed in the A.SW strain was also seen in the F1 mice, but not in B10.S mice. The concentration of mercury in the kidneys as well as the fractional renal deposition (% of WBR) was higher in male A.SW mice than in any other group. The organ depositions of mercury in B10.S mice were lower than in mice from the A.SW strain. Organ deposition in the F1 mice was generally lower than in A.SW mice and higher than in B10.S mice. Susceptibility related to increased mercury deposition seems qualitatively inherited from the male A.SW mice to their F1 offspring, but quantitatively clearly affected by their mother strain (B10.S). As absorption is primarily passive, susceptibility appears related to elimination kinetics.

INTRODUCTION

The kinetics of inorganic mercury has repeatedly been demonstrated to vary between different strains of inbred mice [1, 2]. As the absorption of inorganic mercury following oral exposure is expected to be passive diffusion across the intestinal epithelium, kinetic differences between strains pertain to distribution, organ deposition, and elimination [1, 2]. The deposition of mercury in the kidney, the main target organ for inorganic mercury, varies significantly between strains of mice, thereby giving them different susceptibility to mercury toxicity [3]. Thus, the renal deposition of mercury following ten weeks drinking water exposure to mercuric chloride (5 mg/L) varied from

13 µg/g to 28 µg/g in five different mouse strains [3]. In a comparison between A.SW mice and B10.S mice given 2 mg Hg/L drinking water for ten weeks, the average deposition of mercury in kidney and spleen at week ten was 7000 and 114 ng/g w.w. in male A.SW mice and 1700 and 63 ng/g w.w. in B10.S mice, respectively [4].

Toxicity may, however, not only pertain to traditional renal toxicity, i.e. proximal tubular damage, but may also render some strains more susceptible to other forms of toxicity, i.e. different systemic autoimmune responses [4]. Thus, the systemic autoimmune response induced by inorganic mercury is clearly genetically linked to the configuration of the major histocompatibility complex (MHC) in rodents [5, 6], but regions outside the MHC domain influencing the renal deposition of mercury is also of importance [3]. We have previously demonstrated significant differences in whole-body retention as well as organ deposition of mercury between mice of the A.SW strain and mice of the B10.S strain following prolonged drinking water exposure [4]. Gender related differences were also observed in mercury kinetics in these strains [4]. Whether the mercury kinetics of the F1 generation from a cross-over between A.SW and B10.S mice will be similar to either of the parental strains or something in between is presently not known, i.e. will the increased susceptibility reflected through an increased renal deposition of mercury in the male A.SW mice be present in the male offspring from a crossover between A.SW mice and B10.S mice? Thus, the present study aimed at investigating the inheritance of mercury susceptibility through a comparison of mercury kinetics in A.SW mice, B10.S mice and their F1 generation.

MATERIALS AND METHODS

Animals: A.SW mice, originally obtained from Taconic M&B (Ry, Denmark) and B10.S mice (obtained from Jackson, Bar Harbor, MN) were kept inbred in a high-barrier unit within the facility for experimental animals at the Faculty of Health Sciences in Linköping. Production of F1 (A.SW males × B10.S females) hybrids, and treatment of mice took take place at these facilities. All mice were kept under controlled conditions with free access to standard mouse pellets and drinking water. Drinking water consumption was measured during the experimental period. The ID of each mouse was secured by subcutaneous implantation of a chip which can be monitored externally. F0 and F1 hybrids of both genders were included in the study. The group size was seven and the mice were 8-16 weeks old when included in experiments.

Mercury exposure: The experimental groups were exposed to mercuric chloride in the drinking water (2 mg Hg/L) for six weeks before sacrifice. The mercury was labeled with ^{203}Hg to allow whole-body counting during the experimental period as well as easy determination of organ accumulation of mercury after sacrifice. The experimental model to study kinetics of mercury has been described in detail in Nielsen [1]. Briefly, drinking water consumption was measured and used to calculate mercury intake, and whole-body retention of mercury was measured at regular intervals in live animals throughout the experimental period by use of a whole-body counter (NaI well crystal). To adjust for counting efficiency and radioactive decay, a standard of known intensity (1 mL drinking water) was used at all counting sessions. After six weeks, all animals were killed by cervical dislocation and relevant organs excised and counted in a Perkin Elmer Wizard Automatic gamma counter. The study period was 6 weeks to assure that the whole-body retention of mercury had reached steady state.

Ethics: The study was approved by the Swedish National Board of Ethics of Animal Experiments.

RESULTS

Body weights differed between strains and genders, with the F1 hybrids being significantly larger than the other two strains and male mice being heavier than female mice *(table 1)*. Weight gain was similar in exposed and control animals (data not shown). The average drinking water consumption was close to 3 mL/day/mouse corresponding to a daily intake of 6 μg mercury *(table 1)*. A steady state WBR of mercury was reached after approximately four weeks, and remained at this level with minor fluctuations for the remaining experimental period. After six weeks, WBR in A.SW males was significantly higher than in any other group of both genders *(table 1)*. The gender related difference in WBR observed in the A.SW strain was also seen in the F1 mice, but not in B10.S mice *(table 1)*. Correcting the WBRs for strain-related differences in body weight supports the uncorrected observation that male A.SW is the only group with a WBR significantly different from all other groups. Thus, WBR in male A.SW mice was 50% higher than in females of the same strain, 40% higher than in male B10.S mice, and close to 25% higher than the WBR in male F1 mice *(table 1)*.

Table 1. Drinking water consumption (DWC), body weight (BW) at six weeks, and whole-body retention (WBR) of Hg after 6 weeks drinking water exposure to mercuric chloride (2 mg/L). DWC is given as group average, and BW and WBR are given as mean values (n=7) ± sem.

	A.SW male	F1 Male	B10.S Male	A.SW Female	F1 Female	B10.S female
DWC (mL/day/ mouse)	2.6	3.0	3.5	2.7	3.0	2.7
BW (g)	22.8±1.5	32.1±0.8^{A}	27.0±0.4^{AB}	19.2±0.7^{A}	20.8±0.5^{B}	19.5±0.4
WBR (μg Hg)	4.92±0.28	3.99±0.29^{A}	3.51±0.20^{A}	3.28±0.17^{A}	3.12±0.17^{B}	3.23±0.13

^{A} - significantly different from A.SW males; ^{B} - significantly different from F1 males.

Considering the different drinking water consumptions between groups, it is evident that male A.SW mice with the lowest drinking water consumption and the highest WBR of mercury following six weeks exposure to mercuric chloride have the highest fractional retention of inorganic mercury following oral exposure. Male B10.S mice have the lowest fractional retention of mercury. The fractional retention of mercury in male F1 mice was between the two parental strains, whereas no significant differences were observed between females from the three groups.

The renal deposition of mercury was highest in A.SW mice irrespectively of gender *(fig. 1)*. The other parental strain (B10.S) displayed the lowest renal mercury deposition, and the F1 hybrid showed only slight, insignificantly higher renal depositions than the B10.S strain *(fig. 1)*. The highest concentration of mercury retained in any investigated organ was observed in the kidneys for all groups, reaching average concentrations between 5-600 ng Hg/g tissue in B10.S mice and 2300 ng Hg/g tissue in male A.SW mice *(fig. 1)*. The hepatic deposition of mercury demonstrated the same distributional pattern as for the renal deposition with the highest concentrations observed in A.SW mice followed by the F1 hybrids and with the hepatic concentration in B10.S mice being lowest *(fig. 1)*. However, in contrast to the renal deposition, female mice retained higher hepatic concentrations of mercury than males *(fig. 1)*.

Mercury deposition in the spleen was quantitatively limited, but given the low weight of the organ, the concentrations of mercury measured in the spleen was between 10 and 30 ng/g wet weight *(fig. 1)*. Again, the highest concentrations were observed in A.SW mice of both genders followed by the F1 hybrids and the B10.S strain *(fig. 1)*. The deposition of mercury in the heart demonstrated a similar distribution pattern between groups as for the other organs *(fig. 1)*. The general trend for all organs was that the highest mercury concentration was observed in A.SW mice followed by the F1 hybrids and the lowest concentrations were observed in organs from B10.S mice. Gender related differences were subtle with the exception of the renal deposition in A.SW mice.

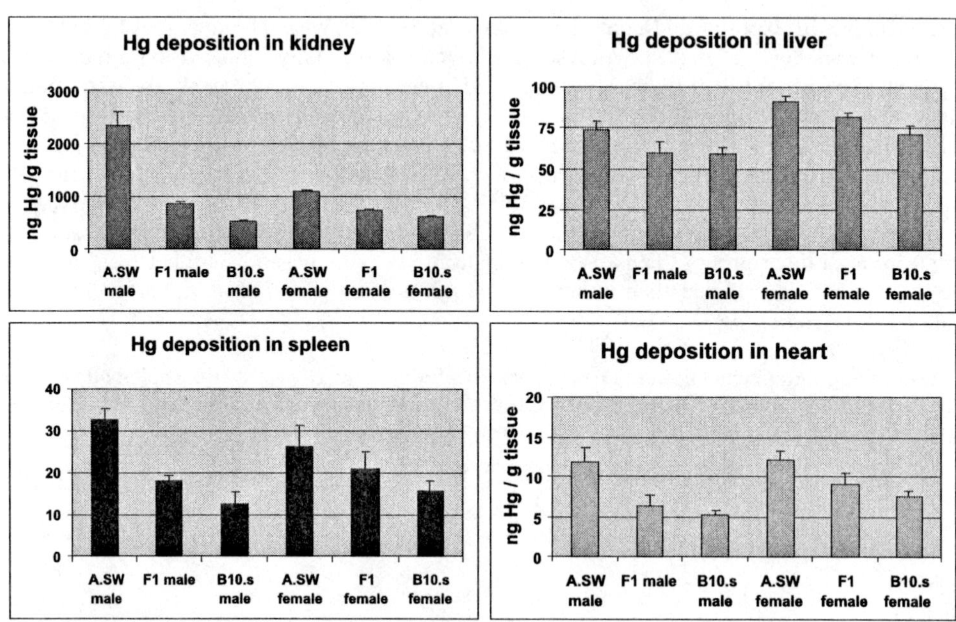

Fig. 1. Organ deposition of mercury in males and females of two inbred mouse strains and their F1 hybrid following six weeks drinking water exposure to mercuric chloride (2 mg Hg/L). Results are given as mean values + 1 sem and expressed in ng mercury/g tissue (wet weight).

DISCUSSION

Higher WBR and organ deposition of mercury following six weeks drinking water exposure in A.SW mice than in B10.S mice is in accordance with our previous study [3]. Likewise, the higher renal mercury deposition observed in male A.SW mice compared to female A.SW mice is reported earlier [4]. A WBR of mercury at six weeks of 3-5 µg and a daily drinking water consumption causing a daily intake of mercuric chloride of close to 6 µg indicate very dynamic kinetics. Adding together the average mercury deposition in the four organs included in this study gives close to 1 µg mercury per mouse. Thus, the majority of the observed WBR of mercury at any time is related to mercury temporarily present as unabsorbed in the gastrointestinal tract. Based on previous experimental studies [1], the fractional intestinal absorption of mercuric chloride is close to 15%. Thus, slightly less than 1 µg mercury is expected to be absorbed daily in these mice indicating a daily renal elimination of the same amount at approximated steady state conditions, i.e. after six weeks exposure. Among the three male groups, the ratios between WBR and DWC indicate that male B10.S and male F1 mice most efficiently eliminate orally absorbed mercury. All female groups have very similar drinking water consumption, weight and WBR indicating that the lower elimination rate observed in male A.SW mice is not only related to the strain but rather to a combination of strain and gender. Considering the higher body weight of F1 males, the WBR/BW ratio in this F1 hybrid (0.12) resembles the ratio in male B10.S mice (0.13) more than A.SW mice (0.22). Thus, the significantly decreased ability to eliminate absorbed inorganic mercury characterising the male A.SW strain is not passed on from the male A.SW mice to their F1 offspring having B10.S mothers. On the contrary, when the significantly higher bodyweight of the F1 male mice is considered, the kinetics of the F1 mice is very similar to the B10.S mice.

Generally, the standard deviations observed for different parameters in the F1 group are not larger than for the parental strains. This indicates that the F1 group does not consist of two sub-groups resembling the strain and gender characteristics of either their mothers or their fathers as this situation would have generated considerable larger standard deviations.

Considering data on WBR as well as organ deposition it appears that the dominating difference between A.SW mice and B10.S mice relates to a decreased ability to eliminate mercury causing an increased renal deposition in male A.SW mice. An increased renal deposition is also seen in the male F1 mice, but not quantitatively comparable to the significantly higher renal deposition in male A.SW mice. Except for this trait, which is qualitatively evident but quantitatively limited and the higher body weight in F1 males compared to both A.SW and B10.S mice, the toxicokinetics of the F1 hybrids resemble much more their mother strain, B10.S.

REFERENCES

1. Nielsen JB. Toxicokinetics of mercuric chloride and methylmercuric mercury in mice. J Toxicol Environ Health 1992; 37: 85-122.
2. Nielsen JB, Hultman P. Strain dependence of steady state retention and elimination of mercury in mice after prolonged exposure to mercury(II) chloride. Analyst 1998; 123: 87-90.
3. Nielsen JB, Hultman P. Experimental studies on genetically determined susceptibility to mercury-induced nephrotoxicity and autoimmune response. Renal Failure 1999; 21: 343-348.
4. Hultman P, Nielsen JB. The effect of dose, gender, and non-H-2 genes in murine mercury-induced autoimmunity. J Autoimmunity 2001; 16: 27-37.
5. Mirtcheva J, Pfeiffer C, De Bruijn JA, Jaquesmart F, Gleichmann E. Immunological alterations inducible by mercury compounds. III. H-2A acts as an immune response and H-2E as an immune “suppression” locus for $HgCl_2$-induced antinuclear antibodies. Eur J Immunol 1989; 12: 2257-2261.
6. Hultman P, Nielsen JB. The effect of toxicokinetics on murine mercury-induced autoimmunity. Environ Res 1998; 77: 141-148.

Therapy

Metal Ions in Biology and Medicine: vol. 9. Eds Maria Carmen Alpoim, Paula Vasconcellos Morais, Maria Amélia Santos, Armando J. Cristóvão, José A. Centeno, Philippe Collery.
John Libbey Eurotext, Paris © 2006 pp. 358-1.

Antitumor Effects of Gallium (III) Tris (Salicylate)-Ethanol on Malignant Cell Lines and Tumor Bearing Swiss Albino Mice

Dina A. Ismail[1], Abdelfattah Badawi[1], Philippe Collery[2], Nadia I. Zakhary[3], Sarah Abdel Raouf[3]

[1]*Applied Surfactant Laboratory, Egyptian Petroleum Research Institute*
[2]*Service de Cancérologie- Polyclinique Maymard, 20200 Bastia, France*
[3]*Cancer Biology Department, National Cancer Institute, Cairo University, Egypt*

ABSTRACT

The gallium (III) tris (salicylate)-ethanol was prepared and characterized through FTIR, mass and H[1]NMR spectra. This complex was found cytotoxic on Earlich Ascitis Carcinoma (EAC) cells and showed antitumor activity in EAC tumor bearing swiss albino mice.

INTRODUCTION

The present study was designed aiming to prepare a new organometallic gallium (Ga) compound, the Gallium (III) tris (salicylate)- ethanol and to evaluate its anticancer effects (inhibitory effects on malignant cells in culture as well as the antitumour effects in tumour-bearing animals).

SYNTHESIS OF Ga SALICYLATE

Freshly prepared 0.97gm of Ga $(OH)_3$ was added to 6.98 salicylic acid dissolved in 150ml of anhydrous ethanol. The suspension was then refluxed on a water bath until all the gallium hydroxide had been reacted. The resulting white colored solution was then filtered and white crystals were deposited by cooling. These were filtered off washed with cold alcohol and air dried to yield 3.2gm of gallium salicylate.

The structure of the prepared compound was confirmed by:

1. Micro elemental analyses (VARIO El Elementar).
2. FTIR spectra (ATI mattson Genesis series FTIR™).
3. Mass spectra (Mass spectrophotometer HP Model GC MS-QPL 000 EX (Shimadeu).
4. The ^{1}HNMR spectra was measured on varian Genini - 200 μHz spectro-photometer, laser unit.

The chemical structure of the prepared compound was studied by IR spectra exhibiting ester c=o at/1703 cm^{-1}, n-OH at-1300 cm^{-1} n-OH aliphatic at 3650 - 3590cm^{-1}, n-CH aliphatic at 2920cm^{-1}, and CH aromatic at 3047cm^{-1}. M.S. spectrum of the compound showed the base peak at m/e 120 (100%) which could be attributed to OH- (C_6H_5) C^+O. The intense peak. at m/e 69 is due to Cu. molecular ion beak. ^{1}HNMR spectrum $(CDCL_3)$; 2s(OH) alcohol; 3.6 t2 (CH_2); 5s(OH) aromatic and 7.4 - 7.8m (5H. ArH).

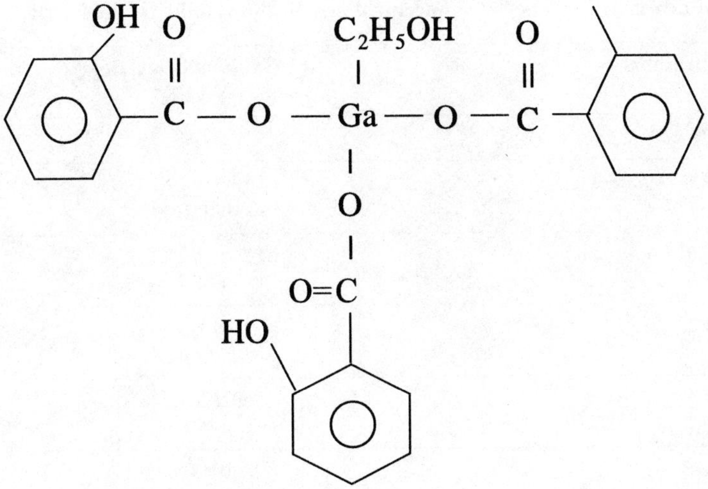

Gallium (III) tris (salicylate) ethanol (M. W = 527.14)

Table 1. Micro analysis of Ga Salicylate.

Compound		Micro analysis %		
		C	H	Ga
Ga sal	Calculated	52.5	3.8	13.25
	Found	52.27	3.68	13.00

ANTITUMOUR EFFECTS

Inhibitory effects on malignant cells in culture

The effect of Ga Salicylate on the viability of EAC cells was studied according to the method of El-Merzabani et al.

The effects of different concentrations of Ga Salicylate on the survival of cultured EAC cells are shown in *table 2*. The concentrations used ranged from 0.8 to 100 mg/ml.

The results shown are expressed as percentage of non viable cells (% NVC). The addition of Ga Salicylate to the culture media of EAC cells showed a dose dependent cytotoxic effect. The cytotoxic effect ranged from 13.7% NVC for a concentration of 0.8 mg Ga Sal/ml to 72.3% NVC when Ga Salicylate was used at a concentration of 100mg/ml.

Antitumour effects on tumour-bearing animals

30 Healthy untreated Female Swiss albino mice weighing 20g each were divided into the following groups:

I. Control group.

II. Ehrlich Ascitic Carcinoma (EAC) group: Mice were i.p. injected with 2.5×10^6 EAC cells.

III. EAC + Ga Sal group: Mice were i.p. injected with 2.5×10^6 EAC cells and the treatment by a dose of 50 mg/Kg body weight of Ga Salicylate was administered at days 2, 4 and 6 after the tumour inoculation.

The survival was compared within the three groups.

Table 2. Effect of different Ga salicylate concentrations on the viability of EAC cells

Concentrations	Gallium Salicylate $\bar{X} \pm SD$*
0	1%
0.8	13.7 ± 1.8 (a) (11-16)#
1.6	26.3 ± 2.1 (a) (24-29)
3.2	41.0 ± 1.3 (a) (39-42)
6.3	50.2 ± 1.5 (a) (48-52)
12.5	57.0 ± 0.89 (a) (56-58)
25.0	64.0 ± 1.5 (a) (62-66)
50.0	69 ± 1.5 (a) (67-71)
100.0	72.3 ± 1.8 (a) (70-73)

(a) Significant from control at P-value <0.001 in Gallium salicylate group and expressed as percent of non-viable cells.
 # Result are expressed as range.
** Mean (SD of 6 experiments).*

BODY WEIGHT

The effects of salicylate complex on body weight of EAC bearing mice have been calculated as percent of change in body weight, taking the starting day as zero percent.

The results are tabulated in *table 3*. The untreated tumor bearing animals showed a progressive increase in their total body weight (B.W.) reaching 94.1% on the 26th day. The changes in body weights of mice in the groups of EAC + Ga Salicylate were 19.9%. and in healthy control 32.4%.

Table 3. Percent of change in body weight of groups of mice under different treatments.

Group \ Day	2	4	6	11	16	21	26	31	36	41	46	51	56
Control	1.2	2.9	4.7	7.1	23.5	31.5	36.5	47.1	52.9	54.4	59.4	65.3	64.7
EAC	0.6	4.7	11.8	46.2	47.1	73.1	94.1						
EAC+Ga Sal.	0.5	1.2	2.3	10.0	9.9	18.4	22.8	27.5	40.4	50.9	63.7	73.4	

% change in body weight of animals = $\frac{w_2 - w_1}{w_1} \times 100$

where w_1 = *average body weight of animal at day one,*
w_2 = *average body weight of animals at another specific day.*
Mice were injected with Ga salicylate on the 2nd, 4th and 6th day post EAC inculation.

ANIMAL SURVIVAL

Survivals of mice in the different groups under investigation were tabulated, continuously, for a period of 45 till the end days and expressed in *table 4*.

Thirty percent of the mice inoculated with EAC and treated with Ga Sal. Survived for 30 days and only 10% survived for 45 days, where as none was cured. Their M.S.T. was 26.5 days.

Table 4. Mean survival time (M.S.T.)

Group	**Survival**			
	M.S.T.	**%M.S.T**	**30 days**	**45 days**
Control			10/10	10/10
EAC	15.4	100%	0/10	0/10
EAC+Ga Sal.	26.5	172%	3/10	1/10

M.S.T. is defined as the sum of survival days of all mice in each group divided by the total number of animals in this group (10 mice).

DISCUSSION

In order to improve the anticancer effects of Gallium (1), the synthesis of a new complex with salicylate has been performed as salicylate salts have also a demonstrated antitumoral effect (2-4). This new Ga compound appears to be active against cancer, but different schedules of treatment need to be tested in order to define the optimal dosages, duration of time and way of administration.

REFERENCES

1. Collery P, Keppler BK, Madoulet S, Desoize B. Gallium in Cancer Treatment. Vol. 42, 2002:283-96.
2. Liu Y EW, Seow-Choen F, Cheah Y. Differential cytostatic effect of sodium salicylate in human colorectal cancers using an individualized histoculture system. Cancer Chemother Pharmacol, Vol. 49, 2002:473-8.
3. Katerinaki E. HJW, Lalla R., Carlson K. E., Yang Y., Hill R. P., Lorigan P. C., Macneil S. Sodium salicylate inhibits TNF-alpha-induced NF-kappaB activation, cell migration, invasion and ICAM-1 expression in human melanoma cells. Melanoma Res. 2006;16:11-22.
4. Li G Fau - Sha Su-Hua SSF-ZE, Zotova E Fau - Arezzo Joseph, Arezzo J Fau - Van de Water Thomas, Van de Water T Fau - Schacht, Jochen, Schacht J. Salicylate protects hearing and kidney function from cisplatin toxicity without compromising its oncolytic action. Lab Invest, Vol. 82, 2002:585-96.

Metal Ions in Biology and Medicine: vol. 9. Eds Maria Carmen Alpoim, Paula Vasconcellos Morais, Maria Amélia Santos, Armando J. Cristóvão, José A. Centeno, Philippe Collery.
John Libbey Eurotext, Paris © 2006 pp. 362-1.

Inhibitory Effects of Cerium (III) Tris (salicylate) Ethanol on Malignant Cell lines and Antitumor Effects in Tumor Bearing Swiss Albino Mice

Abdelfattah M.Badawi[1], Dina A. Ismail[1], Philippe Collery[2], Nadia I. Zakhary[3], Sarah Abdel Raouf[3]

[1]*Applied surfactant laboratory, Egyptian petroleum Research Institute.*
[2]*Service de cancérologie, polyclinique Maymard, 20200 Bastia, France.*
[3]*Cancer Biology Department, NCL, Cairo University.*

INTRODUCTION

Previous studies were carried out to study the effect of organic and inorganic complexes in controlling tumour growth (1, 2).

Cerium (Ce) is a rare earth metal from a lanthionioid group, which acts similarly to gallium as an iron chelating agent. Iron binding agents act as inhibitors of DNA synthesis by blocking animal cells in the G1 phase (3). Ce (IV) Mitoxantrone complex was reported to exhibit a higher lethality to Ehrlich acites (EAC) carcinoma cells than that of free drug and showed stronger inhibition ability on the DNA synthesis of the tumor cell. Thus the Ce (IV) mitoxantrone complex may become a more potent antitumor drug than mitoxantrone itself (4).

Some complexes of cerium (III) and neodymium (III) showed marginal cytotoxic activity against transformed leukemic cell lines (P3 HR1 and THP-1) as compared to the inorganic salts (5, 6).

We synthesized a new Ce compound, a cerium (III) tris (salicylate) ethanol, identified it by elemental analysis (IR, Mass and H1 NMR spectra) and tested its activity on malignant cells in culture and in tumour-bearing animals.

Preparation of Ce Salicylate

Freshly prepared Ce $(OH)_3$ (0.01 moL) was added to salicylic acid (0.05 moL) dissolved in 50 ml of anhydrous ethanol. The suspension was then refluxed on a water bath unit all the cerium hydroxide had been reacted. The resultant white coloured solution was then filtered, and the white crystals were deposited by cooling. These were filtered off, washed with cold alcohol and air dried to yield 3.2 gm of Ce Salicylate.

The structure of the prepared compound was confirmed by:

1. Micro elemental analysis (VARIO EL ELEMENTAR).

2. FTIR Spectra (ATI Mattson Genesis Series FTIRTM).

3. Mass Spectra (Mass Spectro Photomerter HP MODEL GC MS-QPL OOO EX (shimadeu).

4. The H^1NMR Spectra was measured on varian Gemini-200 μH_2 Spectro-Photometer, Laser unit.

The results are expressed in *table 1*.

IR spectra exhibits new absorption bands C-Ce at 635cm^{-1}, C-H (str) at 2919-2851cm^{-1} C-H bending at 1340cm^{-1}, CH_2 at 1450cm^{-1}, C-H Ar at 780 cm^{-1}, C=O at 1703cm^{-1}, O-H Ar at 1310cm^{-1} and O-H at 3590cm^{-1}.

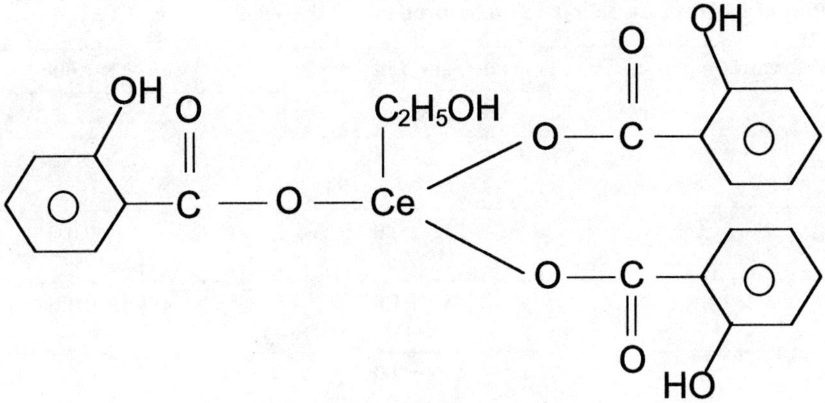

Tri (salicylate) cerium (III) ethanol.

Table 1. Specification of Cerium (III) Tris (Salicylate)

Compound		Micro Analysis %		
		C	H	Ce
Ce. SaL	Calculated	46.23	3.51	23.45
moL. Wt = 597	Found	46.69	3.82	23.85

Effects on malignant cells in culture

The effects of different concentrations of Ce Salicylate on the viability of Ehrlich carcinoma cells (EAC) were studied according to the method of El-Merzabani et al (7) and shown in *table 2*. The concentrations used ranged from 0.8 to 100 mg/ml. The results are expressed as a percentage (mean ± SD of 6 experiments) of non viable cells (% NVC).

The addition of Ce Sal to the culture media of EAC showed a dose dependent cytotoxic effect from. 2% NVC when Ce Salicylate used was 0.8 µg/ml until 88.2% NVC with a concentration of 100 µg Ce Salicylate.

Experimental study in tumor-bearing animals (ascitic tumor)

The antitumour effects of Ce Salicylate were studied using 30 Healthy untreated Female Swiss albino mice weighing 20 g, each were divided into the following groups.

I. Control group.

II. EAC group: Mice were i.p. injected with 2.5×10^6 EAC.

III. EAC + Ce Sal group: Mice were inoculated with 2.5×10^6 EAC and then i.p treated by 100 mg/kg body weight of Ce Salicylate at Days 2, 4 and 6 after the inoculation of tumor cells.

The effects on body weight of EAC bearing mice have been calculated as percent of change in body weight taking the starting day as zero percent.

The results are tabulated in *tables 3, 4*. The untreated tumor bearing animals showed a progressive increase in their total body weight (B.W) reaching 94.1% on the 26th day. The changes in body weights of mice in the groups of EAC+ Ce Salicylate were noted until day 21 as all mice died at the 22nd day.

Table 2. Effect of different Ce Salicylate Concentrations on the Viability of EAC.

Concentration	Cerium Salicylate $\times \pm$ SD•	P-value
0	0	....
0.8	13.2 ± 1.5 (11-15)	< 0.001
1.6	21.3 ± 2.0 (19-24)	< 0.001
3.2	33.3 ± 1.0 (32-35)	< 0.001
6.3	43.3 ± 2.0 (41-46)	< 0.001
12.5	50.0 ± 1.4 (48-52)	< 0.001
25.0	63.0 ± 1.7 (61-65)	< 0.001
50.0	80.0 ± 1.5 (78-82)	< 0.001
100.0	88.2 ± 1.6 (86-90)	< 0.001

Table 3. Percent of Change in Body Weight of Groups of Mice Under Different Treatments

Group \ Day	2	4	6	11	16	21	26	31	36	41	46	51	56
Control	1.2	2.9	4.7	7.1	23.5	31.5	36.5	47.1	52.9	54.4	59.4	56.3	64.7
EAC	0.6	4.7	11.8	46.2	47.1	73.1	94.1						
EAC+ Ce SaL	1.0	2.5	6.5	10.4	30.0	34.3							

% of change in body weight of animals = $\frac{w_2 - w_1}{w_1} \times 100$

where w_1= average body weight of animals at day one w_2 = average body weight of animals at another specific day.

Table 4. Effects of Different Treatments on the percentage of surviving mice and Mean Survival Time (M.S.T) of Mice Under Different Treatments.

Group	% number of surviving mice						Survival			
	3	6	9	12	15	18	M.S.T	% M.S.T	30 days	45 days
Control	2.1	4.7	7.1	5.9	19.1	28.2	100%	100%	10/10	10/10
EAC	2.7	11.8	33.3	51.2	50	51.8	15.4	100%	0/10	0/10
EAC + Ce.SaL	1.8	6.5	10.2	14.2	26.5	32.5	15.8	103%	0/10	0/10

M.S.T is defined as the sum of survival days of all mice in each group divided by the total number of animals in this group (10 mice).

In the group of mice inoculated with EAC and treated with Ce Salicylate, none of them survived till the day 30. Their M.S.T was 15.8 days.

DISCUSSION

It is of interest to search for new agents which act on cells by different mode of action, or those which can modulate the growth rate of tumor and enhance the anticancer activity with the less possible side effects. Ehrlich ascites carcinoma cells, as a model system in this study, was based on the finding that it is an excellent tool for studying the biological behavior of malignant tumors and drug action with the cells (8).

Cerium is a rare earth metal from lanthanoids.Cerium (IV)-mitoxantrone complex exhibits a higher lethality to Ehrlich ascites tumor cells than the free drug and shows stronger inhibition ability on the DNA synthesis of the tumor cells (4). In the present study, EAC cells have been used as an experimental model to evaluate the role of Ce Salicylate as an anticancerous drugs. It was shown that Ce Salicylate showed a cytotoxic effect on EAC cells in culture. The maximum effect observed was 88.2% of NVC at concentration 100 µ/ml. The tumoricidal effect of Ce Salicylate is a dose dependent one. These results agree with those of Xiao et al. (9), who studied that cerium had inhibitory effects on tumor cell growth and that it causes reduction of malignancy. In the present work all mice inoculated with EAC died after 26 days post inoculation, and their M.S.T was 15.4 days. Treating EAC bearing mice with Ce Salicylate did not improve the survival, as all mice died after 22 days only and the M.S.T reached 15.8 days. Treating mice with Ce Salicylate did not change the M.S.T. as compared with EAC treated mice, but it may be due to the schedule of the treatment or to a too low dose.

REFERENCES

1. Osman A.M., Mohommed T.A. and Assem M.M. Effect of ascorbic acid and melphalan on the growth of human melanoma cells in vitro. J. Egypt. Natl. cancer. Inst. 2: 421-425, 1986.
2. El Merzabani M., El-Aser A.A, Osman A.M, Ismail N and Abuel Ela F. Potentation of therapeutic effect of methane-sulphonate and protection against its organ cytotoxicity by vitamin C in Ehrlich Ascites carcinoma bearing mice. J. Pharm. Belg. 44: 877-884, 1989.
3. Ganeshaguru K, Hoffbrand A.V, Grodv R.W and Ceremi A. Effect of various iron chelating agents on DNA synthesis in human cells. Biochem. Pharmacol. 29: 1275-1279, 1980.
4. Wang H, Yang, Tia, Y, Zhang Z and Zhao C. Experimental antitumor achivity of the Ce (IV)-mitoxanxtrone complex and its interaction with deoxyribonucleic acid. J. Inorg. Biochem., 68 (2): 117-121 (1997).
5. Kostova I, Manolov I., Nicolova I., Konstantinov S., Karaivanova M. New lanthanide complexes of 4-methyl-7-hydroxy coumarin and their pharmacological activity. Eur. J. Med. Chem.; 36 339-46, 2001.
6. Manolov I., Kostova I., Netzeva I., Konstantinov S., Karaivanova M. Cytotoxic activity of cerium complexes with coumarin derivatives. Molecular modeling of the ligands. Arch Pharm (weinheim). 333(4): 93-8, 2000.
7. El-Merzaban M.M, El-Aaser A. A. and Attia M.A. Screening system for Egyptian plants with potential antitumor activity. J. Plants Medica. 36: 150-155 (1979).
8. Hamburger A.W. Use of in vitro tests in predictive cancer chemotherapy. J. N. Natl. Cancer. Inst., 66: 981-987, 1981.
9. Xiao B, Ji, Y. and Cui M. Effects of lanthanum and cerium on malignant proliferation and expression of tumor- related gene. Chung. Hug. yu. Fang. I Hsueh. Tsa. Chih., 31 (4): 228-280, 1997.

Metal Ions in Biology and Medicine: vol. 9. Eds Maria Carmen Alpoim, Paula Vasconcellos Morais, Maria Amélia Santos, Armando J. Cristóvão, José A. Centeno, Philippe Collery.
John Libbey Eurotext, Paris © 2006 pp. 366-1.

Thymus, apoptosis and zinc

Lastra MD, Aguilar AE, Munguía N, Saldivar L

School of Chemistry, National University of Mexico
Cd Universitaria, Fac Química, UNAM, México DF, México 04510 lastraa@servidor.unam.mx

INTRODUCTION

Zinc is an essential trace element for humans. Lack of zinc is associated with immunodeficiency conditions that include thymic atrophy and a variety of syndromes affecting particularly T cells response [1, 2, 3, 4]. This is important in perinatal stages when zinc levels are critical in various aspects, particularly in the immune response [5].

It is known that both, lack of zinc, even in marginal deficiencies, as well as zinc excess, cause deleterious effects on various metabolic pathways and particularly, in the immune system.

There is abundant evidence on the actions of zinc supplementation which increases and restores both humoral and cellular immune responses.

OBJECTIVE

In this work we study the effect of *in vivo* zinc supplementation over thymus cells apoptosis in BALB/c mice 21 to 49 days old.

METHODS

The mice received zinc acetate (500 μg/mL) in drinking water administered from the day of mating throughout gestation, lactation and postweaning. Mice were divided into five groups according to age and to Zn administration. Zinc intracellular concentrations were determined by Atomic Absorption Spectrometry (AAS) and apoptosis was assessed by Fluorescence Activated Cell Sorting (FACS).

Cell preparation

Thymus were obtained from BALB/c mice 21 to 49 days old treated with zinc and from controls. Cell suspensions were obtained by gently pressing the thymus through a sieve in RPMI 1640 supplemented medium (Hyclone Utah, USA). The cell suspensions were washed with RPMI by centrifugation (280 g, 5 min, 4°C). The cell pellet was resuspended in 500 μL ammonium solution (0.8 mM EDTA, 15mM NH_4Cl, 0.1 mM $NaHCO_3$, pH 7.4) to eliminate erythrocytes. Finally, the cell pellet was resuspended in 1 mL RPMI. Trypan blue dye exclusion viability test was performed (>95%) (Flow Laboratories Inc, McLean VA USA). The cell suspension was adjusted to 10^7 cell/mL in cold RPMI.

Final RPMI concentration was: fetal bovine serum 10% (Sigma Chem. St. Louis USA), L-glutamine 2mM (Hyclone Road Utah, USA), non essential aminoacids 0.5% (Microlab Mexico), sodium piruvate 0.5%, and penicillin 200U/mL/streptomycin 100 μg/L, respectively.

Apoptosis induction *in vitro*

For the apoptosis induction, 10^6 cells were deposited in RPMI 1 mL with 10^{-7} M dexamethasone (Metax[MR]). Cells were maintained at 37°C in humidified 5% CO_2 environment, during the optimal period according to the induction kinetics of apoptotic cells (4, 6 and 8 hours). At the end of the incubation period apoptotic cells staining was carried out with FITC conjugated Annexin-V.

Apoptotic cells staining with FITC conjugated Annexin-V

For the detection of the apoptotic cells a commercial kit was used (Annexin-V-Fluos Staining, Roche Germany). After incubation with the inducer, 10^6 cells were washed with cold PBS and subsequently centrifuged at 200 g for 5 min, the cellular pellet was resuspended in 100 μL buffer binding solution, Annexin-V-FTC 1 μL and propidium iodide 1 μL were added; cells were incubated for 10 to 15 minutes at room temperature in the dark. The samples were analyzed with a flow cytometer (Becton Dickinson Palo Alto CA ISA) using a CellQuest program version 2.0.

AAS analysis

Cell suspension (20×10^6 cells) samples (1 mL) were digested through a wet-digestion with Suprapur concentrated Nitric Acid 65% (HNO_3 Merck, Darmstadt, Germany), Perhydrol 30% (H_2O_2 Merck, Darmstadt, Germany); the cells were finally taken to a 6 mL volume with deionized water (18 MΩcm Barnstead deionization); reagents blanks were also prepared.

The Zn concentrations were obtained with AAS technique. The detection and quantification limits were quantified [6]. In order to validated the method and results we utilized the NIST (Standard Reference Material, 1577b, bovine liver).

Statistical analysis

ANOVA test was performed for statistical analysis. A *p*-value less than 0.05 was considered significant.

RESULTS

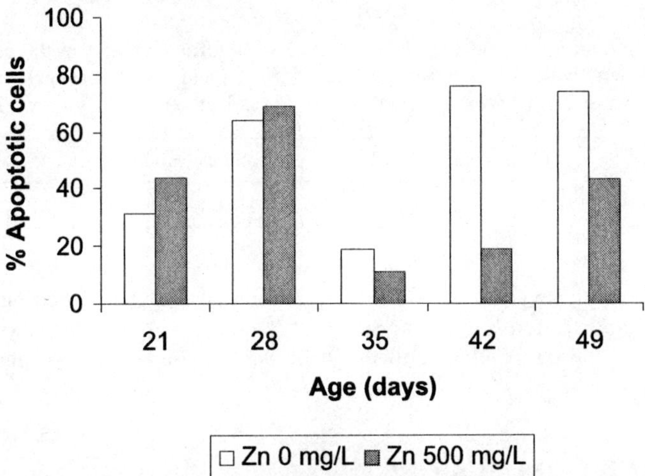

Fig. 1. Effect of Zn supplementation *in vivo* over thymus cells apoptosis in BALB/c mice. Treated mice showed an increase in the apoptotic cells percentage at 21 and 28 days, that became 44.01% and 68.49% respectively; the percentage decreased to 11.05% in mice 35 days old, and to 18.65% and 43.29% in mice 42 and 49 days old, respectively.

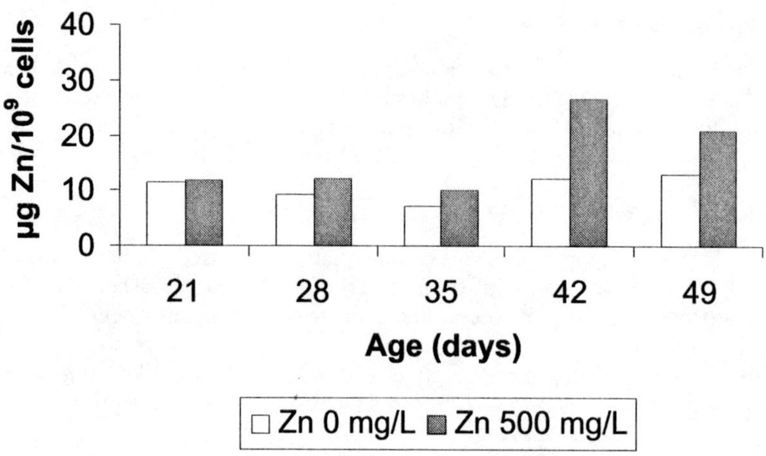

Fig. 2. Zinc intracellular concentrations in thymus cells

Table 1. Zn concentrations in BALB/c mice thymus cells. Zn concentrations increase noticeably in +Zn mice at 42 and 49 days, no important changes were observed in mice 21, 28 and 35 days old.

	-Zn	**+Zn**
Age (days)	**mmol Zn/cell**	**mmol Zn/cell**
21	1.75×10^{-13}	1.8×10^{-13}
28	1.40×10^{-13}	1.86×10^{-13}
35	1.11×10^{-13}	1.52×10^{-13}
42	1.89×10^{-13}	4.05×10^{-13}
49	1.95×10^{-13}	3.2×10^{-13}

Table 2. Values for the standard reference material. The obtained value for the standard reference material is in agreement with the certificated value with a good % of recovery. The detection and quantification limits were 0.011 µg/mL and 0.037 µg/mL respectively.

Element	Certificated Value*	Obtained value	% of recovery
Zn	127 ± 16 µg/g	118 ± 14 µg/g	95.6%

*NIST 1577b

From the methodological viewpoint zinc concentrations data in all analyzed samples were above the detection and quantification limits. The standard reference material values obtained validated the analytical method and the results, confirming the AAS as one of the adequate techniques for these matrix samples.

DISCUSSION AND CONCLUSIONS

There is evidence showing the enhancing capacity of zinc over immune responses during perinatal stages. Rodents moderate zinc deficiency might result in multiple gestational problems including fetus malformations.

Our results suggest that *in vivo* zinc supplementation (500 μg/mL) throughout gestation, lactation and postweaning, delays thymic involution. Thymic involution involves an array of physiological and metabolic changes that result in profound alterations of the immune functions. These phenomena were studied observing thymic cells apoptosis by FACS. One of the findings is the existence of a relationship between the zinc concentration levels and the apoptotic index, particularly in zinc treated mice 35, 42 and 49 days old, where the percentage of apoptotic cells decrease was of 40%, 75% and 40%, respectively. Results showed a clear tendency that relates apoptotic cells number, with zinc intracellular concentration levels.

On view of these findings we conclude that oral zinc supplements should be carefully monitored during perinatal stages.

REFERENCES

1. Chandra RK. Trace elements and immune response. In: Chandra RK, ed. *Trace element in nutrition of children II*, workshop series vol. 23. NY: Nestle Ltd, 1991: 201-214.
2. Li L, Hsu HC, William GE, Stockard CR, Ho KJ, Lott P, Yang PA, Zhang HG and Mountz JD. Cellular mechanism of thymic involution. *Scand J Immunol* 2003; 57: 410-422.
3. Chaplin DD. Overview of the immune response. *J Allergy Clin Immunol* 2003; 111: S442-S459.
4. Gill J, Mail M, Sutherland J, Gray D, Hollander G and Boyd R. Thymic generation and regulation. *Immunol Rev* 2003; 195: 28-50.
5. Lastra MD, Pastelin R, Herrera M, Orihuela VD and Aguilar AE. Increment of immune responses in mice perinatal stages after zinc supplementation. *Arch Med Res* 1997; 28: 67-72.
6. Miller JC y Miller JN. Métodos de calibración en análisis instrumental: regresión y correlación. In: Pearson Educación, ed. *Estadística y Quimiometría para Química Analítica*, 4ª Edición. España: Prentice Hall, 2002: 111-152.

Metal Ions in Biology and Medicine: vol. 9. Eds Maria Carmen Alpoim, Paula Vasconcellos Morais, Maria Amélia Santos, Armando J. Cristóvão, José A. Centeno, Philippe Collery.
John Libbey Eurotext, Paris © 2006 pp. 370-1.

Importance of selenium in iodine deficiency IDD

Melo V., Reyes J., Castrejón E., Salas J., Chavez A.

Metropolitan Autonomous University-Xochimilco. Calzada del Hueso 1100, Edif. Central, 1er piso, Coyoacán, 04960, D.F. México. vmelo@correo.xoc.uam.mx

ABSTRACT

Worldwide, iodine deficiency is one of the most common nutritional disorders, with an estimated 200 million people suffering from goitre, three million from overt cretinism and millions more from intellectual deficit. There is a consensus that near one billion are at risk from living in an environment where iodine has been taking away from soil; this arises by the leaching effects from water and heavy rainfall, which removes iodine from the soil. The lack of iodine in the soil leads to deficiency in all forms of plants and human life, because the continue absence of this metal in diet leads to impaired function of the thyroid gland, and also delay in the growth and severe mental retardation. Selenium element plays an important role in the metabolism of the iodothyronine deiodinase enzyme, which converts the prohormone thyroxine (T_4) to the active form triiodothyronine (T_3). Selenocysteine is also an antioxidant in glutathione peroxidase, which protects the thyroid hormone synthesis. Jumil forest bug consumed in different rural communities of the highlands of Mexico is an insect, which has both metals. The objective of this paper is to analyze iodine and Selenium in Jumil *Atizies taxcoensis* A, captured late January 2006 at Huizteco hill, at Guerrero State, and profile samples of Iodine by titration with thiosulfate and Selenium by Atomic Absorption Spectrophotometer. Data obtained were iodine 0.91 mg/100 g dry basis, and Selenium 55 μg. Jumil insect is temporal available, however, due to its high content in Iodine can be storage without spoilage for more than a year. In conclusion, thyroid disease and severe mental retardation caused by iodine deficiency can be prevented by intake of two or three insects a day.

INTRODUCTION

Iodine is an essential component of the thyroid hormones, which are required for normal calorigenesis, thermoregulation, intermediary metabolism, protein synthesis, reproduction, growth, development, hematopoiesis and neuromuscular function. It is present in small amount in water and plants, and animals such as jumiles, surviving on them [1, 2]. Deficient iodine in soil and water occurs mainly in mountainous regions and in many flood plains [2]. Maternal iodine deficiency causes teratogenic effects in the offspring, referred to as endemic cretinism, with symptoms of dwarfism, hypothyroidism, neuromuscular disturbances, increased embryonic and postnatal mortality, deafness, mental retardation and impaired fertility, all of these affects economic productivity among other important social consequences [3, 4]. Thyroid disease is presented at long-standing iodine deficiency that induces thyroid enlargement and nodule formation that sometimes become permanently, independent of normal control. Jumil forest bug can be found in many states of Mexico and is consumed by population since ancient times [5, 6].

Inorganic soil selenium is utilized by plants for the synthesis of selenomethionine, which is incorporated into plants proteins. When humans and animals consume these proteins, the selenomethionine released in digestion is used non-specifically for the synthesis of tissue proteins. Human and animals also convert selenomethionine to selenocysteine, which is incorporated selectively into enzyme glutathione peroxidase. Proteins that include a selenocysteine residue are called selenoproteins. The objective of this paper is to analyze the importance of selenium in iodine deficiency, iodine absorption and disseminate its consumption in areas where there are deficiencies of this element.

MATERIALS AND METHODS

Jumil forest bugs adults, emerge in autumn, winter and spring, in different habitats wherever there is a shelter, food and suitable nearby sites. Guerrero state was monitored to evaluate available resources of the jumil as well as time for collection. Insects were found since October to May, among the fallen leaves or under the rocks. Samples gathered were kept in a glass container labelled and taken to laboratory to determine nomenclature and metal analysis [2, 7]. Moisture content was measured by drying samples in an oven at 60° C for 24 hrs. Samples were powdered separately in a Willey Mill to 60 mesh size, organic matter destroyed by incineration at 600° C in a muffle furnace and ashes dissolved in dilute HCl. All minerals except iodine and phosphorus were analysed by Atomic Absorption Spectrophotometer. Phosphorus content in the triple acid digested extract and determined colorimetrically. Iodine: liberation of free iodine from insects' powder by addition of H_2SO_4, excess of KI is added to help solubilize the free iodine, and then titrated with thiosulfate. In the titration step, Iodine from insects is consumed by sodium thiosulfate [8, 9, 10].

RESULTS

Table 1. Insects *Atizies taxcoensis* A, year availability.

Season	Winter			Spring			Summer			Autumm		
Months	J	F	M	A	M	J	J	A	S	O	N	D
Atizies taxcoensis A	X	X	X	X	-	-	-	-	-	X	X	X

Table 2. Nomenclature of *Atizies taxcoensis* A

Class	Insecta
Order	Hemiptera
Family	Pentatomidae
Genus	*Atizies*
Specie	*taxcoensis* A
Generic name	Jumil

Morón, M. A., Terrón, R. 1980 [2].

Table 3. Dietetic requirements for Iodine and Selenium elements by RDA and content in Jumiles

Gender/Age	RDA Iodine	Iodine/jumil	RDA Selenium	Selenium/jumil
Males/25-50	120 µg	0.91 mg/100g	40 µg	55 µg
Females/25-50	150 µg		70 µg	

RDA Recommended Dietary Allowance [17].

Table 4. Iodine and Selenium composition of Jumil *Atizies taxcoensis* A in dry basis

Insect	Iodine	Selenium
Atizies taxcoensis A	0.91 mg/100g	55 µg

Assessment of Iodine by thiosulfate titration and Selenium by Atomic Absorption Spectrophotometer [8, 9, 10].

DISCUSSION AND CONCLUSION

Jumil insect can be found almost all year round, mainly in mountainous regions, among dead leaves on soil biomass *(table 1)*. It is easy to collect manually; they are very low in moisture (26%), which means that contents are concentrated [1]. Iodine deficiency is a severe global problem with an estimated population of one billion at risk, because they live in environment where the soil has been deprived from iodine. Iodine disorders are among the most common of humankind [11]. One of these clinical forms is cretinism, when the mother is limited in her own production of thyroid hormone by insufficient iodine ingest. The effect begins in early fetal life and becomes most apparent later, when the neonate may be permanently impaired, especially with regard to neuromuscular and cognitive attainment. Also, a reduced iodine supply produces a compensatory increase in iodine clearance by the gland mediated by increased secretion of thyroid stimulating hormone (TSH), consequently grow of the thyroid goitre occurs and can readily be detected; goitre may obstruct the trachea and oesophagus. Activation and metabolism of thyroid hormone requires of three seleno-enzymes, the iodothyronine deiodinases [12, 13]. This in liver is the major enzyme that converts T_4 to triiodothyronine T_3, and is responsible for most circulating plasma T_3 levels. In selenium deficiency, decreased DII activity results in lower T_3 levels. Selenium dependent deiodinases are also found in specialized tissues, such as brain, pituitary, brown adipose tissue and skin. Its principal physiologic role is for local intracellular production of T_3. In conclusion, thyroid hormone is essential to development, the main secretory product of the thyroid gland, thyroxin T_4, it is converted to the principal metabolically active, species triiodothyronine T_3 and seleno-enzymes are essential in this process. Jumil insect has both iodine and selenium, therefore consumption of it can provide both elements to prevent these metals deficiency [16, 17].

REFERENCES

1. Ancona, H.L. 1932. Los jumiles de Taxco. Tomo IV, Número 2, Instituto de Biología, UNAM. México.
2. Morón, M.A., Terrón, R. 1980. Entomología Práctica. Instituto de Ecología, A. C., Mexico.
3. Reyes, J.J. et al 2005. Elementos Químicos Esenciales para el Organismo. Universidad Autónoma Metropolitana, Mexico.
4. Melo, V., Chavez, A., Chavez, M. 2004. *Atizies taxcoensis* A and *Euchistus sufultus* S, Jumil bugs: Nutraceutic Foodstuff for Iodine deficiency. Collery, Ph. Ed. In chief. Metal Ions in Biology and Medicine. Editions John Libbely Eurotext. France.
5. Menzel, P., D'Alusio, F. 1998. Man Eating Bugs. Ed. Ten Speed Press (Material World Books), Berkeley, CA, USA.
6. Simmons, P.L. 2001. The Curiosities of Food. Ed. Ten Speed Press, Berkeley, CA, USA.
7. Ross, H. 1982. Introducción a la Entomología General y Aplicada. Ed. Omega, España.
8. AOAC. 1995. Official Methods of Analysis. 16th Ed. Association of Official Analytical Chemists, Washington, D. C.
9. Nielsen, S.S. (editor) 1994. Introduction to the Chemical Analysis of Foods. Ed. Jones and Bartlet Publishers International, London, UK.
10. Osborne, D.R., Voogt, P. 1978. The Analysis of Nutrients in Food. Ed. Academic Press Inc., London, UK.
11. Arthur, J.R., Beckett, G.J., Mitchell, J.H. 1999. The interactions between selenium and iodine deficiencies in man and animals. Nutr. Res Rev 12:55-73.

12. St. Germain, D.L., Galton, V.A. 1979. The deiodinase family of selenoproteins. Thyroid 7:655-68.
13. Berry, M.J., Banu, L., Larsen, P.R. 1991. Type 1 iodothyronine doiodinase is a selenocysteine containing enzyme. Nature 349:438-40.
14. Stanbury, J.B., Dun, J.T. 2001. Iodine and iodine defiency disorders. Brown, B. A. Russell, R.M. Eds. ILSI Press. Washington, D.C. USA.
15. Sounde, R.A. 2001. Selenium. Brown, B. A. Russell, R.M. Eds. ILSI Press. Washington, D.C. USA.
16. De Mayer, E. M., Lowenstein, F.W., Thilly, C.H. 1997. The Control of Endemic Goitre. World Health Organization, Geneva, Switzerland.
17. Recommended Dietary Allowances. 1989. National Academic Press, 10th. Edition. Washington, D.C. USA.

Metal Ions in Biology and Medicine: vol. 9. Eds Maria Carmen Alpoim, Paula Vasconcellos Morais, Maria Amélia Santos, Armando J. Cristóvão, José A. Centeno, Philippe Collery.
John Libbey Eurotext, Paris © 2006 pp. 374-1.

Synergistic Effect of Cisplatin and cis-Rhenium(III) Diadamantate on Tumor Growth

Shtemenko Natalia[1], Collery Philippe[2], Shtemenko Alexander[3]

[1]*Dnepropetrovsk National University, 13, Naukoviy by-street, 49050, Dnepropetrovsk, Ukraine ;*
[2]*Service de Cancérologie - Polyclinique Maymard - 20200 Bastia, France ;*
[3]*Ukrainian State Chemical-Technological University, 8, Gagarin avenue, 49005 Dnepropetrovsk, Ukraine*

ABSTRACT

Previous investigations of cluster rhenium compounds made possibility to expect their antitumor properties being revealed in two kinds of experiments: a) with use of substances with cis-configuration of perfect ligands alone; b) with use of rhenium substances together with well-known cytostatics. Both these directions are represented in this work. The aim of the work is to investigate anticancer properties of cis-Rhenium(III) Diadamantate chloride alone and together with cisplatin to find possible synergism. Cisplatin and cis-$[Re_2(AdCOO)_2Cl_4]\cdot 2CH_3CN$ - (Re2), where AdCOO-adamantanecarbonic acid residues, have been tested in the model of rat's specific Guerink (T8) carcinoma. Cluster rhénium compound with adamantanecarboxylic residues and chlorine as ligands (cis-isomer) enhanced the cisplatin action on tumor growth. Together with synergistic effect with cisplatin, the rhenium substance led to increase of quantities of normal forms of RBC during process of tumor growth and prevention.

Key words : Cluster rhenium compound, adamantane ligand, cisplatin, carcinoma Guerink, red blood cells, hemoglobine.

INTRODUCTION

Cluster rhenium compounds with adamantanecarboxylic residues as ligands were synthesized [1] and their structure and chemical properties were studied [2]. These compounds belong to low-soluble in water ones and require liposome forms [3, 4] to be involved in biochemical trials. In these works it was shown that cluster rhenium substances interacted with artificial and natural membranes, some of them displayed themselves as stabilizers of erythrocytic membranes against acidic hemolysis. Especially important observation was made that biological activity of cis-isomers were higher than That of trans-isomers (the analogy with platinides) and chlorine complexes showed more efficiency than bromine ones. In this range of substances the adamantanecarboxylic derivatives are very interesting as adamantane - a frame, steroid-analogical radical has its own biological activity [5]. As anticancer effects of some dirhenium carboxylates were shown and assumed [6, 7] it is reasonable to suppose that antioxidant and all above described properties of cluster rhenium compounds, their low toxicity may have an affect on suppression of tumor growth in two kinds of experiments: a) with use of substances with cis-configuration of perfect ligands alone; b) with use of rhenium substances together with well-known cytostatics. Both these directions are represented in our work.

The aim of the work is to investigate anticancer properties of cis-Rhenium(III) Diadamantate chloride alone and together with cisplatin to find possible synergism.

MATERIALS AND METHODS

Cisplatin and cluster rhenium compound with organic ligand with formula:

cis-$[Re_2(AdCOO)_2Cl_4]\cdot 2CH_3CN$ - (Re2), synthesized according to procedure described in [1], where AdCOO- adamantanecarbonic acid residues, have been tested.

Wistar rats weighting 100-120 g were inoculated by tumor carcinoma Guerink (T8) cells. The cells were taken in the Institute of Oncology and Experimental Pathology by R.E. Kavetskiy (Kiev). The single intraperitoneal administration of Cisplatin at the dose of 8 mg/kg was made on the 9 day after the tumor inoculation according to [8]. The intraperitoneal administration of the Re2 at the dose of 7 μM/kg according to the scheme of antioxidant therapy [9] in liposome forms [4] began on the 3 day after the inoculation of the tumor cells and was repeated every 2 days until day 21. Body weights were measured from day 2 after tumor inoculation, the volume of tumors were assessed from the day 7. On the day 21 animals were sacrified under chlorophormium anesthesia and the tumors were isolated and weighted. Concentrations of hemoglobine (Hb) and quantity of red blood cells (RBC) were measured [10].

Four groups of 15 animals in each were compared: control group; group with introduction of cisplatin; group with introduction of Re2; and group with introduction of cisplatin together with Re2. Wilcoxon non parametric tests were used to compare the tumor volumes according to the absence of treatment and each group of treatment or between 2 treated groups.

RESULTS AND DISCUSSION

Growth of the tumors in control group was very rapid and reached 146000 mm cub and occupied approximately 1/3 of the animal weight. Dynamics of tumor growth is represented on the *figure 1*.

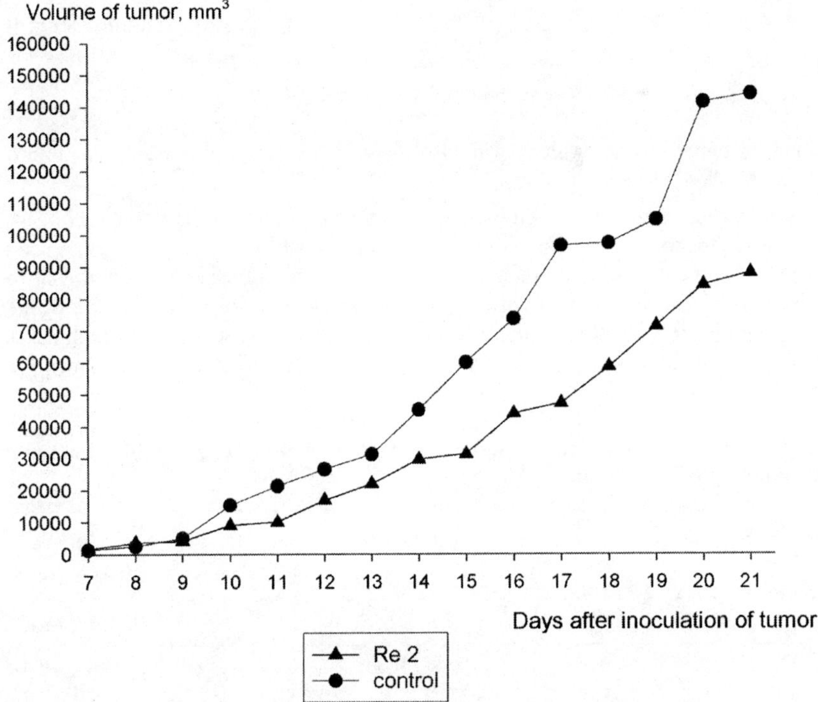

Fig. 1. Dynamics of tumor growth in control group and in group with Re2 treatment.

The treatments by Re2 alone did not prevent tumor growth but caused a little delay in progression of growth.

A significant decrease in measured tumor volumes was shown in cisplatin and cisplatin plus Re2 treated groups of animals *(fig. 2)* in comparison to control group.

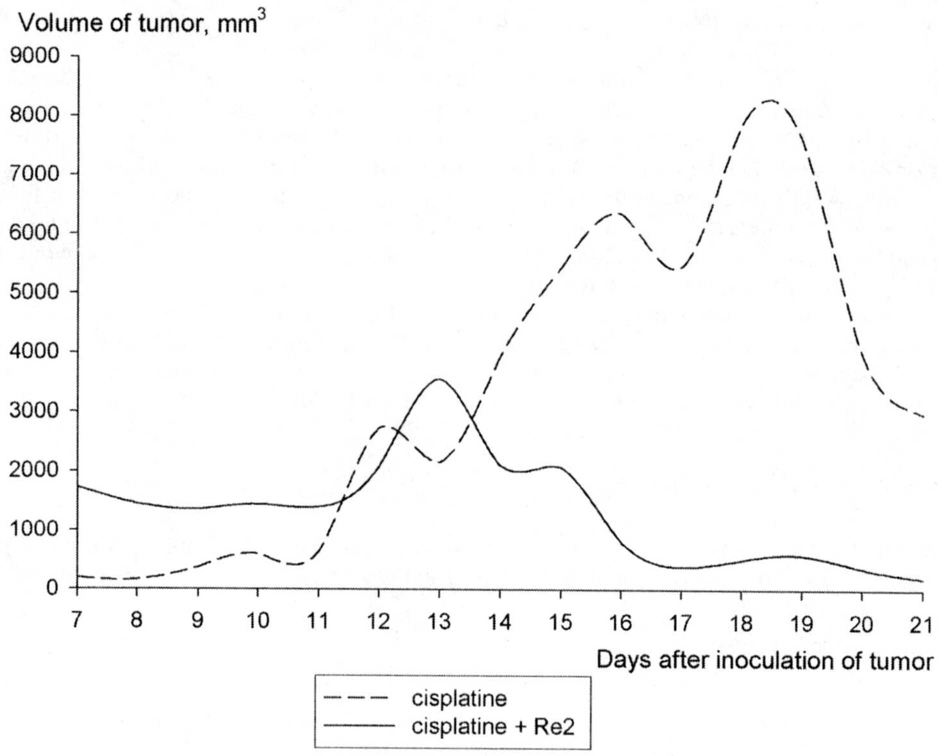

Fig. 2. Dynamics of tumor growth in group with cisplatin and in group with cisplatin plus Re2 treatment.

Especially little sizes of measured volumes of tumors were found on the last stages of these experiments. If compare influence of cisplatin and Re2 on tumor growth, we see a great difference in the area 15-20 days of development of tumor. Also, at the last day 21 the decrease was significant for rhenium group combined with cisplatin in comparison to the treatment by cisplatin alone. Taking into account practically absence of effect for Re2 alone, we may establish synergistic action of both substances.

Weight of isolated tumors and Hb levels in average were the same as in control group as in group treated by Re2 *(table 1)*.

Table 1. Weight of isolated tumors (m, g) and concentration of Hb (Hb, g/l) in blood of animals on the 21 day after tumor cells inoculation

Group	m, g	Hb, g/l
control	44,87 ± 25,19	89,86 ± 10,36
Re2	38,27 ± 16,77	72,02 ± 11,12
cisplatin	9,88 ± 9,90	129,49 ± 12,43
cisplatin + Re2	3,92 ± 2,55	95,75 ± 9,04

Small isolated tumors were found in both next groups, especially under synergistic effect of cisplatin and Re2. There was a significant increase in hemoglobin in cisplatin and cisplatin with Re treated groups of animals in comparison to control group. This may be explained by the efficacy in tumor growth prevention. The rhenium compounds did not significantly modify the hemoglobin values in comparison to the administration of cisplatin alone, but there are additional experimental data, presented in *table 2*, which showed that level of Hb is not the only parameter that may appreciate anemic state of an organism.

Table 2. Morphological forms of RBC in blood of animals on the 21 day after tumor cells inoculation, %

Group	Discocites	Echinocites	Damaged RBC
normal	65,00 ± 6,12	23,30 ± 3,12	11,70 ± 2,16
control	8,47 ± 1,88	52,57 ± 3,66	58,96 ± 4,54
Re2	56,33 ± 4,32	22,14 ± 2,16	21,53 ± 2,34
cisplatin	46,36 ± 3,18	24,99 ± 3,84	28,65 ± 3,98
cisplatin + Re2	60,67 ± 5,54	30,18 ± 4,08	9,15 ± 2,08

Development of malignancy led to morphological shift to the side of damaged forms of RBC and reversible forms - echinocites. You see, introduction of Re2 supported quantities of discocites and ehinocites on a rather high level, nevertheless did not prevent tumor growth. And in the experiment with cisplatin introduction of rhenium substance led to practically normal morphological picture of RBC, even to reduction of quantities of damaged cells.

Presented data concerning normalization of antianemic state by rhenium substances were not surprising as close results have been obtained in the experiments with chemically induced hemolytic anemia [3], where such properties of cluster rhenium compounds were explained by a quadrupol Re-Re bond in the structure of such substances, which may work as a trap for free radicals. In this work we have shown that together with synergistic effect on tumor growth with cisplatin, a rhenium substance supported normal state of RBC that is very important during development of malignancy.

CONCLUSIONS

Cluster rhénium compound with adamantanecarboxylic residues and chlorine as ligands (cis-isomer) enhanced the cisplatin action on tumor growth. Together with synergistic effect with cisplatin, the rhenium substance led to increase of quantities of normal forms of RBC during process of tumor growth and prevention.

REFERENCES

1. Golichenko A.A., Shtemenko A.V. Synthesis and Properties of Binuclear Cluster Rhenium(III) Compounds with Adamantanecarboxylic Acids. Russ. Journal of Coord. Chemistry 2006; 32, N4: 237-46.
2. Shtemenko A.V., Golichenko A.A., Domasevitch K.V. Synthesis of Novel Tetracarboxylato Dirhenium(III) Compounds and Crystal Structure of them. Z. Naturforsch 2002; 56b: 381-5.
3. Shtemenko AV, Shtemenko N.I, Oliynik SA, Zelenuk MA. Lyposome forms of rhenium cluster compounds in models of Haemolytic anemia. In Metal Ions in Biology and Medicine. Eds. Khassanova LK, Collery P, Maymard I, Khassanova Z, Etienne JC. John Libbey Eurotext, Paris 2002; 7: 558-61.

4. Shtemenko A.V., Zelenuk M.A., Shtemenko N.I., Verbytska Ya.S. Spectrophotometric investigation of interaction rhenium complex compounds with phosphatydilholine under the liposomes obtained. Ukr. Biokhim. Journal (Ukr) 2002; 74, n° 6: 38-43.
5. Spasov A.A., Hamidova T.V., Bugaeva L.I., Morosov I.S. Pharmacological and toxicological properties of adamantine derivatives (issue) Chemical-Pharmacological Journal (Rus) 1999; 34, n° 1: 3-9.
6. Eastland G.W., Yang G., Thompson T. Studies of Rhenium Carboxylates as Antitumor Agents. Part II. Antitumor Studies of Bis(μ-Propionato) Diaquotetrabromodirhenium(III) in Tumor-Bearing Mice. Meth and Find Exptl Clin Pharmacol 1983; 5, N7: 435-8.
7. Collery P., Shtemenko N., Shtemenko A., Bourleaud M., Etienne J.C., Maymard I., Loriquet P. Supplementation by rhenium compounds instead of iron compounds during the treatment by erythropoeitin of anemia in cancer patients. In: Metal Ions in Biology and Medicine John Libbey Eurotext Paris 2004; 8: 534-7.
8. Taylor S.K. Is recombinant human erythropoietin (rh-epo) more than just a treatment of anemia in cancer and chemotherapy? Medical Hypothesis 2003; 60, n° 1: 89-93.
9. Meerson F.Z., Evstigneeva M.E., Ustinova E.E. Effect of chronic haemolytic anemia on heart contractile function and increase of its resistance to hipoxia. *Pat. Physiol. and Exp. Therap.(Rus)* 1983; N5: 25-9.
10. Chevary C., Andyal T., Shtrenger Y. Measurement of antioxidant parameters of blood and their diagnostic significance in adult patients. Laboratornoe delo (Rus) 1991; n° 10: 9-13.

Toxicology

Metal Ions in Biology and Medicine: vol. 9. Eds Maria Carmen Alpoim, Paula Vasconcellos Morais, Maria Amélia Santos, Armando J. Cristóvão, José A. Centeno, Philippe Collery.
John Libbey Eurotext, Paris © 2006 pp. 381-1.

Characterization of Metal Bound to Thiol Endogenous Ligands in the Liver of Rats Exposed to Methylmercury and Co-Exposed to Selenomethionine

C.M.L. Carvalho[1], Z. Pedrero[2], A.P.M. Santos[1], M.L. Mateus[1], Y. Madrid[2], C. Cámara[2] and M.C.C. Batoréu[1]

[1]*Centro de Estudos de Ciências Farmacêuticas, Faculdade de Farmácia, Universidade de Lisboa, Portugal (Cristina.Carvalho@ff.ul.pt)*
[2]*Facultad Ciencias Quimicas, Universidad Complutense de Madrid, Espana*

INTRODUCTION

The two major elements under study are very distinct as mercury (Hg) is a toxic heavy metal and selenium (Se) is an essential trace element that becomes toxic at higher doses.

It has been established that the toxicity of mercury is mainly due to its ability to form stable complexes with the sulfhydryl cysteine groups of proteins and non-protein thiols, causing subsequent alterations in enzyme functions. The consequences are the increase in reactive oxygen species (ROS) and oxidative stress induction leading to cellular and organ injury.

Many studies related to Hg toxicity have been performed in the brain or in the kidney, however, the liver is the main organ involved in detoxification and the hepatic function should be implicated in the incorporation and transportation of this element to the target organs.

The liver is also considered the central organ of selenium metabolism. Most ingested selenium enters specific metabolism pathways after the uptake from the portal vein blood or removal from selenomethionine (SeMet) via the transsulfuration pathway, being this Se used for the synthesis of selenoproteins or excreted in urine in the form of metabolites. The selenoproteins that are synthetized by the liver include selenoenzymes that support liver function and Selenoprotein P that is released to the blood.

The selenoenzymes include glutathione peroxidase (GSHPx), glutathione reductase (GSH reductase) and thioredoxin reductases (TRs). Thioredoxin reductases such as TR1 (cytosol TR), thioredoxin glutathione reductase (TGR) and TR3 (mitochondrial TR) have been proven to exist in humans and animal models such as the rat and are responsible for the reduction of the active site disulfide in oxidized thioredoxin (protein thiol redox regulation); thioredoxin is approximately 500-fold more effective as a reducing substrate than GSH (Burk and Hill, 2005).

TGR is a selenoprotein oxidoreductse with specificity for thioredoxin and GSH systems (Sun et al., 2005) and exhibits also broad substrate specificity. Expression of TGR has been proven to be regulated by both selenium and tRNA status in liver. TR1 and TR3 were shown to have high priority for selenium supply, in comparison to stress-related selenoproteins such as GSHPx (Sun et al., 2005).

Selenium protective effects against mercury toxicity have been subject of discussion being the available results still controversial. In this process selenoproteins and glutathione anti-oxidant systems might play a key role in the cellular protection against pro-oxidants and this work aims to contribute for its understanding in relation to methylmercury (MeHg) toxicity.

MATERIALS AND METHODS

In Vivo Study and Experimental Design

Twenty-four male Wistar rats (150-175g) supplied by Charles River Laboratories were kept for 1 week acclimatization period with food and water ad libido. After that they were divided in groups and were i.p. exposed during 2 weeks to 5 doses of 1.5 mg/Kg methylmercury hydroxide (MeHg) (G1), to 2 doses 1.5 mg/Kg MeHg (G2), to 2 doses of 1 mg/Kg selenomethionine from Sigma (SeMet) (G3) and co-exposed to 2 doses 1.5 mg/Kg MeHg and 2 doses of 1 mg/Kg SeMet (G4). Non-exposed rats were used as control (G5). On day 32 of the experiment (12 days after the last exposure) animals were sacrificed and livers were removed and kept at -20°C.

Methylmercury hydroxide was supplied by Alfa Aesar (Johnson Mattey, Germany) and seleno -DL-methionine by Sigma (Portugal).

Determination of Glutathione

To determine the GSH content, 0.5g of rat liver were homogenized with 4.5 ml 0.1M phosphate buffer at pH 7.4. To each homogenate were added 4.5 ml of 4% sulphosalicilic acid followed by vortex mixing and centrifugation for 10 min at 2500 rpm. To 0.5 ml of the supernatant was added 0.05 ml DTNB (5,5-dithiobis-2-nitrobenzoic acid) and 4.5 ml 0.1M phosphate buffer pH 7.4 with vortex mixing; the absorbance at 412 nm was read after 2 min against blank solution of reactants. A standard calibration curve was prepared with 98% GSH solution from Sigma.

Mercury Quantification

Dried liver samples (~100 mg) were digested with 3mL of HNO_3 (65%) and 1mL of H_2O_2 (35%) from Panreac in an analytical microwave oven (CEM, 1000W MSP, Mattheus, NC, USA) with double-walled advanced composite vessels.

The total Hg concentration was determined by external calibration of the signal obtained by the continuous Hg cold vapor system connected to atomic fluorescence spectrometer, AFS (Merlin 10.023, P.S. Analytical Ltd.,UK) for 5 standard solutions.

To extract the inorganic mercury, approximately 100mg of samples were treated with 5ml HCl 5M and then, sonicated for 15 min before being centrifuged for 10 min at 3500 rpm. The liquid phase was separated and diluted to 10ml before analysis by CV-AFS. The difference between the total amount of mercury and the inorganic form is assumed to correspond to the MeHg stored in liver.

Total Selenium Quantification

Dried digested samples as described in (3) were filtered and analyzed by ICP-MS for total selenium quantification. An inductively coupled plasma mass spectrometer (ICP) (HP-4500 Plus, Tokyo, Japan) was used as detector after the separation was performed by an HPLC pump (Milton Roy CM4000). Samples and standards for calibration were all analyzed in triplicate.

Selenium speciation

Samples for Se speciation were weighed in duplicate (100mg) with 20 mg protease type XIV from *Streptomyces griseus* (Sigma) and were added 3 ml 25mM Tris/HCl and 0.1M KCl pH 7.5. Digestion of samples was performed using a focalized sonicator (Bandelin Sonoplus) for 120s with 20% of potency. The solutions were then centrifuged for 20 min with 7500 rpm at 20°C.

An inductively coupled plasma mass spectrometer (ICP) (HP-4500 Plus, Tokyo, Japan) was used as detector after the separation was performed by an HPLC pump (Milton Roy CM4000). The analytical peaks obtained were evaluated in terms of peak area by the standard additions method at m/z 82.

Determination of elemental/protein fractions using SEC

To attain the elemental/protein profile 0.5g of liver samples were added 3ml of 25mM Tris+0.1M KCl at pH 7.5 and homogenized in an ice bath. Homogenates were centrifuged for 30min at 4°C using 14,000 rev/min. The supernatant was decanted and filtrated through 0.22 μm nylon filters. The samples were then kept in ice till chromatographic analysis by ICP-MS with an HP 4500 Plus and HPLC-UV (at 280 and 250 nm using spectrometer 5000 DAD LDC Analytical) for protein profile determination. Mobile phase with 25mM Tris and 0.05 mM KCl was set at pH 6.8 with HCl. Both analytical processes were carried out using a molecular size exclusion column Biosep-Sec-S 2000 from Phenomenex with 300×7.80 mm allowing identification of species in the range 1-300 kD. Calibration of this column with standards led to the following relation between retention time and molecular weight: $\log(MW) = (-0.4773)\, t_R + 5.5112$.

The distribution of Hg, Se and other relevant elements such as Cr, Mn, Fe, Co, Cu, Zn, As, Cd, Pb, S, Mo and Ni in association to proteins was investigated.

RESULTS AND DISCUSSION

The hepatic glutathione (GSH) content was evaluated at the sacrifice of animals *(table 1)*. The detrimental effects of MeHg in the liver are evidenced by the depletion of GSH with G1 presenting 78% and G2 88% of the GSH control content two weeks after the last MeHg administration.

Total Hg accumulated in a dose-dependent manner in the liver and was not detected either by CV-AFS or by ICP-MS analysis in the non-exposed MeHg groups.

Table 1. Hepatic GSH content in the different groups of Wistar rats.

	GSH content (μmol/g liver)	STD	N	% of control
Control (G5)	8.51	0.441	5	100
5 MeHg (G1)	6.62	0.951	4	77.8
2 MeHg (G2)	7.47	0.875	4	87.7
2 SeMet (G3)	7.67	1.09	3	90.1
2 MeHg+2SeMet (G4)	7.69	0.667	5	90.4

Fig. 1 shows that concentrations of Hg in liver 12 days after the last exposure are still high; G1 presented 15.8mg/kg and G2 6mg/kg (slightly above G4). This indicates that MeHg accumulates in liver. The quantification of inorganic Hg was carried out being the values between 0.9-1.8% in G1 and below the detection limit for the other groups. Thus, 98% of the mercury in liver is MeHg.

Total selenium quantification was carried out by ICP-MS and no significant differences were noticed *(fig. 2)* among the different groups, although the groups administered with SeMet displayed higher average values.

Speciation of selenium was also carried out and the only identified species were selenocysteine (SeCys) and SeMet, with SeCys representing 80-87% of total. Besides the area of peaks there were no significant changes in chromatograms and *fig. 3* shows the result obtained for the control group. Quantification results of the two species are displayed in *fig. 4 and 5*.

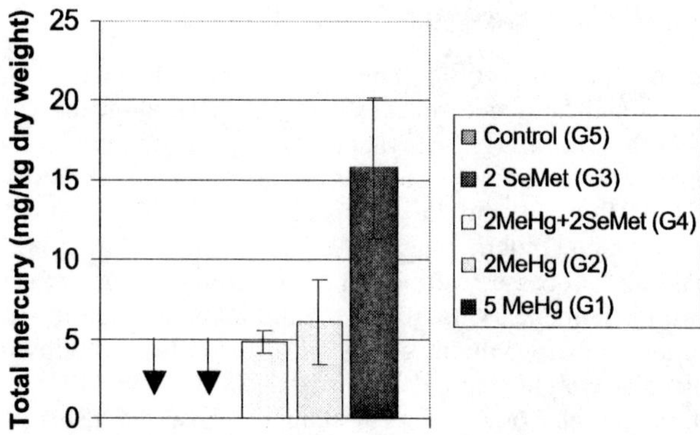

Fig. 1. Total mercury concentration determined in liver using CV-AFS.

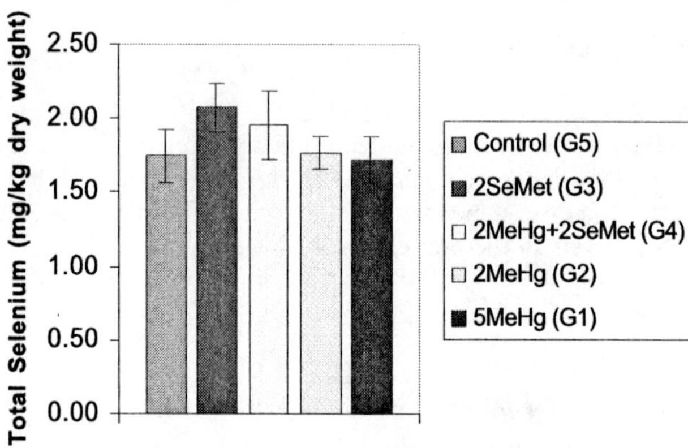

Fig. 2. Total selenium concentration determined in liver by ICP-MS.

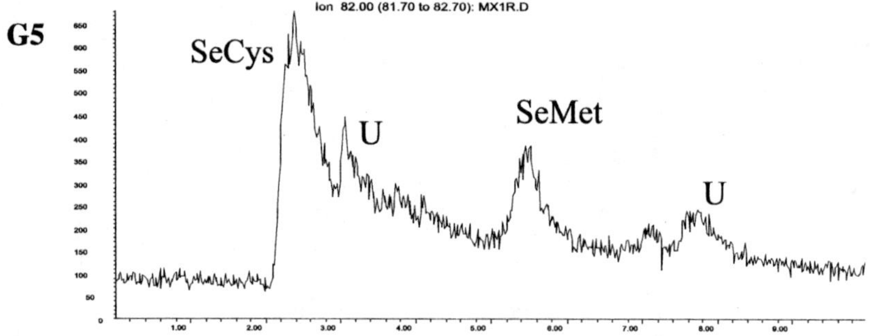

Fig. 3. Chromatogram obtained for the selenium speciation in liver samples of the control group (G5). U represents the non-identified species.

The main variations occur in SeMet concentration *(fig. 4)* with the groups exposed (G1 and G2) or co-exposed (G4) to MeHg presenting a decrease in its content when compared with G5 and G3, respectively. Possible interpretations of these results include: 1) the presence of Se in the form of SeMet promotes the synthesis of selenoenzymes to hinder the detrimental effects of MeHg and increases SeMet consumption; 2) MeHg interacts with the selenol derived from the SeMet and accelerates the rate of conversion of SeMet decreasing its concentration. Previous works support these hypotheses.

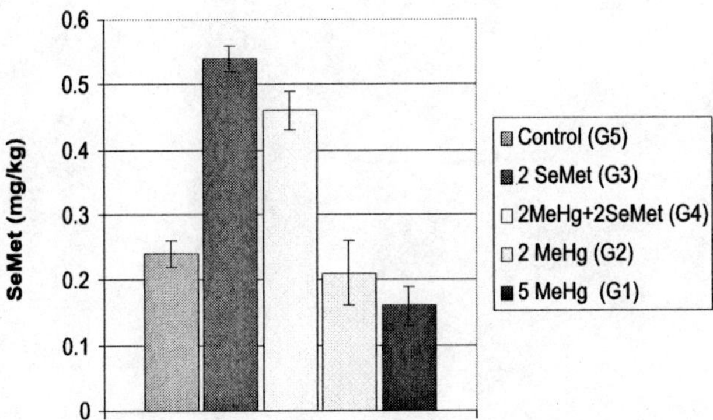

Fig. 4. Concentration of SeMet in the liver obtained by speciation analysis of dried samples by ICP-MS.

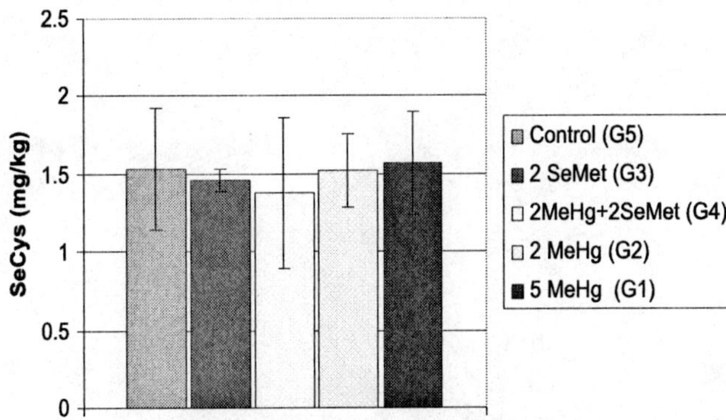

Fig. 5. Concentration of SeCys in the liver obtained by speciation analysis of dried samples by ICP-MS.

The increase of hepatic Se concentration leads to Se induction of detoxificant enzymes such as GSHPx increase in aquatic birds (Hoffman, 2002). On the other hand there are reports that SeMet reacts with MeHg removing it partly (Seppanen et al., 1998).

The proteins profiles attained with SEC and UV detection were similar with protein peaks overlapping. The typical profile is the first chromatogram displayed in *figs 6-9*.

Among the elements studied the patterns of distribution associated with peptide/proteins association changed in some of the experiment groups for sulphur (S), zinc (Zn), Hg and Se.

The distribution of S with the MW of proteins *(fig. 6)* indicates a complex whole of three adjacent peaks that possibly includes the cellular proteins (200-300kD), selenoproteins and selenoenzymes (~50-60kD), and a group of smaller MW proteins 25-13kD that comprises thioredoxin (12kD) and enzymes such as GSHPx (22.2kD), GSH transferase (25.6kD), methionine sulfoxide reductase (19kD) and superoxide dismutase (15.8kD) among others. Small peaks were noticed at 3.5-5.5 kD, which might be metallotioneins.

However, the main difference in S distribution among the different animal groups was for a peak correspondent to a very small MW between 0.6-1.5kD.

This peak is in the limit of SEC column applicability and the MW can not be expressed with more precision. It is displayed by all the groups but increases when there is exposure to MeHg especially in G1 (5 doses). Interestingly, the co-exposed G4 contains more of this low MW specie(s) than G2 that was exposed to the same doses of MeHg.

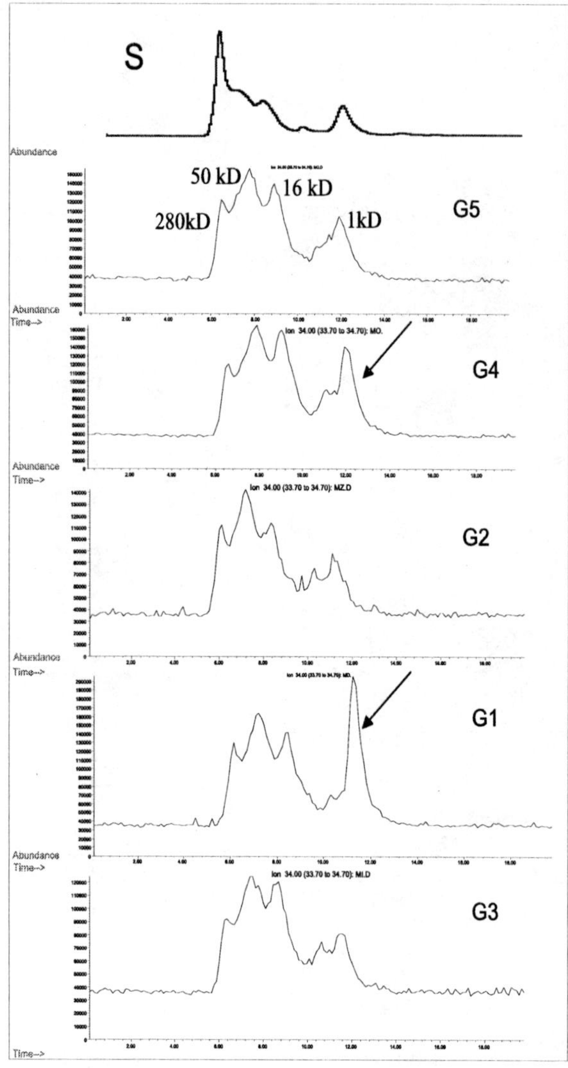

Fig. 6. Chromatograms obtained by ICP-MS for sulphur fractions.

This ≤ 1kD peak can be attributed to GSH (0.3 kD) and to oxiglutathione (GSSG) (MW 0.61 kD), the dominance being to GSSG in G1-G4 since a depletion of GSH was noticed *(table 1)*.

The glutathione conjugates such as CH_3Hg-SG complex (MW 0.49kD), catalysed by GSH-S-transferase, might have been formed in the cytosol of hepatocytes but once formed they are promptly excreted from cells, therefore 2 weeks after exposure they were not detected in liver (see *fig. 8* with Hg chromatograms). The association of the peak to GSSG also explains the increase of the peak in G4 as the reduction of hidroperoxides needs GSHPx (Se-containing enzyme) to form GSSG and the co-administration of SeMet may activate liver GSHPx as mentioned before.

Moreover, it has been reported by other authors the pro-oxidative effects of selenium compounds and SeMet in particular, in rat liver (Farina et al., 2004; Hoffman, 2002) this justifying the synergic effect verified in group 4 towards the increase of GSSG.

Selenium is an essential element and intracellular concentrations of essential elements are normally maintained within a narrow range due to homeostatic control. As discussed above *(fig. 2)* total selenium slightly varies in the different groups but the results are statistically similar. Also the chromatograms obtained with SEC *(fig. 7)* maintain the main characteristics with a single poorly defined peak (s) in the range of 50-60kD.

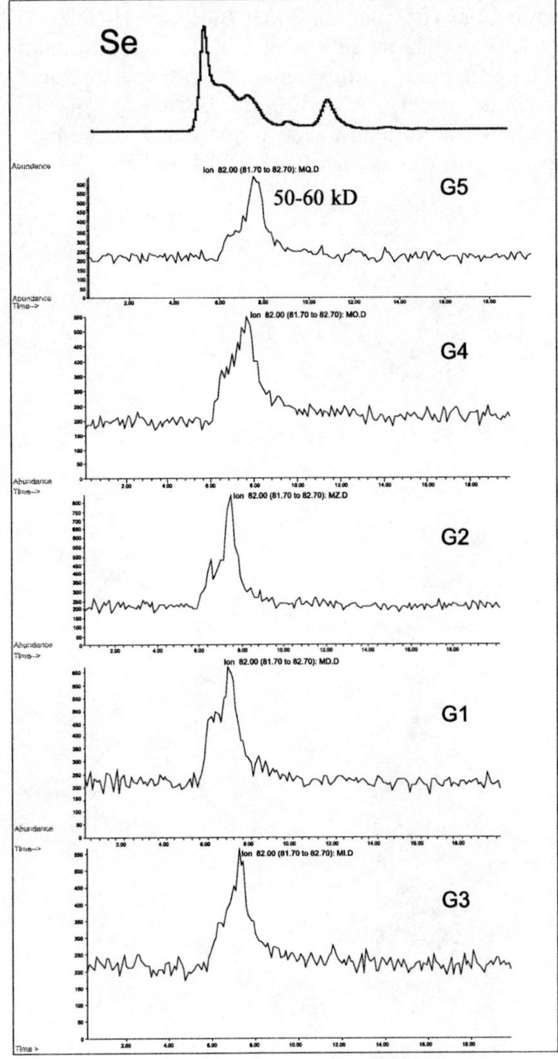

Fig. 7. Chromatograms obtained by ICP-MS for selenium fractions.

Besides Selenoprotein P (50.5kD) and their isoforms, other selenoenzymes that support liver function such as GSH reductase (45.8kD) and thioredoxin reductase, TrxR (58kD) and thioredoxin/glutathione reductase, TGR, (65kD) are also included in this broad range. Some of these selenium-containing enzymes have been reported only in the last few years and their structure as well as their function is not fully known, but they might be a key for some of the detoxification mechanisms involved.

Mercury was not detected in G3 and in G5. In the remaining groups Hg interacts with high to medium MW cellular proteins of 300-40kD *(fig. 8)*.

Again the selenoproteins referred above on Se chromatograms, Selenoprotein P and selenoenzymes (GSH reductase, TrxR and TGR) have compatible MW and may be key proteins for Hg interaction due its high affinity for reduced sulfhydryl groups, including those of cysteine and GSH this being related to its transport by molecular mimicry (Clarkson, 1993; Ballatori, 2002).

The primary structure of selenoprotein P contains many potential redox centers in the form of cysteine (17) and selenocysteine (10) residues and this protein is predominantly produced by the liver with a rapid turn-over in rat plasma. Most authors associated Selenoprotein P with selenium transport but others suggest some anti-oxidant functions (Burk et al., 2003; Burk and Hill, 2005) and explain its rapid turnover to the fact that it could serve as an anti-oxidant molecule that cannot be reduced back to an active form. Due to the high histidine and cysteine content, selenoprotein P seems to be suitable to bind heavy metals such as mercury. According to this it was reported that the co-administration of selenite and mercuric chloride lead to the formation of a complex that binds to Se-P10 but works on that are scarce and still lack confirmation (Burk and Hill, 2005).

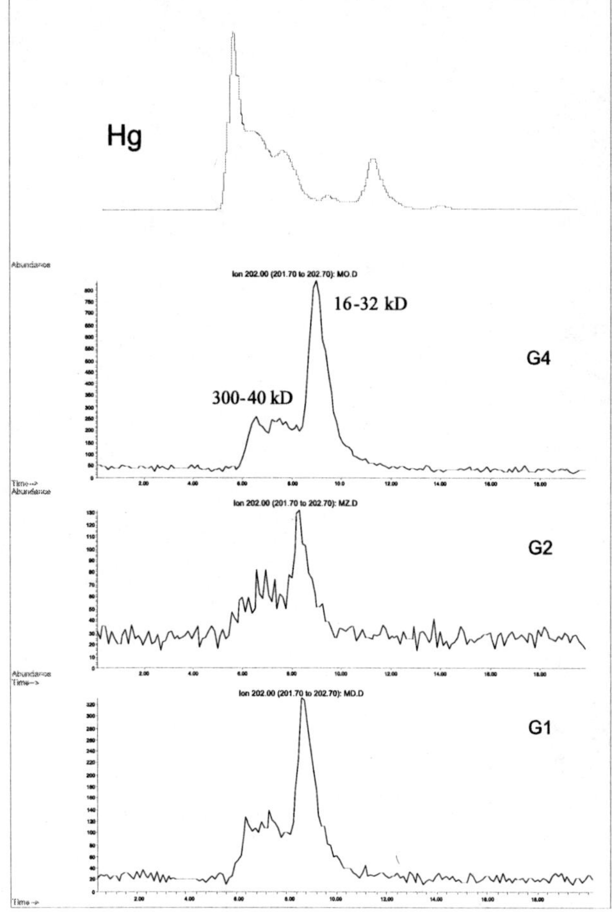

Fig. 8. Chromatograms obtained by ICP-MS for mercury fractions.

The most notorious association of mercury to liver proteins is showed by a sharp peak at 8.4 min for G1 and G2 and 8.8-9.0 for the G4 co-exposed group *(fig. 8)*, hence, the target proteins to MeHg in liver seem to have a MW 16-32kD; in this range emphasis should be given to GSHPx (22.2kD) (hydroperoxide catabolism) and GSH transferase (25.6kD). Also superoxide dismutase (SDO) with 15.8kD and methionine sulfoxide reductase (MSrA) with 18.9kD can be considered.

Until now there is evidence that MeHg inhibits GSHPx and a proposed mechanism is the direct chemical interaction of MeHg with selenolate at the active center of the enzyme, as the selenols(ates) are more reactive toward Hg than thiols(ates) (Farina et al., 2004).

Bando et al., 2005 also noticed that mercury ($HgCl_2$) induced liver responses including significant changes in endogenous antioxidant enzymes such as GSHPx, GR, G6PDH and SODs.

TRs might also be target selenoenzymes to MeHg due to their structure. TR1 (TrxR) in rats is homologous of GSH reductase with a selenocysteine-containing carboxyl-terminal elongation (Zhong et al., 1998) and that SeCys residue forms a redox active bridge with the neighboring Cys residue and such a Cys-SeCys bridge is present in the oxidized form of TrxR. The reduced form presents wide substrate specificity unlike GSH reductase. Inactivation of TrxR has been noted with low MW electrophilic compounds.

Since some of these enzymes are Se-containing proteins and the fact that the administration of SeMet has a synergic effect on oxidative stress justifies the magnitude of the sharp peak in different groups: G1-320; G2-125 and G4-800, although the experiment was not performed with quantifiable purposes but just to identify the species involved.

Concerning the Zn distribution *(fig. 9)* G1 and G2 have a similar profile although different from G3-G5 groups, which chromatograms overlap. The difference is in the peak eluted at 9.6 min that corresponds to a MW around 8.5kD and the profiles show that MeHg administration removes Zn from this group of proteins except when SeMet is supplied. The MW is compatible

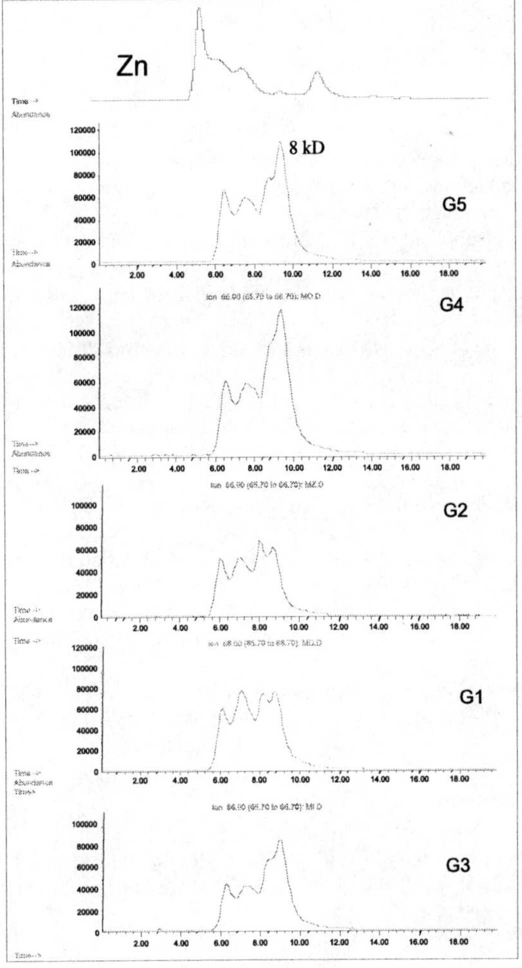

Fig. 9. Chromatograms obtained by ICP-MS for zinc fractions.

with metallothioneins MT1-MT4 with 6 to 10kD. Furthermore, it was established by Leiva-Presa et al., 2004 that $MeHg^{+}$ cation replaces Zn(II) in recombinant mammalian MTs with the concomitant unfolding of MTs. This fact corroborates our observation of Zn displacement from low MW proteins as well as explains the reason why Hg was not found associated to MTs.

CONCLUSIONS

Methylmercury accumulates in liver and cause oxidative stress associated to thiol deplection. Cellular responses of hepatocytes involve the activation of antioxidant defensive mechanisms, such as enzymes, scavengers of radicals or reductants. MeHg seems to interact strategically with some enzymes like GSHPx and GSH reductase, thioredoxin reductases and affect their activity, the result being the overwhelming of antioxidant defense mechanisms. Nevertheless, the role of some selenoproteins and/or seleno-dependent enzymes is not well established nor on the detoxification process or on the protection against oxidative stress. This work reinforces the pro-oxidant effect of MeHg in rat liver and based on the multi-elemental association to proteins proposes some explanations to improve the understanding of molecular mechanisms underlying the toxic effects of MeHg as well as the interference of selenium on this process.

This study is also a start-point for the search of metallomic biomarkers that could be useful to clarify the mechanisms of action and to detect early effects of toxicity.

REFERENCES

Ballatori, N. Transport of Toxic Metals by Molecular Mimicry. *Environ. Health Perspect.* 2002; 110: 689-694.

Bando, I. Reus, M.I.S, Andrés, D. and Cascales, M. Endogenous Antioxidant System in Rat Liver Following Mercury Chloride Oral Intoxication. *J. Biochem. Molec. Tox.* 2005; 19: 154-161.

Burk, R.F., Hill, K.E. and Motley, A.K. Selenoprotein Metabolism and Fuction: Evidence for more than one Function for Selenoprotein P. *J. Nutr.* 2003; 133: 1517S-1520S.

Burk, R. F. and Hill, K. E. Selenoprotein P: An Extracellular Protein with Unique Physical Characteristics and a Role in Selenium Homeostasis. *Annu. Rev. Nutr.* 2005; 25: 215-235.

Clarkson, T.W. Molecular and ionic mimicry of toxic metals. *Annu. Rev. Pharmacol. Toxicol.* 1993; 32: 545-571.

Farina, M., Soares, F.A.A., Zeni, G., Souza, D.O. and Rocha, J.B.T. Additive Pro-oxidative Effects of Methylmercury and Ebselen in Liver from Suckling Rat Pups. *Toxicol. Lett.* 2004; 146: 227-235.

Hoffman, D. J. Role of Selenium Toxicity and Oxidative Stress in Aquatic Birds. *Aquatic Toxicol.* 2002; 57: 11-26.

Kültz, D. Molecular and Evolutionary Basis of the Cellular Cell Response. *Annu. Rev. Nutr.* 2005; 67: 225-257.

Leiva-Presa, A., Capdevila, M., Cols, N., Atrian, S. and González-Duarte, P. Chemical Foundation of the Attenuation of Methylmercury (II) Cytotoxicity by Metallothioneis. *Eur. J. Biochem.* 2004; 271: 1323-1328.

Seppanen, K., Laatikainen, R., Salonen, J.T., Kantola, M., Lotjonen, S., Harri, M., Nurminen, L., Kaikkonen, J. and Nyyssonen, K. Mercury-binding Capacity of Organic and Inorganic Selenium in Rat Blood and Liver. *Biol. Trace Elem. Res.* 1998; 65: 197-210.

Sun, Q., Su, D., Novoselov, S. V., Carlson, B.A., Hatfield, D.L. and Gladyshev, V.N. Reaction Mechanism and Regulation of Mammalian Thioredoxin/Glutathione Reductase. *Biochemistry.* 2005; 44: 14528-14537.

ACKNOWLEDGEMENTS

Project POCTI/41741/ESP/2001 - Risk Assessment of Methylmercury Exposure: Integrated actions through the food chain. Eixo 2, medida 2.3 POCTI do QCA III (componentes Feder e OE) and Portuguese-Spanish Integrated Actions 2004/2005 N°E-40/04

Metal Ions in Biology and Medicine: vol. 9. Eds Maria Carmen Alpoim, Paula Vasconcellos Morais, Maria Amélia Santos, Armando J. Cristóvão, José A. Centeno, Philippe Collery.
John Libbey Eurotext, Paris © 2006 pp. 391-1.

Molecular Mechanisms of Nickel Toxicity and Carcinogenicity

Haobin Chen, Todd L. Davidson, Qin Li, Qingdong Ke, and Max Costa

Dept. of Environmental Medicine, New York University School of Medicine, Tuxedo, NY 10987

ABSTRACT

Both soluble and insoluble nickel compounds have been implicated as human carcinogens. Among several mechanisms proposed to explain nickel carcinogenesis, the hypoxia-mimicking stress and aberrant epigenetic changes distinguish carcinogenic Ni compounds from a number of other known carcinogens. The work conducted in this laboratory indicates that these two distinct mechanisms may be linked by a common thread in involving the interference of Ni ions with iron function. Exposure of cells to soluble nickel compounds results in a decrease of cellular iron levels, which subsequently activate iron regulatory protein (IRP) binding to an iron response element and also lead to an inhibition of aconitase activity, since aconitase moonlights as IRP. This nickel-induced IRP activation subsequently stabilizes and increases transferrin receptor mRNA as well as decreases ferritin protein synthesis, which are both compensatory measures responding to decreased cellular iron levels. Hypoxia inducible factor 1 alpha (HIF-1 alpha) transcription factor is stabilized as a result of the depletion of cellular iron. The primary mechanism by which nickel ions stabilize HIF-1 alpha is by their inhibition of iron- and oxoglutarate-dependent dioxygenases that regulate the stability of HIF-1 alpha. Nickel ions are likely to displace and deplete iron from these enzymes. In addition, nickel ions are found to inhibit a putative iron- and oxoglutarate-dependent histone H3 lysine 9 demethylase *in vitro*, whose inactivation likely results in an increase of global histone H3 lysine 9 dimethylation which eventually triggers the epigenetic silencing of genes. Since this demethylase should utilize the same mechanism to bind iron as the dioxygenases that regulate the stability of HIF1 alpha, nickel ions target these enzymes by interfering with the function of the iron moiety. Collectively, these findings unveil a common mechanism of nickel carcinogenesis that is related to the ability of nickel ions to interfere with iron binding and catalysis of the iron-dependent dioxygenases. These dioxygenases have important roles as diverse as regulating the stability of HIF-1 alpha transcription factor as regulating histone methylation which is the mark for gene silencing.

INTRODUCTION

Nickel (Ni) compounds are important occupational and environmental pollutants. Epidemiological studies have correlated increased incidences of nasal and lung cancers with worksite exposure to water-soluble and -insoluble Ni compounds [1-3]. In animal studies, water-insoluble forms of Ni were proven to be more potent carcinogens than water-soluble Ni [4]. Various mechanisms have been proposed to explain the toxicity and carcinogenicity of Ni compounds, including chromosomal aberrations, DNA strand breaks, excessive reactive oxygen species production, impaired DNA repair, hypoxia-mimicking stress, aberrant epigenetic changes, and signaling cascade activation [4, 5]. Among these mechanisms, the hypoxia-mimic stress and aberrant epigenetic changes distinguish carcinogenic Ni compounds from many other known carcinogens. It was proposed that Ni compounds initiate a hypoxic response in cells by inhibiting several iron-dependent dioxygenases related to hypoxia inducible factor 1 alpha (HIF-1α) [6]. Recently, Trewick et al. (2005)

proposed that iron-dependent dioxygenase(s) may also be involved in the dynamic regulation of epigenetic modifications, such as the removal of methyl groups from histone H3K9 [7]. Theoretically, the inhibition of such enzyme(s) could result in a similar aberrant epigenetic alterations and gene silencing as observed following Ni exposure. Thus, it appeared that interference with iron functions could link these two distinct proposed mechanisms of Ni carcinogenesis, the hypoxia-mimic stress and aberrant epigenetic changes. This article will review the work conducted in this laboratory that describes the effects of soluble Ni compounds on cellular iron homeostasis and the functions of selected iron-containing enzymes, as well as, discuss future directions for studying nickel carcinogenesis.

Interference of nickel ions with cellular iron homeostasis

In tissue culture systems, iron regulatory protein 1 (IRP1) is a major player in cellular iron regulation [8]. Under iron-depleted conditions, IRP1 gains maximum binding activity to iron response elements (IREs) located at the target mRNAs. Conversely, when iron is plentiful, IRP1 loses its IRE binding activity and is converted into cytosolic aconitase by gaining a [4Fe-4S] cluster. To assess the effects of Ni ions on cellular iron regulation, the human A549 lung cells were exposed to soluble $NiCl_2$ for selected time intervals, and the cellular aconitase activity and IRP binding activity were determined. *Figure 1* shows a time-dependent decrease of cellular aconitase activity and a concomitant increase of IRP binding activity following $NiCl_2$ exposure in A549 cells. These results demonstrate that Ni ion exposure disturbs cellular iron regulation and initiates the conversion of cytosolic aconitase to IRP1.

The activated IRP1 can bind to iron responsive elements (IREs) located at 3' untranslated region of the transferrin receptor (Tfr) mRNA, and prevents its mRNA from degradation; the subsequent increase of Tfr protein synthesis results in an elevation of Fe uptake. Meanwhile, the binding of IRP1 to IRE located at 5' untranslated region of some mRNAs, such as ferritin, blocks the assembly of the translation machinery on this mRNA, and thus, decreases ferritin synthesis and iron storage. The increase of Fe import and decrease of Fe storage compensates for the lowered intracellular iron level and re-establishes a new level of cellular iron homeostasis. *Figure 2* shows an increase of Tfr receptor mRNA and the decrease of ferritin protein following $NiCl_2$ treatment in A549 cells. These results demonstrate that Ni-induced IRP binding activity in A549 cells is biologically functional and actively involved in the establishment of a new cellular iron homeostasis.

As aforementioned, an increase in IRP activity primarily reflects a decrease of intracellular iron levels. Thus, the iron levels in A549 cells were determined using atomic absorption following Ni treatment. The results in *figure 3* show a dose- and time-dependent decrease of intracellular Fe levels following 1 mM $NiCl_2$ treatment in A549 cells. Note that at 2 hr following $NiCl_2$ treatment, cellular iron levels begin to decrease, although this decrease is not statistically significant. The time interval that cellular iron levels decrease parallels the observed increase of IRP activity and the decrease in aconitase activity, suggesting a causative role played by the lowered cellular iron levels following Ni treatment. To further investigate the relationship between the decrease of cellular iron levels and the increase of IRP binding activity following Ni treatment, A549 cells were exposed simultaneously to Ni and Fe ions at a ratio of 1:10 of Fe to Ni ions. *Figure 4a* shows a complete block of Ni-induced IRP activation by the addition of Fe ions. The addition of Fe ions has also been found to reverse half of the Ni-induced decrease of aconitase activity, as shown in *figure 4b*. The addition of Fe ions alone to the cells causes a statistically insignificant increase of aconitase activity, and this increase is less remarkable when compared with the ability of Fe ions to reverse the Ni-induced decrease of aconitase activity. Collectively, the observed decrease of cellular iron levels and increase of IRP activity following Ni treatment could have a profound impact on the function of cellular iron-containing enzymes.

The effect of nickel compounds on hypoxia signaling

One of the most significant changes following Ni exposure is the stabilization and activation of transcriptional factor HIF-1α [9]. *Figure 5a* shows a time-dependent increase of HIF-1α protein following 1 mM $NiCl_2$ treatment in A549 cells. This increase of HIF-1α protein is paralleled by the change of cellular Fe levels and IRP binding activity, suggesting a possible connection between these observations. The expression of HIF-1α is primarily regulated at the post-translational level. Under normoxia conditions, HIF-1α protein is hydroxylated at its proline 402 and 564 residues by several Fe(II)- and O_2-dependent prolyl hydroxylases (PHD 1-3). The hydroxylated HIF-1α is then recognized and ubiquitinylated by an ubiquitin ligase complex containing the von Hippel Lindau tumor suppressor protein (VHL), and is subsequently targeted for rapid proteasome-dependent degradation. Under hypoxic conditions, these prolyl hydroxylases are inhibited and HIF-1α is not longer hydroxylated. Thus, a loss of the degradation of HIF-1α leads to the accumulation of protein in cells, since this protein has a half-life in the order of minutes. *Figure 5b* shows that a time-dependent decrease of cellular prolyl hydroxylase activity following Ni treatment in A549 cells as assessed by the *in vitro* VHL assay. In this assay, the HIF-1α protein was allowed to be hydroxylated by the PHDs from the cell extracts under an *in vitro* optimized condition, and the degree of HIF-1a hydroxylation was subsequently assessed by the amount of ^{32}S-labeled VHL protein binding. Therefore, the amount of ^{32}S-labeled VHL protein binding reflects the activity of PHDs in the cell extracts. The decrease of PHDs activity following Ni treatment support the previous hypothesis that nickel compounds increase HIF-1α protein by inhibiting the activity of PHDs.

To further investigate whether Ni compounds inhibits PHDs by interfering with the function of its Fe moiety, A549 cells were exposed to Ni and Fe ions simultaneously. *Figure 6* shows that the addition of Fe ions can substantially reverse the stabilization of HIF-1α protein following Ni treatment. As aforementioned, the addition of Fe ions can also reverse the effects of Ni ions on IRP and aconitase activity. These results support the notion that cellular iron depletion is responsible in part for HIF-1α stabilization and the hypoxia signaling in cells under normal oxygen tension. Additionally, since iron is bound by two histidine residues in PHDs, a small amount of nickel ions that enter cells are also likely to compete effectively with the iron in these enzymes. Using the imidazole ligand to model the binding of Fe^{2+} to the histidine sites of prolyl hydroxylase, the binding strength of Ni^{2+} coordination to two imidazole molecules is found to be three orders of magnitude greater than for Fe^{2+} to bind the same two molecules [10]. Therefore, both cellular iron depletion and competition by Ni compounds are likely factors that result in inhibition of PHDs and subsequent stabilization of HIF-1α. The hypoxic signaling in cells is likely to be an important contributory mechanism in cancer development.

The effects of nickel exposure on histone H3K9 methylation

Although nickel compounds are highly carcinogenic, they exhibit insignificant mutagenic activity in most bacterial and mammalian cell assays [11]. An unusual exception is the G12 transgenic cell line, where Ni compounds caused the inactivation of the transgene via epigenetic mechanisms, rather than gene mutation and deletion [12]. In support of the epigenetic nature of the transgene silencing, the transgene promoter in Ni-induced silenced clones was found to associate with nucleosomes having a decrease in histone H3 and H4 acetylation, as well as an increase in histone H3 lysine 9 (H3K9) dimethylation, DNA methylation and chromatin condensation [12, 13]. Furthermore, the transgene function can be restored following treatment with histone deacetylase trichostatin A or DNA-demethylating agent 5-azacytidine [12, 14]. It has been reported that DNA hypermethylation of tumor suppressor gene p16 existed in all of the malignant fibrous histiocytomas induced by NiS implantation in mice [15], which demonstrates the critical role of epigenetic gene silencing in Ni carcinogenesis.

Among the identified epigenetic modifications in the silenced transgene promoter, H3K9 dimethylation is a critical mark for the establishment of long-term gene silencing [16]. Our recent data suggested that Ni compounds can directly increase global histone H3K9 dimethylation by inhibiting an unidentified Fe-dependent H3K9 demethylase. *Figure 7* shows a dose-dependent increase of global H3K9 dimethylation in A549 cells following $NiCl_2$ treatment. The steady level of H3K9 dimethylation in A549 cells is balanced between a well-studied methylation process and a poorly-understood demethylation process. The histone methyltransferase G9a was found to play a dominant role in H3K9 dimethylation *in vivo* [17]. Knocking out G9a dramatically diminished global H3K9 dimethylation in mouse embryonic stem cells (MES) [17]. To examine the role of G9a in Ni(II)-induced H3K9 dimethylation, MES cells with G9a ablation ($G9a^{-/-}$ MES) and their derivatives that were stably transfected with a wild type G9a vector ($G9a^{-/-}$ + G9a WT MES) were utilized. *Figure 8* shows that Ni ions are still able to increase H3K9 dimethylation in $G9a^{-/-}$ cells, although the basal level of H3K9 dimethylation was much lower in these cells compared to wild type (WT) and ($G9a^{-/-}$ + G9a WT) cells. Therefore, Ni ions increased global H3K9 dimethylation by inhibiting H3K9 demethylation rather than increasing H3K9 methylation by G9a.

Histone H3K9 methylation had long been thought as a permanent modification. Recently, an oxidative demethylation mechanism has been proposed to explain the methylation removal from histone lysine residue and the demethylase responsive for such a process is likely to be a Fe(II)-2-oxoglutarate-dependent dioxygenase(s) [7]. In support of this notion, *figure 9* shows that, besides $NiCl_2$, low oxygen (hypoxia), 2-oxoglutarate analog (dimethyloxalylglycine, DMOG) and iron-depletion (deferoxamine, DFX) all substantially increase global H3K9 dimethylation in A549 cells. Thus, this putative Fe(II)- and 2-oxoglutarate-dependent dioxygenase could be responsible for H3K9 demethylation in mammalian cells.

To further investigate the nature of this demethylation process, an *in vitro* H3K9 demethylation assay was set up to monitor the removal of ^3H-labeled methyl group from methylated H3K9 residue in histone H3 peptide. *Figure 10* demonstrates the activity of H3K9 demethylase as observed with an *in vitro* assay. Such a H3K9 demethylase activity depends on the presence of iron and 2-oxoglutarate, and the addition of $NiCl_2$ inhibits this activity *(fig. 10)*. Note that a small decrease of H3K9 methylation was still present without the addition of exogenous Fe ions or 2-oxoglurate. These observations were likely due to the presence of cellular-derived iron and 2-oxoglutarate in the nuclear extract, since the demethylation activity was completely blocked by the addition of the iron chelator deferoxamine. In support of our findings, JHDM1 was recently discovered to utilize the same oxidative demethylation mechanism to remove the methyl group specifically from methylated H3K36 residue [18]. Since this group of histone demethylase belongs to the Fe(II)-2-oxoglutarate dioxygenase family, a similar mechanism (2-His-1-carboxylate triad motif in sequence) is utilized to bind iron as in PHDs. Thus, nickel exposure could inhibit the activities of these histone demethylases by both iron depletion and competition with the enzyme iron binding site. Future work should be directed at identifying these proposed histone demethylases.

In conclusion, nickel compounds were found to disturb cell iron homeostasis and inhibit the activities of several iron-containing enzymes. As a consequence of these iron-containing enzyme inhibitions, cells experience a state of hypoxia under normal oxygen tension as well as an increased steady state levels of H3K9 dimethylation. These events are involved in the alteration of gene expression during Ni exposure in cells, and thus the disturbance of cellular Fe functions is likely to be an important contributory mechanism underlying Ni toxicology and carcinogenesis.

REFERENCES

1. Roberts RS, Julian JA, Muir DC, Shannon HS: Cancer mortality associated with the high-temperature oxidation of nickel subsulfide. *IARC Sci Publ* 1984; 23-35.
2. Roberts RS, Julian JA, Muir DC, Shannon HS: A study of mortality in workers engaged in the mining, smelting, and refining of nickel. II: Mortality from cancer of the respiratory tract and kidney. *Toxicol Ind Health* 1989; 5: 975-93.

3. Polednak AP: Mortality among welders, including a group exposed to nickel oxides. *Arch Environ Health* 1981; 36: 235-42.
4. Kasprzak KS, Sunderman FW, Jr., Salnikow K: Nickel carcinogenesis. *Mutat Res* 2003; 533: 67-97.
5. Costa M, Salnikow K, Cosentino S, Klein CB, Huang X, Zhuang Z: Molecular mechanisms of nickel carcinogenesis. *Environ Health Perspect* 1994; 102 Suppl 3: 127-30.
6. Epstein AC, Gleadle JM, McNeill LA, Hewitson KS, O'Rourke J, Mole DR, Mukherji M, Metzen E, Wilson MI, Dhanda A, Tian YM, Masson N, Hamilton DL, Jaakkola P, Barstead R, Hodgkin J, Maxwell PH, Pugh CW, Schofield CJ, Ratcliffe PJ: C. elegans EGL-9 and mammalian homologs define a family of dioxygenases that regulate HIF by prolyl hydroxylation. *Cell* 2001; 107: 43-54.
7. Trewick SC, McLaughlin PJ, Allshire RC: Methylation: lost in hydroxylation? *EMBO Rep* 2005; 6: 315-20.
8. Papanikolaou G, Pantopoulos K: Iron metabolism and toxicity. *Toxicol Appl Pharmacol* 2005; 202: 199-211.
9. Salnikow K, Davidson T, Costa M: The role of hypoxia-inducible signaling pathway in nickel carcinogenesis. *Environ Health Perspect* 2002; 110 Suppl 5: 831-34.
10. Davidson TL, Chen H, Toro DMD, D'Angelo G, Costa M: Soluble nickel inhibits HIF-Prolyl-Hydroxylases creating persistent hypoxic signaling in A549 cells. *Mol Carcinog* 2006; In press.
11. Klein CB, Costa M: DNA methylation, heterochromatin and epigenetic carcinogens. *Mutat Res* 1997; 386: 163-80.
12. Lee YW, Klein CB, Kargacin B, Salnikow K, Kitahara J, Dowjat K, Zhitkovich A, Christie NT, Costa M: Carcinogenic nickel silences gene expression by chromatin condensation and DNA methylation: a new model for epigenetic carcinogens. *Mol Cell Biol* 1995; 15: 2547-57.
13. Yan Y, Kluz T, Zhang P, Chen HB, Costa M: Analysis of specific lysine histone H3 and H4 acetylation and methylation status in clones of cells with a gene silenced by nickel exposure. *Toxicol Appl Pharmacol* 2003; 190: 272-7.
14. Sutherland JE, Peng W, Zhang Q, Costa M: The histone deacetylase inhibitor trichostatin A reduces nickel-induced gene silencing in yeast and mammalian cells. *Mutat Res* 2001; 479: 225-33.
15. Govindarajan B, Klafter R, Miller MS, Mansur C, Mizesko M, Bai X, LaMontagne K, Jr., Arbiser JL: Reactive oxygen-induced carcinogenesis causes hypermethylation of p16(Ink4a) and activation of MAP kinase. *Mol Med* 2002; 8: 1-8.
16. Peterson CL, Laniel MA: Histones and histone modifications. *Curr Biol* 2004; 14: R546-51.
17. Tachibana M, Sugimoto K, Nozaki M, Ueda J, Ohta T, Ohki M, Fukuda M, Takeda N, Niida H, Kato H, Shinkai Y: G9a histone methyltransferase plays a dominant role in euchromatic histone H3 lysine 9 methylation and is essential for early embryogenesis. *Genes Dev* 2002; 16: 1779-91.
18. Tsukada YI, Fang J, Erdjument-Bromage H, Warren ME, Borchers CH, Tempst P, Zhang Y: Histone demethylation by a family of JmjC domain-containing proteins. *Nature* 2006; In press.

ACKNOWLEDGEMENT

We thank Dr. Yoichi Shinkai for providing mouse embryonic stem cell wild type (WT), G9a knockout ($G9a^{-/-}$) and $G9a^{-/-}$ stably transfected with a wild type G9a vector ($G9a^{-/-}$ + G9a WT) cells. This work was supported by grant numbers ES00260, ES10344, and T32-ES07324 from the National Institute of Environmental Health Sciences, and CA16087 from the National Cancer Institute.

Metal Ions in Biology and Medicine: vol. 9. Eds Maria Carmen Alpoim, Paula Vasconcellos Morais, Maria Amélia Santos, Armando J. Cristóvão, José A. Centeno, Philippe Collery.
John Libbey Eurotext, Paris © 2006 pp. 396-1.

Pathology of kidney and liver caused by inhaled dimethyl selenide

Cherdwongcharoensuk D[1,2], Henrique R[3], Upatham S[2], Pereira AS[1], and Águas AP[1]

[1] *Department of Anatomy, ICBAS (Abel Salazar Institute for Biomedical Sciences), University of Porto, Lg. Prf.Abel Salazar,2, 4099-003 Porto, Portugal.*
[2] *Department of Medical Science, Faculty of Science, Burapha University, Thailand.*
[3] *Department of Pathology, Portuguese Oncology Institute, Porto, Portugal.*
E-mail address: duangrud@yahoo.com or duangrud@hotmail.com

ABSTRACT

Accidental inhalation of selenium (Se) is harmful to the respiratory system and possibly to other organs of the body. These accidents may occur in smelter, refinery, and glass bangle industries. The putative pathology of kidney and liver caused by inhaled Se has not been defined so far. We have investigated the cellular pathology of CD-1 mice kidney and liver after a single intratracheal instillation of Se as dimethyl selenide (DMSe) 0.05 and 0.1 mg Se/kg BW. The animals were sacrificed 1, 7, 14, and 28 days after either one of the two DMSe treatments. Kidney and liver samples were studied by light microscopy. In the kidney, acute tubular damage characterized by swelling and vacuolation of epithelial cells of proximal tubules was observed after treatment with the low dose of DMSe. These lesions were transient and recovery was seen by day 14. The low dose of DMSe also caused damage to centrolobular hepatocytes expressed by swollen and vacuolized liver cells. After the instillation of the higher dose of DMSe, the mice showed sustained liver and kidney focal necrosis. Our data show that inhalation of DMSe results in: (i) acute tubular injury of the kidney and damage to centrolobular liver cells, (ii) this systemic pathology induced by DMSe is a dose-dependent phenomenon.

INTRODUCTION

Selenium (Se) is one of the toxic agents that is widely used in smelter, refinery, and glass bangle industries (Clayton and Clayton, 1994). Humans can accidentally be harmed by Se through several routes, one of them being inhalation. We have shown before that inhaled Se can damage the respiratory tissues (Cherdwongcharownsuk *et al.*, 2003, 2004). However, few investigations have been focused on the pathology of kidney and liver after Se inhalation.

Ingestion or drinking of supplements containing Se has been investigation by a number of scientists. Jacobs and Forst (1981) studied the toxicology of drinking water supplements containing 1, 4, 8, 16, 32 and 64 ppm of selenium as sodium selenide in Swiss mice and found that mice present liver and kidney congestion and liver necrosis after the treatment. Dagalla and Adam (1986) addressed the toxicity of diet containing 0.5, 1 and 3 ppm sodium selenite in 7-day-old hybro-type chicks for 4 weeks. Focal necrosis, congestion and fibroplasia were seen in the liver; and degeneration, congestion and necrosis were observed in the kidney. Mensink and others (1990) reported that high concentrations of selenium were found in liver of kidney of sow herd piglets that were born with an abnormal horn formation. Later on, Meotti and his coworkers (2003) investigated hepatic and renal toxicities of diphenyl diselenide, diphenyl ditelluride and Ebselen in rats and mice and found that intraperitoneal injection of diphenyl diselenide (160, 320 and 500 μmol/kg) in mice and rats did not increase the activity of the hepatic injury markers (serum alanine aminotransferase and aspertate aminotransferase) and the level of renal injury markers (serum urea and creatinine).

Inhalation or intratracheal instillation of Se has been studied by a few investigators. Medinsky *et al.* (1981) concluded that inhaled selenious acid is absorbed into blood faster than elemental Se. This is consistent with the findings of Weissman *et al.* (1983) reporting that inhaled selenious acid was more rapidly absorbed to blood circulation than aerosol Se; these metal substances were then distributed to liver, kidney, spleen and heart. The continuous inhalation of Se at threshold limit value leads to Se accumulation in the lung, liver, and blood with the values of 22,000, 1,200 and 440 ng S/g, respectively (Medinsky *et al.*, 1985).

There is limited information on the pathology of kidney and liver caused by inhaled Se. We have investigated here the histopathology of kidney and liver of CD-1 mice after a single intratracheal instillation of Se as dimethyl selenide (DMSe).

MATERIALS AND METHODS

Selenium. DMSe (C_2H_6Se) in liquid form, at analytical grade, was purchased from Fluka Chemical Co (ref. no. 41572) with a purity greater than 99%.

Animals. 64 one-month-old CD-1 mice (Charles River strain), weighing about 20 g, were kept under standard housing conditions. Six mice per each group were exposed to intratracheal instillation of DMSe [0.05 or 0.1 mg Se/kg of body weight (BW)]. Additional 16 mice were used as controls.

Intratracheal Instillation of DMSe. The CD-1 mice were anesthetized by intramuscular injection of 4.0-8.0 mg/kg BW of ketamine (Ketalar, Parke-Davis Co., Barcelona, Spain), and of 0.8-1.6 mg/kg BW of xilazine (Rompun, Bayer Co., Amadora, Portugal). Intratracheal instillation of DMSe in mice has described before by Cherdwongcharownsuk *et al.* (2003 and 2004). Six mice for each selenium dose and control were sacrificed at 1, 7, 14 and 28 days after the treatment. Kidneys and livers were rapidly removed and fixed in Bouin's solution. The tissue samples were processed, cut and stained with haematoxylin-eosin (HE) and Masson's trichrome and viewed by light microscopy.

RESULTS

Histopathology caused by the low dose of DMSe

Kidney. 9 of 24 mice show swelling and vacuolation of epithelial cells of proximal renal tubules after 1 day (5 of 6), 7 days (3 of 6) and 14 days (1 of 6) of treatment. The cytoplasm appeared poorly stained with different sizes of vacuoles; the cells were enlarged *(fig. A)*. After 14 and 28 days of Se treatment, kidneys showed again a normal morphology.

Liver. Cell swelling was the major change observed in livers 1 day (2 of 6), 7 days (6 of 6), 14 days (5 of 6) and 28 days (6 of 6) after instillation *(fig. B)*. A few focal necrosis were observed 1 (1 of 6) and 14 days (1 of 6) after treatment *(fig. C)*.

Histopathology caused by the high dose of DMSe

Kidney. After instillation, 9 out of 24 mice showed cell swelling and vacuolation of proximal tubule epithelium [day-1 (6 of 6), day-7 (2 of 6) and day-14 (1 of 6)] *(fig A)*. More severity of tubular necrosis was found only one mouse after treatment 7 days. Kidneys of mice at days 14 and 28 of Se treatment had recovered from the injury.

Liver. 14 of 24 mice had cell swelling 1 day (1 of 6), 7 days (4 of 6), 14 days (6 of 6) and 28 days (3 of 6) after treatment *(fig. B)*. Focal necrosis was also seen in 2 mice at day-1, 2 mice at day-7 and 1 mouse at day-28 after treatment *(fig. C)*. In addition, the condensation of nuclear chromatin was observed in 2 mice at day-28 after Se instillation *(fig. D)*.

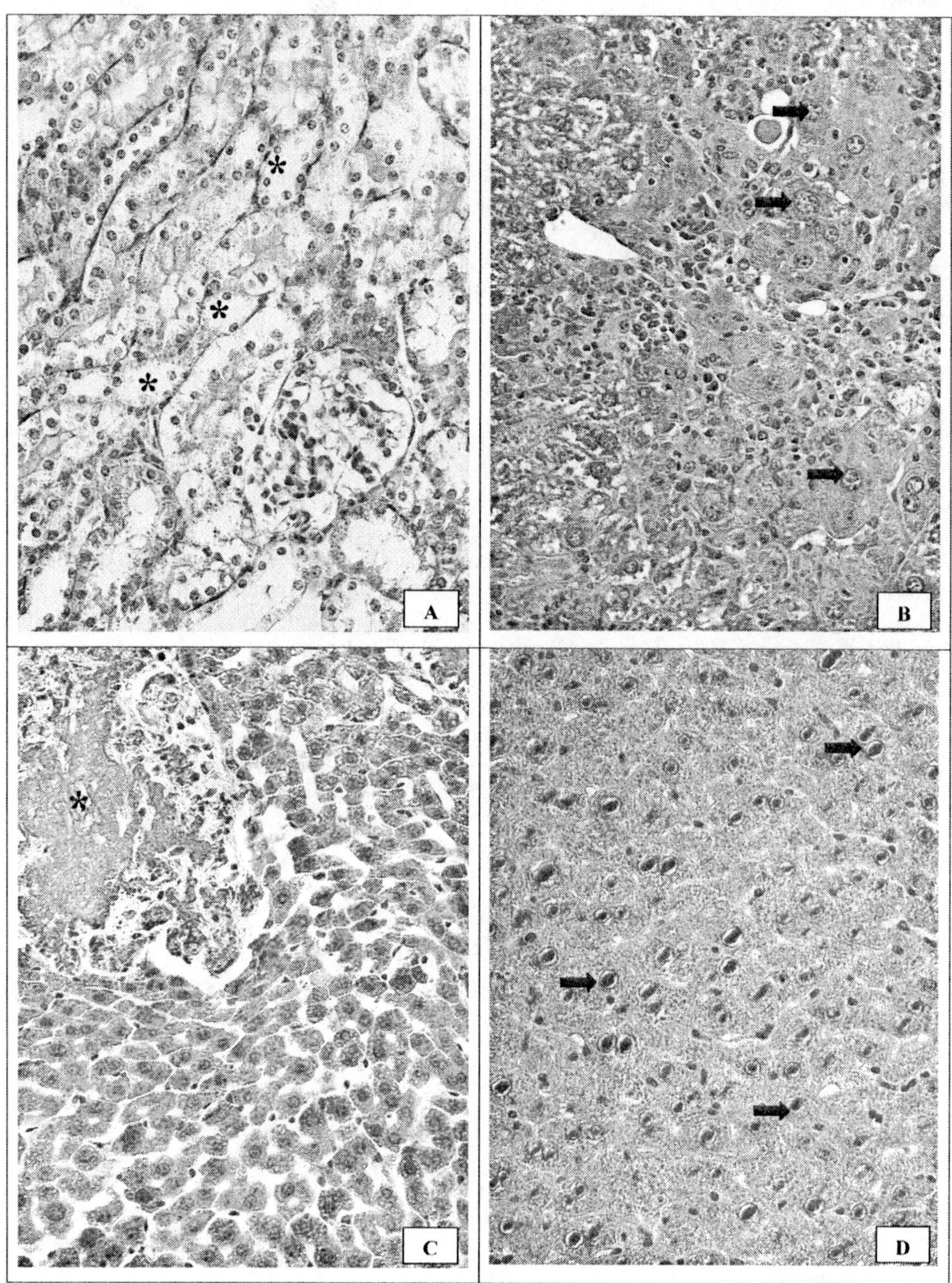

Figures. Light micrographs of CD-1 mice after instillation of the higher dose of DMSe. (A) Kidney showing tubular swelling, vacuolation and necrosis (*) after 7 days of Se treatment. (B) Liver showing cell swelling (→) after 28 days of Se treatment. (C) Liver showing focal necrosis (*) after 7 days of Se treatment. (D) Liver showing condensation of nuclear chromatin (→) after 28 days of Se treatment (HE staining x400).

DISCUSSION

The single intratracheal instillation of Se as DMSe at a dose of 0.5 or 0.1 mg Se/kg BW caused swelling, vacuolation and necrosis of the kidney, and swelling, necrosis and nuclear chromatin condensation of the liver of CD-1 mice. In addition, the higher dose of DMSe resulted in more severity of kidney tubular necrosis and focal necrosis and nuclear chromatin condensation of the liver. These data indicate the pathology induced by DMSe is dose-depended. The kidney showed recovery 14 and 28 days after the inhalation, whereas liver injuries were seen until 28 days after the treatment.

The herein kidney and liver lesions caused by inhalation of Se as DMSe resemble the changes investigated in mice that drank water containing sodium selenide (Jacobs and Forst, 1981), and also in 7-day-old hybro-type chicks that ingested a diet containing sodium selenite (Dagalla and Adam,1986). Our data are in contrast with the results of Meotti and his coworkers (2003) that did not find any changes of the activity of the hepatic injury markers (serum alanine aminotransferase and aspertate aminotransferase) and the level of renal injury markers (serum urea and creatinine) caused by diphenyl diselenide in rat.

Our observations are in accordance with the data of Mensink and others (1990) that concluded that the high concentrations of selenium identified in liver of kidney of the sow herd piglets were associated with an abnormal itis such as horn formation. Also, Medinsky *et al.* (1981 and 1985) and Weissman *et al.* (1983) found that inhaled Se and its compounds were absorbed into blood circulation and distributed to liver, kidney, spleen and heart. Inhalation of Se at threshold limit value can lead Se accumulating in the lung, liver, and blood (Medinsky *et al.*, 1985). In conclusion, inhaled Se as DMSe was absorbed into the blood circulation after a single intratracheal instillation, and it was distributed and accumulated in liver and kidney where Se triggering cell injury.

REFERENCES

1. Cherdwongcharoensuk D, Águas AP, Henrique R, Upatham S, Sousa Pereira A. Toxic effects of selenium inhalation: acute damage of the respiratory system of mice. *Hum Exp Toxicol* 2003; 22: 551-7.
2. Cherdwongcharoensuk D, Upatham S, Oliveira JC, Pereira AS, Águas AP. Changes in bronchoalveolar lavage cells after intratracheal instillation of dimethyl selenide in mice. *Toxicol Pathol* 2004; 32: 345-50.
3. Clayton GD, Clayton FE. *Patty's industrial hygiene and toxicology, part D: toxicology*. 4th ed. New York: Wiley-Insterscience, 1994.
4. Dafalla R, Adam SE. Effects of various levels of dietary selenium on hybro-type chicks. *Vet Hum Toxicol* 1986; 28: 105-8.
5. Jacobs M, Forst C. Toxicological effects of sodium selenite in Swiss mice. *J Toxicol Environ Health* 1981; 8: 587-98.
6. Medinsky MA, Cuddihy RG, McClellan RO. Systemic asorption of selenious acid and elemental selenium aerosols in rats. *J Toxicol Environ Health* 1981; 8: 917-28.
7. Medinsky MA, Cuddihy RG, Griffith WC, Weissman SH, McClellan RO. Projected uptake and toxicity of selenium compounds from the environment. *Environ Res* 1985; 36: 181-92.
8. Mensink CG, Koeman JP, Veling J, Gruys E. Haemorrhagic claw lesions in newborn piglets due to selenium toxicosis during pregnancy. *Vet Rec* 1990; 126: 620-2.
9. Meotti FC, Borges VC, Zeni G, Rocha JB, Nogueira CW. Potential renal and hepatic toxicity of diphenyl diselenide, diphenyl ditelluride and Ebselen for rats and mice. *Toxicol Lett* 2003; 143: 9-16.
10. Weissman SH, Cuddihy RG, Medinsky MA. Absorption, distribution, and retention of inhaled selenious acid and selenium metal aerosols in beagle dogs. *Toxicol Appl Pharmacol.* 1983; 67: 331-337.

ACKNOWLEDGMENTS

The authors are very grateful to Mr. Antonio Costa e Silva, Mr. Emanuel Monteiro, Dr. Madalena Costa, and Mrs. Alexandrina Ribeiro for technical assistance. This work was supported by a FCT grant (POCTI/BSE/36188/2000), Portugal.

Metal Ions in Biology and Medicine: vol. 9. Eds Maria Carmen Alpoim, Paula Vasconcellos Morais, Maria Amélia Santos, Armando J. Cristóvão, José A. Centeno, Philippe Collery.
John Libbey Eurotext, Paris © 2006 pp. 400-1.

Nickel sulfate genotoxic activity in germline and somatic cells of WR mice

M.G. Domschlak[1], N. Yu. Vorobyova[2], A.L. Elakov[3], A.N. Osipov[2,3]

[1]*Institute of Occupational Health Russian Academy of Medical Science, Moscow 105275, Russia;* [2]*N.N. Semenov Institute of Chemistry Physics RAS, Moscow 11991, Russia, e-mail: nuv.rad@mail.ru;* [3]*Scientific and Industrial Association "Radon", Moscow 119121, Russia.*

ABSTRACT

The results of the investigation of $NiSO_4$ genotoxic activity in dose range of 0.5-5.0 mg/kg on germline and somatic cells of WR mice are presented and discussed in this report. It was shown that $NiSO_4$ *per os* administration at a dose range of 1.0-5.0 mg/kg induce statistically significant increasing of dominant lethal mutation's. The most expressed genetic effect was seen in germ cells on late spermatocyte stage after 5.0 and 1.0 mg/kg ($p<0.01$). $NiSO_4$ uptake at dose of 0.5 mg/kg does not increase dominant lethal mutations frequency in germ cells at any stage of spermatogenesis comparing with control. There is no statistically significant increasing of DNA double strand breaks total level in sperm exposed on the late spermatocyte stage. At the same time, it was pointed out significant increasing of cell percentage with a highly fragmentized DNA (supposedly apoptotic) under $NiSO_4$ uptake in doses of 0.5 and 1.0 mg/kg.

INTRODUCTION

Nowadays the researcher's interest is focused on the hazard of the environmental pollution by heavy metals including nickel and its compounds. A particularly hazardous situation characterizes the regions of nickel mining and processing. For example a medical hygienic study at the Apatit nickel-processing factory has shown that the factory workers were exposed to nickel at concentrations of 0.183-0.087 mg/m^3 (maximum permissible dose - 0.005 mg/m^3, electrolysis department). However, literature data show that male reproductive function suffers more from these effects whereas high risk of the nickel impact on female reproduction is more connected to the conditions of work in Zapolyar'e and to lifting heavy weights [1]. Thus, further epidemiological and experimental investigation of the situation is expedient.

The data on impairment of DNA structure by nickel salts are scarce. An introduction of $NiSO_4$ in vivo in cell culture was shown to lead to DNA - protein cross-links (DPCs) [2], oxidative lesions [3], and repression of DNA repair [4]. The formation of DPCs and DNA breaks was demonstrated in BALB/c3T3 cells upon nickel exposure [5]. The high level of DNA breaks may indicate nucleic acid fragmentation, which is a key step of apoptosis (genetically programmed cell death).

Thus, the results of *in vitro* and *in vivo* studies suggest that nickel compounds can induce genotoxic effects. All of the above evidence involve only somatic cells and cannot be extrapolated to cells determining progeny quality.

Analysis of the published studies on mutagenic effects of nickel compounds shows that they used these compounds at relatively high dose (concentration).This doesn't permit estimating the minimum threshold level (LOAEL) or nonobservable genetic level (NOAEL) of the effect of these substances.

The aim of the present work was to study the molecular and genetic changes in germline and somatic cells of WR mice upon exposure to nickel sulfate at low doses.

We choose nickel sulfate as a test agent because it causes more marked toxic effect then the other soluble nickel compounds [6].

MATERIALS AND METHODS

We used mice of the single-locus strain WR (genotype aa $+w^y$). These mice were derived from a cross between females of strain 129 (R-c X/129), genotype Aw Aw, cchp/cch p and male?6, heterozygous at gene W^y. The dominant W^y gene causes regular white spotting and reduced pigmentation in heterozygous state. The manifestation of W^y gene in the WR strain background is the characteristic of the unstable genes. W^yW^y homozygotes die after birth from anemia. WR mice are characterized by the high level of mosaicism, resulting from mutation Dominant spotting viable (W^y) at the W locus of chromosome 5 [7]. This mutation alters the oncogene of the receptor tyrosine kinase c-kit gene. Mutations at the W locus are pleiotropic, affecting to a certain extend pigmentation, the development of germline cells, and hematopoiesis. The c-kit gene is involved in proliferation and differentiation of neural, far and male germline cells. This gene is located in human chromosome 4 which allows for more correct extrapolation of experimental data [8].

The LD50 of nickel sulfate (100 mg/kg) was estimated in preliminary experiments. Nickel sulfate was administrated to male and female mice endogastrially at doses of 5.0 (Ni-1.04mg/kg), 1.0 (Ni-0.21mg/kg) and 0.5 (Ni-0.10 mg/kg) mg/kg.

Immediately after nickel sulfate administration, intact females SHK (1♂ × 3♀♀) were placed with the nickel treated males (three female per male) each week during 5 weeks and in 2 months for estimating DLM during the whole cycle of spermatogenesis, including stem spermatogonia. In the latter case, the ratio off four females per male was used (1♂ × 4♀♀).

The DLM frequency was estimated at day 18 after pregnancy according to the published protocols [9] on the basis of postimplantation embryonic lethality (the ratio of the number of dead embryos to the number of the implantation sites) and induced lethality:

100% × (postimplantation lethality in the experiment/ postimplantation lethality in the control). This parameter eliminates "natural background" - the embryonic lethality in the control group, which permits to analyze DLM frequency, induced exactly by the mutagen tested. Females were administrated the nickel salt on days 10-11 of pregnancy, since the most mutation events take place during this developmental stages of the embryos, which contain 150 melanocytes [10].

The frequency of gene mutations was estimated from the number of black spots on the skin of heterozygous (F1) on the 2 and 4 weeks after birth.

For the estimation of double-strand break frequency in sperm, DNA comet technique modified by Singh and Stephens [11] was used.

DNA comets in sperm were examined visually using a fluorescent microscope Micmed-2 (Russia). For each mouse 100 comets were analyzed using the system proposed by Collins et al. [12]. According to their shape they were assigned to one of the five classes from 0 to4 (0 and 4 indicates the lack and the maximum DNA damage respectively). The average DNA comet index was calculated from the formula: $ACI= (0{\cdot}n0 + 1{\cdot}n1 + 2{\cdot}n1 + 3{\cdot}n3 + 4{\cdot}n4)/ \Sigma$, where n1 - n4 - number of comets in classes 1-4, $H\Sigma$ - is the sum of all the comets scored, including those in class 0 comets.

Statistical analysis of the data was performed using Statistica 6.0.

RESULTS AND DISCUSSION

As seen from the data presented in *table 1*, nickel sulfate at a dose of 5.0mg/kg (1/20 LD50) induced a marked mutagenic effect, i.e., increased the dominant lethal mutation (DLM) frequency

Table 1. Frequency of dominant lethal mutations induced by nickel sulfate in germline cells of WR mice at different stages of spermatogenesis

Dose, mg/kg	Stage of spermato-genesis	Number of		Male fertility, %	Number of			Post-implantation lethality	
		male	Pregnant female		Implantation sites	embryos		% (M±m)	with correction by control, % (M+m)
						alive	dead		
5.0	Spermatozoa	12	28	77.8	232	197	46	15.1±2.3 $p \leq 0.01$	11.0±2.6
1.0		12	25	69.4	237	210	27	11.4±2.1 $p \leq 0.01$	6.6±2.5
0.5		8	20	83.3	149	136	13	8.8±2.3	4.2±2.6
control		12	30	83.3	233	222	14	4.8±1.4	-
5.0	Late spermatids	12	25	69.4	228	198	23	11.0±2.0 $p \leq 0.05$	6.1±2.6
1.0		12	25	69.4	239	216	23	9.7±1.9	4.8±2.4
0.5		8	20	83.3	134	125	9	6.7±2.1	1.7±2.6
control		12	25	69.4	230	218	12	5.2±1.5	-
5.0	Early spermatids	11	31	93.9	240	211	29	12.1±2.1 $p \leq 0.01$	7.2±2.5
1.0	12	26	72.2	224	199	25	11.4±2.1 $p \leq 0.02$	7.0±2.5	
0.5	8	20	83.3	144	132	12	8.4±2.4	2.3±2.8	
control		11	27	75	225	216	12	5.3±1.5	-
5.0	Late spermatocy-tes	10	23	76.7	169	142	27	16.0±2.8 $p \leq 0.001$	12.6±3.2
1.0		12	28	77.8	217	182	14	16.1±2.5 $p \leq 0.001$	12.7±2.9
0.5		8	21	87.5	156	150	6	4.0±1.6	-
control		11	25	75.8	183	175	8	4.4±1.64	-

Table 1. Suite

Dose, mg/kg	Stage of spermato-genesis	Number of		Male fertility, %	Number of			Post-implantation lethality	
		male	Pregnant female		Implantation sites	embryos		% (M±m)	with correction by control, % (M+m)
						alive	dead		
5.0	Early spermatocy-tes + β-spermato-gonia	10	21	70	152	127	25	16.5±3.0 $p \leq 0.001$	12.3±3.3
1.0		11	25	75.8	185	178	7	3.8±1.4	-
0.5		8	18	75	149	145	4	2.7±1.3	-
control		11	25	75.8	191	181	10	5.2±1.6	-
5.0	stem spermatogo-nia	10	30	75.0	206	187	19	10.0±2.1 $p \leq 0.05$	5.5±2.5
1.0		11	30	68.18	202	183	19	10.0±2.2 ≤ 0.05	5.5±2.6
0.5		8	26	81.25	193	183	10	5.2±1.3	0.5±1.9
control		11	34	72.27	232	221	11	4.8±1.4	-

at all stages of spermatogenesis. The effect of nickel sulfate at a dose 1.0 mg/kg (1/100 LD50) was observed in spermatozoids, early spermatids late spermatocytes, and stem spermatogonia. To estimate the non observable adverse effect level, the mice were administrated nickel sulfate at a dose 0.5mg/kg (1/200 LD50). Salt exposure on this level did not increase the DLM frequency in germline cells at any of the stage of spermatogenesis as compared with the control level.

Thus, the nonobservable effect level of nickel sulfate estimated by the DLM frequency (NOAEL) was1/200 DL50 and the threshold level (LOAEL), 1/100 DL50.

These results indicate that the most sensitive to nickel sulfate spermatogenesis stages in the interval of 5.0 to 0.5 mg/kg doses are spermatozoids, early spermatids, and late spermatocytes and stem spermatogonia.

Today the attention of researchers is focused on the absence of the linear relationship upon the effect of physical and chemical mutagens at low dose levels. It was shown that upon irradiation at low doses, the dose-effect relationship is bimodal, which is explained by the absence of inducible repair or its incomplete character [13].

A nonlinear relationship was also shown upon exposure to toxic pharmaceutical compounds at low doses. In this case, the relationship curve can also be bimodal; inverted (the effect higher at low doses than at high ones); V-shaped; including hyperlinear, sublinear, and linear segments. This relationship is characteristic of groups that inhabit ecologically hazardous regions [14].The increase of DLM frequency in stem spermatogonia, albeit small ($p<0.05$), should be taken into account, because repopulation of these cells provides restoration of spermatogenic epithelium. An induced increase in mutation frequency in stem cells at these stages can be preserved during the reproductive period.

Fig. 1 represents the relationship between the DNA comet index in sperm and the dose of nickel sulfate. A statistically significant increase of the mean sperm comet index was shown to be absent 4 weeks after the administration of nickel sulfate (exposure at the stage of late spermatocytes). At the same time a significant ($p<0.05$) increase in the percentage of cells with a very high DNA fragmentation level (supposedly apoptotic cells) was recorded at doses of 0.5 and 1.0 mg/kg. The following mechanisms may underlie this phenomenon:(1) because of possible low effectiveness of induced DNA repair, the exposure to nickel sulfate at low doses leads to the appearance of mutations in germline cells, which are subsequently eliminated by apoptosis;

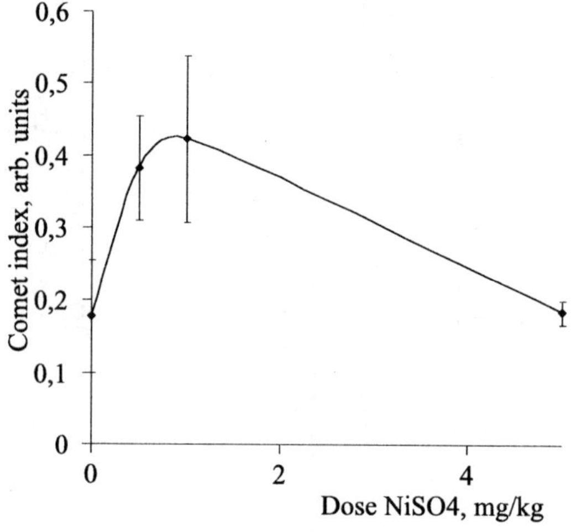

Figure 1. Changes in the mean index of DNA comets in sperm of mice upon intraperitoneal administration of nickel sulfate at different doses at the late spermatocyte stage.

(2) elimination of cells with genetic load is faster upon exposure to nickel sulfate at higher doses.

These results support the view that apoptosis plays an important role in selection of germline cells at all stages of spermatogenesis [15]. To explain the mechanisms of apoptosis in germline cells, two alternative theories have been advanced. According to the first theory, DNA fragmentation is caused by disturbed activity of endogenous nucleases (in particular, topoisomerase II) that produce DNA breaks [16]. The second theory implies the participation in this process of a surface protein, Fas, which is similar to the tumor necrosis factor and apoptosis mediators (Fas protein binding to Fas ligand or anti-Fas antibodies results in cell death) [17].

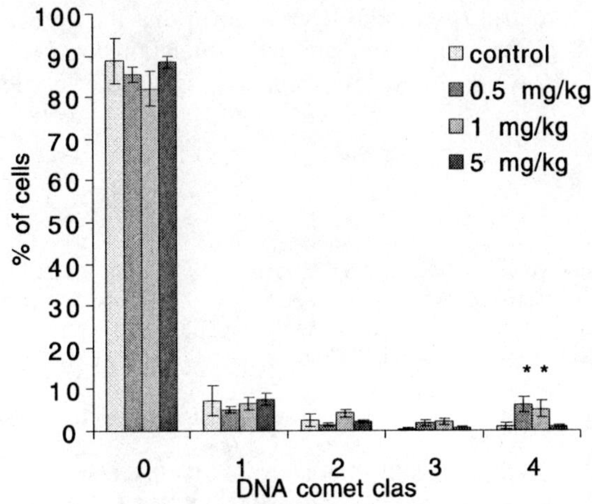

Figure 2. Distribution of spermatozoa by DNA comet classes in mice upon intraperitoneal administration of nickel sulfate at different doses at the late spermatocyte stage. *P < 0.01.

The effect of nickel sulfate at a dose 5.0 (1/20 ΛΔ50) and 1.0 (1/100 LD50) mg/kg induced the increase the expression of c-kit gene in pigment cells of (F1) heterozygous WR mice as compared to the control level ($p \leq 0.001$). The Wy frequencies upon exposure to nickel sulfate at those doses was practically the same. To estimate the threshold level (LOAEL) the mice were administrated nickel sulfate at a dose of 0.5mg/kg (1/200 LD50). As shown in *table 2*, nickel sulfate at that dose did not increase the mutation frequency over the control level.

Consequently, genetic sensitivity of germline (based on the frequency dominant lethal mutations) and somatic (based on the frequency of gene mutations - Wy) cells to nickel sulfate at low doses (1/20 LD50 (1/200 LD50) is similar.

WR mice show a high frequency of mosaics (occurrence of spots with abnormal pigmentation in heterozygous individuals). This seems to explain an increase in frequency of coat-colour mosaics in F1 mice upon treatment with NiSO4 at low doses.

Table 2. Gene mutation frequency induced by nickel sulfate in somatic cells of first-generation WR mice

Dose, mg/kg (level)	Number of scored heterozygous F1 mice	Number of coat-color mosaics	Gene mutation frequency, % (M+m)
5.0 (1/20 LD50)	57	24	42.1±5.6. $p \leq 0.001$
1.0 (1/100 LD50)	58	23	39.7±5.5. $p \leq 0.001$
0.5 (1/200 LD50)	58	15	28.9 ±4.7
CONTROL	467	95	20.3±1.7

In summary, the results of the present study indicate that the spermatogenesis stages most sensitive to nickel sulfate (at a dose of 1.0 mg/kg) are spermatozoids, early spermatids, late spermatocytes and stem spermatogonia. There was no detected a statistically significant increase in the total DNA breaks level in spermatozoids 4 weeks after exposure (expose on the late spermatocyte stage). At the same time, a significant ($p<0.05$) increase in percentage of cells with an extremely high level of DNA fragmentation (supposedly apoptotic cells) was observed upon the exposure at a dose of 0.5 and 1.0 mg/kg. This indirectly indicates an important role of apoptosis in elimination of impaired germline cells. Nickel sulfate at doses 5.0 and 1.0 mg/kg induced a marked increase in the c-kit gene expression in pigmental cells of heterozygous first generation WR mice as compared to control ($p<0.001$). It was shown that the no observable adverse effect level (NOAEL) of nickel sulfate on the dominant lethal mutations frequency and gene mutations (NOAEL) was 1/200 LD50, while the lowest observable adverse effect level (LOAEL) - 1/100 LD50.

REFERENCES

1. Toxicological Profile for Nickel (Update). *US Department of Health & Human Services Public Health Service, Agency for Toxic Substances and Diases Registry* 1997; 51-52, 82, 124-129.
2. Patierno SR, Sugiyama M, Basilion JP, Costa M. Preferential DNA-Protein Crosslinking by NiCl2 in Magnesium-Insoluble Regions of Fractionated Chinese Hamster Ovary Cell Chromatin. *Cancer Res* 1985; 45: 5787-94.
3. Kasprzak KS. The Role of Oxidative Damage in Metal Carcinogenicity. *Chem Res Toxicol* 1991; 4: 604-15.
4. Hartwig A, Mullenders LHF, Schlepegrell R, et al. Nickel(II) Interferes with the Incision Step in Nucleotide Excision Repair in Mammalian Cells. *Cancer Res* 1994; 54: 4045-51.
5. Lei YX, Chen JK, Wu ZL. Detection of DNA Strand Breaks, DNA-Protein Crosslinks, and Telomerase Activity in Nickel-Transformed BALB/C 3T3 Cells. *Teratogen Carcinogen Mutagen* 2001; 21(6): 463-71.
6. Mastromatteo E. Jant Memorial Lecture: Nickel. *Am Ind Hyg Assoc J* 1986; 47: 589-01.
7. Malashenko AM, Surkova NI. WR, A New Mouse Line Highly Sensitive to the Cytogenetic Effect of ThioTEP. *Tsitol Genet* 1979; 13: 387-91.
8. Yang-Feng TL, Ulrich A, Franke A. The Oncogene c-kit (KIT) Is Located on Man Chromosome 4 and Mouse Chromosome 5. *Cytogenet Cell Genet* 1987; 46: 723.
9. Ehling UH, Machemer L, Buselmaier W, et al. Standard Protocol for the Dominant Lethal Test on Male Mice. *Arch. Toxicol* 1978; 39: 173-85.
10. Fahrig R. A Mammalian Spot-Test: Induction of Genetic Alterations in Pigment Cells of Mouse Embryos with X-Rays and Chemical Mutagens. *Mol Gen Genet* 1975; 138(4): 309-14.
11. Singh NP, Stephens RE. X Ray-Induced DNA Double-Strand Breaks in Human Sperm. *Mutagenesis* 1998; 13 (1): 75-9.
12. Collins AR, Ma AG, Duthie SJ. The Kinetics of Repair of Oxidative DNA Damage (Strand Breaks and Oxidized Pyrimidine Dimers in Human Cells). *Mutat Res* 1995; 336(1): 69-7.
13. Burlakova EB. Distant Consequences of the Integral Effect of Low Doses and Damaging Environmental Factors on Population Viability. *Budushchee natsii (Future of the Nation).* Moscow. 1995; part 2: 64-6.
14. Svendsgaard D, Calabrase EJ. U-Shaped Dose Response Relationships in Toxicology. *XXI Medichen Congr* (18-21 October 1994, Melbourne) 1994: 106-24.
15. Sakkas D, Mariethoz E, Manicardi G. et al. Origin of DNA Damage in Ejaculated Human Spermatozoa. *Rev Reprod* 1999; 4: 31-37.
16. McPherson SMG, Longo FJ. Chromatin Structure Function Alterations during Mammalian Spermatogenesis: DNA Nicking and Repair in Elongating Spermatids. *Eur J Histochem* 1993; 37: 109-28.
17. Lee J, Richburg JH, Younkin SC, Boekelheide K. The Fas System Is a Key Regulator of Germ Cell Apoptosis in the Testis. *Endocrinology* 1997; 138: 2081-88.

Metal Ions in Biology and Medicine: vol. 9. Eds Maria Carmen Alpoim, Paula Vasconcellos Morais, Maria Amélia Santos, Armando J. Cristóvão, José A. Centeno, Philippe Collery.
John Libbey Eurotext, Paris © 2006 pp. 407-1.

Uranium-induced oxidative stress in kidney and testis of rats

Linares V[1,2], Bellés M[1,2], Albina ML[1,2], Sirvent JJ[3], Sánchez DJ[1,2], Gómez M[1], Domingo JL[1,*]

[1]*Laboratory of Toxicology and Environmental Health,*
[2]*Physiology Unit and*
[3]*Pathology Unit,, School of Medicine, "Rovira i Virgili" University, San Lorenzo 21, 43201 Reus, Spain, *joseluis.domingo@urv.net*

INTRODUCTION

Uranium occurs naturally in the earth's crust as well as in surface and ground waters. Military use of uranium as depleted uranium (DU) is likely to have any significant impact on the environmental levels of this heavy metal. At sites where DU munitions were used, measurements of uranium indicate only localized contamination at the ground surface. However, in some circumstances the levels of contamination in food and ground water could rise after some years and there is a reasonable possibility of significant quantities of DU entering the food chain [1]. DU is toxic based on the findings in animals exposed to natural uranium, with the kidney being the main target organ [2].

There is an increasing concern on the role of environmental contaminants on male reproduction of wildlife and humans. An important role in the decline of quality and quantity of human semen [3] has been noted with some environmental contaminants, which have shown to induce ROS generation in both intra- and extracellular spaces of cells or individuals leading to cell death and tissue injury [4]. Previous studies have shown that environmental pollutants may alter antioxidant system in the testes of the rat [5]. Although the effects of uranium have been studied in experimental animals, the mechanism of action of this element has not been elucidated yet.

On the other hand, it is also well known that physiological and biochemical alterations are common response to stress [6]. Information on the combined effects of simultaneous exposure to metals and stress is rather scarce. However, it is evident that humans can be potentially exposed to different environmental levels of uranium, while they can be also concurrently subjected to various types of stress. The aim of the present study was to evaluate in male rats the effects of uranium on the induction of oxidative stress in reproductive tissues (and also in the kidney as the target organ), as well as the potential influence of stress on these effects.

METHODS

Chemical. Uranium was administered as uranyl acetate dihydrate (UAD), which was purchased from E. Merck (Darmstadt, Germany). UAD was dissolved in tap water and given orally at 10, 20 and 40 mg/kg/day. These doses are approximately equal to 1/20, 1/10, and 1/5 of the acute oral LD_{50} of UAD in adult rats [7].

Treatment. Sexually mature male and female Sprague-Dawley rats (220-240g) were obtained from Criffa (Barcelona, Spain). Animals were housed in plastic cages in a climate-controlled facility with a constant day-night cycle (light: 08.00-20.00h) at a temperature of 22±2°C, and a relative humidity of 50±10%. After a quarantine period of 14 days, male rats were orally exposed to UAD for 3 months. Food (Panlab rodent chow, Barcelona) and drinking water were available *ad libitum*. Male rats were randomly divided into eight groups and received the following treatments. Animals in six groups drank solutions of UAD at 10, 20, and 40 mg/kg/day for 3 months. Animals in three of these groups were also subjected to restraint for 2 h/day during the same period. For it, rats were immobilized in metacrilate cylindrical holders (Letica Scientific Instruments, Panlab, Barcelona) [6]. Two control groups included restrained and unrestrained male rats not exposed to UAD.

At the end of the experimental period, male rats were euthanized with ketamine-xylazine. Testes and kidneys were removed, cleared of the adhering tissues and weighed. The activities of superoxide dismutase (SOD), catalase (CAT), glutathione reductase (GR) and glutathione peroxidase (GPx), as well as the levels of oxidized glutathione (GSSG), reduced glutathione (GSH) and lipid peroxidation (TBARS) were determined in both tissues. Uranium concentrations were determined by inductively coupled plasma-mass spectrometry (Perkin Elmer, Elan 6000) according to previously reported methods [8].

Statistics. Homogeneity of variances was analyzed employing Levene's test. If variances were homogeneous ANOVA was used followed by the Tukey method to evaluate all dose groups simultaneously. The Kruskal-Wallis test was used when variances were not homogeneous. Differences between control and uranium-treated groups were analyzed using the Mann-Whitney U-test. Statistical significance was set at $P < 0.05$.

RESULTS

The results of the current study showed a positive correlation ($P < 0.01$) between increased uranium exposure and renal injury, which was evidenced by an increase in lipid peroxidation (TBARS) when compared with the corresponding control group *(fig. 1, A)*. Although an increase in some biochemical parameters such as GSSG and SOD activity was observed, an association between renal uranium content and these parameters was not found (data not shown).

In uranium treated rat testis, SOD activity was significantly enhanced while GR, GSH and CAT decreased in the male reproductive tract (data not shown). However, only GSH levels and SOD activity were significantly associated with an increase of uranium concentrations in testes *(fig. 1, B and C* respectively).

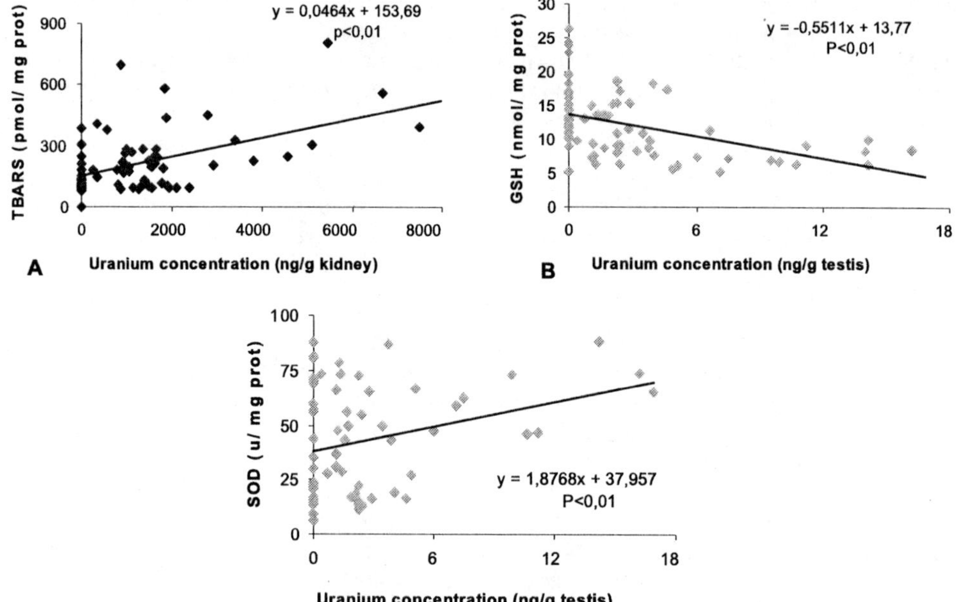

Figure 1. Correlations between uranium concentrations and the levels of TBARS in kidney (A) and GSH levels and SOD activity in testis (B and C, respectively).

Histopathological examination of the kidney revealed differences between control and uranium-exposed animals *(fig. 2)*. A progressive angiomatose transformation in uranium-exposed animals was observed.

Any of those parameters was significantly affected by restraint stress.

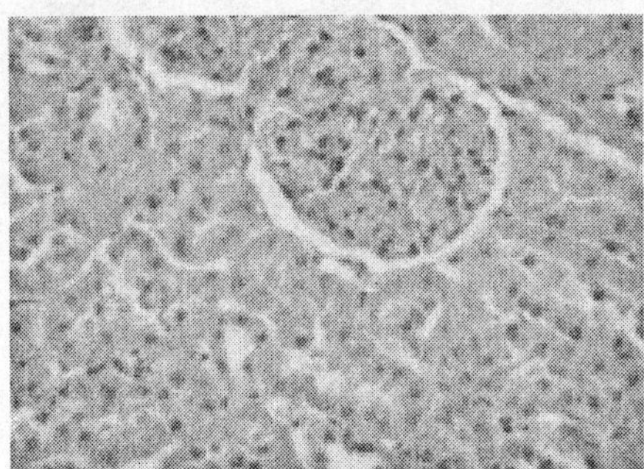

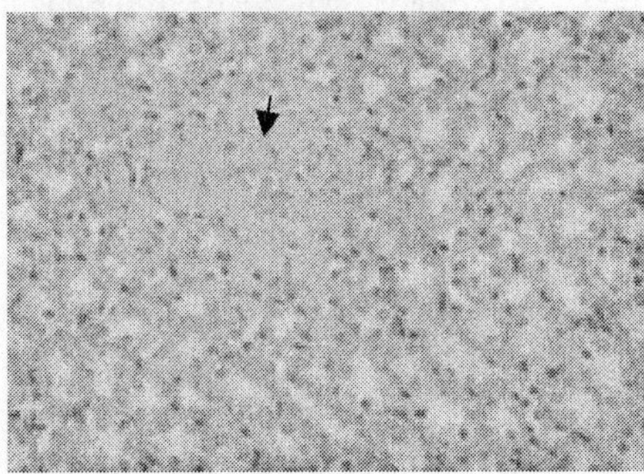

Figure 2. Histological sections of kidneys stained with H/E under light microscopy. The difference between a normal kidney section (left) and an angiomatose transformation in uranium-exposed animals is noted (right).

CONCLUSIONS

The above results indicate that oral exposure to uranium causes toxicity in rat kidney and testis. Graded doses of uranium elicit depletion of the antioxidant defence system of the rat and induce oxidative stress in both examined tissues. Although at the current uranium doses, restraint stress scarcely showed additional adverse effects, its potential influence should not be underrated.

REFERENCES

1. World Health Organization (WHO). Depleted Uranium. Sources, Exposure and Health Effects. Department of Protection of the Human Environment. Report No:WHO/SDE/PHE/01.1. WHO, 2001, Geneva, Switzerland.
2. Domingo JL., 2001. Reproductive and developmental toxicity of natural and depleted uranium: a review. *Reprod. Toxicol.* 2001; 15: 603-9.
3. Colborn T., vom Saal FS., Soto AM., 1993. Developmental effects of endocrine-disrupting chemicals in wildlife and humans. *Environ. Health Perspect.* 1993; 101: 378-4.
4. Chitra KC., Latchoumycandane C., Mathur PP., 2003. Induction of oxidative stress by bisphenol A in the epididymal sperm of rats. *Toxicology* 2003; 185: 119-27.
5. Latchoumycandane C, Chitra KC, Mathur PP, 2002. Induction of oxidative stress in the rat epididymal sperm after exposure to 2,3,7,8-tetrachlorodibenzo-p-dioxin on the antioxidant system in mitochondrial and microsomal fractions of rat testis. *Toxicology* 2002; 171: 127-35.
6. Colomina, M.T., Albina, M.L., Domingo, J.L., Corbella, J., 1997. Influence of maternal stress on the effects of prenatal exposure to methylmercury and arsenic on postnatal development and behavior in mice: A preliminary evaluation. *Physiol. Behav.* 1997; 61: 455-9.
7. Domingo, J.L., Llobet, J.M., Tomas, J.M., Corbella, J., 1987. Acute toxicity of uranium in rats and mice. *Bull. Environ. Contam. Toxicol.* 1987; 39: 168-74.
8. Sánchez, D.J., Bellés, M., Albina, M.L., Sirvent, J.J., Domingo, J.L., 2001. Nephrotoxicity of simultaneous exposure to mercury and uranium in comparison to individual effects of these metals in rats. *Biol. Trace Elem. Res.* 2001; 84: 139-54.

ACKNOWLEDGEMENTS

Financial support for this study was provided by the "Fondo de Investigación Sanitaria", Ministry of Health, Spain, through grant no. PI030254. The authors thank the "Servei d'Anatomia Patològica", Hospital Joan XXIII, for valuable technical assistance.

Metal Ions in Biology and Medicine: vol. 9. Eds Maria Carmen Alpoim, Paula Vasconcellos Morais, Maria Amélia Santos, Armando J. Cristóvão, José A. Centeno, Philippe Collery.
John Libbey Eurotext, Paris © 2006 pp. 411-1.

Prenatal exposure of female rats to lead acetate. Effect on their progeny

Nemmiche Said[1], Chabane-Sari Daoudi[2]

[1]*Department of Biology, Faculty of Sciences, University of Mostaganem BP 227, 27000 Mostaganem, Algeria. snemiche@hotmail.com*
[2]*Department of Biology, Faculty of Sciences, University of Tlemcen BP 119, Tlemcen 13000, Algeria*

ABSTRACT

The contamination of the pregnant woman's organism by toxic metals poses a serious risk of the some quantitative degree of contaminating the organism of the child developing in her womb. Qualitative changes may be much more serious in the fetus as they affect young structures, intensively developing, with no well-formed defense mechanisms. Multidirectional studies evaluating the environmental pollution contribute to the prophylaxis of toxicological threats. The aim of this paper is to see if it exist changes of the neurochemical parameters during developmental related to chemical dose treatment of female rats. METHODS: Female Wistar rats (3 weeks of age) were given to experiments during 90 days, were treated by lead acetate tri hydrate (2000ppm) dissolved in drinking water. These female rats were mated with an unprocessed male. Their progeny was used in this survey. The dosage of the neurochemicals parameters: choline acetyltransferase activity (CAT) and glutamic acid decarboxylase (GAD) was achieved. RESULTS: The level of the blood lead (PbB) of descendants varies from 15 to 24 μg/dl. The weight of young rats doesn't record any significant difference ($P < 0.05$) in relation to control group for a postnatal development of 14 days. However, a significant difference ($P < 0.05$) for a postnatal development of 28 days. This is how the lead exposure caused a reduction of 34% of the CAT activity, specific enzyme of neurons cholinergics, in relation to control group, in the hippocampus (postnatal 14 days). This reduction attain 40% in the 28th days (postnatal 28 days), which indicate a reduction in the expression of the enzyme in the cellular bodies of neurons or in the number of their cells. In addition we note a significant effect on the expression of the GAD, a GABAergic neuron marker enzyme, in this region of the brain, for the development postnatal 28th days (a reduction of the GAD activity of 25% in relation to control group). Conclusions: It confirms that prenatal exposures with PbB of 20 μg/dl induce a significant reduction in the Septal cholinergic muscarinic receptors during the period of the postnatal development.

Keys Words: Choline acetyltransferase, Glutamic acid decarboxylase, Lead exposure, Rats, Postnatal development.

INTRODUCTION

Lead is an environmental pollutant which has received much attention, partly because of the particular sensitivity of children to this element. Exposure to lead can result in significant adverse health effects to multiple organ systems. Nowadays, motor transport industry is the dominating source of lead entering into the environment (Semczuk and Semczuk-Sikora, 2001). The central nervous system is one of the most important targets of Pb^{+2}-mediated toxicity. The neurobehavioral effects of chronic and acute exposure to Pb^{+2} during development are well known (Bellinger et *al.*, 1984; Needleman et *al.*, 1996; Jett et *al.*, 1997; Moreira et *al.*, 2001; Carpenter et *al.*, 2002). In addition, data obtained from epidemiological studies implicate a causal link between low-level chronic exposure to Pb^{+2} and deficiencies in intelligence quotients in children (Needleman et *al.*, 1990; Schwartz, 1994; Wasserman et *al.*, 2003). Functional impairment of the developing brain has been reported at blood lead levels as low as 10-15 µg/dl (Bellinger and *al.*, 1987; Davis and *al.*, 1990). Childhood exposure to low levels of lead causes cognitive functioning deficit and a reduction in intelligence through a direct action on the hippocampus and cortex (Petit et *al.*, 1992; Wilson et *al.*, 2000). Deficits in cognitive function are the undisputed effects of childhood lead (Pb2+) intoxication (Bellinger, 2004). Although the exact molecular mechanisms of these Pb2+ effects are not fully understood, antagonism of the N-methyl-d-aspartate receptor (NMDAR), an ionotropic glutamate receptor, is emerging as a principle mechanism of Pb2+ neurotoxicity (Toscano et *al.*, 2005). Others studies point to an interaction between the glutamatergic neurotransmitter system and inorganic lead neurotoxicity, the interaction of glutamate and Pb+2 results in increased neuronal cell death via mechanisms that involve an increase in reactive oxygen species (ROS) production, a decrease in intracellular glutathione (GSH) defense against oxidative stress and probably T-type voltage-sensitive calcium channels (VSCCs) (Loikkanen et *al.*, 2003). Accumulating evidence has shown that lead causes oxidative stress by inducing the generation of ROS and weakening the antioxidant defense system of cells [Lawton and Donaldson, 1991; Adonaylo and Oteiza, 1999). Malondialdehyde (MDA) levels were strongly correlated with lead concentration in the brain of lead-exposed rats (Villeda-Hernández et *al.*, 2001). The activity of antioxidant enzymes such as superoxide dismutase (SOD), catalase, and glutathione reductase (GR) was decreased in lead-exposed rats. The aim of the present study was to see if it exist changes of the neurochemical parameters during developmental related to chemical dose treatment of female rats.

MATERIALS AND METHODS

Animal exposure protocol

Two groups of female Wistar rats aged 3 weeks were treated during 3 months by a dose of 0 ppm or 2000 ppm lead acetate tri hydrate in the drinking water, respectively. From the offspring, a total of 20 lead exposed (exits of female treated by a dose of 2000ppm mated to an unprocessed male) and 10 control pups (male and female) were used for this study and examination at postnatal days 14-28.

Determination of lead in blood and tissue samples

Blood and brain tissues were collected of lead analysis from control and lead-exposed rats at postnatal days 14 and 28. Following exsanguinations, the brain was rapidly removed and stored frozen at -20°C. Lead in blood and brain tissue samples was measured by graphite furnace atomic absorption spectrophotometer (SP9 Unicam).

Dosage of the neurochemicals parameters

Choline acetyltransferase (CAT) activity was measured according to Fonnum (1969) and glutamic acid decarboxylase (GAD) activity was determined as described by Miller and *al.* (1978).

Statistical analysis

The values in the figures are means ± SEM. The comparison of the data was done by one way variance analysis, and $P < 0.05$ was considered significant.

RESULTS

The level of the blood lead (PbB) of descendants varies 15 to 24µg/dl. The weight of young rats doesn't record any significant difference ($P<0.05$) in relation to control group for a postnatal development of 14 days against a significant difference ($P<0.05$) for a postnatal development of 28 days *(fig. 1)*. However the lead exposure caused a reduction of 34% of the choline acetyltransferase activity *(fig. 2)*, specific enzyme of neurons cholinergics, in relation to control group, in the hippocampus (postnatal 14 days); this reduction attain 40% to the 28th days (postnatal 28 days), indicatory of a reduction in the expression of the enzyme in the cellular bodies of neurons or a reduction in the number of these cells.Besides one notes a significant effect on the expression of the GAD *(fig. 3)*, a GABAergic neuron marker enzyme, in this region of the brain, for the development postnatal 28th days (a reduction of the GAD activity of 25% in relation to control group).

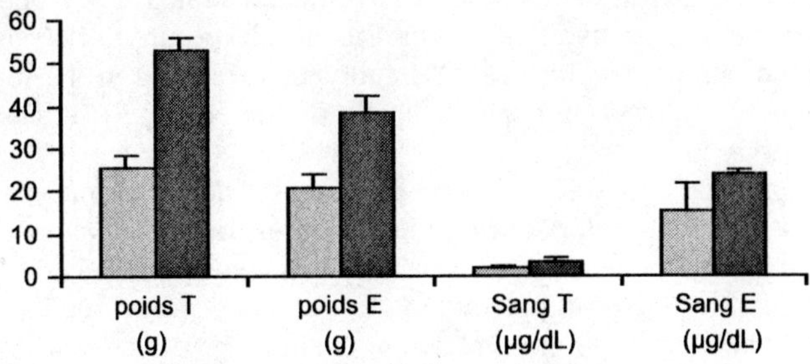

Figure 1. Body weight in control group rats and in rats exposed to lead, exits of female treated mated with an unprocessed male, and dosage of their blood lead

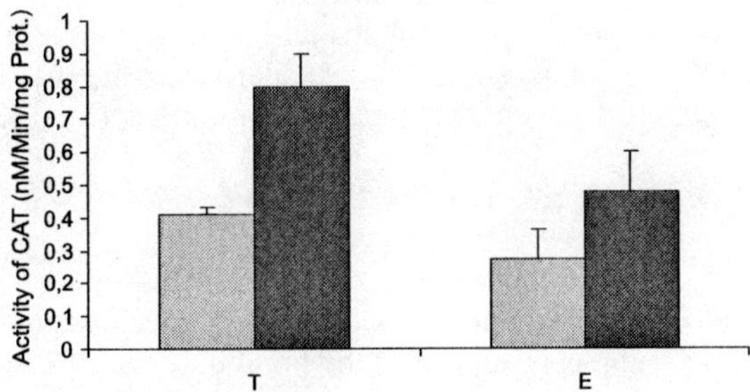

Figure 2. Postnatal development of Choline Acetyl Transferase Activity in rat brain (hippocampus region) of control rats (T) and exposed group (E)

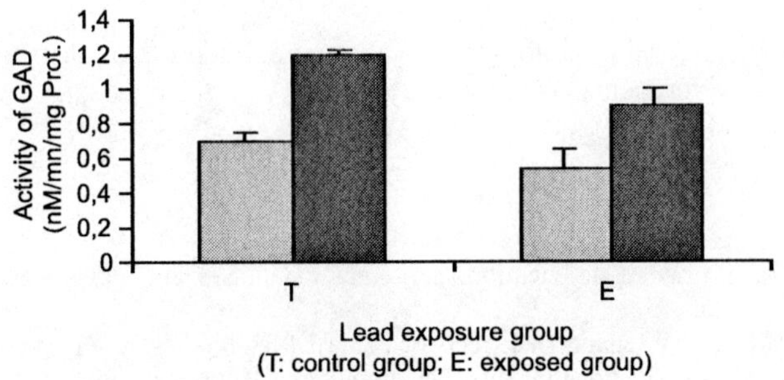

Figure 3. Activity of glutamic acid decarboxylase in rat brain (hippocampus region)

DISCUSSION

Some similar results are found by Bielarczyk et *al.* (1994) that worked with pregnant Sprague-Dawley rats, treated with 0.2% of lead acetate via the water of drink, show that in contrast to the significant reduction of CAT activity, find no effect of the expression of GAD in either brain region. The authors speculated that such a septal cholinergic hypo function produced by Pb^{+2} could result in an up regulation of postsynaptic sites, possibly M2 sites in the hippocampus.

Cory-Slechta (1995), reported decreases of in vivo acetylcholine turnover rate of 35-54% in cortex, hippocampus, midbrain, and striatum in rats exposed to Pb lactationally.

An increase in blood lead from 10 to 20μg/dl was associated with a decrease of 2.6 IQ points in the Meta analysis (Schwartz, 1994). A similar level of exposure with a PbB of 10-15 μg/dl measured at children of an age group of 3 months to 2 years, is associated with a deficit of 2-3 points of the index of the mental development (Davis et *al.*, 1990) or 5.8 points in the WISC-R-full-Scale IQ (Bellinger et *al.*, 1992). Experimental studies have demonstrated that blood levels of 10μg/dl interfere with broad range of cognitive function in primates. Exposure to Pb^{+2} during development alters the expression and proportion of NMDAR subtypes expressed in the hippocampus of rats exhibiting environmentally relevant blood Pb^{+2} levels (Nihei et *al.*, 2000; Toscano et *al.*, 2002; Zhang et *al.*, 2002).

It confirms that a prenatal exposure with PbB of 20 μg/dl induce a significant reduction in the Septal cholinergic muscarinic receptors during the period of the postnatal development. Lead interferes with GABAergic and dopaminergic neurotransmission. It has been shown to bind to the NMDA receptor and inhibit long-term potentiation in the hippocampal region of the brain.

An integral role for cholinergic systems in learning/memory processes is widely accepted (Cory-Slechta, 1995). Learning and memory are affected by the chronic exposure to lead (Needleman et *al.*, 1990). Several studies have shown that Pb^{2+} - induced inhibition of NMDA receptors during development and subsequent changes is emerging as a mechanism underlying the deficits in synaptic plasticity and learning caused by this metal (Toscano et *al.*, 2002; Guilarte et *al.*, 2003). Animals exposed to Pb^{+2} also express deficits in spatial learning and hippocampal long-term potentiation (LTP) (Toscano et *al.*, 2005). Another molecular target that has been recently reported to be affected in vitro by Pb^{2+} is mitogen-activated protein kinases (MAPKs) (Leal et *al.*, 2002).

CONCLUSIONS

Lead (Pb^{2+}) is widely recognized as a neurotoxicant whose mechanisms of action are not completely established. The hippocampus is an area of the brain necessary for spatial learning. A large number of studies have reported negative associations between lead exposure and cognitive development in children at lead concentrations once considered normal. A role for cholinergic hypo function as a factor in behavioral neurotoxicity of Pb^{2+} has been implicated by the observation that maternal lead exposure result in a significant reduction in acetylcholine turnover in the hippocampus of suckling rats.

A central issue in behavioral teratology or developmental neurotoxicology is the establishment of prenatal causes of developmental behavioral disorders.

REFERENCES

Adonaylo, V. N. Oteiza, P.I. Lead intoxication: antioxidant defenses and oxidative damage in rat brain. Toxicology 1999; 135: 77-85.

Altmann L., Gutowski M., and Wiegand H. Effects of maternal lead exposure on functional plasticity in the visual cortex and hippocampus of immature rats. Developmental Brain Res 1994; 81: 50-56.

D.C. Bellinger, Lead, Pediatrics 2004; 113: 1016-1022.

Bellinger, D.C., Needleman, H.L., Bromfield, R., Mintz, M. A follow-up study of the academic attainment and classroom behaviour of children with elevated dentine lead levels. Biol Trace Elem Res 1984; 6: 207-214.
Belliger D., Leviton A., Watermaux C., Needleman HL., and Rabinowitz M. Longitudinal analyses of prenatal and postnatal lead exposure and early cognitive development. N Engl J Med 1987; 316: 1037-43.
Bellinger D., A. Leviton, C. Waternaux, H. Needleman and M. Rabinowitz. Low-level lead exposure, social class, and infant development. Neurotoxicol Teratol 1989; 10: 497-503.
Bellinger D. C., Stiles K. M., and Needleman H. L. Low-level lead exposure, intelligence and académic achievement: A long-term follow-up study. Pediatrics 1992; 90(6): 855-861.
Bielarczyk H., Tomsing J. L., and Suszkiw J. B. Perinatal low-level lead exposure and the septo-hippocampal cholinergic system: selective reduction of muscarinic receptors and cholineacetyltransferase in the rat septum. Brain Research 1994; 643: 211-217.
Carpenter, D.O., Hussain, R.J., Berger, D.F., Lombardo, J.P., Park, H.Y. Electrophysiologic and behavioral effects of perinatal and acute exposure of rats to lead and polychlorinated biphenyls. Environ Health Perspect 2002; 110 (Suppl. 3): 377- 386.
Cory-Slechta D.A. Relationships between Lead-induced Learning Impairments and changes in Dopaminergic, Cholinergic, and Glutamatergic Neurotransmetter System Functions. Annu Rev Pharmacol Toxicol 1995; 35: 391-415.
S.A. Counter, M. Vahter, G. Laurell, L.H. Buchanan, F. Ortega, S. Skerfving, High lead exposure and auditory sensory-neural function in Andean children, Environ Health Perspect 1997; 105: 522-526.
Davis J.M., D.A. Otto, D.E. Weil and L. D. Grant, The comparative developmental neurotoxicity of lead in humans and animals. Neurotoxicol Teratol, 1990; 12: 215-229.
Fonnum F. Radiochemical micro assay for the determination of choline acetyltransferase. Biochem J 1969; 115: 465-472.
T.R. Guilarte, C.D. Toscano, J.L. McGlothan, S.A. Weaver, Environmental enrichment reverses cognitive and molecular deficits induced by developmental lead exposure, Ann Neurol 2003; 53: 50-56.
Jett, D.A., Kuhlmann, A.C., Farmer, S.J., Guilarte, T.R., Age-dependent effects of developmental lead exposure on performance in the Morris water maze. Pharmacol Biochem Behav 1997; 57: 271-279.
A.C. Kuhlmann, J.L. McGlothan, T.R. Guilarte, Developmental lead exposure causes spatial learning deficits in adult rats, Neurosci Lett 1997; 233: 101-104.
Lawton, L. J., Donaldson, W. E. Lead-induced tissue fatty acid alterations and lipid peroxidation. Biol Trace Elem Res 1991; 28: 83-97.
G.-H. Lianga, L. Järlebarka, M. Ulfendahla, J.-T. Bianb, E.J. Moore. Lead (Pb2+) modulation of potassium currents of guinea pig outer hair cells. Neurotoxicology and Teratology 2004; 26: 253-260.
R.B. Leal, F.M. Cordova, H. Lynn, L. Bobrovskaya, P.R. Dunkley, Lead-stimulate P38mapk-dependent Hsp27 phosphorylation, Toxicol Appl Pharmacol 2002; 178: 44- 51.
Loikkanen J, Naarala J, Vahakangas KH, Savolainen KM. Glutamate increases toxicity of inorganic lead in GT1-7 neurons: partial protection induced by flunarizine. Arch Toxicol 2003 Dec; 77(12): 663-71.
Miller LP., Martin D.L., Mazumder A., and Walters J.R. Studies on the regulation of GABA synthesis: substrate-promoted dissociation of pyridoxal-5'-phosphate from GAD. J Neurochem 1978; 30: 361-369.
R.G. Morris, E.I. Moser, G. Riedel, S.J. Martin, J. Sandin, M. Day, C. O'Carroll, Elements of a neurobiological theory of the hippocampus: the role of activity-dependent synaptic plasticity in memory, Philos Trans R Soc London, B Biol Sci 2003; 358: 773- 786.
Moreira, E.G., Vassilieff, I., Vassilieff, V.S. Developmental lead exposure: behavioral alterations in the short and long term. Neurotoxicol Teratol 2001; 23: 489-495.
Needleman, H.L., Schell, A., Bellinger, D., Leviton, A., Allred, E.N. The long-term effects of exposure to low doses of lead in children. An 11-year follow-up report. N Engl J Med 1990; 322: 83-88.
Needleman, H.L., Reiss, A., Tobin, M.J., Beisecker, G.E., Greenhouse, J.B. Bone lead levels and delinquent behavior. JAMA 1996; 275: 363-369.
M.K. Nihei, N.L. Desmond, J.L. McGlothan, A.C. Kuhlmann, T.R. Guilarte, N-methyl-d-aspartate receptor subunit changes are associated with lead-induced deficits of long-term potentiation and spatial learning, Neuroscience 2000; 99: 233-242.
Petit, T. L, LeBoutillier J C, Brooks, WJ. Altered sensitivity to NMDA following developmental lead exposure in rats. Physiol Behav 1992; 52: 687-693.
Semczuk M., A. Semczuk-Sikora. New data on toxic metal intoxication (Cd, Pb, and Hg in particular) and Mg status during pregnancy. Med Sci Monit 2001; 7(2): 332-340.
Schwartz J. Low-level lead exposure and children's IQ: A meta analysis and search for a threshold. Environm Res 1994; 65: 42-55.

K.C. Staudinger, V.S. Roth. Occupational lead poisoning. Am Fam Phys 1998; 57: 719-726.
Thoreux-Manlay A., G. Pinon-Lataillade, H. Coffiny, J.C. Soufir, R. Masse. Prenatal or lactational exposure of male rats to lead acetate. Effect on reproductive function. Bull Environ Contam Toxicol 1995; 54: 266-272.
Toscano D. Christopher, James P. O'Callaghan, Toma's R. Guilarte,T. Calcium/calmodulin-dependent protein kinase II activity and expression are altered in the hippocampus of Pb2+-exposed rats. Brain Research 2005; 1044: 51-58.
C.D. Toscano, H. Hashemzadeh-Gargari, J.L. McGlothan, T.R. Guilarte, Developmental Pb2+ exposure alters NMDAR subtypes and reduces CREB phosphorylation in the rat brain, Dev Brain Res 2002; 13: 217-226.
Villeda-Hernández, J., Barroso-Moguel, R., Méndez-Arment, M., Nava-Ruíz, C. Huerta-Romero, R. Rios, C. Enhanced brain regional lipid peroxidation in developing rats exposed to low level lead acetate. Brain Res Bull 2001; 55: 247-251.
Wasserman, G.A., Factor-Litvak, P., Liu, X., Todd, A.C., Kline, J.K., Slavkovich, V., Popovac, D., Graziano, J.H. The relationship between blood lead, bone lead and child intelligence. Neuropsychol Dev Cogn, Sect C, Child Neuropsychol 2003; 9: 22-34.
Wilson, M.A., Johnston, M.V, Goldstein G.W. Blue, ME. Neonatal lead exposure impairs development of rodent barrel field cortex. Proc Natl Acad Sci U.S.A. 2000; 97: 5540-5545.
X.Y. Zhang, A.P. Liu, D.Y. Ruan, J. Liu, Effect of developmental lead exposure on the expression of specific NMDA receptor subunit mRNAs in the hippocampus of neonatal rats by digoxigenin-labeled in situ hybridization histochemistry Neurotoxicol Teratol 2002; 24: 149-160.

Metal Ions in Biology and Medicine: vol. 9. Eds Maria Carmen Alpoim, Paula Vasconcellos Morais, Maria Amélia Santos, Armando J. Cristóvão, José A. Centeno, Philippe Collery.
John Libbey Eurotext, Paris © 2006 pp. 417-1.

Arsenic trioxide induced oxidative stress in Sprague-Dawley rats

Anita K. Patlolla[1] and Paul B. Tchounwou[1]

[1]*Molecular Toxicology Research Laboratory, NIH - Center for Environmental Health, College of Science, Engineering, and Technology, Jackson State University, Jackson, MS, USA.*

ABSTRACT

Arsenic is a known human carcinogen and induces a variety of human diseases in addition to cancers of the lung, skin, bladder, kidneys and liver. The mechanism, by which arsenic induces cancer, however remains poorly understood. Although multiple pathways such as inhibition of DNA repair, methylation status, and cocarcinogenesis with other environmental toxicants have been proposed, recent studies have pointed out that arsenic toxicity is associated with the formation of reactive oxygen species, which has a role in the pathogenesis of arsenic-induced diseases. The main aim of the present investigation was to determine the concentration of malondialdehyde (MDA), as an indicator of lipid peroxidation in the serum of Sprague-Dawley rats. Four groups of six male rats each weighing approximately 60 ± 2 g, were injected intraperitoneally, once a day for five days with doses of 5, 10, 15, 20 mg/kg body weight (BW) of arsenic trioxide dissolved in distilled water. A control group was also made of six animals injected with distilled water without chemical. Following anaesthetization, blood specimens were immediately collected in tubes containing EDTA as an anticoagulant, and the concentration of malondialdehyde (MDA), a convenient index of lipid peroxidation in serum samples was determined using by colorimetry (Calbiochem). Arsenic trioxide (As_2O_3) exposure significantly ($p \leq 0.05$) increased the concentration of MDA in the treated groups [8.0-22.3 μM] compared to the control group [7.3 μM], showing a gradual increase in lipid peroxidation with increasing doses of arsenic. These findings indicate that oxidative stress plays a role in arsenic-induced cellular damage in Sprague-Dawley rats.

INTRODUCTION

Arsenic is of significant environmental concern worldwide because millions of people are at risk of drinking water contaminated by arsenic [1]. Acute exposure due to accidental uptake or intentional administration (in cases of suicidal or homicidal attempts) is rare and may result in gastrointestinal discomfort, vomiting, coma and sometimes even death. However, it is chronic poisoning which is of prime concern to environmental toxicologists; it causes a wide range of toxic effects involving multiple organ systems of the body. One of the important signs of chronic arsenic toxicity in humans is occurrence of skin lesions, characterized by hyper-pigmentation, hyperkeratosis and hypo-pigmentation [2]. Oxidative deterioration of polyunsaturated fatty acids by a process known as lipid peroxidation has been widely accepted as a general mechanism of action for cellular injury and toxic effects of arsenic [3-5]. It is well reported that arsenic induced lipid peroxidation and generation of reactive oxygen species is the main cause of genotoxicity in laboratory animals [6, 7]. In addition, it has been suggested that arsenic has a co-clastogenic effect, which in turn may be attributed to its ability to interfere with DNA repair pathways [8].

Analyzing the toxic effects of arsenic is complicated because; the toxicity depends on its chemical state. Inorganic arsenic in its trivalent form is more toxic than penatvalent arsenic. The toxicity of arsenic also depends on the exposure dose, frequency and duration, the biological species, age, and gender, as well as on individual susceptibilities, genetic and nutritional factors. By binding to thiol or sulfhydryl groups on proteins, As (III) can inactivate over 200 enzymes. This is the likely mechanism responsible for arsenic's widespread effects on different organ system. As (V) can replace phosphate, which is involved in many biochemical pathways. The major metabolic pathway for inorganic arsenic in humans is methylation. Arsenic trioxide is methylated to two major metabolites via a non-enzymatic process to monomethylarsonic acid (MMA), which is further methylated enzymatically to dimethyl arsenic acid (DMA) before excretion in the urine [9].

Although research over the past decade strongly endorsed the role of free radical species in the pathogenicity of arsenic-induced diseases, their molecular effects to be elucidated. Therefore, the specific aim of this study was to determine the concentration of malondialdehyde (MDA), as an indicator of lipid peroxidation in the serum of Sprague-Dawley rats, which may be useful as a biomarker of sensitivity and effect associated with arsenic exposure.

MATERIALS AND METHODS

Animal maintenance and treatment

Healthy adult male Sprague-Dawley rats (8-10 weeks of age, with average body weight (BW) of 60 ± 2 g) were used in this study. They were obtained from Harlan-Sprague-Dawley Breeding laboratories in Indianapolis, Indiana, USA. The animals were randomly selected and housed in polycarbonate cages (three rats per cage) with steel wire tops and corn-cob bedding. They were maintained in a controlled atmosphere with a 12h:12h dark/light cycle, a temperature of 22 ± 2°C and 50-70% humidity with free access to pelleted food and fresh tap water. The animals were supplied with dry food pellets commercially available from PMI Feeds Inc. (St. Louis, Missouri). They were allowed to acclimate for 10 days before treatment.

In this investigation, a total of 30 animals were used, 5 groups including one control. Each group had 6 animals per dose. Arsenic trioxide was administered to the animals by intraperitoneal injection once a day for 5 days. At the end of treatment period, rats were anesthetized using 95% CO_2 for 70 seconds and then decapitated by cervical dislocation. Immediately following anaesthetization blood specimens were collected using EDTA syringes to prevent clotting, and the serum was separated by centrifugation at 2000 g for 10 min. Serum samples were evaluated for malondialdehyde (MDA) concentration using a colorimetric assay protocol provided by Calbiochem (San Diego, CA).

Assay for Lipid peroxidation

Lipid peroxidation is a well-established mechanism of cellular injury in both plants and animals. This process leads to the production of lipid peroxides and their by-products and ultimately the loss of membrane function and integrity. Malondialdehyde (MDA) is an end product derived from peroxidation of polyunsaturated fatty acids and related esters. Measurement of such aldehydes provides a convenient index of lipid peroxidation. The colorimetric assay from Calbiochem (San Diego, CA, USA) was used in this study; this assay kit takes advantage of a chromogenic reagent, R1, which reacts with MDA at 45°C. Condensation of one molecule of MDA with 2 molecules of reagent R1 yields a stable chromophore with maximum absorbance at 586 nm.

H O + 2 Ph N → N Ph Ph N+

MDA : R = OH
4-hydroxyalkenal : R= hydroxyalkyl

Max = 586 nm

RESULTS

Figure 1 represents a linear graph constructed between mean MDA equivalents for each standard [X-axis] versus the corresponding spectrophotometer reading [Y-axis]. The concentration of MDA equivalents in nmol/ml in specimen are determined by intrapolation from the standard curve.

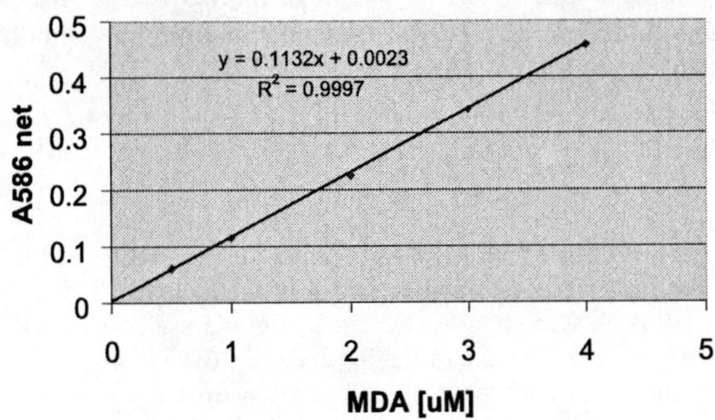

Figure 1. Malondialdehyde (MDA) Standard Curve.

Lipid Peroxidation

Figure 2 presents the experimental data obtained from the analysis of malondialdehyde (MDA) in the serum of Sprague-Daley (SD) rats. Arsenic trioxide (As_2O_3) exposure significantly ($p \leq 0.05$) increased the concentration of MDA in the treated groups [8.0-22.3 μM] when compared with the control group [7.3 μM], indicating a gradual increase in lipid peroxidation with increasing doses [5, 10, 15 & 20 mg/kg body wt] of arsenic.

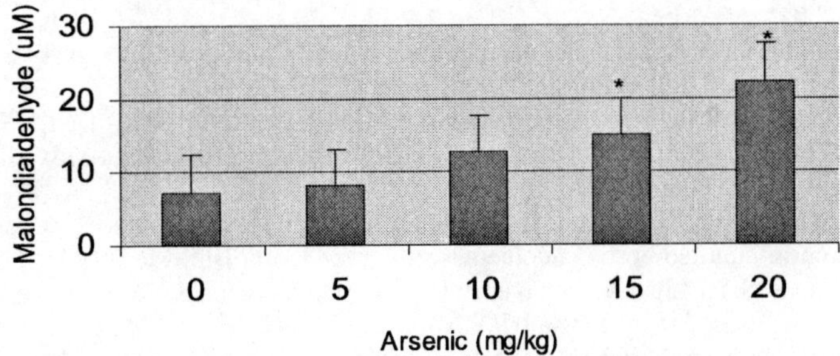

Figure 2. Effect of arsenic trioxide on the concentration of malondialdehyde in serum of Sprague-Dawley rats.

DISCUSSION

The data obtained from this study clearly show that arsenic trioxide significantly increased the concentration of malondialdehyde (MDA); an indicator of lipid peroxidation, in a dose-dependent manner in Sprague-Dawley rats. Lipid peroxidation is only one of the reactions set into motion as a consequence of the formation of free radicals in cells and tissues. Arsenic causes damage to biological system because of its ability to generate oxidative stress in the cells. Arsenic is known to generate ROS and free radicals like hydrogen peroxide [10-13] hydroxyl radical [10], nitric oxide [14], superoxide anion [11, 15], dimethyl arsenic peroxy radical [16, 17] and dimethylarsinic radical [17, 18] in living systems. In its trivalent form, arsenic binds with high affinity to GSH, restricts its antioxidant activity and inhibits various enzymes, which require GSH as cofactor.

Arsenic in other studies [19, 20] has been shown to induce lipid peroxidation of membranes and formation of lipid peroxide both in animal models and in human subjects exposed to arsenic. The initial biochemical evidence of these studies was increase in intracellular oxidative stress and oxidative damage, subsequent to the reduction of glutathione level and antioxidant enzymes.

It has been suggested that lipid peroxidation of cellular membranes, as a common mechanism in a large number of pathologic conditions and even in many clinical diseases. Our findings therefore indicate that malondialdehyde (MDA) an indicator of lipid peroxidation may be useful as a biomarker for arsenic-induced oxidative stress.

REFERENCES

1. Tchounwou P.B., Centeno J.A., and Patlolla A.K. Arsenic toxicity, mutagenesis, and carcinogenesis - A health risk assessment and management approach, Mol Cell Biochem 2004, 255, 47-55.
2. Tchounwou P.B., Patlolla A.K, Centeno J.A. Carcinogenic and systemic health effects associated with arsenic exposure - A critical review, Toxicol Pathol 2003, 31(6), 575-88.
3. Gutteridge J.M.C., Quinlan G.J. Malondialdehyde formation from lipid peroxides in thiobarbituric acid test: the role of lipid radicals, iron salts, metal chelators. J. Appl. Biochem 1983, 5, 293-299.
4. Halliwell B. Oxygen radicals: a commonsense look at their nature and medical importance. Med. Biol 1984, 62(2): 71-7.
5. Del Razo L.M., Qintanilla-Vega B., Brambila-Colombres E., Calderon-Aranda E.S., Manno M., Albores A. Stress proteins induced by arsenic. Toxicol Appl Pharmacol. 2001, 177(2), 132-48.
6. Nordenson I., Beckman L. Is the genotoxic effect of arsenic mediated by oxygen free radicals? Hum Hered. 1991, 41(1), 71-3.
7. Yager J.W., Wiencke J.K. Inhibition of Poly (ADP-ribose) polymerase by arsenite. Mut. Res 1997, 386(3), 345-51.
8. Gebel T.W. Genotoxicity of arsenical compounds. Int J Hyg Environ Health. 2001, 203, 249-262.
9. Patlolla A.K., Tchounwou P.B. Cytogenetic evaluation of arsenic trioxide toxicity in Sprague-Dawley rats. Mut. Res. 2005, 587, 126-133.
10. Wang T.S., Kuo C.F., Jan K.Y. Arsenite induces apoptosis in Chinese hamster ovary cells by generation of reactive oxygen species. J Cell Physiol. 1996, 169(2), 256-68.
11. Barchowsky A., Roussel R.R., Klei, L.R., James P.E., Ganju N., Smith K.R., Dudek E.J. Low levels of arsenic trioxide stimulate proliferative signals in primary vascular cells without activating stress effectors pathways. Toxicol. Appl. Pharm. 1991, 159, 65-75.
12. Barchowsky A., Dudek E.J., Treadwell M.D., Wetterhahn K.B. arsenic induces oxidant stress and NF-kappa B activation in cultured aortic endothelial cells. Free Radic Biol Med. 1996, 21, 783-790.
13. Chen Y.C., Lin-Shiau S.Y., Lin J.K. Involvement of reactive oxygen species and caspase 3 activation in arsenite induced apoptosis. J. Cell Physiol 1998, 177(2), 324-33.
14. Gurr J.R., Liu F., Lynn S., K.Y. Jan. Calcium-dependent nitric oxide production is involved in arsenite-induced micronuclei, Mut. Res. 1998, 416, 137-148.
15. Lyn S., Gurr J.R., Lai H.T., Jan K.Y. NADH oxidase activation is involved in arsenite induced oxidative DNA damage in human vascular smooth muscle cells. Cir. Res. 2000, 86, 514-519.
16. Yamanaka K., Hasegawa A., Sawamura R., Okada S. Cellular response to oxidative damage in lung induced by administration of dimethylarsinic acid, a major metabolite of inorganic arsenic in mice. Toxicol Appl. Pharmacol. 1991, 108, 205-213.
17. Yamanaka K., Hayashi M., Tachikawa M., Kato K., Hasegawa A., Oku N., Okada S. Metabolic methylation is a possible genotoxicity enhancing process of inorganic arsenic. Mut.Res. 1997, 394, 95-101.
18. Yamanaka K., Mizol M., Kato K., Hasegawa A., Nakano M., Okada S. Oral administration of dimethylarsinic acid, a main metabolite of inorganic arsenic, in mice skin tumorigenesis initiated by dimethyl benz(a)anthracene with or without ultraviolet B as a promoter. Biol Pharm Bull 2001, 24(5), 510-4.
19. Maiti S., Chatterjee A.K. Differential response of cellular antioxidant mechanism of liver and kidney to arsenic exposure and its relation to dietary protein deficiency. Environ Toxicol Pharmacol 2000, 8, 227-235.
20. Ramanathan K., shila S., Kumaran S., Panneerselvam C. Ascorbic acid and alpha-tocopherol as potent modulators on arsenic induced toxicity in mitochondria. J. Nutr. Biochem 2003, 14, 416-420.

ACKNOWLEDGMENTS

This research was financially supported by the NIH-RCMI Grant No. 1G12RR13459. The authors thank Dr. Ronald Mason Jr., President, and Dr. Abdul Mohamed, Dean of the JSU-College of Science, Engineering and Technology, at Jackson State University, for their technical support of this project.

Metal Ions in Biology and Medicine: vol. 9. Eds Maria Carmen Alpoim, Paula Vasconcellos Morais, Maria Amélia Santos, Armando J. Cristóvão, José A. Centeno, Philippe Collery.
John Libbey Eurotext, Paris © 2006 pp. 422-1.

Serum Alkaline Phosphatase as a Biomarker of Arsenic-Induced Hepatobiliary or Cholestatic Effect in Sprague-Dawley Rats

Anita K. Patlolla and Paul B. Tchounwou

Molecular Toxicology Research Laboratory, NIH-Center for Environmental Health, CSET, Jackson State University, Jackson, MS, USA

ABSTRACT

Recent studies in our laboratory have demonstrated that arsenic trioxide is hepatotoxic and able to biochemically induce a significant increase in the activities of serum aminotransferases in Sprague-Dawley rats [Tchounwou et al., Metal Ions in Biology & Medicine Vol. 8:284-288, 2004]. In humans chemically induced hepatocellular toxicity has also been linked to obstructive cholestasis involving the hepatobiliary system. The mechanisms involved in drug-induced cholestasis are poorly understood. One of the major reasons for this deficiency is a lack of animal model. It is possible, however to produce cholestatic effects in animals with selected bile acids, some steroids and certain chemicals that have no therapeutic utility. The aim of this study was to conduct biochemical analysis to determine the effect of arsenic trioxide on the activity of alkaline phosphatase (ALP), an important liver enzyme that may be released from hepatocytes as a result of cholestatic injury. Four groups of six male rats each weighing approximately 60 ± 2 g were used in this study. Arsenic trioxide was intraperitoneally administered to the rats at the doses of 5, 10, 15, 20mg/kg body weight (BW), one dose per 24 hour given for five days. A control group was also made of 6 animals injected with distilled water without chemical. Following anaesthetization, blood specimens were immediately collected using heparinized syringes, alkaline phosphatase identification and quantification was performed in serum samples by spectrophotometry. Arsenic trioxide exposure significantly increased the activity of alkaline phosphatase (ALP). Optical density readings of 0.163 ± 0.014, 0.239 ± 0.023, 0.242 ± 0.010, 0.303 ± 0.024, 0.399 ± 0.049 (ALP) were recorded for 0, 5, 10, 15, and 20 mg/kg, respectively; indicating a gradual increase in phosphatase activity with increasing doses of arsenic. Our results indicate that alkaline phosphatase is a candidate biomarker for arsenic-induced hepatobiliary or cholestatic effect in Sprague-Dawley rats.

INTRODUCTION

Inorganic arsenic is a common environmental pollutant and a high priority hazardous substance for human exposure both in the US and around the world. The general population is exposed to inorganic arsenicals primarily through contaminated drinking water, food and soil while occupational exposure is usually from arsenic inhalation in a number of industrial settings [1]. Drinking water contamination by arsenic remains a major public health problem. Acute and chronic arsenic exposure via drinking water has been reported in many countries of the world, where a large proportion of drinking water is contaminated with high concentrations of arsenic. General health effects that are associated with arsenic exposure include cardiovascular and peripheral vascular disease, developmental anomalies, neurologic and neuro-behavioural disorders, diabetes, hearing loss, portal fibrosis, hematologic disorders (anemia, leucopenia and eosinophilia) and multiple cancers: significantly higher standardized mortality rates and cumulative mortality rates for cancers of the skin, lung, liver, urinary bladder, kidney, and colon in many areas of arsenic pollution [2].

The liver is clearly a target of arsenic in humans and arsenic exposure is associated with development of hepatocellular carcinomas as well as other toxic lesions [3-6]. Evidence indicates that inorganic arsenic in drinking water can target the liver in animal model systems. Arsenic and its compounds have been shown to induce toxic lesions such as fatty infiltration [6], hyperplasia [7] hepatocellular proliferative lesions including neoplasia in rodents [8]. Thus, it appears the liver can be a potential target of arsenic carcinogenesis in both humans and non-human species. High alkaline phosphatase activity usually means that liver has been damaged; it can also be due to blockage of bile ducts leading to cholestatic effect. Recent studies in our laboratory demonstrated that other liver enzymes AST and ALT activities were high indicating the effect being hepatotoxic [9].

One of the major mechanisms by which arsenic exerts its toxic effect is through an impairment of cellular respiration by inhibition of various mitochondrial enzymes, and the uncoupling of oxidative phosphorylation. Most toxicity of arsenic results from its ability to interact with sulfhydryl groups of proteins and enzymes, and to substitute phosphorus in a variety of biochemical reactions. Although the evidence of carcinogenicity of arsenic seems strong, the mechanism by which it produces tumors is not completely understood [10].

In humans chemically induced hepatocellular toxicity has also been linked to obstructive cholestasis involving the hepatobiliary system. The mechanisms involved in drug-induced cholestasis are poorly understood. One of the major reasons for this deficiency is a lack of animal model. It is possible, however to produce cholestatic effects in animals with selected bile acids, some steroids and certain chemicals that have no therapeutic utility [11, 12]. The aim of this study was to conduct biochemical analysis to determine the effect of arsenic trioxide on the activity of alkaline phosphatase (ALP), an important liver enzyme that may be released into the bloodstream due to blockage in the bile duct as a result of cholestatic injury in Sprague-Dawley rats.

MATERIALS AND METHODS

Animal maintenance and treatment

Healthy adult male Sprague-Dawley rats (8-10 weeks of age, with average body weight (BW) of 60 ± 2 g) were used in this study. They were obtained from Harlan-Sprague-Dawley Breeding laboratories in Indianapolis, Indiana, USA. The animals were randomly selected and housed in polycarbonate cages (three rats per cage) with steel wire tops and corn-cob bedding. They were maintained in a controlled atmosphere with a 12h:12h dark/light cycle, a temperature of 22 ± 2°C and 50-70% humidity with free access to pelleted food and fresh tap water. The animals were supplied with dry food pellets commercially available from PMI Feeds Inc. (St. Louis, MO, USA). They were allowed to acclimate for 10 days before treatment.

In this investigation, a total of 30 animals were used, 5 groups including one control. Each group had 6 animals per dose. Arsenic trioxide was administered in the animals by intraperitoneal injection once a day for 5 days. At the end of treatment period, rats were anesthetized using 95% CO_2 for 70 seconds and then decapitated by cervical dislocation. Immediately following anaesthetization blood specimens were collected using EDTA syringes to prevent clotting, and the serum was separated by centrifugation at 2000 g for 10 min. Serum samples were evaluated for enzyme (alkaline phosphatase) identification and quantification using colorimetric method.

Enzyme analysis

To determine the activity of alkaline phosphatase in serum a method by Kay [13] was followed, it was measured using a Diagnostic kit from Sigma (St. Louis, MO, USA). Alkaline phosphatase is also known as orthhophosphoric monoester phosphohydrolase, ALP. It is a prototype of those enzymes that reflect pathological reductions in bile flow. This enzyme has been extensively employed in experimentally induced hepatic dysfunction. Alkaline phosphatase refers not to a single enzyme but to a family of enzymes with different physico-chemical properties and broad overlapping substrate specificities.

The procedure for alkaline phosphatase depends upon the hydrolysis of p-nitrophenyl phosphate by the enzyme, yielding p-nitrophenol and inorganic phosphate. When made alkaline, p-nitrophenol is converted to a yellow complex readily measured at 400-420 nm. The intensity of color formed is proportional to phosphatase activity.

The reaction for ALP is as follows:

$$\text{Orthophosphoric monoester} + H_2O \xrightarrow{\text{ALP}} \text{alcohol} + H_3PO_4$$

RESULTS

Alkaline phosphatase

Figure 1 presents the experimental data obtained from the analysis of alkaline phosphatase (ALP). The results yielded optical density readings of 0.163 ± 0.014; 0.239 ± 0.0023; 0.242 ± 0.010; 0.303 ± 0.024; 0.399 ± 0.049 (ALP) for 0, 5, 10, 15, and 20 mg arsenic trioxide/kg bodywt (BW). As shown in this figure, arsenic trioxide exposure significantly increased the activity of alkaline phosphatase (ALP). Our results indicate that ALP is a candidate biomarker for arsenic-induced hepatobiliary or cholestatic effect in Sprague-Dawley rats.

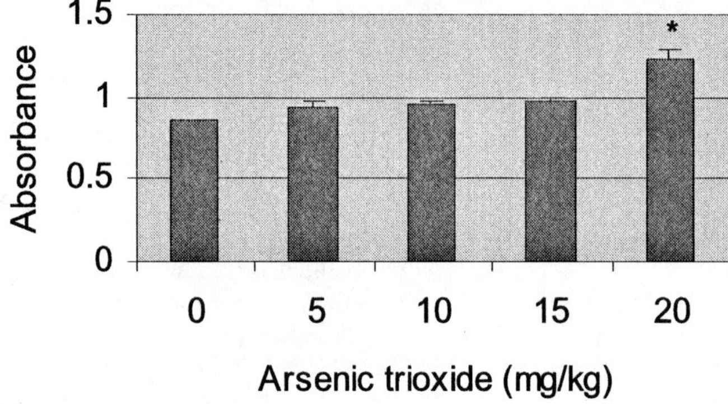

Figure 1. Effect of Arsenic trioxide on serum alkaline phosphatase in Sprague-Dawley rats

DISCUSSION

The data obtained from this study clearly show that arsenic trioxide significantly increased the activity of serum alkaline phosphatase in a dose-dependent manner. Alkaline phosphatase of the liver is produced by the cells lining the small bile ducts (ductoles) in the liver. If the liver disease is primarily of an obstructive nature (cholestatic) i.e., involving the biliary drainage system, the alkaline phosphatase will be the first and foremost enzyme that is found to increase. Serum activity of the enzyme has been reported to increase and is indicative of an impaired hepatic clearance (cholestasis).

Studies conducted by other investigators [14, 15] have also reported elevated levels of serum alkaline phosphatase following arsenic toxicity. The initial biochemical evidence of these studies was predominantly conjugated hyperbilirubinemia and increase serum ALP activity which were related to the concentration of total arsenic (TA) suggesting the presence of cholestasis in arsenic exposed individuals [14, 15].

It has been suggested that hepatocyte injury following metal exposure may be due to binding in the inner membrane and accumulation in the mitochondria, leading to the collapse of the mitochondrial membrane, followed by plasma membrane depolarization and cell death [16]. Our data therefore indicate that alkaline phosphatase may be useful as biomarker for arsenic-induced hepatobiliary or cholestatic effect in Sprague-Dawley rats.

REFERENCES

1. Tchounwou P.B., Wilson B.A., Ishaque A. Important considerations in the development of public health advisories for arsenic and arsenic containing compounds in drinking water, Rev Environ Hlth 1999, 14 1-19.
2. Tchounwou P.B., Patlolla A.K., Centeno J.A. Carcinogenic and systemic health effects associated with arsenic exposure-A critical review, Toxicol Pathol 2003, 31(6), 575-88.
3. IARC. Monographs World Health Organization. IARC scientific publications, IARC, Lyon (Suppl. 7), 1987, pp.100-106.
4. National Research Council (NRC). Arsenic in drinking water. National Academy Press, Washington, D.C, p.310.
5. Chen C.J., Yu M.W., Liaw Y.F. Epidemiological characteristics and risk factors of hepatocellular carcinoma. J.Gastroenterol. Hepatol 1997, 12, 294-308.
6. Liu J., Liu Y., Goyer R.A., Achanzar W., and Waalkes M.P. Metallothionein-I/II null mice are more sensitive than wild-type mice to the hepatotoxic and nephrotoxic effects of chronic oral or injected inorganic arsenicals. Toxicol Sci 2000, 55, 460-467.
7. Kotsanis N., and Iliopoulou-Georgudaki J. Arsenic induced liver hyperplasia and kidney fibrosis in rainbow trout (Oncorhynchus mykiss) by microinjection technique: a sensitive animal bioassay for environmental meatl-toxicity. Bull. Environ. Contam. toxicol 1999, 62, 169-178.
8. Waalkes M.P., Keefer L.K., and Diwan B.A. Induction of proliferative lesions of uterus, testes and liver in Swiss mice given repeated injections of sodium arsenate; possible estrogenic mode of action. Toxicol Appl Pharmacol 2000, 166, 24-35.
9. Tchounwou P.B., Patlolla A.K., Centeno J.A. Serum aminotransferases as biomarkers of arsenic-induced hepatotoxicity in Sprague-Dawley rats. Metal Ions in Biol and Med. 2004, 8, 284-288.
10. Tchounwou P.B., Centeno J.A., and Patlolla A.K. Arsenic toxicity, mutagenesis, and carcinogenesis - A health risk assessment and management approach, Mol Cell Biochem 2004, 255, 47-55.
11. Plaa G.L., Priestly b.G. Intrahepatic cholestasis induced by drugs and chemicals. Pharmacol Rev 1976, 28, 207-273.
12. Plaa G.L. Toxic responses of the liver. In: Amdur MO, Doull J, Klaassen CD, eds. Casarett and Doull's Toxicology, 4Th ed. New York: Pergamon Press, 1991, 334-353.
13. Kay H.D., Plasma phosphatase. I. Method of determination. Some properties of the enzyme. J Biol Chem 1930, 89, 235.
14. Santra A., Maiti A., Das S., Lahiri S., Charkaborty S.K., Mazumder D.N. Hepatic damage caused by chronic arsenic toxicity in experimental animals. J Toxicol Clin Toxicol 2000, 38(4), 395-405.
15. Hernandez-Zavala A., Del Razo L.M., Aguilar C., Garcia-Vargas G.G., Borja V.H., Cebrian M.E. Alteration in bilirubin excretion in individuals chronically exposed to arsenic in Mexico. Toxicol Lett 1998, 99(2), 79-84.
16. Chang L.W., Suzuki T. Toxicology of Metals. CRC Press. Boca Raton. Fl, 1996, pp. 885-899.

ACKNOWLEDGMENTS

This research was financially supported by the NIH-RCMI Grant No. 1G12RR13459. The authors thank Dr. Ronald Mason Jr., President, and Dr. Abdul Mohamed, Dean of the JSU-College of Science, Engineering and Technology, At Jackson State University, for their technical support of this project.

Metal Ions in Biology and Medicine: vol. 9. Eds Maria Carmen Alpoim, Paula Vasconcellos Morais, Maria Amélia Santos, Armando J. Cristóvão, José A. Centeno, Philippe Collery.
John Libbey Eurotext, Paris © 2006 pp. 426-1.

Oral aluminum exposure: effects on locomotor activity and spatial learning in a transgenic mouse model of Alzheimer's disease

Ribes D[a,b], Torrente M[a,b], Vicens P[a,b], Colomina MT[a,b], Domingo JL[b,*]

[a]*Department of Psychology, Psychobiology Unit and*
[b]*Laboratory of Toxicology and Environmental Health, School of Medicine, "Rovira i Virgili" University, San Lorenzo 21, 43201 Reus, Spain. joseluis.domingo@urv.net*

INTRODUCTION

Aluminum (Al), a non-essential element, is ubiquitous in industrialized societies. Because of its supposed biological inert properties and its low absorption after oral exposure, its use on foodstuffs, beverage cans, and pharmacological and cosmetic compounds is very common. However, it is well established that Al is neurotoxic, and when ingested orally can access into the brain. Notwithstanding, the amounts deposited are low in comparison to the relatively large quantities ingested. Moreover, Al is associated to various diseases such dyalisis encephalopathy, osteomalacia, microcytic anemia and severe neurodegenerative disorders. In particular, the relationship between Al exposure an Alzheimer disease (AD), a multifactorial disease in which both genetical and environmental factors play an important role, has been suggested. In this sense, it has been reported that gastrointestinal absorption of Al is greater in AD patients than in controls [1], while high Al concentrations in neurofibrillary tangles have been also found. However, the relation between Al and Alzheimer disease (AD) is still a controversial question.

Some epidemiological studies have indicated a possible relationship between water Al content and AD [2], whereas exposed workers to Al showed impaired cognitive functions [3]. On the other hand, experimental studies have shown that intracerebroventricular infusions of Al in rabbits and cats induced neurofibrillary tangles [4]. More recent investigations have demonstrated that Al is linked to beta amyloid deposition in vivo and in vitro (see review by Kawahara et al. [5], induces oxidative stress in the brain [6, 7], increases beta amyloid deposits in rodents (Pratico et al., 2002) and induces neuropathological changes in brains [8, 9].

On the other hand, experimental studies conducted in rodents to evaluate behavioral changes after oral Al exposure have provided results ranging from none to moderate effects, it can be due to a reduced sensitivity to generate neurodegenerative processes in the strains evaluated. However, advances in generating transgenic mice models more prone to neurodegeneration can help to elucidate the relationship between Al and neurodegeneration. Some studies conducted with transgenic models of AD have already provided evidences to link Al and AD [7]. It has been demonstrated that transgenic mice models of AD are particularly well-suited to such studies.

The aim of the present study was to assess the behavioral effects of Al in an animal model which carries a transgene coding for the 695-amino acid isoform of human Alzheimer β-amyloid (Aß) precursor protein derived from a Swedish family with early-onset Alzheimer's disease (AD). The main objective was to evaluate whether low doses of Aluminum intake could accelerate behavioral and spatial learning deficits observed in transgenic mice.

MATERIALS AND METHODS

Subjects and treatment

Sixteen transgenic male (Tg 2576) and 15 wild control mice (Taconic Europe, Denmark) were used. Animals were quarantined for 7 days after shipping and individually housed in plastic cages in an animal room, which was maintained at a temperature of 22 ± 2 °C, a relative humidity of $50 \pm 10\%$, and a 12-h light/dark automatic light cycle (light: 0800-2000 h). All animals were allowed free access to food and water. Control mice received normal chow and aluminum treated mice were fed rodent chow (Harlam, Barcelona, Spain) supplemented with Al lactate at 0 or 1 mg/g, during 120 days. The experimental groups (n=7-8) were distributed as follows: Control wild, Al-treated wild, Control Transgenic (Control Tg), and Al-treated transgenic (Aluminum Tg).The use of animals and the experimental protocol were approved by the Animal Care and Use Committee of the "Rovira i Virgili" University (Tarragona, Spain).

Behavioral assessment

At three months of oral Al exposure (9 months of age at testing), a functional observational battery was performed. Activity in an open-field and learning in a water maze were also evaluated.

Functional Observation Battery (FOB). The protocol used in this study consisted of eighteen endpoints that evaluated different aspects of nervous system function [10, 11]. After a brief assessment of each mouse in its home cage, the animal was removed and held in the observer's hand to score reactivity and to observe general appearance. Afterwards, the mouse was placed in an exploratory white box (60cm × 90 cm), where the observer analyzed CNS activity (arousal, rearing), CNS excitability (easy of removal, handling reactivity, clonic and tonic movements), autonomic effects (palpebral closure, urination, defecation, lacrimation, piloerection), muscle tone and equilibrium (gait, mobility, righting reflex, inverted screen), and sensoriomotor reactivity (approach response, click response, touch response). Data were recorded on standardized sheets and conducted between 09.00 and 14.00 h.

Open field activity. General motor activity was measured in an open-field apparatus, consisting of a wood 1 × 1 m square surrounded by a 47 cm-high dark colored wall. During the test, mice were allowed to move freely for 15 min. The video tracking program Etho-Vision® was used to measure the distance traveled.

Water maze test. The water maze consisted of a circular tank (diameter: 1m; high: 60 cm), divided into four quadrants. A escape platform was located 1 cm below the water surface in the target quadrant. Data were analyzed by the video tracking program Etho-Vision®. Mice were subjected to 3 trials/day for 5 consecutive days. Trial duration was 60 s and each trial was separated by a 30 s inter-trial interval. If the animal did not locate the platform within 60 s, the animal was placed on the platform for 30 additional seconds. Immediately after the last trial, a probe trial was performed consisting of a 60 s free swim without the escape platform. The latency to find the escape platform during the training sessions, as well as the total time spent in the target quadrant during the probe trial were analyzed.

Statistics

Behavioral data were analyzed by a two-way (nature × Al treatment) and one-way ANOVA. When appropriate a DMS post hoc test was also used for multiple group comparisons. Significance was set at $P<0.05$.

RESULTS

Functional Observation Battery. In its home cage a diminished activity was noted through mice groups. Al-exposed wild mice and Al-exposed transgenic mice showed less activity (decreased climbing) [p<0.05] than control wild and control transgenic mice. Al-exposed wild mice and Al-exposed and unexposed transgenic mice showed also a lower eating/drinking behavior [p<0.05] *(fig. 1)*. Piloerection was also noted [p<0.05] in wild and transgenic mice exposed to Al when compared to wild and transgenic controls *(fig. 1)*. Finally, there were differences in sensoriomotor reactivity. Al-exposed transgenic mice showed an increased reaction to approach and click stimulus [p<0.05] *(fig. 2)*.

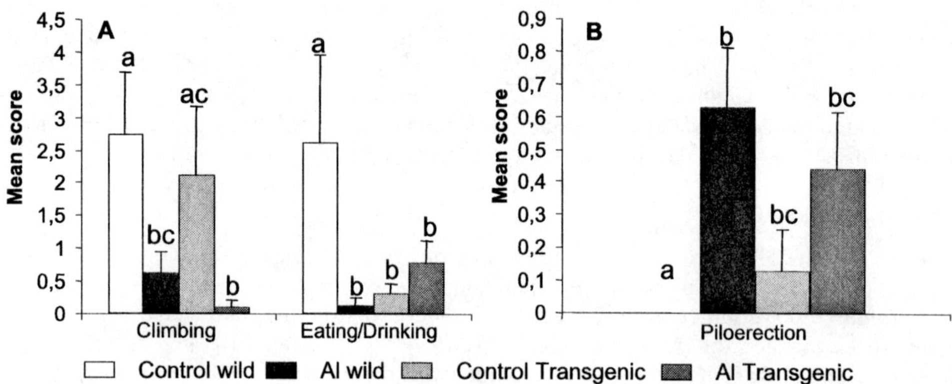

Figure 1. Functional Observation Battery, **A**) assessment in its home cage. **B**) General appearance. Groups not sharing a common letter a,b,c are significantly different at p<0.05. Data are expressed as mean ± S.E.M.

Open field activity. No significant differences in general motor activity were observed. However, significant differences between groups [F(3,30)= 4,241, p= 0.014] were noted in distance moved at center using the ratio distance moved in the center/total distance moved. DMS test showed a lower activity in the center of the apparatus in Al-treated transgenic mice compared with control wild animals *(fig. 2)*.

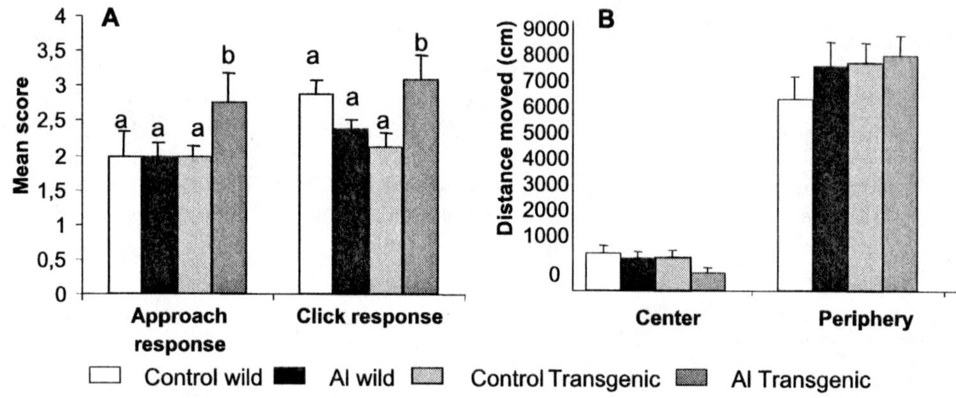

Figure 2. A) FOB, assessment in exploratory box. B) Total distance moved in an open field in center and periphery. Different letters indicate significant differences between groups at p<0.05. Data are expressed as mean ± S.E.M.

Water maze. An overall effect of Al in retention probe trial was observed [F(1,26)= 6,838, p= 0.015]. However, the differences between groups did not reach the level of statistical significance (p= 0.056).

DISCUSSION

After 3 months of oral Al exposure a Functional Observational Battery evidenced general neurotoxic signs. In the home cage general activity was diminished in wild mice exposed to Al and in transgenic mice, exposed or not to Al. Moreover, an increased reaction to stimulus was only observed in Al-exposed transgenic mice. On the other hand, general activity evaluated in an open-field did not show significant differences between groups. However, a more detailed analysis to investigate activity in the center and periphery of the open field indicated that transgenic Al exposed mice were less active in the center of the open-field, which is considered an axiogenic location. This finding was not previously found in Al-exposed non-transgenic rodent models evaluated in our laboratory [12, 13]. The current results indicating a more exacerbated response to sensory stimulus and the decreased center activity in an open-field are compatible with an increased anxiety levels due to Al exposure in transgenic mice. An increased anxiety may occur in up to 70% of AD patients during the course of the illness. Moreover, anxiety symptoms are also significantly correlated with impairments in activities of daily life [14].

Although only punctual differences were observed in water maze acquisition, retention of Al-exposed mice was impaired, which is indicated by an overall effect due to Al exposure. Probably, a more prolonged exposure might better have evidenced the Al effects on spatial tasks. In conclusion, the present results indicate that transgenic mice (model 2576) and wild type mice used in this experiment are sensitive to Al neurotoxic effects even administered at low doses of this element.

REFERENCES

1. Moore PB, Day JP, Taylor GA, Ferrier IN, Fifield LK, Edwardson JA. Absorption of aluminium-26 in Alzheimer's disease, measured using accelerator mass spectrometry. Dement. Geriatr. Cogn. Disord. 2000; 11: 66-9.
2. Rondeau V. A review of epidemiologic studies on aluminum and silica in relation to Alzheimer's disease and associated disorders. Rev. Environ. Health 2002; 17: 107-21.
3. Rifat SL, Eastwood MR, McLachlan DR, Corey PN. Effect of exposure of miners to aluminum powder. Lancet 1990; 336: 1162-65.
4. Savory J, Huang Y, Herman MM, Reyes MR, Wills MR. Tau immunoreactivity associated with aluminum maltolate-induced neurofibrillary degeneration in rabbits. Brain Res. 1995; 669: 325-9.
5. Kawahara M. Effects of aluminum on the nervous system and its possible link with neurodegenerative diseases. J. Alzheimers Dis. 2005; 8: 171-82.
6. Esparza JL, Gómez M, Romeu M, Mulero M, Sánchez DJ, Mallol J, Domingo JL. Aluminum-induced pro-oxidant effects in rats: protective role of exogenous melatonin. J. Pineal Res. 2003; 35: 32-9.
7. Praticò D, Uryu K, Sung S, Tang S, Trojanowski JQ, Lee VM. Aluminum modulates brain amyloidosis through oxidative stress in APP transgenic mice. FASEB J. 2002; 16: 1138-40.
8. Fattoretti P, Bertoni-Freddari C, Balietti M, Giorgetti B, Solazzi M, Zatta P. Chronic aluminum administration to old rats results in increased levels of brain metal ions and enlarged hippocampal mossy fibers. Ann. NY Acad. Sci. 2004; 1019: 44-7.
9. Szutowicz, A. Aluminum, NO, and nerve growth factor neurotoxicity in cholinergic neurons. J. Neurosci Res. 2001; 66: 1009-18.
10. Sills RC, Valentine WM, Moser V, Graham DG, and Morgan DL. Characterization of carbon disulfide neurotoxicity in C57BL6 mice: behavioral, morphologic, and molecular effects. Toxicol. Pathol. 2000; 28: 142-48.
11. Golub MS, Germann SL, Lloyd KCK. Behavioral characteristics of a nervous system-specific erbB4 knock-out mouse. Behav. Brain Res. 2004; 153: 159-70.
12. Colomina M T, Roig J L, Torrente M, Vicens P, Domingo J.L. Concurrent exposure to aluminum and stress during pregnancy in rats: Effects on postnatal development and behavior of the offspring. Neurotoxicol. Teratol. 2005; 27: 565-74.

13. Roig JL, Fuentes S, Colomina MT, Vicens P, Domingo JL. Aluminum, restraint stress and aging: Behavioral effects in rats after 1 and 2 years of aluminum exposure. Toxicology 2006; 218: 112-24.
14. Cummings JL, Nadel A, Masterman D, Cyrus PA. Efficacy of metrifonate in improving the psychiatric and behavioral disturbances of patient with Alzheimer's disease. J.Geriatr. Psychiatry Neurol. 2001; 14: 101-8.

Metal Ions in Biology and Medicine: vol. 9. Eds Maria Carmen Alpoim, Paula Vasconcellos Morais, Maria Amélia Santos, Armando J. Cristóvão, José A. Centeno, Philippe Collery.
John Libbey Eurotext, Paris © 2006 pp. 431-1.

Combined action of uranium and restraint stress in pregnant rats: developmental and behavioral effects in the offspring

Sánchez DJ[1,2], Bellés M[1,2], Albina ML[1,2], Gómez M[1], Linares V[1,2], Domingo JL[1,*]

[1]Laboratory of Toxicology and Environmental Health and [2]Physiology Unit, School of Medicine, "Rovira i Virgili" University, San Lorenzo 21, 43201 Reus, Spain, [*]joseluis.domingo@urv.net

INTRODUCTION

Uranium (U) exposure can result in both chemical and radiological toxicity. Depleted uranium (DU) is a by-product of the nuclear industry used in nuclear weapons production [1]. General population may be exposed to low levels of U by ingestion or inhalation of airborne U-containing dust particles or aerosols. Studies in rodents on the reproductive and developmental toxicity of natural U compounds indicate that this element is potentially toxic to reproductive tissues and teratogenic to the developing fetus at high levels of exposures [2]. Humans can be potentially exposed to U from different sources, while they can be also concurrently subjected to various types of stress (home, occupational, environmental). In relation to this, it is well known that behavioral changes together with physiological and biochemical alterations are common responses to stress [3, 4]. The aim of the present investigation was to assess the influence of stress on the adverse behavioral effects of U in gestational rats, as well as the individual effects of U exposure on physical and neurobehavioral changes in the offspring.

MATERIALS AND METHODS

Animals and treatment

Male Sprague-Dawley rats (220-240 g) were mated with females (1:2). Six groups of plug-positive females received uranyl acetate dihydrate (UAD) in the drinking water at 0, 40 and 80 mg/kg/day during twelve weeks. One-half of animals in each group was concurrently subjected to restraint stress during 2 h per day throughout the study. Restraint was administered by placing the animals in metacrilate cylindrical holders (Letica Scientific Instruments, Barcelona, Spain). On gestation day 14, one-half of rats were euthanized. Maternal toxicity and gestational parameters were evaluated. Pups born from the remaining rats were evaluated for physical development, neuromotor maturation, as well as for behavioral effects. Uranium concentrations in brain, kidney and bone were determined by inductively coupled plasma-mass spectrometry spectrometry (Perkin Elmer, Elan 6000) [5].

Behavioral tests

• *Passive avoidance:* The recent memory of animals was tested in a passive avoidance conditioning task. The apparatus consisted of a shuttle box (Ugo Basile model 7550, Comerio, Italy) equipped with a door to restrict access between equal-sized illuminated and dark compartments. In the acquisition trial, rats were individually placed in the illuminated compartment. After 30 seconds, the door separating the two compartments was opened. Following some seconds (T1), the animal entered the dark compartment. The door was shut 1 second after the crossing, and the rat was given a 0.5 mA/3 seconds duration foot shock. Twenty-four h later (retention trial), the same procedure was repeated without delay period to open the door and without electric foot shock. The time elapsed to enter the dark compartment was recorded as T2. A latency of entry greater than 5 min was the criterion for successful learning [6].

• *Morris water maze test.* Spatial learning and retention were tested in a water maze according to a modified procedure of Morris (1984). The movements of the animal in the tank (160 cm diameter and 60 cm height) were monitored with a video tracking system (Etho-Vision®).

• *Reference memory test.* The animals were tested in blocks of five trials during three consecutive days (each trial started from one of four points assigned on different arbitrary quadrants of the circular tank). The total distance traveled and the latency time before reaching the platform were recorded. The maximum trial latency to reach the platform was 60 seconds. The rat climbed the platform (or the rat was placed on the platform if the animal did not find it in 60 seconds). Once there remained for 30 seconds and then was returned to the cage. The intertrial interval was 60 seconds.

• *Probe test.* At the fourth day, a single probe trial was conducted. The platform was removed from the pool and each rat was allowed to swim for 60 seconds in the maze. The time and the distance that the animal swam in the quadrant in which the platform had been located was recorded.

Statistical analysis

A two-way (uranium dose x restraint) analysis of variance (ANOVA) was used to evaluate the data. The homogeneity of variances was analyzed employing the Levene's test. The homogeneous variables were analyzed by one-way ANOVA followed by the Tukey method for multiple comparisons. The non-homogeneous variables were evaluated using the using the Kruskal-Wallis and the Mann-Whitney U-test. A P value of < 0.05 was accepted as significant.

Table 1. Effects of uranium, restraint and combined uranium and restraint on body weight of young rats on postnatal days 1, 4, 12 and 21

Uranium (mg/kg/day)	0	0	40	40	80	80
Types of stress	None	Restraint	None	Restraint	None	Restraint
N° of dams	8	8	8	8	8	8
Body weight (g) day 1						
Males[2]	7.35±0.30	7.35±0.58	6.92±0.34	7.68±1.14	7.43±0.88	7.40±0.47
Females[2]	7.60±1.45	6.86±0.38	6.77±0.42	7.45±0.89	7.22±0.58	7.01±0.69
Body weight (g) day 4						
Males[2]	11.97±1.79[a]	12.11±1.09 [ab]	11.00±1.11[b]	12.07±1.66 [ab]	11.84±1.60 [ab]	12.11±1.31 [ab]
Females[2]	12.82±2.55[a]	11.46±0.83 [ab]	10.58±1.07[b]	11.56±1.59 [ab]	11.68±1.11 [ab]	11.72±1.28 [ab]
Body weight (g) day 12						
Males[1]	33.37±6.70[a]	29.70±1.89[b]	28.22±3.36[c]	28.27±3.56[c]	31.24±2.35[b]	30.27±1.42 [bc]
Females[2]	35.00±7.36[a]	28.69±1.14[b]	28.31±2.04[b]	27.03±3.54[b]	30.55±2.27[b]	29.06±1.93[b]
Body weight (g) day 21						
Males[2]	63.80±12.2 0[a]	55.68±1.17[b]	55.63±4.37[b]	54.19±3.12[b]	55.98±3.57[b]	55.76±2.05[b]
Females[2]	64.55±12.6 5[a]	54.22±0.94[b]	54.34±3.49[b]	53.46±1.46[b]	56.40±3.88[b]	56.68±4.61[b]

Results are expressed as mean values ± SD.
Statistics: [1]Kruskal-Wallis and U Mann-Whitney test. [2]ANOVA and Tukey test.
[a,b,c]Values in the same row not showing a common superscript are significantly different at $P<0.05$.

RESULTS AND DISCUSSION

In all treated groups, U concentrations in kidney and bone were significantly higher than those in brain. These concentrations were not affected by restraint stress (data no shown). The effects of administration of U and restraint on the body weight of young rats on postnatal days 1,4,12 and 21 are summarized in *table 1*. In general terms, U-treated animals showed a significantly reduction on body weight on days 12 and 21 in comparison with values in the control group. This effect was noted in both male and female young rats.

On the other hand, no significant effects of restraint stress were noted at any U dose.

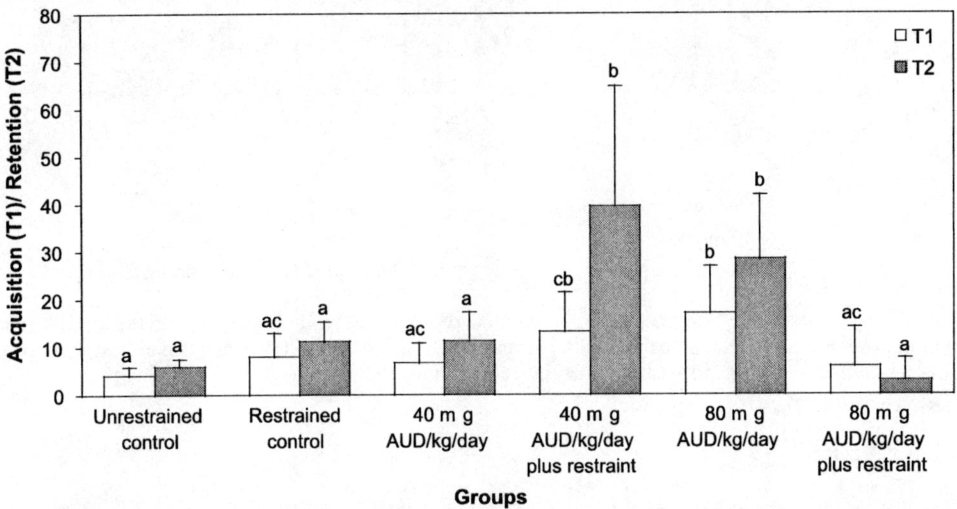

Figure 1. Passive avoidance acquisition (T1) and retention 24 h later (T2). Data are expressed as means ± SD. Statistics: Kurskal-Wallis and Mann-Whitney U-test. Groups not showing a common letter (a,b,c) were significantly different at P<0.05.

Passive avoidance acquisition (T1) and retention (T2) are summarized in *figure 1*.

Restraint significantly modified the retention time in the passive avoidance test at 40 mg/kg/day but not at 80 mg/kg/day. Only the highest U dose increased significantly the acquisition and retention in comparison with those in the control group. Notwithstanding, no significant sex effect was found in any of the tested groups.

The mean total distance traveled (cm) in the Morris water maze is showed in *figure 2*.

Although some differences were observed on days 1, 2 and 3, restraint did not affect significantly the results at any U dose. In previous studies, similar results in the offspring were found when male rats were treated with different concentrations of U during 60 days [4]. With regard to behavior of the offspring, no significant differences among groups, or between the experimental groups and the restrained and unrestrained control groups, could be observed on the passive avoidance acquisition and the mean distance traveled in the Morris water maze. The influence of restraint stress on the few uranium-induced effects was, in general, not significant.

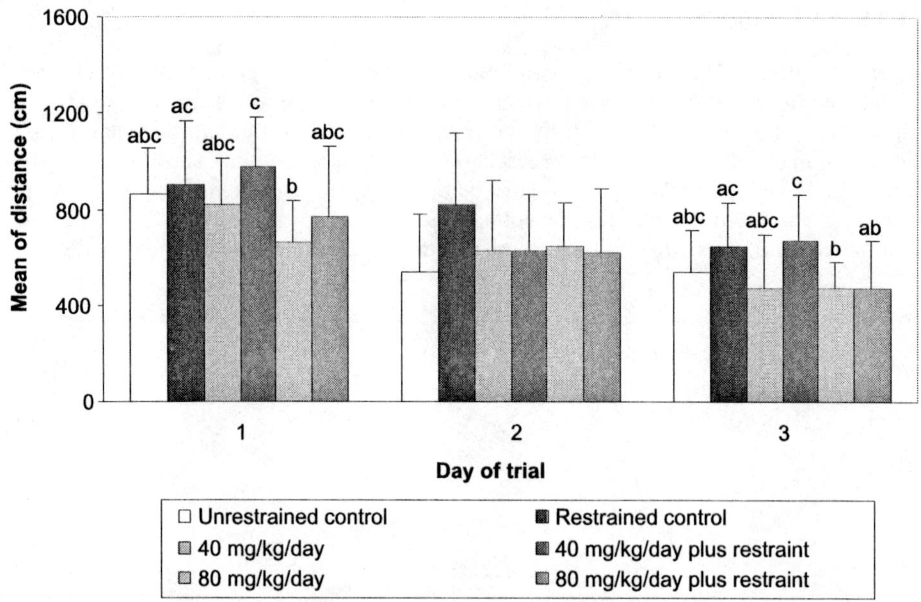

Figure 2. Effects of exposure of female rats to uranium and/or restreint in their offspring on the mean distance traveled in a water maze. Data are expressed as means ± SD. Statistics: ANOVA and Tukey test. Groups not showing a common letter (a,b,c) were significantly different at P<0.05.

REFERENCES

1. Monleau M, Bussy C, Lestavel P, Houpert P, Paquet F, Chazel V. Bioaccumulation and behavioural effects of depleted uranium in rats exposed to repeated inhalations. *Neurosci. Lett.* 2005; 390: 31-6.
2. Domingo JL. Reproductive and developmental toxicity of natural and depleted uranium: a review. *Reprod. Toxicol.* 2001; 15: 603-9.
3. Vogel WH. The effect of stress on toxicological investigations. *Hum. Exp. Toxicol.* 1993; 12: 265-71.
4. Albina ML, Bellés M, Linares V, Sánchez DJ, Domingo JL. Restraint stress does not enhance the uranium-induced developmental and behavioral effects in the offspring of uranium-exposed male rats. *Toxicology* 2005; 215: 69-79.
5. Sánchez DJ, Bellés M, Albina ML, Sirvent JJ, Domingo JL. Nephrotoxicity of simultaneous exposure to mercury and uranium in comparison to individual effects of these metals in rats. *Biol. Trace Elem. Res.* 2001; 84: 139-54.
6. Colomina MT, Roig JL, Sánchez DJ, Domingo JL. Influence of age of exposure on aluminum-induced neurobehavioral effects and morphological changes in the brain of rats. *Neurotoxicology* 2002; 40: 142-9.

ACKNOWLEDGEMENT

Financial support for this study was provided by the “Fondo de Investigación Sanitaria”, Ministry of Health, Spain, through grant no. PI030254.

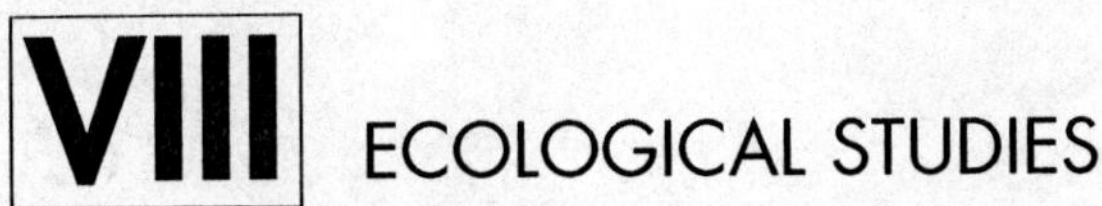

VIII ECOLOGICAL STUDIES

Metal Ions in Biology and Medicine: vol. 9. Eds Maria Carmen Alpoim, Paula Vasconcellos Morais, Maria Amélia Santos, Armando J. Cristóvão, José A. Centeno, Philippe Collery.
John Libbey Eurotext, Paris © 2006 pp. 437-1.

The fitoremediation approach for the control of hydric pollution

Dias, V.[1]; Gomes, A. R.[1]

(1) Gaiagreen, Estudos e Serviços de Engenharia Ambiental, Lda. Rua Quirino da Fonseca, 4, 2º Dto. 1000-252 Lisboa, Portugal
E-mails : verdis@gaiagreen.pt; anaritagomes@gaiagreen.pt

ABSTRACT

This paper focuses on the control of hydric pollution by means of fitoremediation/constructed wetland (CW) systems, which are based on the morphology and biogeochemistry of natural wetlands. An overview of contaminant removal mechanisms as they occur in such areas is given, namely in what concerns organic compounds, nitrogen and phosphorus, metals and pathogens. Several kinds of wastewater are nowadays and throughout the world treated using CW technology: municipal, industrial and agricultural wastewater, run-offs, landfill leachates, acid-mine drainage waters as well as sludges. A synthesis of available information regarding the number of existing CW in portugal and worldwide is presented. Finally, research needs such as long term monitoring studies, kinetics and balancing of different wastewater constituents, land area, influence of temperature and knowledge about plant species are identified.

ECOSYSTEM BACKGROUND

Fitoremediation technologies for the control of hydric pollution are designed using natural wetlands morphology and biogeochemistry as a model.

Wetland biogeochemical cycles feature a combination of chemical transformations and chemical transport processes not shared by other ecosystems (Kadlec & Knight, 1996; Mitsch & Gosselink, 2000). Wetland soils are formed when oxygen is cut off due the presence of water, causing reduced conditions and, in many ways, an environment physiologically harsh with different stresses, including anoxia and the wide salinity and water fluctuations.

Organisms living in the wetlands should have specific adaptations to this environment. To counter anoxia, one important structural adaptation in vascular plants is the development of pore space in the cortical tissues, which allows oxygen to diffuse from the aerial parts of the plant to the roots to supply root respiratory demands. Part of this oxygen diffuses also to the surrounding space, creating a thin layer of oxidized soil (Vymazal *et al.*, 1998; Cooper *et al.*, 1996) *(fig. 1)*.

FITOREMEDIATION VERSUS CONSTRUCTED WETLANDS

Although there can be differences between the two concepts, in this paper it's assumed that fitoremediation is equivalent to constructed wetland.

Plants play a key role in depuration/remediation processes, hence being used as a structuring factor both in fitoremediation and in constructed wetlands.

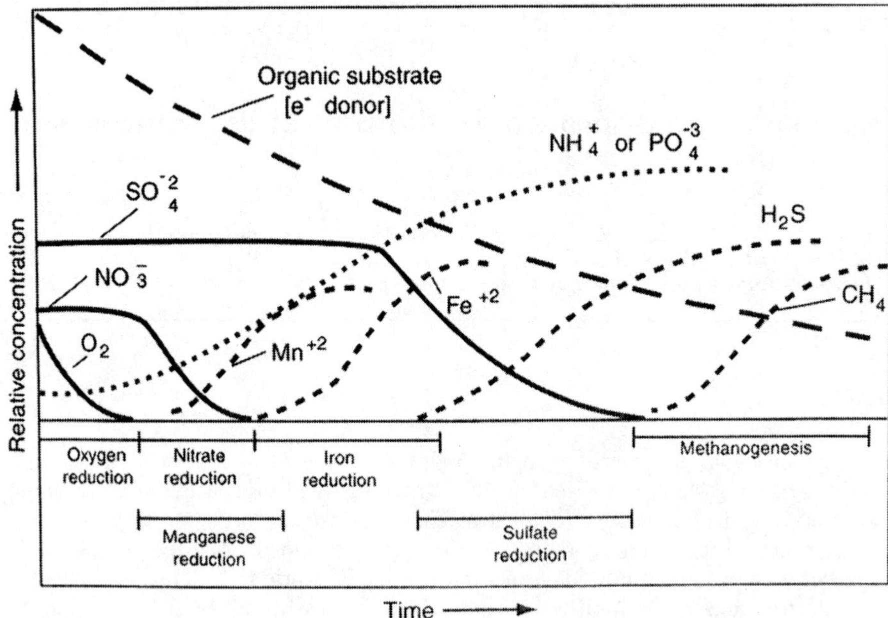

Fig. 1. Sequence in time of transformations in wetland soils after flooding (after Ready D'Angelo *in* Mitsch & Gosselink, 2000).

NUTRIENT REMOVAL AND TRANSFORMATION MECHANISMS

Organic compounds

Settleable organics are rapidly removed in wetland systems under quiescent conditions by deposition and filtration. Attached and suspended microbial growth is responsible for removal of soluble organics. Organic compounds are degraded both aerobically and anaerobically.

Aerobic degradation of soluble organic matter is governed by the aerobic heterotrophic bacteria according to the following reaction (Vymazal *et al.*, 1998):

$$(CH_2O) + O_2 \text{ fi } CO_2 + H_2O$$

Anaerobic degradation is a multi-step process that occurs within constructed wetlands in the absence of dissolved oxygen (Cooper *et al.* 1996). The process can be carried out by either facultative or obligate anaerobic heterotrophic bacteria. Anaerobic degradation of organic compounds is much slower than aerobic degradation. However, when oxygen is limiting at high organic loadings, anaerobic degradation will predominate (Cooper *et al.*, 1996) *(fig. 2)*.

Nitrogen transformations

The major nitrogen transformations in wetlands are presented in *fig. 3*. The various forms of nitrogen are continually involved in chemical transformations from inorganic to organic compounds and back from organic to inorganic. Some of these processes require energy (typically derived from an organic carbon source) to proceed, and others release energy, which is used by organisms for growth and survival. All of these transformations are necessary for wetland ecosystems to function successfully, and most chemical changes are controlled through the production of enzymes and catalysts by the living organisms they benefit (Kadlec & Knight, 1996; Vymazal *et al.*, 1998).

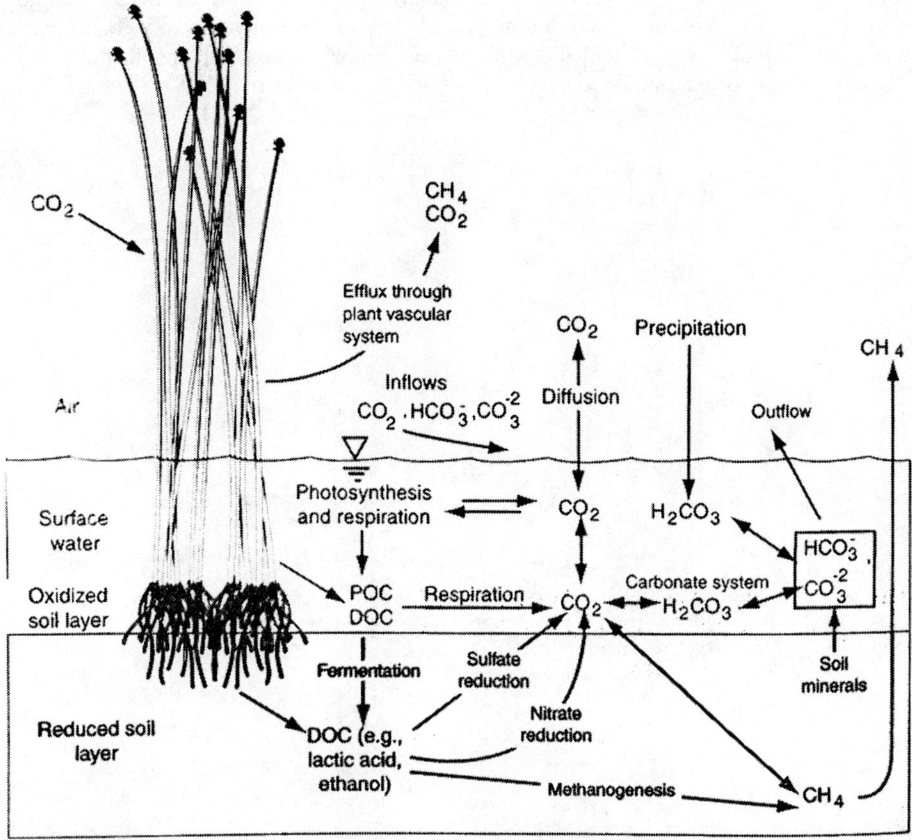

Fig. 2. Carbon transformations in wetlands. POC indicates particulate organic carbon; DOC indicates dissolved organic carbon (after Ready D'Angelo *in* Mitsch & Gosselink, 2000).

Phosphorus transformations

The wetlands provide an environment for the interconversion of all forms of phosphorus (phosphorus transformations and cycling in wetlands are shown in *fig. 4*).

Soluble reactive phosphorus is taken up by plants and converted to tissue phosphorus or may become sorbed to wetland soils and sediments. Organic structural phosphorus may be released as soluble phosphorus if the organic matrix is oxidized. Insoluble precipitates form under some circumstances, but may redissolve under altered conditions (Kadlec & Knight, 1996).

Metals

The processes of metal removal in constructed wetlands include sedimentation, filtration, adsorption, complexation, precipitation, cation exchange, plant uptake, and microbially-mediated reactions, especially oxidation (Watson *et al.* 1989).

Metals occur in either the soluble or particulate associated forms, with the former representing the most bioavailable form, particularly when the metal is present as either an ionic or weakly complexed species. The distribution between particulate and dissolved phases is determined by physico-chemical processes such as sorption, precipitation, complexation, sedimentation, erosion and diffusion. Certain metals such as Cd or Zn have been shown to have a stronger affinity for the dissolved phase whereas Pb tends to be predominantly particulate associated (Morrison *et al.*

1984). Specific parameters which control the sediment-water partitioning of metals include flow/suspended solids ratio, oxic/anoxic conditions, ionic strength, pH value, dissolved and particulate organic carbon contents, organic and inorganic ligand concentrations and metal mobilisation by biochemically-mediated reactions (Cooper *et al.* 1996; Vymazal *et al.*, 1998).

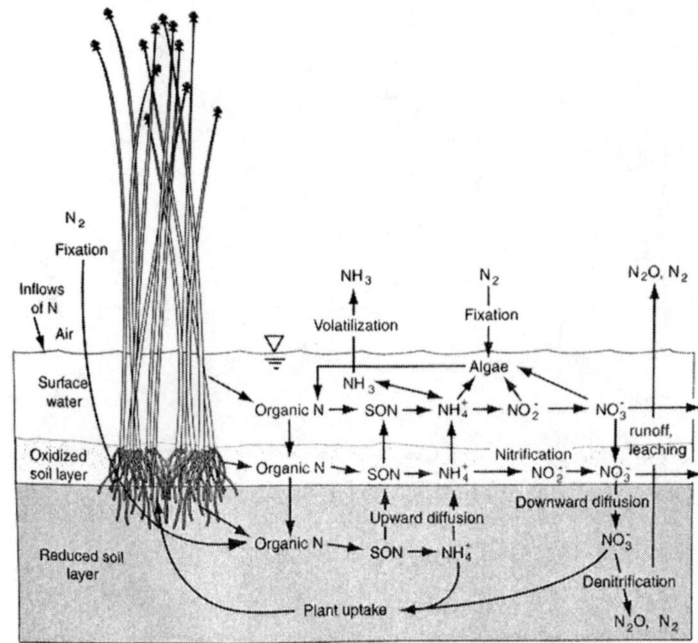

Fig. 3. Nitrogen transformations in wetlands for wastewater treatment; SON indicates soluble organic nitrogen (after Ready D'Angelo *in* Mitsch & Gosselink, 2000).

Pathogens

Constructed wetlands offer a suitable combination of physical, chemical and biological factors for the removal of pathogenic organisms. Physical factors include mechanical filtration and sedimentation. Chemical factors include oxidation, UV radiation, exposure to biocides excreted by some plants and adsorption to organic matter. Biological removal mechanisms include antibiosis, predation by nematodes, protists and zooplankton, attack by lytic bacteria and viruses and natural die-off (Seidel *et al.*, 1978, Hyde & Ross, 1984, Gersberg *et al.*, 1989, Cooper *et al.*, 1996).

CONSTRUCTED WETLANDS FOR WASTEWATER TREATMENT

The analyses of the current distribuiton of CW in the world reveals that this kind of system can be used to treat almost all types of wastewater. Full-scale wetland treatment systems are being used routinely to treat municipal, industrial and agricultural wastewaters; agricultural and urban run-off, landfill leachate; and acid-mine drainage waters (Kadlec & Knight, 1996). The treatment of sludge is also in use (dehydration, mineralization, decontamination) in treatment wetlands.

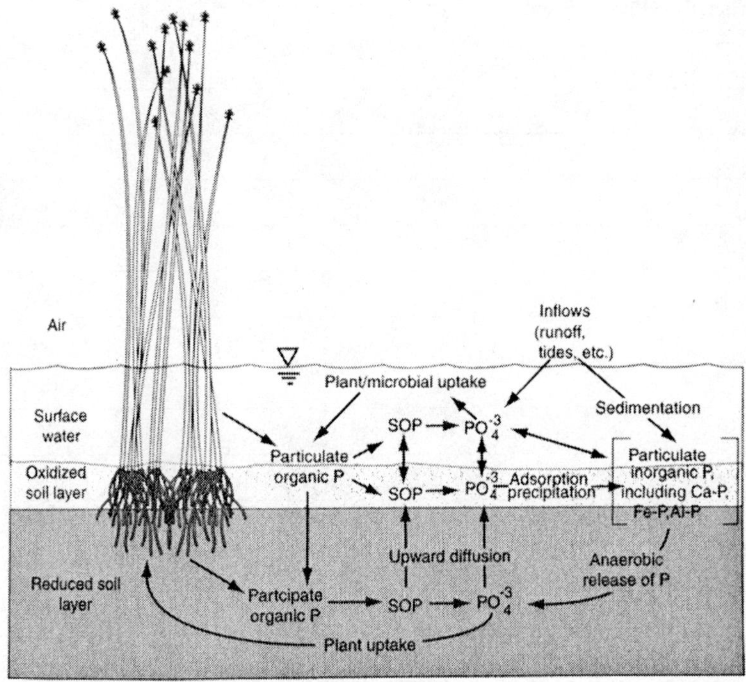

Fig. 4. Phosphorus transformations in wetlands; SOP indicates soluble organic phosphorus (after Ready D'Angelo *in* Mitsch & Gosselink, 2000).

EXISTING CW SYSTEMS

Portugal

Currently there are over 200 constructed wetlands in Portugal. About one-fifth of Portuguese CW are privately owned and the remaining are public systems owned by the municipalities.

The average area for Portuguese constructed wetland is about 900 m^2 with the largest area being 13,000 m^2 and the smallest one 5 m^2. The size of CW according to PE ranges between 3 and 13,000 (average PE $\cong$ 600) (Dias, 2002).

Worldwide

Table 1 depicts a synthesis of available information (bibliography and personal communications) concerning the number of constructed wetland systems already in functioning in several countries.

FUTURE OF CW SYSTEMS FOR WASTEWATER TREATMENT - RESEARCH NEEDS

The value of wetlands for the control of water pollution has been "rediscovered" in the past 30 years; these systems have proven abilities to control hydric pollution. Still, it is essential to remember that many questions concerning the functioning of these systems are still unanswered and must therefore be studied and addressed in order to allow the optimization of the processes that provide the depuration of wastewater.

Table 1. Constructed wetland systems

Country	Number of CW Systems
Austria	180
Check republic	120
Germany	5000
Denmark	134
France	200
Norway	20
Poland	100
Sweden	20
Switzerland	100
Holland	75
United kingdom	700
South africa	100
North america (incluind canada)	2000

Future demands for the depuration of wastewater discharging to small and sensitive water bodies imply the refinement of CW; further research is needed to continue improving the design and engineering criteria of these systems in order to achieve higher levels of contaminant removal.

Currently, there is research concerning a number of issues, particularly in what concerns the optimization of land area, and the influence of temperature (important in countries with very cold winters).

Since this is a relatively new technology there is also great interest in the long term performance of the systems and in kinetics and balancing of different wastewater constituents. Therefore, the need exists for monitoring studies, which follow chemical and other parameters such as vegetation and hydraulics.

Knowledge about plant species, living communities and their particular and global functions in CW also requires further investigation and monitoring so as to accomplish not only the improvement of constructed wetlands but also to rehabilitate natural wetlands.

REFERENCES

1. Cooper, P. F. & de Maeseneer, J. 1996. Hybrid systems - what is the best way to arrangement for the vertical and horizontal-flow stages? IAWQ Specialist Group on the Use of Macrophytes for Water Pollution Control Newsletter No. 15, 8-13.
2. Dias, V., 2002. The Biota of Natural and Constructed Wetlands in Portugal, Proceedings from the 8th International Conference on Wetland Systems for water Pollution Control.
3. Hammer, D. A, 1989. Constructed wetlands for wastewater treatment: municipal, industrial, and agricultural. Lewis Publishers, Michigan.
4. Hyde, H.C. & Ross, R.S. 1984. Technology assessment of wetlands for municipal wastewater treatment. U.S. EPA Municipal Environment. Research Laboratory, Cincinnati, Ohio.
5. Kadlec, R. H & Knight, R. L. 1996. Treatment wetlands. Lewis Publishers, New York.
6. Mitsch, W. J & Gosselink, J. G. 2000. Wetlands, John Wiley &Sons, Inc.

7. Morrison, G. M. P., Revitt, D. M., Ellis, J. B., Balmer, P. & Stevenson, G. 1984. Heavy metal partitioning between the dissolved and suspended solids phases from stormwater runoff in residential areas. Science Tot. Environment, 33, 287-296.
8. Moshiri, G. A. 1993. Constructed wetlands for water quality improvement. Lewis Lewis Publishers, Michigan.
9. Rivera, F., Warren, A., Ramirez, E., Decamp, O., Bonilla, P., Gallegos, E., Calderon, A. & Sanchez, J. T. 1995. Removal of pathogens from wastewaters by the root zone method (RZM). Water Science and Technology, 32, 211-218.
10. Seidel, K., Happel, H. & Graue, G. 1978. Contribution to revitalization of waters. Limnologische Arbeitsgruppe, Max-Plank-Gesellschaft.
11. Vymazal, J., Brix, H., Cooper, P.F., Green, M.B., Haberl, R. (ed). 1998 Constructed wetlands for wastewater treatment in Europe. Backhuys Publishers, Leiden.
12. Watson, J. T., Reed, S. C., Kadlec, R. H., Knight, R. L. & Whitehouse, A. E. 1989. Performance expectations and loading rates for constructed wetlands. In: Hammer,D.A. (ed). Constructed Wetlands for Wastewater Treatment. pp. 319-358. Lewis Publishers, Chelsea, Michigan.
13. Watson, J. T. & Hobson, J. A. 1989. Hydraulic design considerations and control structures for constructed wetlands for wastewater treatment. In: Hammer, D.A. (ed), Constructed Wetlands for Wastewater Treatment. pp. 379-391. Lewis Publishers, Chelsea, Michigan.

Metal Ions in Biology and Medicine: vol. 9. Eds Maria Carmen Alpoim, Paula Vasconcellos Morais, Maria Amélia Santos, Armando J. Cristóvão, José A. Centeno, Philippe Collery.
John Libbey Eurotext, Paris © 2006 pp. 444-1.

Radon daughters survey in the atmosphere of Athens and the correlation with increase of vehicles of gasoline combustion in circulation

K. Grigoropoulos, Ferendinos G.

University of Patras - Greece Environmental Geology - air pollution

ABSTRACT

In this paper we have done a continuous measuring of Radon daughters (^{218}Po, ^{216}Po, ^{214}Po, ^{212}Po, for a period of thirty months (June 2003-Dec 2005) in the atmosphere environment.

The area of this study was at a main avenue of the city of Athens, which is very hectic during the whole day. We used an active detector, whose function is based on a-spectroscopy method. The results of our measurements were correlated with the data obtained from the counters (which count CO,NOX,SO2), of the Greek Environmental Ministry,division air pollution which were placed in several parts of the city. The results of this survey are very interesting, because at the normal days traffic, our values do not exceed the 25 -40 Bq.But when there were taxi-strikes (15.000 taxi vehicles out of circulation and duplication of the private cars in the road) in some days of the months, June, September, October November and December the values increased 150 Bq and more.

At the same time we observed an increase to the values of the air polluters, CO, NOX SO2 at detectors of the air pollution division of our Environmental Ministry.

We deduct, that the increase of private cars exhausts (gasoline consumption), increased immediately the quantity of the radon daughters in atmosphere enviroment.

INTRODUCTION

Many studies in the past have connected the human lung cancer with radon and his decay daughters. Those nuclides with respiration arrive to the lungs, which decay and damage the DNA of the cells, with the consequence of the pathogenesis of lung cancer (Lung cancer Beir. 1999).

Most of the measurements until now have been done in old houses, constructions in places whose ground is rich of Uranium deposits and more in mines in use, where the hazard is in direct contact (aerosols) with the employed personnel. Several other researchers have investigated radon in schools, waters, caves ventilated or not, then in air, soil and underground measourings, some times arrive even five meters deep.

In atmosphere enviroment they make predictions of earthquakes by measuring radon, and/or the change of the underground water temperature variations. Moreover, there are several studies about eruptions of volcanos which liberated radon in air (Etna-Sicily, Dall'Aglio 1994).

We have to take into consideration that measurements of radon in the atmosphere are prevented by the wind, which does not permit serious concentrations of radon in atmosphere. That is the reason that the researchers are cautious with the mesurements in the enviroment. They can certainly try to detect radon with active detectors, when there is no wind.(calm). Our results have particular importance because they have been done for a period of two and a half years continuous monitoring and most of them without wind (under complete calm). Therefore we conclude that the increase of vehicles number (gasoline consumption) in circulation due to the taxi-strikes increase immediately the values of Radon daughters.

Radon problem and the several air polluters, as cars exhausts and industrial combustions have put in scepticism all the researchers since the 1950's when they discovered that statistically the most admissions in European hospitals usually refered in cardio-respiratory failures. In fact a serious percentage index of arrhythmias and heart-infarts are caused by the combustion products (CO, SO2, NOX, TSM).Many papers about these issues have been published the last fifty years.

London lethal cases (1952/1991) comparison (Michelle Bell,Devra Lee Davis).

Particulate matters, Sulfur dioxide and daily mortality in Chongqing-China (Scott Venners, Binyan Wang, Zhonggui peng, Yu Xu. 2003).

This association of Rn daugthers and traffic air-borne aerosols in atmosphere must be taken into serious consideration in the future not only by medical doctors but also by all those scientists who are occupied with the enviromental health morbidity.

We hope that the **Kyoto** protocol (February 2005) will be firmed and respected by all those countries which really care for the human health future.

METHODOLOGY

The city of Athens is localized in the region Attica basin and have (3.000.000 popul.) The town is connected to the seaside by three avenues with Southwest direction. These avenues are daily full of traffic due to people commuting to the center of the city, most of them going to work. The total number of vehicles circulating in the city is 1.800000 private cars,gasoline combustion 97%, 15.000 taxis, 84% diesel), 177.000 light trucks, 50.900 heavy trucks and 6.940 public buses (Data from Greek Environmental Ministry - Division Air pollution).

In this research we use an active detector in which the sampled air volume is sucked through a filter that is analyzed continuously by a Si-detector.

(The detector is acompanied with certificate of calibration.) Nuclides samples on the surface of the filter are analyzed with respect to their alpha decay energy by alpha spectroscopy. In the end of the measurements, we can obtain PAEC, ERC, absorbed dose and Rn daughters ^{212}Po, ^{214}Po, ^{216}Po, ^{218}Po. We choose one of the main four avenues, which is 3.5 km long and 12 m. large, of double direction and 30 m. high from sea level. We have calculated (at the point where the measurements took place and between 06.00-10.00 a.m.-peak time) an amount of 3.600 vehicles approximately every hour.

Our detector was placed in the chosen avenue at a distance of 2 km from the seaside and 4 meters above the ground well protected from solar light. The measurements began in June 2003 and were of continuous radon monitoring for two and a half years, with small intervals during the windy days. Few of our measurements (as pilot index) in our study, were made in an old house (constructed in 1958) which was completely closed during the counts. There the concentration of Radon is in fact very high and reaches more than 500 Bq/m3 (214Po) and more than 100Bq/m3 (218 Po).

In this research we have taken into account the atmospheric parameters, such as temperature humidity, barometric pressure, air condutivity, wind speed and direction daily. The detector filter was being replaced according to the factory instructions. The official dates of the taxi strikes have been collected from the Athens federation of taxi owners. The values of CO, NOX, SO2 are from the Greek Enviroment Ministry detectors.

MEASUREMENTS ANALYSIS

We started our measurements in atmosphere the first days of June 2003 and in the middle of the month, the Athens federation of taxi owners proclaimed 48 ours strike.

Our measurements, continued during the taxi strike and we noted an increase during the morning (max concentration between 06.00-09.00 a.m.) of radon daughters 218Po (30-70 Bq/m3) and 214 Po (50-350 Bq/m3) which diminished with the end of strike.

In the days without strikes the values do not exceed 8-15 Bq/m3 and 30-40 Bq/m3 in correspondence. In the meantime we also noted an increase on the detectors of the air pollution which they counted CO, NOX, SO2. At first that surprised us, but we had the opportunity to observe a repetition of the phenomenon again, because we had more strikes. In fact during the next two strikes in September, we noted the same increase of values as those of June. The same happened again in month October (four days strike), November (one day) and December (seven days strike).

The following tablet is the map of the Attika basin with the positions of the pollution counters in five several stations around the city. Number six position is our Radon station.

BASIN ATTIKA MAP

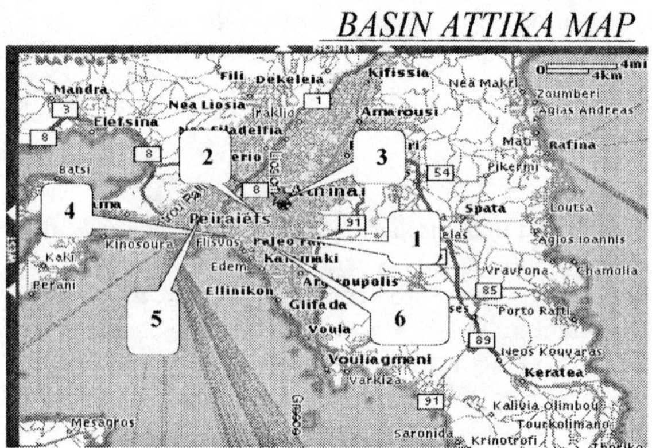

At the following tablets we observe in the diagrams the results of several pollution counters stations (in different parts of Athens) in corellation with the results of our Radon station.

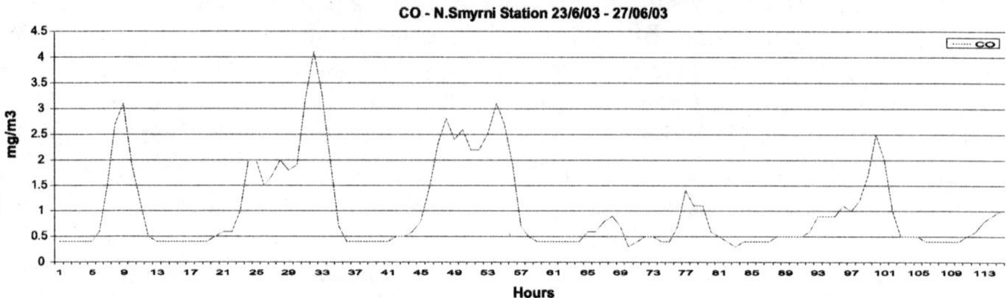

Ne Sm station: The CO during the strike arrives at 4 mg/m3 at 09.00 a.m. Nime o'clock is the 32h of the tablet in the first day of the strike. In normal conditions in the summer the CO does not exceed the 2,5 mg/m3.

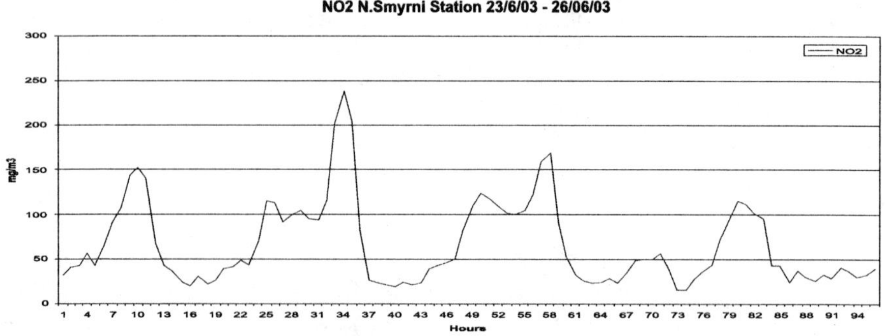

Ne Sm station: NO2 during the strike is more than 150 μg/m^3 at 09.00 a.m. (34h of the tablet). In normal conditions during the year is 60-90 μg/m3.

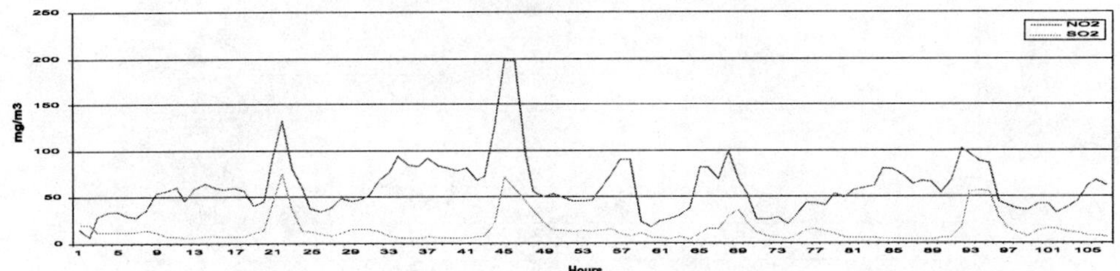

Geo station: at 09.00 a.m. (22h of tablet) SO_2 has a peak of 76 μg/m3 when in summer normal days does not exceed 20μg/m3.At the same time NO_2 has a peak of 200μg/m3 (normal values during the year 60-90μg/m3.

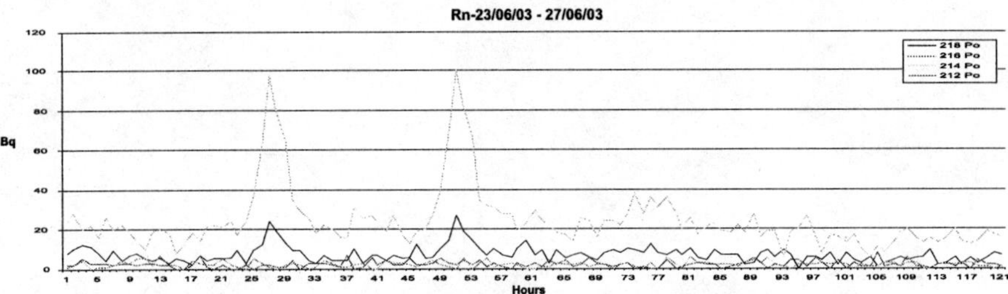

In this tablet is the monitoring of our Radon station between 23/6/03-27/6/03.
We observe an increase of 214Po at 100Bq/m3 and 218Po at 23-26 Bq/m3.
With the end of the strike the values are 20-25Bq/m3 and below 10 Bq/m3.
The other daughters do not present any particular change.

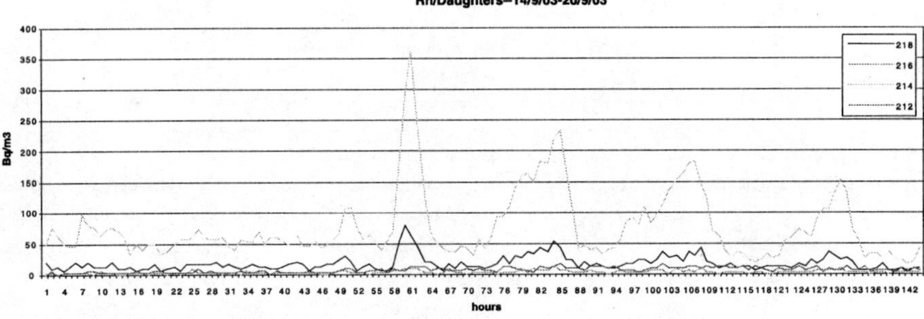

In September we have a new strike at 17, 18, 22, 23, 24 and 25. The following tablet is a monitoring between 14-9-03 until 20-9-03. In comparison with June's strike, we have an increase of the values.

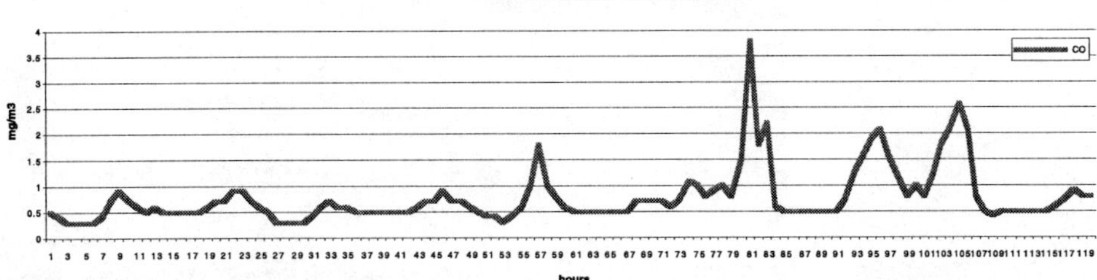

Ne Sm CO station.

The registration is from 15/9/03 until 18/9/2003. The strike is in 17 and 18 September. High concentrations are at 9.00 am. Nine o'clock of the first day strike corresponds to the 57th hour of the table and at the second day to the 81st hour. The values of the first day are not high but the second day arrive at 4mg/m3 like in June's strike.

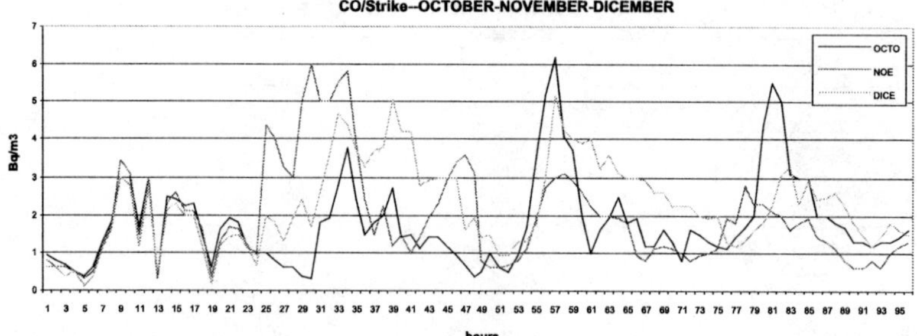

Values of three months are more than 5mg/m3 during strikes.

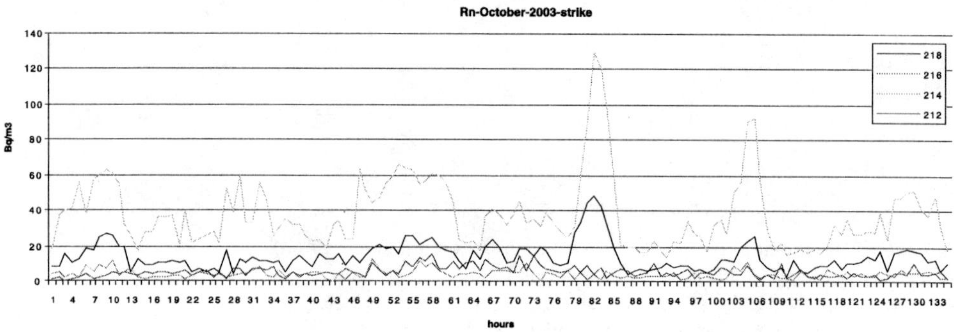

The strike starts after the 76th hour of the table. 214Po arrives more 120Bq and 218Po more than 40Bq/m3.

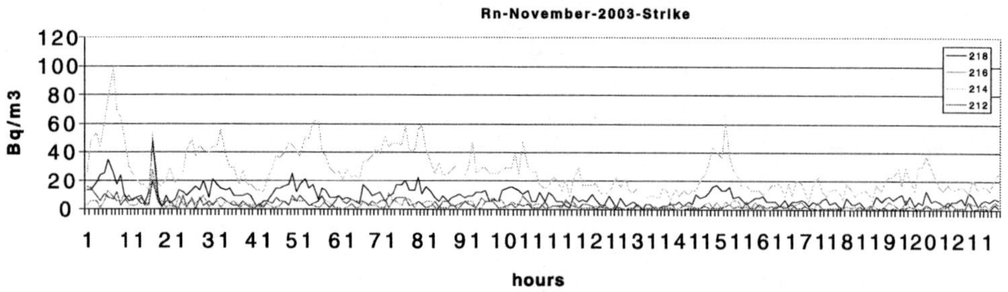

The first 10 hours of table is the strike of 24 h. duration. 214Po arrives 100Bq and 218Po arrives quite 40Bq.

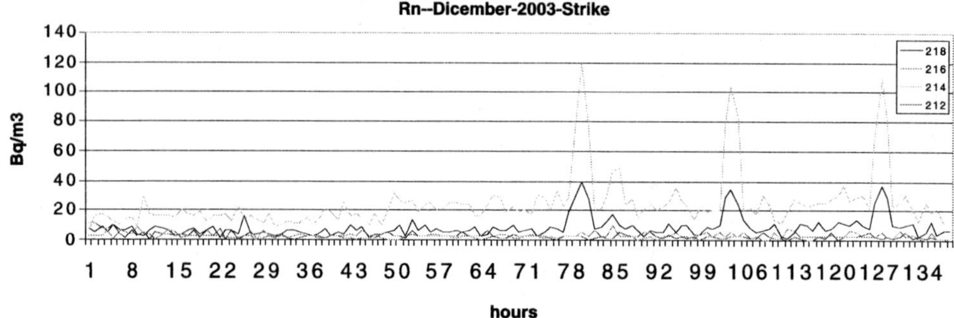

Three days of strike registration. Start of the strike at 80h.The concentrations are more than 100Bq (214Po) and 40Bq (218Po).

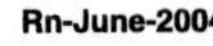

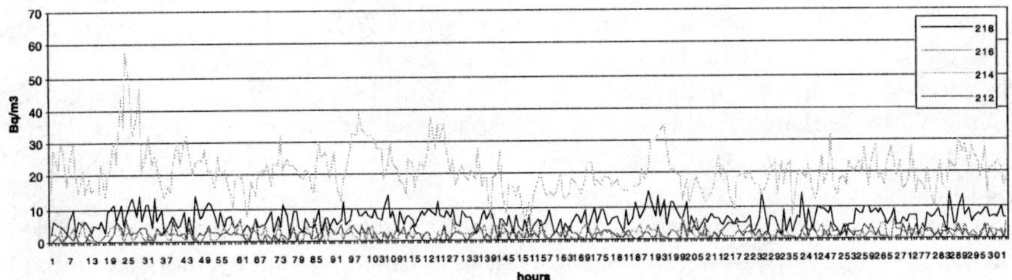

One year later a twelve days monitoring of radon daughters without a strike.

DISCUSSION-CONCLUSION

This research has been done in a principal road where the atmosphere is rich of car exhausts during the early morning hours, when the city's population goes to work.

During the strike we noted an enorme increase of radon daughters and the several air polluters in the atmosphere, which does not happen in the rest of the normal traffic days.

After those results we proceeded for twenty four months monitoring (7 to 12 days registrations) in diverse seasons of the years 2004 and 2005, but without to observe a repetition of the strike fenomenum.

In the end of measurements our counts were classified in three groups.

First is during the normal day hours and weekends (no high traffic) ^{218}Po 6-9Bq/m^3, ^{214}Po 10-12 Bq/m^3). The second is, in early morning time (time to go for work-High traffic), ^{218}Po 8-12, ^{214}Po 20-25 Bq/m^3.

And the third group are days of strike (very high traffic ^{218}Po 40-50 Bq/m^3, ^{214}Po 120-350 Bq/m^3) in which we obtained the maximum values of Radon daughters because we had an increase of private cars number in circulation due to the taxis strike.

It is very importan to note that there were no restrictions in circulation of vehicles during the strike (government restrictions in circulation start in 1985).

Our city geograficaly is surrounded by mountains except in the south where is open to the seaside. That is the reason for the permanent remain of a lot of nocive air molecular substancies in our enviroment. The air pollution problem in Athens, emerged/sorge in the 80's decade with a logarithmic increase of the automobiles number in the following twenty years.

That is the reason why our government (1985) tried to apply restrictions at the cars onwers. So an alternative solution was to permit in circulation the 50% of the total number existing cars daily. Moreover they gave motives to the population for the substitution of autos, with the new tecnology anti-Pb gasoline, but not an evidential change has been registrated.

Between 2001-2004 we had the metro extension and four new electric-tram lines. After that we expected a migliorament at the quality atmosphere but the main problem has not been really resolved. Today approximately every family has in possesion at least three automobiles, comparing to one in early 1980's.

The 1980 restrictions in circulation are also still valid today, but the morbidity epidemiologicaly in cardio-respiratory diseases, continues to occupy all the clinical phycisians (cardiologist, internists pneumonologists and oncologists) in our hospitals with a high statistic index of deaths (lung cancers, leukemias, heart infarts, brain strokes).

Several researchers in the past,have dimostrate direct correlation of radon air propagation with polluters as CO, CO2, NOX, SO2 (Brager, Revzan 1991, Nazaroff and Nero 1988). Radon and CO (Biagi A. Morelli D. 2000). Radon and air polluters (Avino P. Broco D. Lepore L. 2003). Is already know from epidemiological statistics the origine of lung cancer from those polluters (Radon, CO, CO2, Benzene).

Ischemic heart diseases, acute bronco-respiratory, cardio-respiratory diseases and cardiac arrhythmias and many deaths have correlated with CO and NOX (Man, Tager, Lurmann, Segal, others, Epidemiology department, UCLA 2002).

For the moment no one has registered, for so long period (two years) during the last 20 years, the association of those daughters in our city atmosphere with the exhausts (vehicular-aerosols) in circulation and we hope than this research will influence to investigate more and lengthy this our city serious incovenience.

The main question which immerges, is what are the consequencies for the public health and what is the epidemiology response (Pathogenesis of lung cancer or other tumors and other clinico-pathological disorders) of the inhabitants in this area,when the inhalated radon daughters in association with the exhausts polluters, develop a nocive molecular "cluster" which expanding and spreading - traveling for (more than two hours remain) unknow time in this investigated by us atmosphere on our city of Athens.

We express our grateful for the assistance of division air pollution (Greek environmental ministry) and the Athens federation taxis owners.

Out team is already under investigation of some unexpected physical - electric factors (similar to those mentioned by prof. Henshaw 1993) which are probably responsible for the expansion of radon and they have not been investigated in the past.

REFERENCES

Avino, Brocco, Lepore Pareti. (Ann. Chim 2003)
BEIR. (1988)
Brager, Revzan. (Atmosph. Environment 1991)
Nazaroff, Nero 1988
Man, Tager, Lurman, Segal - others. (Epidemiology Dpt UCLA 2002)
Michelle Bell, Devra Lee Davis. London lethal cases (1952/1991) comparison
Scott Venners, Binyan Wang, Zhonggui Peng Yuxu. (Environm. Health Perspect 2003
Biagi A. Morelli D. (Radon and CO pollution. American institute of Physics 2000)

Metal Ions in Biology and Medicine: vol. 9. Eds Maria Carmen Alpoim, Paula Vasconcellos Morais, Maria Amélia Santos, Armando J. Cristóvão, José A. Centeno, Philippe Collery.
John Libbey Eurotext, Paris © 2006 pp. 451-1.

Marine sponge *Cliona celata* as a potential bioindicator

Marques, D.[1], Esteves, A.I.[1], Xavier, J.[3,4], Almeida, M.[1,2], Humanes, M.[1]

[1]*Centro de Química e Bioquímica - Departamento de Química e Bioquímica da Faculdade de Ciências da Universidade de Lisboa, Edifício C8, Campo Grande, 1749-016 Lisboa, Portugal (mmhumanes@fc.ul.pt)*
[2]*Instituto de Tecnologia Biomédica, Faculdade de Medicina Dentária da Universidade de Lisboa, 1649-003 Lisboa, Portugal (mmalmeida@fc.ul.pt)*
[3]*Institute for Biodiversity and Ecosystem Dynamics, University of Amsterdam, Mauritskade 57, 1092 AD Amsterdam, The Netherlands*
[4]*Departamento de Biologia, Universidade dos Açores, Rua Mãe de Deus, Apartado 1422, 9501-855 Ponta Delgada, Portugal*

The analytical studies of sponges have recently become a matter of interest, since they have been reported to accumulate high levels of particular elements including metals, which may have an anthropogenic origin, allowing their application as environmental pollution indicators. Variations of individual antioxidants are difficult to predict and they often vary according to class of chemicals, species sensitivity and several environmental and biological factors. To contribute to this global aim, we studied the variation of the well known biomarkers glutathione peroxidase and the reduced/ oxidized glutathione ratio in the cosmopolitan sponge *Cliona celata*. Specimens were collected from pre-selected sites considered undisturbed in terms of pollution, although some anthropogenic activities can occur.The main goals of this work are to check if these biomarkers are present in the sponge, to determine the normal range value and to check for eventual differences in the collection sites.

INTRODUCTION

Coastal and estuarine ecosystems and their inhabitants are subject to increased stress associated with the huge human population growth in these areas. This situation requires careful monitoring of biological resources and development of strategies to minimize the impacts. The critical issues involve determining if the organisms that should live and thrive in a habitat are adversely affected, and identifying the effects of chronic stress on biotic health.

Compensatory mechanisms may function to sequester, detoxify, or ameliorate the effects of stressors - so, exposures do not always translate into adverse effects. In other cases, individual stressors or combinations of stressors may cause chronic stress that can compromise basic physiological functions, including reproduction, so long-term population dynamics and sustainability are endangered. Therefore, sensitive tools are needed to recognize when habitat conditions adversely affect biotic integrity, before the effects are irreversible or very hard to remedy [1].

Cellular biomarker responses provide one of the best tools for identifying when conditions have exceeded compensatory mechanisms and the individuals (and populations) are experiencing chronic stress, which may severely effect the ecosystem level. In biomedical applications these parameters are routinely used as diagnostic tools, as early warning signals of disease conditions, for prognosis, and for drug evaluation. These kinds of tests can be applied to marine organisms as a means of characterizing habitat quality. Sponges, as filter feeding organisms inhabiting all the oceans, seas, rivers and lakes, without differentiated organs, seem to meet all the qualifications for a sentinel species. But, surprisingly, there is not a lot published on this subject [2-4].

The sponge we choose for this work, *Cliona celata*, is a cosmopolitan sponge, commonly called yellow boring sponge, because it bores into soft limestone, using an acid digestion technique. The sponge can also bore into mollusc and barnacle shells and they are considered highly detrimental, in oyster farms [5].

One of the attributes of cellular response assays is thatthey should be readily applicable to a wide range of organisms, with fairly minor modifications. To do this effectively, requires a sound basis for interpreting cellular data, including expected values and an appreciation of the potential variation. In the biomedical context, this is analogous to defining the normal range of responses.

Glutathione (γ-glutamilcysteinylglycine-GSH) is a low molecular weight intracellular thiol [6, 7] that is an important overall modulator of cellular homeostasis and serves numerous essential functions including detoxification of metals and oxy-radicals [8, 9]. While exposure to pollutants or stressful conditions can result in elevated GSH levels, there is evidence that adverse effects are associated with GSH depletion in marine bivalves [10, 11] as well as mammalian systems [12]. Organisms may also be more susceptible to additional stressors when GSH is depleted [13] and GSH status has been proposed as a potential risk factor in human-based risk assessments [14]. The oxidized glutathione (GSSG) is formed in the redox reactions involving the glutathione and can accumulate, at cellular level, as a result of the increase of the oxidative processes. It has been proposed that the GSH/GSSG ratio may function as a very sensitive indicator of oxidative stress [15]. Another useful biomarker is glutathione peroxidase (GPx) that catalyses the reduction of hydroperoxides, using glutathione as a hydrogen donor and producing water, the respective alcohol and oxidized glutathione.

Experimental

Biological material - Specimens of *Cliona celata* (n = 21) were collected by scuba diving, in several areas of two Portuguese Marine Natural Reserves (Arrábida and Berlengas), and in Graña-Ferrol, Spain, from 2001 to 2004 *(fig. 1)*. After collection, the specimens were transported to the laboratory in isothermal containers, frozen and stored at -20°C. Voucher specimens have been kept in 96% ethanol for taxonomical analysis.

Sample preparation - Since marine sponges possess several organisms associated with them, prior to any use, the biological material was cleaned from any macro organisms (such as small algae or crustacean) or even alien bodies, like sediments or rocks. Samples were homogenized with a blender in fifteen volumes of ice-cold sodium phosphate buffer (0.1M, pH=8.0) in the presence of 25% HPO_3 (4mL per 15mL buffer solution) for two minutes. The solution was stirred for 30 min, at 4°C to increase the extraction efficiency; immediately after the insoluble residues were separated by centrifugation (100000g, 30 min., 4°C). The supernatants were filtered and became ready for analysis.

Stability, repeatability, reproducibility and accuracy studies - In order to perform stability, repeatability, reproducibility and accuracy studies one sponge specimen was randomly chosen

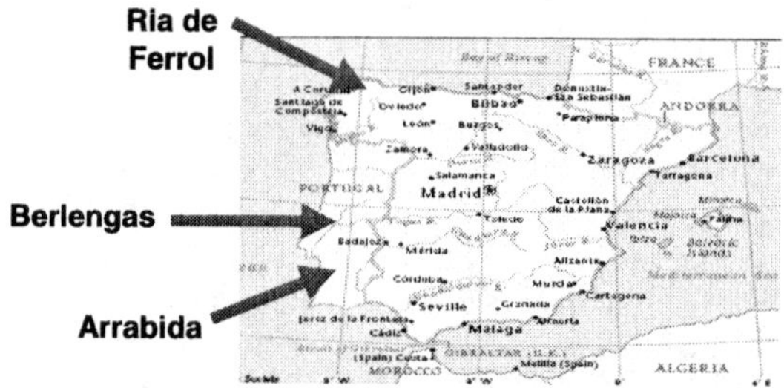

Fig. 1. Location of the collection sites

(B33) and 100 ml of sample homogenate were obtained and divided into thirteen vials. From these thirteen vials, eight were placed at -20° C in order to test stability at this temperature during ten days, four were kept at - 80° C to perform reproducibility studies of the methods tested and the remaining vial was used for repeatability and accuracy studies. For repeatability studies, ten replicates were used for each researched method. The remaining tests used three replicates.

Determination ofthe reduced (GSH) and oxidizedforms of glutathione - A fluorimetric method, previously described was used [16, 17].

Determination of glutathione peroxidase activity - A spectrophotometric method was used [18,19].

Determination of proteins - Lowry method was used for protein quantification [20].

Results and discussion

Sponges, independently of their class or order, in the adult stage, are filter-feeding organisms. The flow of water through the sponge is unidirectional, driven by the beating of flagella that line the surface of chambers connected by a series of canals. These animals do not have organs, or even differentiated tissues. For many organisms, tested as bioindicators, we have to consider the several organs. We can consider the sponge as a whole, but it must be kept in mind that we are dealing with a complex matrix. In these circumstances, the analytical methods should be tested for interferences, reproducibility and accuracy.

The fluorimetric method for the determination of the ratio GSH/GSSG was chosen because of its very high specificity; the interference of other substances present in the analytical media can be minimized using small samples.

For glutathione peroxidase, the method used was checked for repeatability and reproducibility, in one of the samples (B33), randomly chosen. The uncertainty determined ($[0.46 \times 10^{-1}; 2.78 \times 10^{-1}]U/mgP_{GPx}$) was of the same order of the measured; in these circumstances, the values obtained should be treated with care, since they are very susceptible to variations in measuring conditions.

The results obtained for the samples are summarized in *table 1*.

The statistical treatment of the results shows that the population considered presents an asymmetrical distribution for the glutathione peroxidase, similar to the χ^2 probability distribution function. This behaviour suggests the presence of *outliers* (elements with values outside the interval barriers where all the values of a normal population should be contained) and, indeed we found that the GPx value for the sponge A03/7 (0.205U/mg_{Prot})should be considered an *outlier*.

The distribution of GSH/GSSG ratio presents a symmetrical shape of a normal probability distribution function without any *outliers (fig. 2B)*.

We can say that normal range values for reduced/oxidized glutathione in the sponge *Cliona celata* should be in the interval [0.31 - 2.21] whereas the values of glutathione peroxidase in the same organism should be in the range [0 - 0.201] U/mg Prot.

Normal ranges must be determined based on data from unpolluted sites. Although 21 samples is not an extraordinary big sample, it is enough to start. The robustness of the normal range values will be dependent on the size of the data set, but at some point, the values should not change very much with additional data. The use of normal ranges is an important value to investigators that are not limited to evaluating the effects at one unknown site to those of only one or a few reference sites, but can compare any unknown site to a broader array / database of reference sites, thereby reducing uncertainty. In this way, decisions about whether or not the organisms from a site are stressed can be made with greater confidence. All sites designated *a priori* as degraded or polluted should be removed, and means and standard deviations calculated [1].

Following these statements, specimens studied in this work were collected from pre-selected sites considered undisturbed in terms of pollution, although in Arrabida (Rampa da Secil and Arflor) and in Ria de Ferrol (Punta Fornelos) some anthropogenic activities can occur. But, with one exception, all the values are within the normal range and we cannot distinguish between the

Table 1. Characteristics of the sites where samples were collected and values obtained for the reduced/ oxidized glutathione and glutathione peroxidase.

Sample	Collection site	Collection date	Depth (m)	GSH/GSSH	GPx (U/mg Prot)
A03/06	Arrábida (Rampa da Secil)	15/05/2003	10-20	1.06	0.090
A03/07				1.22	0.205
A03/08				1.17	0.055
A03/70	Arrábida (Cabo Espichel)	16/07/2003	7	0.30	0.077
A03/71				1.32	0.097
A03/75	Arrábida (Arflor)	28/07/2003	7	1.49	0.022
B33	Berlengas	04/07/1998	4	0.99	0.162
B418	Berlengas (Furado Grande)	22/07/2003	4	1.53	0.008
B124		12/08/1998	2	1.10	0.089
B173		10/08/1999	7	1.28	0.082
B277		22/07/2000	4	1.17	0.109
B341		30/06/2001	4-5	0.96	0.079
B350		30/06/2001	4-5	1.08	0.054
B357		30/06/2001	4-5	0.38	0.042
B373		30/06/2001	4-5	1.51	0.067
B400	Berlengas, Farilhões (Rabo d'Asno)	22/07/2003	25-29	1.31	0.009
B401				0.69	0.053
B109	Berlengas (Estela)	11/08/1998	13	1.42	0.081
FE01	Ria de Ferrol (Punta Segano)	22/05/2003	5-16	1.74	nd
FE03	Ria de Ferrol (Punta Fornelos)	23/05/2003	5-16	2.16	nd
FE04	Ria de Ferrol (Ensenada Carino)	23/05/2003	5-16	1.72	nd

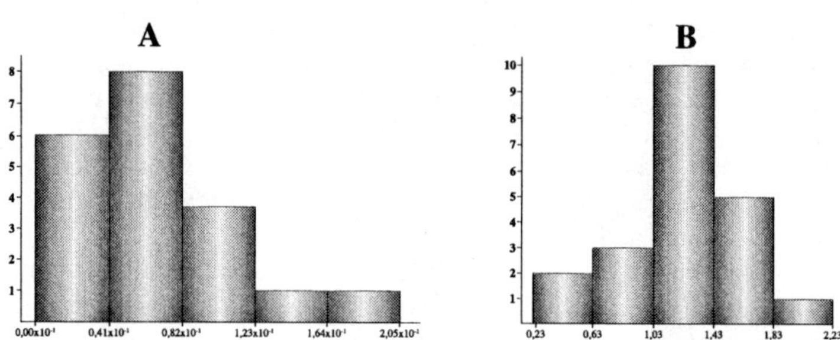

Fig. 2. Histogram of the distribution of the 21 samples (A-glutathione peroxidase values; GSH/GSSH ratio)

two types of sites. Another possible explanation is that these organisms do not reflect oxidative stress on these particular parameters, or the response is small.

To validate the usefulness of sponges as biological indicators it is necessary to test the response of these parameters (reduced/oxidized glutathione and glutathione peroxidase) versus the concentration of stressors. With other organisms, as mussels, crabs or fishes it is usually done in controlled conditions, i.e., using aquaria. Sponges are organisms extremely difficult to keep in aquarium and, even if we succeed, the stress imposed, even in the "blank", can drastically affect the results. It must be kept in mind that all population stresses are necessarily preceded by a biochemical response, whilst biochemical responses need not be associated with a population stress [21].

Environmental determinations *in loco* seem to be the only solution. These determinations should relay basically on the sediments, since sponges feed on particulate matter.

The comparison of the sediment elemental composition, as far as metals are concerned have been done in one of the stations of Berlengas (Furado Grande). The composition of non-polluted sediments - average shale and mean sediment - clearly indicates the absence of any metallic pollutants in the area. In fact, the concentrations of the "anthropogenic" metals are extremely low, under the values measured in the Portuguese continental shelf sediments [22]. Unfortunately, this was not done in the other locations.

With this work we establish the methods for the determination of reduced/oxidized glutathione ratio and glutathione peroxidase, validated the methods and got a basic "normal range" for these two parameters.

REFERENCES

1. Rindwood A H, Hoguet J, Keppler C J, Gielazyn M L, Ward BP, Rourk A R. Cellular Biomarkers (Lysosomal Destabilization, Glutathione & Lipid Peroxidation) in Three Common Estuarine Species: A Methods Handbook. 2003 Marine Resources Research Institute, South Carolina Department of Natural Resources, p. 4-5.
2. Perez T, Wafo E, Fourt M, Vacelet J. Marine sponges as biomonitor of polychlorobiphenyl contamination: concentration and fate of 24 congeners. *Environ Sci Technol.* 2003; 37; 2152-8.
3. Wiens M, Koziol C, Hassanein H M A, Batel R, Schröder H C, Müller W E G, Induction of gene expression of the chaperones 14-3-3 and HSP70 by PCB 118 (2,3',4,4',5-pentachlorobiphenyl) in the marine sponge *Geodia cydonium*: novel biomarkers for polychlorinated biphenyls. *Mar Ecol Prog Series.* 1998; 165; 247-267.
4. De Flora S, Bagnasco M, Bennicelli C, Camoirano A, Bojnemirski A, Kurelec B. Biotransformation of genotoxic agents in marine sponges. Mechanisms and modulation. *Mutagenesis.* 1995; 10(4); 357-64.
5. Rosell D, Uriz M J, Martín D. Infestation by excavating sponges on the oyster (Ostrea edulis) populations of the Blanes littoral (North-Western Mediterranean Sea). *J Mar Biol Ass U.K.* 1999; 79; 409-413.
6. Kosower, N.S., Kosower, E.M. The glutathione status of cells. *Int Rev in Cytol* 1978; 54; 109-160.
7. Mason, A.Z., Jenkins, K.D. Metal detoxification in aquatic systems. In: Metal Speciation and Bioavailability in Aquatic Systems. 1996 A. Tessier and D.R. Turner, eds. John Wiley & Sons, Chicester. p. 479-608.
8. Meister A, Anderson M E. Glutathione. *Ann Rev Biochem* 1983; 52; 711-760.
9. Christie N T, Costa M. *In vitro* assessment of the toxicity of metal compounds. IV. Disposition of metals in cells: interactions with membranes, glutathione, metallothionein, and DNA. 1984. *Biol Trace Elements Res* 6; 1139-1158.
10. Viarengo A L, Canesi L, Pertica M, Poli G, Moore M N, Orunesu M. Heavy metal effects on lipid peroxidation in the tissues of *Mytilus galloprovincialis* Lam. *Comp Biochem Physiol* 1990; 97; 32-42.
11. Ringwood A H, Conners D E, Keppler C J, DiNovo A A. Biomarker studies with juvenile oysters *(Crassostrea virginica)* deployed *in situ. Biomarkers* 1999; 4; 400-415.
12. Dudley R E, Klaassen C D. Changes in the hepatic glutathione concentration modify cadmium-induced hepatotoxicity. *Toxicol ApplPharmacol.* 1984; 72; 530-538.
13. Conners D E, Ringwood A H. Effects of glutathione depletion on copper cytotoxicity in oysters *(Crassostrea virginica). Aquat Toxicol.* 2000; 50; 341-349.

14. Jones D P, Brown L S, Sternberg P. Variability in glutathione-dependent detoxication *in vivo* and its relevance to detoxication of chemical mixtures. *Toxicol.* 1995; 105; 267-274.
15. Lomaestro B M, Malone M. Glutathione in health and disease: pharmacotherapeutic issues. *The Annals of Pharmacotherapy*. 1995; 29, 1263-73.
16. Hissin P, Hilf R. A Fluorimetric Method for Determination of Oxidized and Reduced Glutathione in Tissues. *Anal Biochem* 1976; 74; 214-226.
17. Cohn V, Lyle J. A Fluorimetric Assay for Glutathione. *Anal Biochem* 1966; 14; 434-440.
18. Paglia D E, Valentine W N. Studies on the quantitative and qualitative characterization of erythrocyte glutathione peroxidase. *J Lab & ClinMed* 1967; 70-1; 158-169.
19. OXItek (2004) Total Glutathione Peroxidase Assay Kit. ZMC Catalog #: 0805002.
20. Bensadoun A, Weinstein D. Assay of Proteins in the Presence of Interfering Materials. *Anals Biochem* 1976; 70; 241-250.
21. Rees T J. Glutathione S-Transferase as a Biological Marker of Aquatic Contamination. PhDThesis, 1993, Portsmouth University, UK.
22. Araújo M F, Conceição A, Barbosa T, Lopes M T, Humanes M M. Elemental composition by EDXRF of marine sponges from the Berlengas Natural Park - Western Portuguese coast. *X-ray Spectrometry*, 2003, 32, 428-433.

Metal Ions in Biology and Medicine: vol. 9. Eds Maria Carmen Alpoim, Paula Vasconcellos Morais, Maria Amélia Santos, Armando J. Cristóvão, José A. Centeno, Philippe Collery.
John Libbey Eurotext, Paris © 2006 pp. 457-1.

Impact of metals in bivalve species from guadiana river and estuary

Serafim, A., Company, R., Cravo, A. & Bebianno, M.J.

CIMA, Faculty of Marine and Environmental Sciences, University of Algarve, Campus de Gambelas, 8000 Faro, Portugal.
E-mails : aserafim@ualg.pt, rcompany@ualg.pt, acravo@ualg.pt, mbebian@ualg.pt.

The Guadiana River basin has a total drainage area of 67 840 km^2 of which 11 580 km^2 are located in southeastern Portugal. It constitutes one of the three main drainage units of the Iberian Peninsula shared between Portugal and Spain. The main water problems within the river basin are caused by agricultural runoff, and fragmentation by dams. Point source pollution from industries, mining, sewage treatment plants, landfills, and others also cause major environmental problems.

To assess the impact of metal inputs in this river, several bivalve species were collected along Guadiana River, in a total of 9 sampling sites. These bivalves included the freshwater clam *(Corbicula fluminea)* that occurs in the upper estuary, the common mussel *(Mytilus galloprovincialis)*, the peppery furrow shell *(Scrobicularia plana)* and the Portuguese oyster *(Crassostrea angulata)* collected mainly in the middle-lower estuary of Guadiana.

The concentrations of cadmium (Cd), copper (Cu), lead (Pb) and zinc (Zn) were determined in the whole tissue of the four bivalve species as well as the levels of metallothioneins (MT) and lipid peroxidation (LPO).

A marked spatial gradient of the toxic metals Pb and Cd was observed in the bivalves (mainly *C. fluminea* and *M. galloprovincialis*) along the Guadiana River and Estuary, suggesting an influence of old mining areas in the dispersal of these contaminants. The essential metals Cu and Zn in the tissues of these bivalves were regulated. MT levels seem to follow the pattern of Cd concentrations in *M. galloprovincialis*, while LPO increases with Cu concentrations in *C. fluminea*.

INTRODUCTION

The Guadiana River is one of the longest rivers of the Iberian Peninsula, with a total length of 810 km, of which 550 km is in Spanish territory, 150 km in Portugal and 110 km serves as a border between the two countries [1]. This river begins in Spain, at Campo de Montiel, in the province of Ciudad Real, and drains to the sea between Vila Real de Santo António and Ayamonte. Guadiana has the fourth largest drainage basin of the Iberian Peninsula, 67 840 km^2 in area [2], of which 11 580 km^2 are located in southeastern Portugal, and about 75% is artificially regulated by more than 40 dams [3]. Although the urban pressure along the upper estuary is small and the industry is scarce [4], the main contamination in this area rise from abandoned mining areas of the South Iberian Pyritic Belt, a vast mining area with 250 km length, from Vale do Sado to Vale do Guadalquivir in Spain [5, 6], pesticides as result of agriculture runoff, landfills and sewage treatment plants. Even though mining extraction in Minas de S. Domingos ceased in 1966, it was a central site for the extraction of several precious metals such as Au, Cu and Ag during ancient Roman civilization, and for the exploration of massive Cu deposits along with less abundant metals Zn and Pb and reduced amount of As, Co, Cd, Hg, Ag, Se, Au during the XIX and XX centuries. In this context, metals are one of the most important classes of contaminants in the aquatic systems due to their persistence, toxicity and accumulation through the food chain [7]. Both essential and non-essential metals are known to be toxic to organisms depending of the concentration and time of exposure, and this toxicity is usually associated to the disruption of essential functional groups and/or change in the conformation of biological molecules [8]. Several bivalve species have been extensively studied worldwide to assess metal contamination and dispersion of toxic metallic compounds in marine and estuarine areas, and are often designated by bioindicators species. However, the knowledge concerning metal contamination in water, sediments and organisms from the Guadiana River is still scarce. Therefore, the purpose of this study was to assess the impact of metals in four bivalve species from Guadiana River and Estuary, along with the study of a biomarker of metal exposure and one of effect/damage, the cysteine-rich metal binding protein, metallothionein and the oxidative deterioration of lipids in cellular membranes by the action of reactive oxygen species, called lipid peroxidation (LPO), respectively.

MATERIAL AND METHODS

Four bivalve species *(Corbicula fluminea, Mytilus galloprovincialis, Scrobicularia plana* and *Crassostrea angulata)* were collected along the Guadiana River in a total of 8 sampling sites during the INTERREG-UPTPIA Project in summer 2005. The organisms were clean from sediment residues and depurated during 48 hours in separate aerated aquaria (20 litres). After the depuration period, 10 organisms were dissected and frozen at -80°C until the quantification of metals, MT and LPO. Both toxic (Cd and Pb) and essential metals (Cu and Zn) were determined in the whole bivalve tissues by flame atomic absorption spectrophotometry (AAS) after wet digestion with nitric acid. Metal concentrations are expressed as $\mu g\ g^{-1}$ dry weight tissue. MT levels were determined in the heat treated cytosol by differential pulse polarography (DPP) according to the method described by [9]. MT levels are expressed as $mg\ g^{-1}$ total proteins. LPO in the cytosol was evaluated in terms of production of malondialdehyde (MDA) and 4-hydroxyalkenals (4-HNE) due to decomposition of polyunsaturated fatty acids [10]. Lipid peroxidation is expressed as nmol of MDA and 4-HNE g^{-1} of total protein concentrations. Total protein concentrations in bivalve samples were determined according to [11] and expressed in $mg\ g^{-1}$ wet weight.

RESULTS

Metal Concentrations

Metal concentrations in the organisms collected along the Guadiana River and estuary are present in the *figures 1 and 2* and showed the existence of a metal gradient along the river that was metal dependent. In general, concentrations of both essential and non-essential metals in the species collected along the Guadiana Estuary decrease downstream.

Cadmium levels in the tissues of the freshwater clam *C. fluminea* were significantly higher in sites 1 and 3, two important areas of mining extraction and ore transport, when compared to the other sites in the upper river area. However, Cd concentrations in the estuarine mussel *M. galloprovincialis* were higher between the four species, and the levels decreased significantly toward the river mouth (sites 6 to 8), reflecting the inputs near the densely populated cities of Vila Real de Santo António and Ayamonte, and possible discharges from the international bridge *(fig. 1A).*

Similarly, Pb concentrations in the tissues of *C. fluminea* were also significantly higher in site 1, where the influence of old mining areas is more important, and remained relatively unchanged in the other upper river sampling sites, except in site 4 where a seasonal frequented fluvial beach exist. Higher concentrations of Pb were found in the *C. fluminea* and *S. plana* which is probably associated to the sediment burying behaviour of these two species. Contrarily, the levels of Pb in the filter feeding species *M. galloprovincialis* and *C. angulata* were significantly lower, varying from non detected values to 0.04 $\mu g\ g^{-1}$ d.w. *(fig. 1B).*

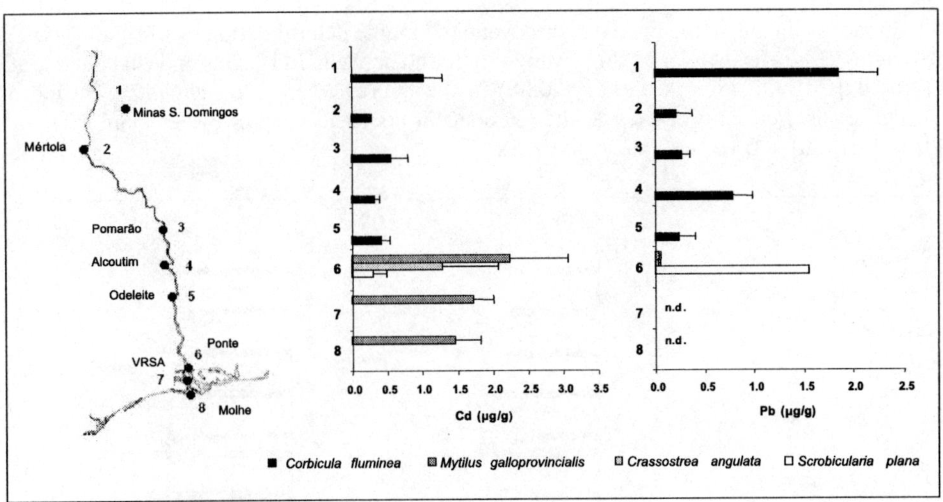

Fig. 1. Levels of non-essential metals in four bivalve species from Guadiana River: (A) Cd concentrations; (B) Pb concentrations.

The concentration of Cu in the clam *C. fluminea* varied along Guadiana upper estuary sites, however these fluctuations were lower than those observed for the non-essential metals (Cd and Pb). In *M. galloprovincialis* the levels of Cu were significantly lower compared to those in *C. fluminea* and remained unchanged in the lower estuary sites *(fig. 2A)*. This suggests that both species are able to regulate the levels of this essential metal in their tissues, like other bivalves. In the oyster *C. angulata* Cu levels were 3-fold and 10-fold higher compared to *C. fluminea* and *M. galloprovincialis* respectively *(fig. 2A)*.

Similarly, Zn concentrations in the tissues of *C. fluminea* remained unchanged along the upper river sites suggesting that, as occurred with Cu, this metal is regulated by this clam *(fig. 2B)*. The levels of Zn in *M. galloprovincialis* increased significantly toward the river mouth, contrarily to what was observed for Cd distribution *(fig. 2B)*.

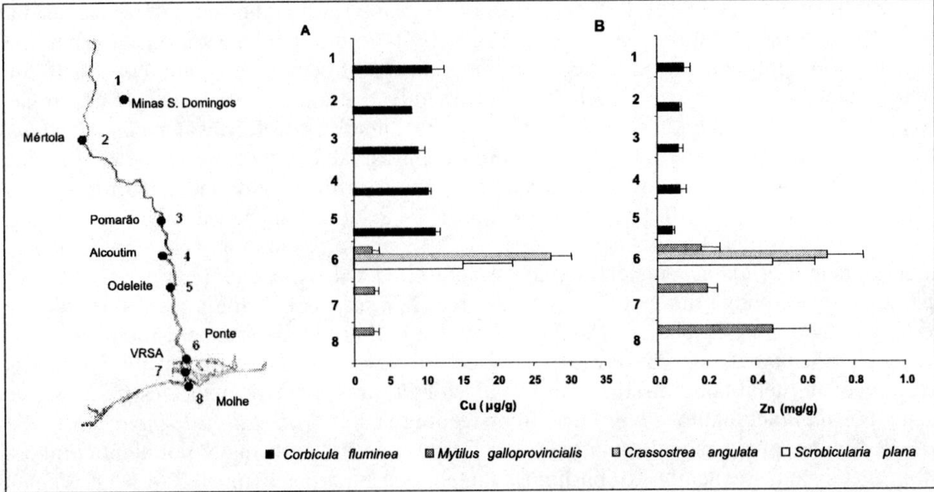

Fig. 2. Levels of essential metals in four bivalve species from Guadiana River: (A) Cu concentrations; (B) Zn concentrations.

Biochemical responses

The impact of metals in the bivalves was evaluated by the determination of MT and LPO levels *(fig. 3A and B)*. Significant relationships were only found between MT levels and Cd concentrations ([MT] = 2.87[Cd] + 2.45; r = 0.917; p>0.05) in the mussel *M. galloprovincialis*. On the other hand, LPO levels were only related to the Cu concentrations in the freshwater clam *C. fluminea* ([LPO] = 1.01[Cu] + 0.18; r = 0.927; p>0.05).

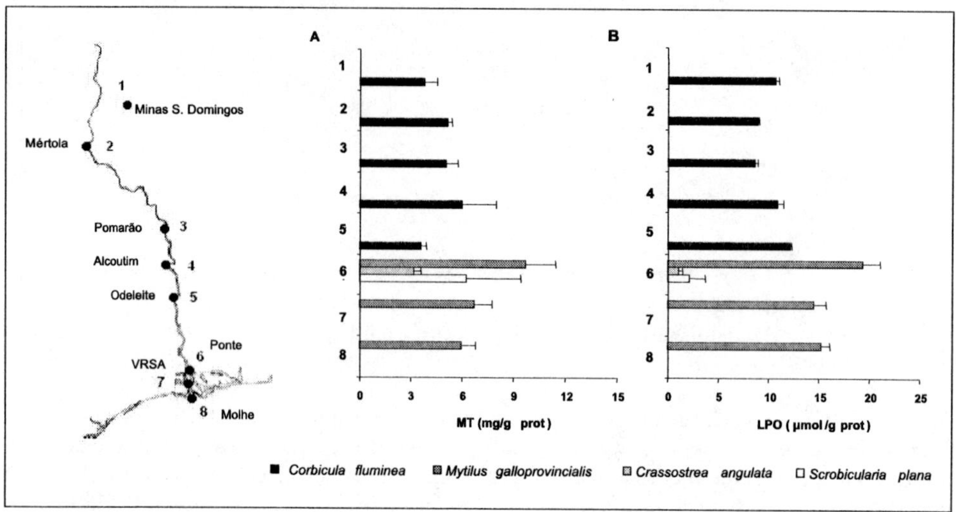

Fig. 3. Levels of biomarkers in four bivalve species from Guadiana River: (A) MT (mg g^{-1} total protein) and (B) LPO (µmol g^{-1} total protein).

DISCUSSION AND CONCLUSIONS

Although Guadiana River is one of the most strategic and economically important rivers in South Portugal and Spain, very little is know about metal inputs to this aquatic system and also their impact in the local fauna. Probably one of the most important sources of metals in the Guadiana River comes from the extensive mining activity in the Iberian Pyritic Belt. Therefore, it is likely that some influence from these old mining areas still occurs and could contribute for the entrance of metals in the upper Guadiana River, mainly for non-essential metals, which can be observed in the relatively higher levels of Cd and Pb found in the freshwater clam *C. fluminea (fig. 1)*, however not particularly high in magnitude. This bivalve, a recently introduced species in Portugal, has been widely used as a bioindicator organism in freshwater and estuarine systems to assess metal pollution [12]. Surprisingly, no significant relationship between MT levels and Cd concentrations was found for this species *(fig. 3)*. Although other authors report the evidence of MT induction in *C. fluminea* under laboratory controlled Cd exposures [13], the present work suggests that, even though more studies are required, MT may not be the most proper biomarker for Cd contamination in the clam *C. fluminea* collected in this aquatic system. Moreover, although sediments along Guadiana River were not analysed, this compartment may contribute for some of the differences in metal concentrations, especially for Pb, found between species living buried in sediments *(C. fluminea* and *S. plana)* and filter-feeding species *(M. galloprovincialis* and *C. angulata)*. Sediments in rivers and estuaries often function as sinks for many pollutant compounds, including metals and frequently exhibit higher metal concentrations compared to what is found in the water column. However, *M. galloprovincialis* a filter-feeding bivalve living in the rocks in lower Guadiana estuary had significantly higher Cd concentrations compared to both *C. fluminea* and *S. plana (fig. 1)*, and is probably related to the vicinity of two densely populated cities (Vila Real de Santo António and Ayamonte) at the river mouth, as well as runoff from the international bridge with intense traffic. The increase of Cd levels in *M. galloprovincialis* is coincident with the decrease of Zn concentrations in this mussel, suggesting a competition between these two metals. Morevoer, metallothionein levels in *M. galloprovincialis* were positively correlated to Cd concentrations, suggesting that this metal binding protein is a good biomarker for Cd contamination in this species, as reported in earlier studies in the same mussel [14]. On the other hand, metals have also been implicated in lipid peroxidation in bivalves by increasing the production of reactive oxygen species, like hydroxyl radicals, superoxide radicals and hydrogen peroxide inside the cells [15]. Although this effect/damage biomarker is not specific for metals, as it can be significantly enhanced by other toxic compounds, it has been used to assess the toxicity of metals in many bivalve species. In the present work, LPO levels increased significantly with the increase of Cu concentrations only in the tissues of *C. fluminea* collected in the upper estuary sites. Although this species seems to regulate Cu levels in their tissues, small changes in Cu concentrations are proportional to lipid damages. In fact, Cu is considered a redox-active metal and is a well-known catalyst of hydroxyl radical production, one of the most powerful inductors of LPO in biological systems. Therefore, this biomarker seems a promising tool to monitor the physiological status of the freshwater clam *C. fluminea* exposed to Cu in the field.

The final conclusions of this preliminary work can be summarized as follows:

• Metal concentrations and levels of biomarkers seem to be species dependent, suggesting different metal susceptibility and accumulation patterns.

• Long time abandoned mines can even nowadays contribute as a source of non-essential metals like Cd and Pb in the upper streams of Guadiana.

• In the lower estuary of Guadiana, the inputs of metals are likely to arise from densely populated urban discharges and probably water contamination from the international bridge traffic.

• Sediments along the Guadiana River and Estuary should be analysed for metal content, as they can be the source of metal contamination for some bivalve species that live in the upper layers of the sediment.

• Metallothioneins seems to be a good bioindicator of Cd contamination in the mussels *M. galloprovincialis* but not in the freshwater clam *C. fluminea*.

• Lipid peroxidation seems to respond to Cu levels in the clam *C. fluminea* and its potential as a future biomarker in this species should be further investigated.

REFERENCES

1. Domingues R.B, Barbosa A, Galvão H. Nutrients, light and phytoplankton succession in a temperate estuary (the Guadiana, south-western Iberia). *Estuarine, Coastal and Shelf Science*, 2005; 64 (2-3): 249-260.
2. Rocha JS, Ferreira JP. A erosão hídrica na bacia do Rio Guadiana e o assoreamento da albufeira de Alqueva. Laboratório Nacional de Engenharia Civil, Lisboa, 1980; pp. 19 (in Portuguese).
3. Morales JA. Evolution and facies architecture of the mesotidal Guadiana River delta (S.W. Spain-Portugal). *Mar Geol*, 1997; 138: 127-148.
4. Chícharo MA, Chícharo LM, Galvão H, Barbosa A, Marques MH, Andrade JP, Esteves E, Miguel C, Gouveia I. Status of the Guadiana Estuary (south Portugal) during 1996-1998: an ecohydrological approach. *Aquatic Ecosystem Health and Management*, 2001; 4: 73-89.
5. Barriga FJAS. Metallogenesis in the Iberian pyrite belt, in Dallmeyer, R.D.; Martinez Garcia, eds., Pre-Mesozoic geology of Iberia. Berlim: Springer-Verlag, 1990, p. 369-379.
6. Sáez R, Pascual F, Toscano M, Almodóvar JR. The Iberian type of volcano-sedimentary massive sulfide deposits. *Mineralium Deposita*, 1999; 34: 549-570.
7. Hernandez-Hernadez F, Medina J, Ansuategui J, Conesa M. Heavy metal concentrations in some marine organisms from the Mediterranean sea (Castellon, Spain): metal accumulation in different tissues. *Scientia Marina*, 1990; 54(2): 113-129.

8. Mason AZ, Jenkins KD. Metal detoxication in aquatic organisms. In: Tessier A, Turner DR (eds.), Metal speciation and bioavailability in aquatic systems, Vol 3. Wiley & Sons, Chichester, 1995, pp. 469-608.
9. Bebianno MJ, Langston WJ. Quantification of metallothioneins in marine invertebrates using differential pulse polarography. *Portugaliae Electrochimica Acta*, 1989; 7: 59-64.
10. Erdelmeier I, Gerard-Monnier D, Yadan JC, Acudiere J. Reactions of N-methyl-2-phenylindole with malondialdehyde and 4-hydroxyalkenals. Mechanistic aspects of the colorimetric assay of lipid peroxidation. *Chem Res Toxicol* 1998; 11: 1184-1194.
11. Lowry OH, Rosenbrough NJ, Farr AL, Randall RJ. Protein measurement with the Folin phenol reagent. *J Biol Chem* 1951; 193: 265-275.
12. Inza B, Ribeyre F, Boudou A. Dynamics of cadmium and mercury compounds (inorganic mercury or methylmercury): uptake and depuration in *Corbicula fluminea.* Effects of temperature and pH. *Aquat Toxicol*, 1998; 43(4): 273-285.
13. Legeay A, Achard-Joris M, Baudrimont M, Massabuau JC, Bourdineaud JP. Impact of cadmium contamination and oxygenation levels on biochemical responses in the Asiatic clam *Corbicula fluminea. Aquat Toxicol*, 2005; 74(3): 242-253.
14. Serafim MA, Company RM, Bebianno MJ, Langston WJ. Effect of temperature and size on metallothionein synthesis in the gill of *Mytilus galloprovincialis* exposed to cadmium. *Mar Environ Res* 2002; 54: 361-365.
15. Géret F, Jouan A, Turpin V, Bebianno MJ, Cosson R.P. Influence of metal exposure on metallothionein synthesis and lipid peroxidation in two bivalve mollusks: the oyster *(Crassostrea gigas)* and the mussel *(Mytilus edulis). Aquat Living Resour*, 2002; 15(1): 61-66.

ACKNOWLEDGEMENTS

This study was supported by the Project INTERREG-UTPIA and the Centre for Marine and Environmental Research of the University of Algarve (CIMA).

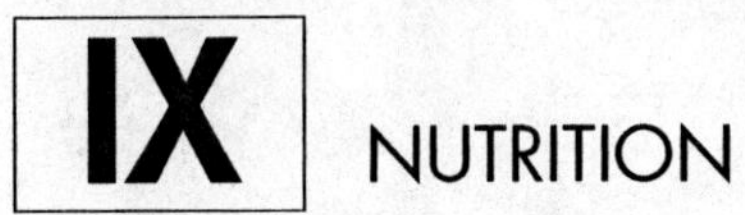

IX NUTRITION

Metal Ions in Biology and Medicine: vol. 9. Eds Maria Carmen Alpoim, Paula Vasconcellos Morais, Maria Amélia Santos, Armando J. Cristóvão, José A. Centeno, Philippe Collery.
John Libbey Eurotext, Paris © 2006 pp. 465-1.

Heavy metals contents in some food from Romania

Carmen Hura, B.A. Hura

Institute of Public Health, Iassy, Street V. Babes nr. 14, Romania.
chura@iasi.mednet.ro

ABSTRACT

Heavy metals toxicity is the result of their interactions with the enzymatic systems from the animal cells or some constituents of cells membranes. The interactions of heavy metals with usual elements from diet (Pb, Cd) have an important role in acute and chronic toxicity. Population can be contaminated with heavy metals by ingestion of contaminated or polluted food or water. The concentration of heavy metals in food products is varied, depending on their origin, storage conditions and progressing technologies.

The study presents the results obtained in 2005 year of some metals (Pb, Cd) in the food (meat, milk, vegetables, juice, diets), in Romania area. Trace elements concentrations were analyzed by atomic absorption spectrophotometer, using a Carl Zeiss Jena, Model AAS-1N, with flame air-acetylene.

In all analyzed samples these metals were found. Generally, a wide variation between individual samples was observed.

INTRODUCTION

Exposure to heavy metals is an important problem of environmental toxicology. Most of these metals are toxic to humans, animals and plants. From the sanitary point of view the presence of all alien substances in food products raises many problems because, with few exceptions, these substances have a certain level of toxicity [1, 2, 3, 4].

The levels of the concentrations of these compounds in food are regulated by the sanitary legislation of each country. For Romania, these levels are indicated in the Health Ministry order 141/2004, in conformity with European Directive. During 1999 we continued the determination of the content of metals in some food products: vegetables, meat and dairy products, fish, meals [5, 6, 7, 8, 9, 10]. The food products were harvested from Romania area. The aim of this study was the evaluation of the heavy metals contents in the food of Romania.

MATERIAL AND METHOD

The study presents the results obtained in 2005 year of some metals [Pb, Cd] in the 1869 samples in which: 750 vegetables samples, 469 meat samples, 283 cereals samples, 162 juice samples and 205 diets samples, from Romania area. Trace elements concentrations were analyzed by atomic absorption spectrophotometer, using a Carl Zeiss Jena, Model AAS-1N, with flame air-acetylene.

RESULTS

In all analyzed samples these metals were found. Generally, a wide variation between individual samples was observed *(fig. 1)*.

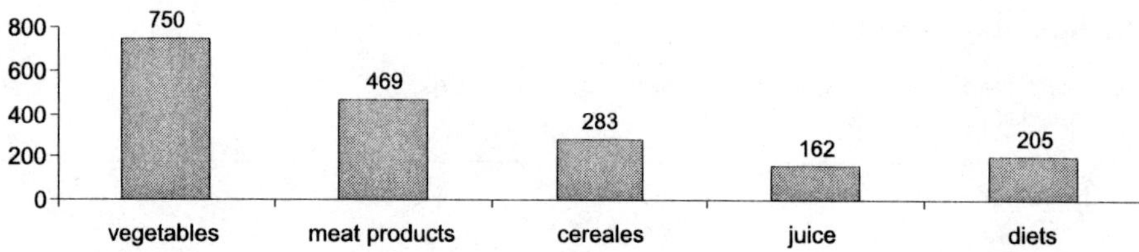

Fig. 1. The distribution of the food samples for the heavy metals, on products category, in Romania, 2005.

1. Vegetables: *Table 1* and *table 2* presents the mean levels of metals from vegetables in Romania (750 samples) from Ardeal, Banat, Moldova, Muntenia districts. The mean levels of Pb in the vegetables samples analyzed were 0.06 mg/kg lead and varied between 0.03 mg/kg (Moldova district) and 0.09 mg/kg (Muntenia district). The mean levels of Cd in the vegetables samples analyzed were 0.02 mg/kg cadmium and varied between 0.01 mg/kg (Banat district) and 0.03 mg/kg (Ardeal district).

Table 1. The mean levels of metals in vegetables from Romania, on districts (mg/kg)

District	**Pb**					**Cd**				
	Samples analyzed	**Samples inadequate**		**Mean**	**min/max**	**Samples analyzed**	**Samples inadequate**		**Mean**	**min/max**
		Nr.	**%**				Nr.	%		
Ardeal	197	15	7.6	0.07	nd - 1.42	**197**	4	2.0	0.03	nd -1.02
Banat	50	2	4	0.06	nd - 0.8	**50**	-	-	0.01	nd - 0.11
Moldova	220	1	0.5	0.03	nd - 0.53	**220**	8	3.6	0.02	nd - 0.3
Muntenia	283	11	3.9	0.09	Nd - 0.53	**228**	6	2.6	0.02	nd - 0.315
Romania	**750**	**29**	**3.9**	**0.06**	**nd - 1.42**	**695**	**18**	**2.6**	**0.02**	**nd - 1.02**

Table 2. The mean levels of metals in vegetables from Romania, on products (mg/kg)

Vegetables	**Pb**					**Cd**				
	Samples analyzed	**Samples inadequate**		**Mean**	**Min/ max**	**Samples analyzed**	**Samples inadequate**		**Mean**	**Min/ max**
		Nr.	**%**				Nr.	%		
Lettuce	190	11	5.8	0.08	nd - 1.42	**174**	2	1.1	0.02	nd - 1.02
Spinach	174	8	4.6	0.06	nd - 0.97	**160**	1	0.6	0.02	nd - 0.3
Potatoes	113	3	2.7	0.06	nd - 0.46	**108**	5	4.6	0.03	nd - 0.35
Carrot	114	4	3.5	0.07	nd - 0.8	**109**	-	-	0.02	nd - 0.11
Apples	159	3	1.9	0.06	nd - 1.21	**144**	10	6.9	0.02	nd - 0.6
Total	**750**	**29**	**3.9**	**0.06**	**nd - 1.42**	**695**	**18**	**2.6**	**0.02**	**nd - 1.02**

Fig. 2 and *fig. 3* present the mean contents of heavy metals (Pb, Cd) from some vegetables consumed in Romania area. The mean levels of Pb in the vegetables samples analyzed were 0.06 mg/kg lead and varied between 0.06 mg/kg (spinach, potatoes, and apples) and 0.08 mg/kg (lettuce). The mean levels of Cd in the vegetables samples analyzed were 0.02 mg/kg cadmium and varied between 0.02 mg/kg (spinach, lettuce, carrot, apples) and 0.03 mg/kg (potatoes).

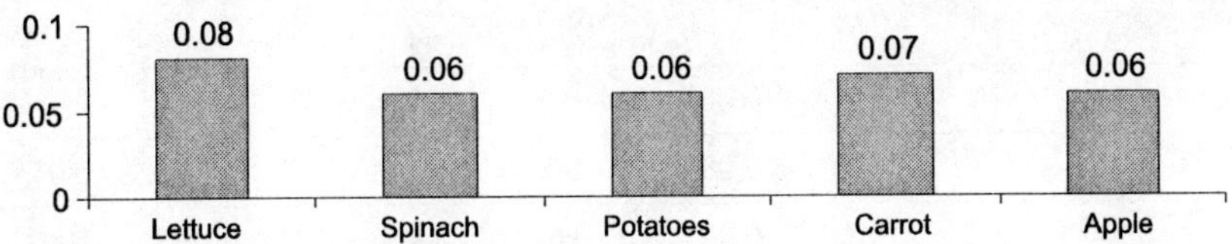

Fig. 2. The mean levels of lead from **vegetables** in Romania, mg/kg.

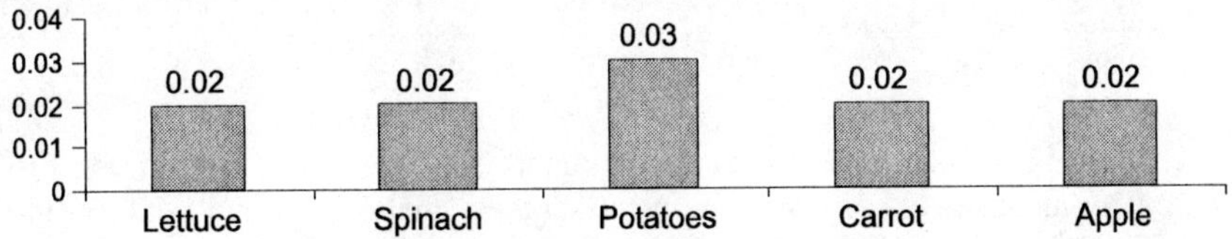

Fig. 3. The mean levels of cadmium from **vegetables** in Romania, mg/kg.

2. Meat: *Table 3* and *table 4* presents the mean levels of metals (Pb, Cd) from meat products in Romania. The mean levels of Pb and Cd in the meat samples analyzed were 0.08 mg/kg lead respectively 0.07 mg/kg cadmium. The mean levels of Pb in the meat samples analyzed were 0.08 mg/kg lead and varied between 0.05 mg/kg (Moldova district) and 0.10 mg/kg (Banat and Muntenia districts). The mean levels of Cd in the meat samples analyzed were 0.07 mg/kg cadmium and varied between 0.03 mg/kg (Ardeal district) and 0.10 mg/kg (Banat district).

Table 3. The mean levels of metals in meat products/districts, from Romania, 2005 (mg/kg)

District	Pb					Cd				
	Samples analyzed	Samples inadequate		Mean	min/max	Samples analyzed	Samples inadequate		Mean	min/max
		Nr.	%				Nr.	%		
Ardeal	126	11	8.7	0.06	nd - 0.62	**128**	4	3.1	0.03	nd - 0.6
Banat	49	-	-	0.1	0.01 - 0.5	**54**	-	-	0.1	nd - 1.0
Moldova	181	1	0.6	0.05	nd - 0.55	**181**	-	-	0.07	nd - 1.0
Muntenia	113	7	6.2	0.1	nd - 0.6	**95**	5	5.3	0.06	nd - 0.95
Total	**469**	**19**	**4.1**	**0.08**	**nd - 0.62**	**458**	**9**	**2.0**	**0.07**	**nd - 1.0**

Table 4. The mean levels of metals in meat products, from Romania, 2005 (mg/kg)

Meat products	Pb					Cd				
	Samples analyzed	Samples inadequate		Mean	Min/ max	Samples analyzed	Samples inadequate		Mean	Min/ max
		Nr.	%				Nr.	%		
Beef	87	3	3.7	0.06	nd - 0.5	**86**	1	1.2	0.01	nd - 0.11
Pork	85	3	3.5	0.08	nd - 0.6	**83**	4	4.8	0.01	nd - 0.32
Chicken	79	12	15.2	0.09	nd - 0.62	**74**	2	2.7	0.008	nd - 0.32
Liver	116	1	0.9	0.08	nd - 0.55	**112**	-	-	0.04	nd - 0.9
Kidney	102	-	-	0.1	nd - 0.6	**103**	2	1.9	0.3	nd - 1.0
Total	**469**	**19**	**4.1**	**0.08**	**nd - 0.62**	**458**	**9**	**2.0**	**0.07**	**nd - 1.0**

Fig. 4 and *fig. 5* presents the mean levels of metals (Pb, Cd) from some meat products in Romania area. The mean levels of Pb in the meat samples analyzed varied between 0.06 mg/kg (beef) and 0.10 mg/kg (kidney). The mean levels of Cd in the meat samples analyzed varied between 0.008 mg/kg (chicken meat) and 0.3 mg/kg (kidney).

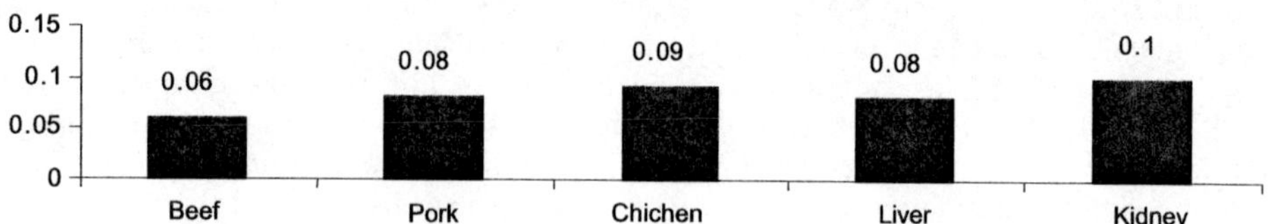

Fig. 4. The mean levels of Lead in meat products from Romania, 2005 (mg/kg).

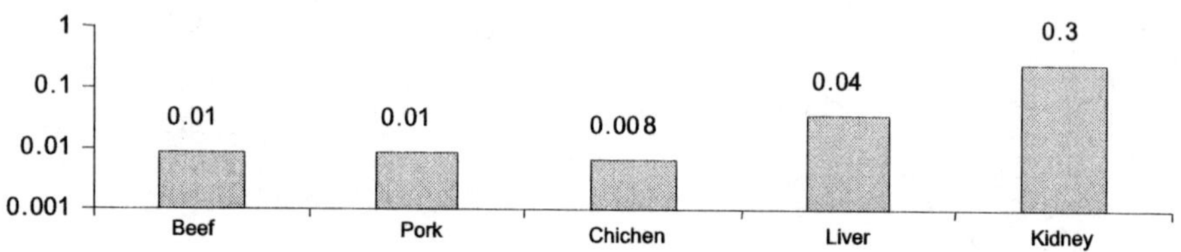

Fig. 5. The mean levels of Cadmium in meat products from Romania, 2005 (mg/kg).

3. Cereals: *Table 5* presents the mean levels of metals from cereals products (283 samples) from Romania area. The mean levels of Pb and Cd in the cereals products samples analyzed were 0.06 mg/kg lead respectively 0.02 mg/kg cadmium.

Table 5. The mean levels of metals in cereals products from Romania, 2005 (mg/kg)

Cereals products	Pb					Cd				
	Samples analyzed	Sample inadequate		Mean	min/max	Samples analyzed	Samples inadequate		Mean	min/max
		Nr.	%				Nr.	%		
Wheaten flour	181	11	6.1	0.06	nd - 0.8	**184**	1	0.5	0.02	nd - 0.4
Maize	102	2	2.0	0.06	nd - 0.42	**102**	-	-	0.01	nd - 0.2
Total	**283**	**13**	**4.6**	**0.06**	**nd - 0.8**	**286**	**1**	**0.3**	**0.02**	**nd - 0.4**

4. Juice: *Table 6* presents the mean levels of metals from juice products (162 samples) from Romania area. The mean levels of Pb and Cd in the juice products samples analyzed were 0.03 mg/kg lead respectively 0.01 mg/kg cadmium.

Table 6. The mean levels of metals in juice products from Romania, 2005 (g/kg)

Juice	Pb					Cd				
	Samples analyzed	Samples inadequate		Mean	min/ max	Samples analyzed	Samples inadequate		Mean	min/ max
		Nr.	%				Nr.	%		
Natural Juice	115	8	7.0	0.5	nd - 9.7	**116**	-	-	0.02	nd - 0.3
Nectar	47	2	4.3	0.04	nd - 0.5	**36**	-	-	0.0005	nd - 0.01
Total	**162**	**10**	**6.2**	**0.3**	**nd - 9.7**	**152**	**-**	**-**	**0.01**	**nd - 0.3**

5. Diets: *Table 7* presents the mean levels of metals from daily diets from Romania (205 samples) from Ardeal, Banat, Moldova, Muntenia districts.

The mean levels of Pb and Cd in the daily diets samples analyzed were 0.5 mg/kg lead respectively 0.01 mg/kg cadmium.

Table 7. The mean levels of metals in daily diets from Romania, 2005 (mg/kg)

District	Pb					Cd				
	Samples analyzed	Samples inadequate		Mean	min/ max	Samples analyzed	Samples inadequate		Mean	min/max
		Nr.	%				Nr.	%		
Ardeal	40	-	-	0.04	nd - 0.31	**40**	-	-	0.007	nd - 0.037
Banat	40	-	-	0.1	0.029-0.3	**40**	-	-	0.03	nd - 0.15
Moldova	60	-	-	0.01	nd - 0.14	**60**	-	-	0.01	nd - 0.06
Muntenia	65	-	-	0.2	nd - 0.92	**65**	-	-	0.01	nd - 0.1
Total	**205**	**-**	**-**	**0.5**	**nd - 0.92**	**205**	**-**	**-**	**0.01**	**nd - 0.15**

CONCLUSION

• The presence of metals in all samples of food products analyzed, some in concentrations which exceeded the maximum allowed limits (MAC) requires the continuation of the determination of these metals in food products In all area of the country for the supervision and monitoring of the chemical pollution and also for to protect the general population's state of health as it is daily exposed to a high number of pollutants in the environment.

• Determinations of these chemical contaminants in food are important in environmental monitoring for the prevention, control and reduction of pollution as well as for occupational health and epidemiological studies.

REFERENCES

1. Dudka, S., and Adriano, D. C. 1997. "Environmental impacts of metal ore mining and processsing: A review" *J. Environ. Quality* 26 (3), 590-602.
2. "Methodology for exposure assessment of contaminants and toxins in food" World Health Organization Food Safety Programme.
3. Report "consultations and Workshops: GEMS/Food Total Diet Studies" WHO/SDE/FOS/ 99.9.
4. Trace Elements in Human Health World Health Organization, Geneva, 19965.
5. Hura C. - *Chemical contaminants in food and human body (in English)*, Publishing House "CERMI", Iasi, 2002, 138 p. (ISBN 973 - 8188-01-6).
6. Hura C. - *Contaminarea chimica a alimentelor în România, 2001, volumul 1*, Publishing House "CERMI", Iasi, 2002, 323 p. (ISBN 973 - 8188 -19 - 9).
7. Hura C. - *Contaminarea chimica a alimentelor în România, 2002, volumul 2*, Publishing House "CERMI", Iasi, 2003, 267 p. (ISBN 973 - 8188 - 90 - 3).
8. Hura C. - *Contaminarea chimica a alimentelor în România, 2003, volumul 3*, Publishing House "CERMI", Iasi, 2004, 235 p. (ISBN 973 - 667 - 079 - 1).
9. Hura C. - *Contaminarea chimica a alimentelor în România, 2004, volumul 4*, Publishing House "CERMI", Iasi, 2005, 164 p. (ISBN 973 - 667 - 142 - 9).
10. Hura C. - *Contaminarea chimica a alimentelor în România, 2005, volumul 5*, Publishing House "CERMI", Iasi, 2006, in press.

Metal Ions in Biology and Medicine: vol. 9. Eds Maria Carmen Alpoim, Paula Vasconcellos Morais, Maria Amélia Santos, Armando J. Cristóvão, José A. Centeno, Philippe Collery.
John Libbey Eurotext, Paris © 2006 pp. 471-1.

Daily food rations used in the soldiers nutrition as a source of calcium

Klos Anna, Bertrandt Jerzy, Stezycka Elzbieta

Military Institute of Hygiene and Epidemiology, 4 Kozielska St., 01-163 Warsaw, Poland

INTRODUCTION

Calcium plays crucial role in building and keeping proper hardness of the bones and teeth. Together with phosphorus and magnesium calcium undergoes crystallization and is a part of osseous tissue causing its hardness. Therefore calcium is really the most important mineral salt of the skeleton [1]. Human organism is able to keep the calcium level in the blood on the specific level even if its amount delivered with food is variable or when organism demands increase. Calcium content in the blood plasma is controlled by:

- increase of reabsorption through kidneys
- decrease of excretion through kidneys
- reserves in bones mobilization

These processes are regulated by vitamin D, parathormone and calcitonin [2].

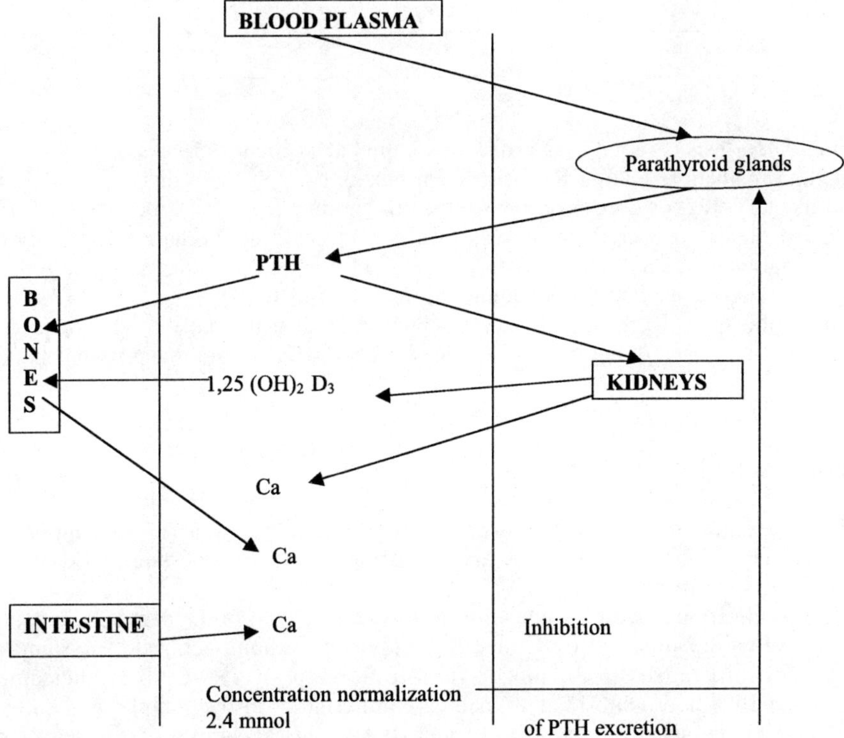

Fig. 1. Regulation of calcium concentration in blood plasma by parathormone (PTH).

Calcium supply with food has the biggest influence on calcium content in the human organism. The fundamental calcium source in average European and American diets is milk and dairy products. It is estimated that these products deliver about 80% of this element. Plants of the cabbage family and leguminous plants are underestimated, but mentioned in the literature, sources of calcium. Although comparing to the dairy products calcium content is relatively low but its bioavailability is by approx. 10% higher. Good source of calcium are sea fish, especially eaten together with skeleton, nuts or almonds [3]. Calcium absorption degree depends mainly on organism needs and bioassimilability depends on the diet components, sex or physiological status.

Table 1. Influence of nutritional elements on calcium absorption, excretion and balance [4].

Nutritive elements	**Absorption**	**Excretion**	**Balance**
Lactose	↑	→	+
Vitamin D	↑	→ ↑	+
Potassium and (or) carbohydrates	→	↓	+
Proteins	→ ↓	↑	-
Cellulose	↓	→	-
Fats	↓	→	-
Coffee	→	↑	-
Alcohol	↓	↑	-

Calcium homeostasis is kept during positive calcium balance in the organism. Negative calcium balance in the organism is caused by insufficient calcium supply with diet, reduced absorption from the alimentary tract or excessive loss with stool and urine.

Quantitative dietary indiscretions such as over-consumption or shortage of not only calcium but other mineral elements as well may cause reduction of health potential and may influence on different kind of diet-depending degeneration chronic diseases [5, 6].

The aim of the work was estimation of calcium content in the daily food rations given for consumption to young men doing military service in the Air Cavalry unit and to male students of MUT in Warsaw.

MATERIAL AND METHODS

Material for examinations consisted of 260 daily food rations given for consumption to men doing military service in the land forces and 39 rations given for consumption to students of Military University of Technology.

The daily food rations given for consumption were collected in the canteens in accordance to the norms obligatory in army [6]. Collected samples were homogenized. The sample weighing 5g was dry mineralized in the muffle furnace in temp. of 450° C. Then the sample was dissolved in the 10% hydrochloric acid. The calcium content in the sample was indicated by the atomic-absorptive spectrometry using the Pye Unicam apparatus of the wavelength of 422,7 nm [7].

RESULTS AND DISCUSSION

It was found that average calcium content in the daily food rations given for consumption in the land forces was 1246.3±162.4 mg. Higher content was found in the rations given to students (1364.9±139.4 mg).

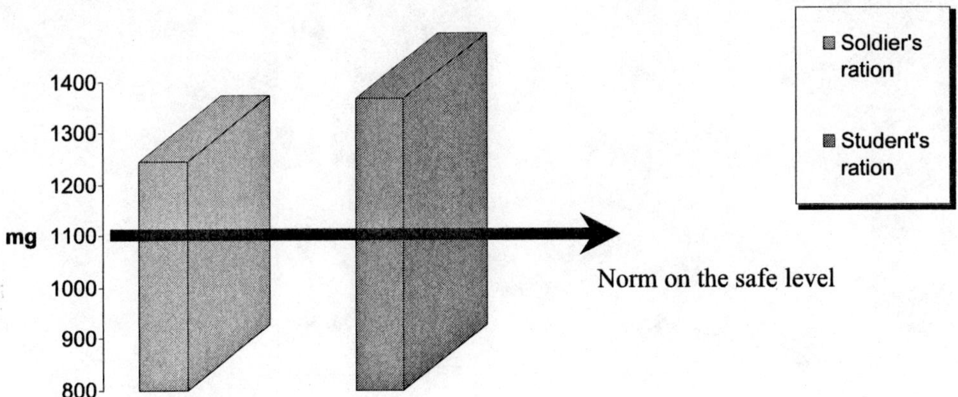

Fig. 2. Calcium content in the food rations given for consumption (mg).

Calcium content in the rations given for consumption met the requirements obligatory in Poland on the safe level [8]. Calcium content in the examined rations used in nutrition of soldiers from the land forces in particular months ranged from 919,9 mg in January to 1429,0 mg in August. Despite the average calcium content was included in the norm and even exceeded it, in the winter months it did not reach the required level *(fig. 3)*.

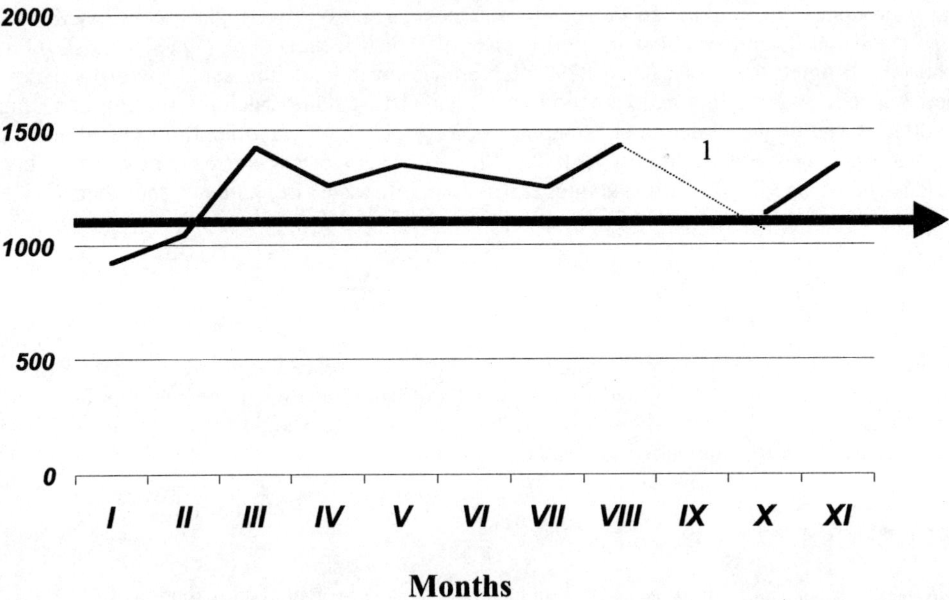

Fig. 3. Calcium content in the daily food rations given for consumption to land forces soldiers in particular months.

Calcium content in the daily food rations given for consumption to MUT students ranged from 1096.9 mg in February to 1595.4 mg in October.

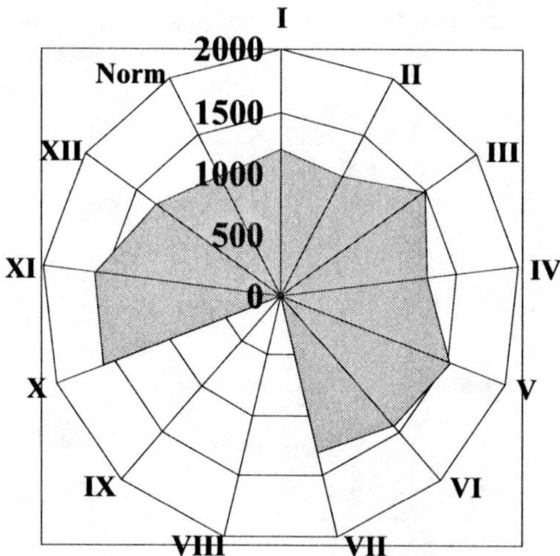

Fig. 4. Calcium content in the daily food rations given for consumption to students in particular months in mg.

Examinations of students from Academy of Physical Education in Kraków carried out in 2000-2002 revealed that average calcium content in the rations was 709 mg. This value was diverging from the recommended norm what with excessive phosphorus supply (1703 mg) caused unprofitable Ca:P ratio [9]. Low calcium content (621±254 mg) was found in the food rations served to students of Medical Academy in Bialystok, what might have been caused by low consumption of milk and dairy products [10]. Schlegel-Zawadzka & co found low calcium supply (522 mg) in the diets of Polish men [11]. The EPOLOS researches [12] showed significant decrease of dairy products consumption in Poland. Researches carried out by Rogalsk-Niedzwiedz & co. [13] showed that calcium content in food rations of Polish teenagers amounted to 502-760 mg, and norm fulfillment did not exceed 82%. Researches on the calcium supply with food rations carried out as a part of international program revealed that daily calcium consumption ranged 800-900 mg. The highest calcium consumption of 1100-1200 mg was found in Finland and Denmark and the lowest (609-680 mg) in Italy [14, 15]. Average calcium content in the diets of American males, aged 20-29, was 990 mg. It was found that 20% of examined indicated very low calcium level <50% RDA, and 14,7% very high one >150% RDA [16].

CONCLUSIONS

1. High average calcium content in the daily food rations served to young men doing military service or to student have been found what is beneficial from nutritional and health point of view.
2. Differences in calcium supply found in particular months should be leveled to include the supply in the norms recommended in Poland.

REFERENCES

1. Agebro P., Andersen H. F. W świecie witamin i minerałów. AMM Warszawa 1997, 93-96.
2. Brzozowska W. Składniki mineralne. w Gawęcki J., Hryniewiecki L. Żywienie człowieka. Podstawy nauki o żywieniu. PWN Warszawa 2000, 207-211.

3. Ziemlański Ś. Podstawy prawidłowego żywienia człowieka. PWN Warszawa 1998, 43-44.
4. Ziemlański Ś. Normy żywienia człowieka. Fizjologiczne podstawy. PZWL Warszawa, 2000, 314-336.
5. WHO. Diet, nutrition and the prevention of chronic diseases. Raport of a WHO Study Group. Technical Report. Series 797, WHO Geneva 1990.
6. Lorenc R.S., Kaczmarkiewicz E. Znaczenie prawidłowego zaopatrzenia w wapń dla ogólnego zdrowia organizmu. Medycyna 2000, 29, 14-19.
7. Ostrowska A., Gawliński S., Szczubiałka Z. Metody analizy i oceny właściwości gleb i roślin. Inst. Ochr. Środ. Warszawa, 1991.
8. Ziemlański Ś. Normy żywienia dla ludności w Polsce. Nowa Medycyna 1995, 5, 20-22.
9. Gacek M. The content of basic nutritive components in daily alimentary rations of Physical Academy students in Cracow. Żyw. Człow. Metab. 202, 29, 170-173.
10. Czapska D., Ostrowska L., Karczewski J. Zawartośc wybranych biopierwiastków w całodziennej racji pokarmowej studentów Akademii Medycznej w Białymstoku. Roczn. PZH. 2000, 4, 353-359.
11. Schlegel-Zawadzka M., Przysławski J., Bertrandt J., Kłos A. The intake of Ca and Mg in the Polish habitual diet and their relation to socio-economic factors. Metal Ions in Biology and Medicine, 2002, 7, 476-479.
12. Skorupa E., Wyszomirski T., Karczmarewicz E. i wsp. Wpływ spożycia wapnia na parametry metabolicznego obrotu kostnego w populacji polskiej. SAS Forum, Warszawa 2003.
13. Rogalska-Niedźwiedź M., Charzewska J., Chwojnowska Z. Zawartość wapnia w dietach młodzieży. Żyw. Człow. Metab. 1992, 19, 244-252.
14. Szajkowski Z. Badania nad zawartością i wzajemnymi relacjami wybranych składników mineralnych w całodziennych racjach pokarmowych wytypowanych populacji z regionu Wielkopolski. Żyw. Człow. Metab. 1996, 23, 55-65.
15. Kardinaal A. F. M., Ando S., Charles P., Charzewska J. et al. Dietary calcium and bone density in adolescent girls and young women in Europe. J. Bone. Miner. Res. 1999, 14, 583-592.
16. Kersitetter J. E., O'Brien K. O., Insogna K. L. Dietary protein, calcium metabolism, and skeletal homeostasis revisited. Am. J. Clin. Nutr. 2003, 78, 848-925.

Metal Ions in Biology and Medicine: vol. 9. Eds Maria Carmen Alpoim, Paula Vasconcellos Morais, Maria Amélia Santos, Armando J. Cristóvão, José A. Centeno, Philippe Collery.
John Libbey Eurotext, Paris © 2006 pp. 476-1.

Vegetables and fruits as a source of vitamins and mineral elements in the daily food rations of different social groups collectively fed

Klos Anna, Bertrandt Jerzy

Military Institute of Hygiene and Epidemiology, 4 Kozielska St., 01-163 Warsaw, Poland

INTRODUCTION

Vegetable and fruit production and their processing are very important part of the food economy in Poland but unfortunately consumption level of these products is one of the lowest in Europe [1]. Vegetables and fruits are first of all a source of many mineral elements and antioxidants. Mineral elements contained in vegetables and fruits show predominance of cations over anions thus may play role of antacid agents. They are factors affecting the acid-base balance and moving it towards basic direction [2]. Vegetables and fruits are a source of cellulose and organic acids [2]. It should be added that vegetables and fruits are products of low energetic value [3]. Moreover these products diversify daily menus by their colors, smell and taste. Therefore it is necessary to assure presence of these products and their variety in the menus while planning daily nutrition, especially collective one [4].

Vegetables and fruits are considered as important and indispensable elements of the diet. Their importance consist in prevention of deviations in the health state and some diseases caused by improper nutrition, what results from the fact that fruits and vegetables are source of many nutritive elements and antioxidants. It is recommended to increase amount of fruits and vegetables in the daily food rations because of the health profits resulting from these products consumption. Optimal daily consumption of these products resulting from the recommendation of so-called "pyramid of proper nutrition", amounts about 300 g fruits and 500 g vegetables. As it is presented by different authors [5, 6, 7] average daily vegetable consumption in Poland is approx. 340g, and fruits 140g only. Fruits consumption in Poland was 35% in 1991 and in 2005 only 40% of amounts eaten in the EU countries [4]. It is considered that regular fruits and vegetables consumption as well as their products significantly decreases risk of occurrence of diseases caused by improper nutrition such as arteriosclerosis, cardiovascular system diseases or some types of neoplasm. For many years epidemiological researches have showed that diet rich in fresh fruits and vegetables decreases risk of become ill from alimentary tract malignant neoplasm. Increase of fresh fruits and vegetables consumption is probably one of the most important nutritional factors that affected, during the last several dozen years, significant decrease of stomach cancer cases in many countries around the world [8]. It should be underlined that bioflavonids contained in fruits and vegetables significantly affects keeping good health state [9].

The aim of the work was estimation of fruits and vegetables supply in the daily food rations planned for nutrition of young and elderly people collectively fed. Percentage of meeting the requirements for mineral elements delivered with vegetables and fruits was assessed as well.

MATERIAL AND METHODS

Total of 100 daily menus were the base for examination based on which the nutrition of young men doing military service, MUT students and elderly people, MPH inmates, was planned. Based on the menus the amount of fruits and vegetables planned for consumption was calculated as well as mineral elements delivered by these products. Percentage participation of mineral elements delivered by fruits and vegetables in the daily norm, provided for examined social groups, was assessed as well.

RESULTS AND DISCUSSION

Menus analysis allowed stating that for men doing military service amount of planned fresh or processed vegetables and fruits amounted as follows: 528.4±145.6g vegetables and 291.0±115.4g fruits. For MUT students: 560.8±102.6g vegetables and 188.2±82.4g fruits were planned daily. But for inmates of the MPH the planned amount was as follows: 409,5±128.1 g vegetables and 202.8±149.6g fruits. Planned for young men and students amounts of vegetables were in accordance to the recommended norms. Food rations planned for elderly people met only 81,9% recommended amount for vegetables.

Amounts of fruits planned in food rations were lower than recommended norm.

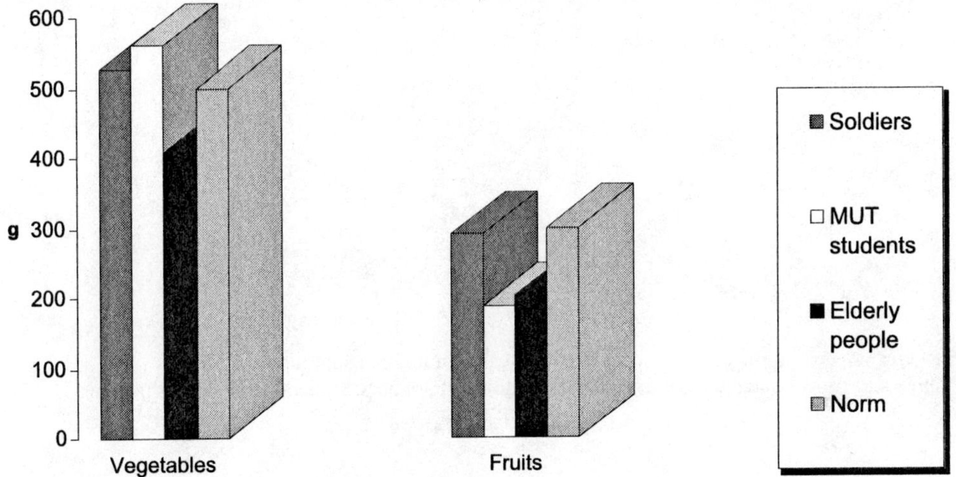

Fig. 1. Amount of vegetables and fruits planned in daily food rations.

For years vegetables consumption in Poland has indicated increasing tendency however it is still lower comparing to the countries applying Mediterranean diet [5, 10]. All-Poland researches on Poles' nutrition habits showed that women eat vegetables more often than men. It was found that elderly people ate vegetable more often than young ones. Predilection for particular kind of vegetables has been changing together with the age. M/a researches revealed that women ate fruits more willingly than men and the amount of eaten fruits increased together with age [11]. Researches carried out among students of Medical Academy in Poznan showed that 30% of examined young people ate fruits and vegetables two times daily [12, 13]. Up to 80% of examined persons participating in the poll conducted by the family doctors revealed too low consumption of these products [14]. It was found that only 7,3% of helicopter pilots doing military service in the Polish Army declared fruits and vegetables consumption more often than 3 times a day. But in menus of 51.2% of examined pilots m/a products occurred only once [15, 21].

Change of consumption model is very important in promotion of proper nutrition rules to reduce incidence of so-called non-infectious nutrition-depending diseases. One of many factors affecting creation of these diseases is incompatible with recommendations consumption of vegetables and fruits. Increased consumption of fruits and vegetables means increased delivery of mineral elements that participates in metabolism and allows organism's proper functioning. Mineral elements are contained in enzymes coordinating protein, fats and carbohydrates decomposition in human organism. Vegetables and fruits declared in the daily food rations of men doing military service met the requirements on the safe level on the highest degree for sodium (129.2%), potassium (99.2%) magnesium (59.6%), iron (55.6%) and copper (51.7-41.4%). Fruits and vegetables in students' rations met the requirements on the higher degree for sodium (65.4%), phosphorus (54.1%) and iron (55.5%). Described products in pensioners' rations met the requirements in amounts from 74.3% for sodium to 19% for calcium *(fig. 2, 3, 4)*.

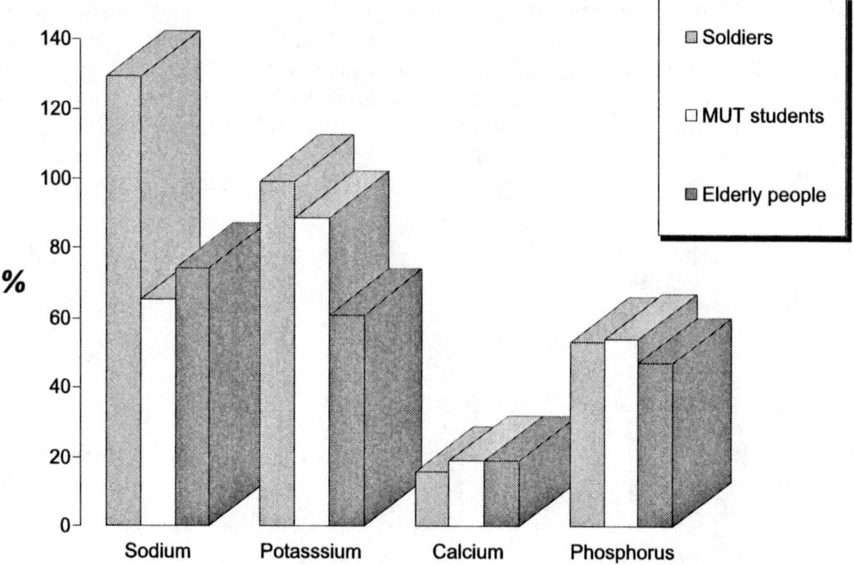

Fig. 2. Percentage of norm for sodium, potassium, calcium and phosphorus fulfillment on the safe level by vegetables and fruits contained in the daily food rations of soldiers, students and elderly people.

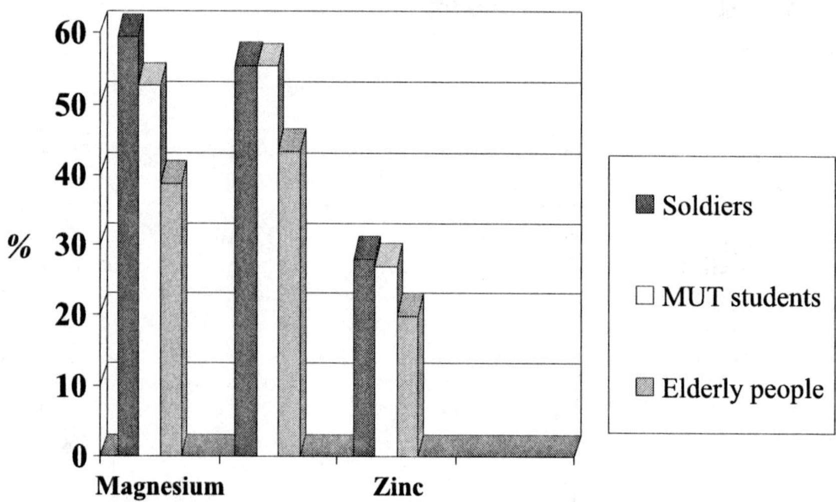

Fig. 3. Percentage of norm for magnesium, iron and zinc fulfillment on the safe level by vegetables and fruits contained in the daily food rations of soldiers, students and elderly people.

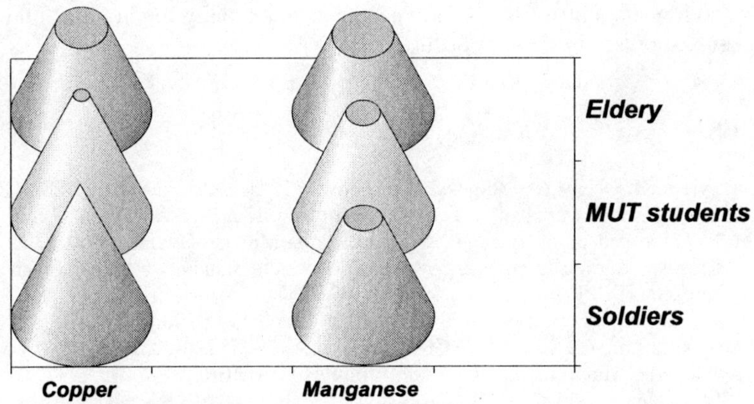

Fig. 4. Percentage of norm for copper and manganese fulfillment on the safe level by vegetables and fruits contained in the daily food rations of soldiers, students and elderly people.

Table 1. Mineral elements delivered by vegetables and fruits in the daily food rations of young men doing military service, MUT students and elderly people

Mineral elements delivered by vegetables and fruits in the daily food ration	Young men doing military service in Polish Army (mg)	Students of Military University of Technology	**Polish norm for mineral elements for young people, aged 19-25 (mg)**	Inmates of the Military Pensioner House (mg)	**Polish norm for mineral elements for elderly people (mg)**
Sodium	807.8±575.7	4089±294.3	**625**	427.5±194.2	**575**
Potassium	3472.7±1092.5	3113.1±488.4	**3500**	2145.2±664.9	**3500**
Calcium	174.4±58,6	208.3±48.7	**1100**	152.2±47.6	**800**
Phosphorus	424.8±134,2	433.3±63.9	**800**	307.1±106.4	**650**
Magnesium	208.8±55,9	184.5±29.6	**350**	135.7±43.8	**350**
Iron	6.12±1.8	6.11±1,13	**11**	4.78±1.71	**11**
Zinc	3.93±1.1	3.8±0.61	**14**	2.79±0.8	**14**
Copper	1.03±0.34	0.91±0.11	**2.0-2.5**	0.63±0.18	**2.0-2.5**
Manganese	1.94±0.5	1.95±0.27	**5**	**1.45±0.47**	**5**

Researches carried out previously among women studying in Military University of Technology showed that regardless of collective nutrition, women bought additionally 215.1±209.0g of different vegetables and fruits and only then the nutrition norms obligatory in Poland were fulfilled [20].

CONCLUSIONS

1. Planned in the daily food rations amounts of fruits and vegetables for young men and MUT students were in accordance to the Polish norms. Food rations served to the elderly people contained only 81.9% of optimal recommended amounts.

2. Planning too low amounts of fruits and vegetables in the daily food rations may be a reason of mineral elements shortage in the diet occurrence.

REFERENCES

1. Halicka E., Kowrygo B. Ocena zmian spożycia owoców w Polsce. Przem Spoż., 2002, 10, 26-28.
2. Nadolna I., Szponar L. Soki warzywne i owocowe a zdrowie. IŻŻ Warszawa, 1988, 7-29.
3. Babicz-Zielińska E. Propedeutyka żywienia. Wyższa Szkoła Morska, Gdynia, 2000, 117-131.
4. Frańczuk H., Kłos A., Karpińska H. Warzywa i owoce źródło składników mineralnych i błonnika w należności żywnościowej Z. Przegl. Kwat., 1987, 4, 74-77.
5. Kaźmierczak R. Spoÿcie warzyw i owoców w Polsce w latach 1993-2002. Wybrane problemy nauki o żywieniu człowieka u progu XXI wieku. SGGW, Warszawa 2004, 220-225.
6. Somer E. Encyklopedia witamin i składników mineralnych. AMBER Warszawa 1997.
7. Gulbicka B. Wyżywienie polskiego społeczeństwa w ostatniej dekadzie XX wieku. IERiGŻ, Warszawa, 2000.
8. Jarosz M. Żywienie a nowotwory złośliwe. Fizjologiczne uwarunkowania postępowania dietetycznego. SGGW, Warszawa cz. 1, 310-315.
9. Kunachowicz H., Nadolna I., Wojtasik A., Przygoda B. Żywność wzbogacana a zdrowie. IŻŻ, Warszawa, 2004, 113-137.
10. Halicka E. Influence of UE common intervention mechanisms on the growth of fruit and vegetables consumption in Poland. Konsument żywności i jego zachowania w warunkach polskiego członkostwa w Unii Europejskiej. SGGW, Warszawa, 2005, 223-229.
11. Sznajder M., Przywecka R. Konsument owoców i warzyw. Wybrane problemy nauki o żywieniu człowieka u progu XXI wieku. SGGW, Warszawa 2004, 376-381.
12. Maruszewska M., Przysławski J., Bolesławska I. Preferencje młodzieży akademickiej w zakresie spożycia owoców. Symp. Żywność- Lek-Zdrowie, 2000, Łódź 21-22. 09.,56-57.
13. Maruszewska M., Przysławski J., Bolesławska I. Preferencje młodzieży akademickiej w zakresie spożycia owoców. Symp. Żywność- Lek-Zdrowie, 2000, Łódź 21-22. 09.,58- 59.
14. Marcinkowski J., Palicka E., Stachowska M. Selected factors of nourishment in opinions of general practitionier's patients. Nowiny Lek. 2005, 74, 4, 434-439.
15. Rozmysł E., Bertrandt J., Kłos A., Kobos Z., Bieniek R. Assessment of military helicopter pilot nutrition taking into consideration frequency of particular food product consumption. Nowiny Lek. 2005, 74, 4, 472-476.

Metal Ions in Biology and Medicine: vol. 9. Eds Maria Carmen Alpoim, Paula Vasconcellos Morais, Maria Amélia Santos, Armando J. Cristóvão, José A. Centeno, Philippe Collery.
John Libbey Eurotext, Paris © 2006 pp. 481-1.

Metals in three species of edible insects in Mexico

Melo V., Reyes J., Castrejón E., Salas J., Nogueda N.

Metropolitan Autonomous University-Xochimilco. Calzada del Hueso 1100, Edif. Central, 1er. piso, Coyoacán, 04960, D.F. México. vmelo@correo.xoc.uam.mx

ABSTRACT

Insects have been source of nutrients for different ethnic groups all over the World since ancient times and consumption in rural communities is emerging from the past and extended at urban cities. Ant eggs, grasshoppers, grubs, larva stages of moths or butterflies, rounded off with different kind of ingredients produce local traditional dishes or exotic ones. Nutritional value of these organisms is well known regarding macronutrients but there is little information about metal ions and their role in health. It is only recently that the metal elements in food began to receive attention on human nutrition and metabolism, since metal ions regulate essential physiological mechanisms with specificity and selectivity. Three species of popular edible insects in Mexico grasshoppers sample 1) *Sphenarium purpurascens* Ch, escamoles ant eggs sample 2) *Liometopum apiculatum* M and maguey white grub larvae stage of a moth sample 3) *Aegiale hesperiaris* K were studied and mineral analysed in dry basis, macrominerals Na, K, Ca, P and microminerals Fe, Cu, Zn, I, by Atomic Absorption Spectrophotometer all of them, except iodine assessed by titration with thiosulfate and phosphorus determined colorimetrically, of a triple acid digested extract. The data obtained were: Macrominerals Na: 1) 1.98 mg/100g; 2) 1.01 mg/100g; 3) 1.15 mg/100g; K: 1) 1560 mg/100g; 2) 1450 mg/100g; 3) 1400 mg/100g; Ca: 1) 258 mg/100g; 2) 215 mg/100g; 3) 198 mg/100g; P: 1) 480 mg/100g; 2) 320 mg/100g; 3) 317 mg/100g. Microminerals Fe: 1) 4.15 mg/100g; 2) 5.56 mg/100g; 3) 8.01 mg/100g. Cu: 1) 0.49 mg/100g; 2) 0.52 mg/100g; 3) 0.55 mg/100g; Zn: 1) 1.93 mg/100g: 2) 1.99 mg/100g; 3) 1.68 mg/100g. None of the insects analysed have iodine. In conclusion the figures given on the metal content in these organisms are the total concentration of these elements, the significance of the chemical species of metals in nutrition and health must be biologically available, however, insects are a source of some minerals for population in rural communities and urban cities.

INTRODUCTION

Insects have played an important role in the history of human nutrition all over the world since ancient times [1, 2, 3].

Years back, their consumption was mainly by cultural tradition and sensory characteristics and not by the nutritional value of these organisms or biological function in the body to maintain healthy individuals. Macronutrients in insects are well known, however, in regard of minerals, there is little information, maybe because they are not consider as nutrients, although, human body contains a great variety of metals that are part of molecules to regulate, transmit and control several metabolic functions, such as: Na and K maintenance of body fluid compartments; Ca and P bone structure; Fe transports oxygen and as component of some proteins; Cu catalyzes reactions, component of enzymes; Zn component of enzymes involved in nucleic acids and protein synthesis; I essential component of thyroid hormones [4, 5, 6, 7, 8]. The consequences of lack of metals have severe results in human nutrition. The aim of this paper is to analyze the content of some metals in popular edible insects in Mexico [9, 10, 11].

MATERIALS AND METHODS

Samples of three species of insects in different metamorphosis stages; escamoles ant eggs of *Liometopum apiculatum* M, maguey grubs larva stage of *Aegiale hesperaris* K and grasshoppers adult stage of *Sphenarium purpurascens* Ch were collected and studied from a semi-desertic region with a xerophyte's thicket vegetation at 2100 meters above sea level, during first week of February 2006 near a rural community at Hidalgo State [12, 13]. Ant eggs near maguey cactus in nests under the ground; larvae grubs from moths gathered from inside maguey leaves and adult grasshoppers in the bush vegetation of the zone. Moisture content was measured by drying samples in an oven at 60° C for 24 hrs. Samples were powdered separately in a Willey Mill to 60 mesh size, organic matter destroyed by incineration at 600° C in a muffle furnace and ashes dissolved in dilute HCl. All minerals except iodine and phosphorus were analysed by Atomic Absorption Spectrophotometer. Phosphorus content in the triple acid digested extract and determined colorimetrically. Iodine: liberation of free iodine from insects' powder by addition of H_2SO_4, excess KI is added to help solubilize the free iodine, and then titrated with thiosulfate. Iodine from insects is consumed by sodium thiosulfate in the titration step [9, 10, 11].

RESULTS

Table 1. Insects *Sphenarium purpurascens* Ch, *Liometopum apiculatum* M, *Aegiale hesperiaris* K, year availability

Season	Winter			Spring			Summer			Autumm		
Months	J	F	M	A	M	J	J	A	S	O	N	D
Sphenarium purpurascens Ch	X	X	X	-	-	-	X	X	X	X	X	X
Liometopum apiculatum M	-	X	X	X	X	-	-	-	-	-	-	-
Aegiale hesperiaris K	-	X	X	X	X	X	-	-	X	X	-	-

Table 2. Nomenclature of insects sample species

Class	Insecta	Insecta	Insecta
Order	Orthoptera	Hymenoptera	Lepidoptera
Family	Acrididae	Formicidae	Megathymidae
Genus	*Sphenarium*	*Liometopum*	*Aegiale*
Specie	*purpurascens* Ch	*apiculatum* M	*hesperiaris* K
Generic name	Grasshoppers	Escamoles	Maguey white grub

Morón, M. A., Terrón, R. 1980. Ross, H. 1982 [12,13]

Table 3. Mineral composition of grasshoppers *Sphenarium purpurascens* Ch, escamoles *Liometopum apiculatum* M, and maguey white grub *Aegiale hesperiaris* K, mg/100g dry basis

Mineral	*Sphenarium purpurascens* Ch 1)	*Liometopum apiculatum* M 2)	*Aegiale hesperiaris* K 3)
Na	1.98	1.01	1.15
K	1560.00	1450.00	1400.00
Ca	258.00	215.00	198.00
P	480.00	320.00	317.00
Fe	4.15	5.56	8.01
Cu	0.49	0.52	0.55
Zn	1.93	1.99	1.68
I	-	-	-

Table 4. Dietetic requirements by RDA of Escamoles, Grasshoppers, Maguey white grub

Mineral	RDA Adult male mg/day	Insect		
		Grasshoppers	Escamoles	Maguey white grub
Na	500/3000	1.98	1.01	1.15
K	900/2700	1560.00	1450.00	1400.00
Ca	800/1000	258.00	215.00	198.00
P	700	480.00	320.00	317.00
Fe	10	4.15	5.56	8.01
Cu	1.5	0.49	0.52	0.55
Zn	12	1.93	1.99	1.68

RDA Recommended Dietary Allowance [14, 15]

DISCUSSION AND CONCLUSION

Edible insects have been the source of macronutrients minerals for population all over the world [1, 2, 3]. The organisms studied are not available throughout the year for rural communities *(table 1)*. However, consumption must of the times are prepared with other foodstuff which increase metal content [1, 3]. Restaurants in urban cities include insects through the year because they refrigerate or freeze them for consumption out of season. The data on mineral analysis reveal that the three investigated insects do not show significant difference in the content, since material samples were gathered on the same area and insects obtain minerals contained in the soil and water metabolized from plants. Nevertheless, samples captured in another region must show differences against these.

Table 3, shows, in regard to RDA recommendations, that insects for themselves do not cover the dietetic requirements but for cooking, salt is added; K is in between the rank. Ca is also very low, however, consumption is with tortilla, which is very high in Ca. Fe, Zn and Cu interact among themselves, because these elements share the same pathways and high concentration of one metal may interfere with the absorption of another *(table 4)* [14, 16]. Iodine was not present in any of these insects. Natural food is better than fortified supplements, since the last ones are not available for all individuals.

REFERENCES

1. Simmons, P.L. 2001. The Curiosities of Food. Ed. Ten Speed Press, Berkeley, CA, USA.
2. Menzel, P., D'Alusio, F. 1998. Man Eating Bugs. Ed. Ten Speed Press (Material World Books), Berkeley, CA, USA.
3. Sahagún, F.B. 1980. Códice Florentino. Archivo General de la Nación. Reproducción Facsimilar. Libro III, Mexico.
4. Hopkins, J. 1999. Strange Foods. Ed. Periplus Editions Ltd., Singapore.
5. Reyes, J.J. et al 2005. Elementos Químicos Esenciales para el Organismo. Universidad Autónoma Metropolitana, Mexico.
6. Fraústo da Silva, J.J. 2001. The biological Chemistry of the Elements. Ed. Oxford University Press, Oxford, UK.
7. Conor, R. 2004. The Nutrition Trace Elements. Blackwell Publishing Ltd., Oxford, UK.
8. Tololen, M. 1995. Vitaminas y Minerales en la Salud y la Nutrición. Ed. Acribia, S. A., España.
9. AOAC. 1995. Official Methods of Analysis. 16th Ed. Association of Official Analytical Chemists, Washington, D. C.
10. Nielsen, S.S. (editor) 1994. Introduction to the Chemical Analysis of Foods. Ed. Jones and Bartlet Publishers International, London, UK.
11. Osborne, D.R., Voogt, P. 1978. The Analysis of Nutrients in Food. Ed. Academic Press Inc., London, UK.
12. Morón, M.A., Terrón, R. 1980. Entomología Práctica. Instituto de Ecología, A. C., Mexico.
13. Ross, H. 1982. Introducción a la Entomología General y Aplicada. Ed. Omega, España.
14. Shils, M.E., Olson, J.A., Shike, M., Ross. A.C. 2002. Nutrición en Salud y Enfermedad. Ed. Mc Graw-Hill/Interamericana, Mexico.
15. Mahan, L.K., Escote-Stump, S. 2001. Nutrición y Dietoterapia de Krause. Ed. Mc Graw-Hill/Interamericana, Mexico.
16. De Mayer, E. M., Lowenstein, F.W., Thilly, C.H. 1997. The Control of Endemic Goitre. World Health Organization, Geneva, Switzerland.

Metal Ions in Biology and Medicine: vol. 9. Eds Maria Carmen Alpoim, Paula Vasconcellos Morais, Maria Amélia Santos, Armando J. Cristóvão, José A. Centeno, Philippe Collery.
John Libbey Eurotext, Paris © 2006 pp. 485-1.

Natural antioxidant vitamin and trace element intakes in healthy and asthmatic Hungarian adolescents

I. Sziklai-László[1], R. Szoke[1], I. Kovács[2], N. Adányi[3], D. Majchrzak[4], M. Á. Cser[5]

[1]*KFKI Atomic Energy Research Institute, 1525 Budapest, P.O.Box 49, Hungary, isziklai@sunserv.kfki.hu,*
[2]*Bethesda Children's Hospital, Budapest, Hungary,*
[3]*Central Food Research Institute, Budapest,*
[4]*Institute of Nutritional Sciences, University of Vienna, Austria,*
[5]*Heim Pál Children's Hospital, Budapest, Hungary*

SUMMARY

The prevalence of bronchial asthma remarkably increased in Hungary in the last decades, it reached 5-6% in childhood. The potential role of diet in respiratory diseases has been recognized and recent studies suggest that an association may exist between the low intake of dietary antioxidants, certain micronutrients and lung diseases including asthma. The aim of the study was to measure the daily intakes of some microelements and carotenoids in asthmatic adolescents compared to their healthy siblings. In addition, blood selenium (Se) and carotenoid status in both groups were also measured. 7-15 year old asthmatic children were investigated (n=25) and 29 healthy age and sex matched children served as controls. Total daily duplicate food samples were collected over eight consecutive days. At the same time blood sampling was also performed. The concentrations of the microelements in food samples were determined by instrumental neutron activation analysis (INAA). Blood selenium (Se) was measured by atomic absorption spectroscopy (AAS). Provitamin and non-provitamin-A carotenoids were determined by HPLC. Blood Se levels and the sum of serum provitamin-A carotenoids were significantly lower in asthmatics compared to healthy children. The sum of non-provitamin-A carotenoid intake was significantly higher in asthmatics ($p<0.05$) compared to the healthy group. The total non-provitamin-A carotenoids were higher in the healthy group, but asthmatics had only the half amount of that. Microelement intakes were similar in the two groups, Fe, Zn and Cr intakes reached by only 45, 49 and 75% of RDA values; however selenium intakes were significantly lower than RDA values in both groups. In spite of their higher dietary carotenoid intakes, asthmatic patients have lower blood carotenoid status than the healthy children. These results may suggest that asthma, as a disease associated with chronic inflammations requires higher antioxidant carotenoid consumption than that in healthy children. The antioxidant status in blood could indicate to the severity of the disease.

INTRODUCTION

Asthma bronchiale is a multifactorial disease with genetic, allergic, environmental, infectious and nutritional components. Oxidative processes are recognized as contributing significantly to the inflammatory pathology of bronchial asthma [1]. Selenium is an essential component of gluthathione peroxidase (GSH-Px), which protect against oxidative damage like inflammation of lung tissues [2]. It has been suggested that lowered GSH-Px activity due to a low intake of Se may play a role in asthma [3-5]. Low dietary intake of vitamin A inversely associated with airflow limitation [6]. Deficient antioxidant capacity may also play a role in the pathogenesis and outcome of asthma

[7]. The potential role of diet in respiratory diseases has been recognized and recent studies suggest that an association may exist between the low intake of dietary antioxidants, certain micronutrients and lung diseases including asthma [8, 9]. The aims of this study were firstly, to measure blood Se parameters and serum provitamin-A, non provitamin-A levels in asthmatic and healthy children. Secondly, we aimed to measure the concentrations of carotenoids and some microelements in asthma compared to healthy controls, in relation to dietary intakes.

MATERIALS AND METHODS

Carotenoid Analysis

Twenty-five, 7 to 15 years old asthmatic children with stable asthma were investigated and 29 healthy age and sex matched children served as controls. Blood samples were taken from all children in morning fasting state between 7-9 a.m. Total daily duplicate-food samples were collected over eight consecutive days. Food sampling and recording was completed by trained dietitians during a summer camp. The concentrations of serum and food β-carotene, α-carotene, β-cryptoxanthin (provitamin-A carotenoids), lycopene, lutein, and zeaxanthin (non provitamin-A carotenoids) were determined by HPLC method according to the slightly modified method of Jakob and Elmadfa [10]. All parameters were quantified by determining peak areas in the HPLC chromatograms calibrated against known amounts of external standards.

Microelement Analysis

Blood selenium concentrations (in erythrocytes, whole blood and in plasma) were determined by AAS. Intakes of microelements were studied by INAA. Samples together with flux monitors were irradiated for 48 hours at the Budapest Research Reactor. After a decay period of about 20-30 days, the samples were counted and the radionuclide ^{51}Cr, ^{59}Fe, ^{75}Se and ^{65}Zn were measured. Gamma-spectrometric measurements were performed with the aid of a PC based Canberra type spectrometer with a Canberra HPGe detector with energy resolution of 1.74 keV and efficiency of 13.6% for the 1332.5 keV ^{60}Co line. The gamma-ray spectra were evaluated by the program HY-PERMET-PC. The quantitative evaluation of the INAA multi-element measurements was based on the k_0 standardization method using gold and zirconium reference comparators co-irradiated with the samples.

Statistical analysis: SPSS for Windows was used for all statistical procedures. Results were expressed as mean value ± SD. T-test and Mann-Whitney U-test have been used for comparison of the results of healthy and asthmatic groups of children.

RESULTS AND DISCUSSION

There was no difference in the age and sex of the healthy controls compared to the asthmatics. Mean daily caloric, total protein, carbohydrate and lipid intakes were not different in the two groups. The erythrocyte, whole blood and plasma Se levels in asthmatic patients and control subjects are shown in *fig. 1*. There was little difference between these two groups in blood or plasma selenium, but erythrocyte selenium concentration was significantly lower in the asthmatic than the healthy group.

The sum of serum provitamin-A carotenoids was significantly lower in asthmatics (43 ± 42, median 27 mcg/L) compared to healthy children (194 ± 115, median 161 mcg/L). The sum of non-provitamin-A carotenoids were in the healthy group (68 ± 30, median 64 mcg/L), but asthmatics had only the half amount of that (38 ± 25, median 33 mcg/L) shown in *fig. 2*.

The total daily carotenoid intakes calculated from the duplicate food sample analysis are shown in *table 1*. There was no relationship between dietary intake and blood levels of carotenoids in the asthmatic or the control groups.

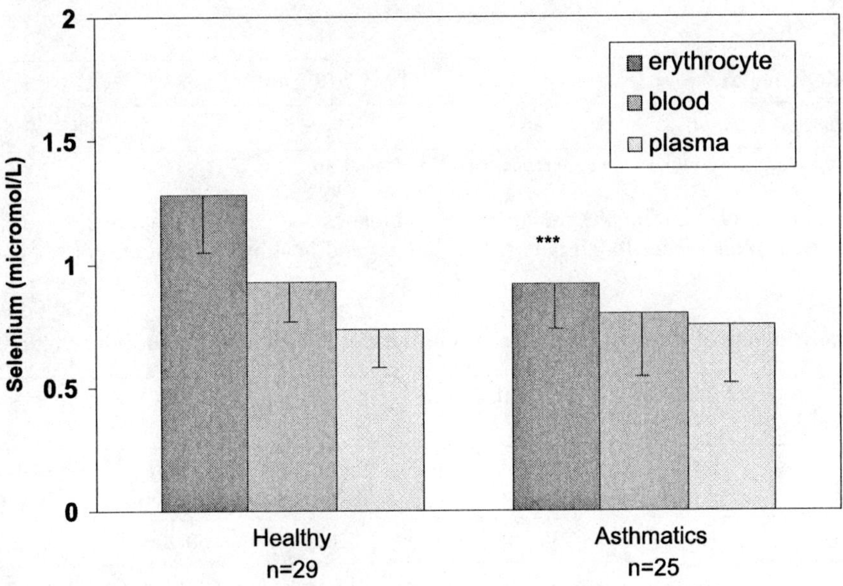

Fig. 1. Blood selenium parameters in healthy and asthmatic children aged 7-15 years.
***p<0.001 asthmatics compared to healthy.

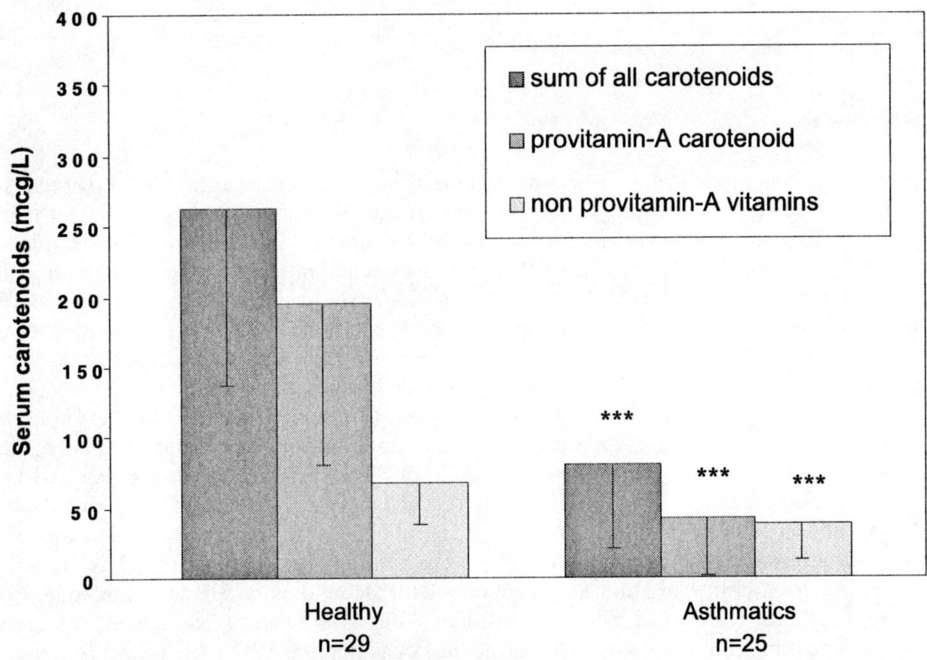

Fig. 2. Comparison of serum carotenoids in healthy and asthmatic children.
***p<0.001 asthmatics compared to healthy.

Table 1. Daily intake of total provitamin-A and non provitamin-A carotenoids in healthy and asthmatic children

Age (7-15 years)	Asthmatics	Healthy
	n=25	n=29
Provitamin-A (mg/d)	5.76 ± 2.46***	0.61 ± 0.86
Non provitamin-A (mg/d)	5.94 ± 6.28*	2.81 ± 2.17

Level of significance in comparison to healthy children. *=p<0.05; ***p<0.001.

The daily microelement intakes are given for asthmatics and controls in *table 2*. No differences in micronutrient intake were found between asthmatic and healthy children except for chromium and zinc.

Table 2. Daily intakes of essential trace elements in the diet of asthmatic and healthy children

	Asthmatics N=25	Healthy n=29	RDA Ref. 14, 15		
Elements			**Adult Males**	**Adult Females**	**Children 7-10 years**
Cr (mcg/d)	12 ± 25	35 ± 18**	50-200	50-200	50-200
Fe (mg/d)3.5 ± 1.3	4.5 ± 2.4	10	15	10	
Se (mcg/d)	31 ± 8	33 ± 8	70	55	30
Zn (mg/d)	3.0 ± 0.7	4.9 ± 3.4*	15	12	10

Level of significance in comparison to asthmatics. *p<0.05; **p<0.01.

CONCLUSION

We found that the blood status of Se was decreased in patients with asthma in agreement with other publications [11, 12]. A negative association between asthma and serum Se content in children aged 4 to 16 years has been demonstrated in the National Health and Nutrition Examination Survey (USA) (NHANES III), with an SD increase in selenium being associated with a 10% reduction in asthma prevalence [13]. Recent epidemiologic studies have confirmed the benefit of selenium supplementation on the clinical prevalence of asthma [2]. Serum provitamin-A carotenoids as the best sources for vitamin A and retinol were lower in asthmatics, than that of healthy children. Serum non-provitamin-A carotenoids were much lower in the asthmatic patients compared to the healthy controls. The food carotenoid intakes were higher in the asthmatic group than in the healthy controls. In spite of their higher dietary carotenoid intakes, asthmatic patients have lower blood carotenoid status than the healthy children. The daily intakes of Fe, Zn and Cr in healthy children compared to USA RDA values reached only 45, 49 and 75%. Asthmatics had lower Cr, Fe and Zn intakes than healthy children. Se intakes were significantly lower than RDA values both in asthmatics and in healthy children. The findings for selenium may have important implications for food policy in Hungary, a country with a low dietary selenium intake and high prevalence of asthma. These results may suggest that asthma, as a disease associated with chronic inflammations requires higher antioxidant carotenoid consumption than that in healthy children. Antioxidant nutrients appear to be necessary in asthma treatment, the antioxidant blood status could indicate to the severity of the disease.

REFERENCES

1. Wood LG, Gibson PG, Gary ML. Biomarkers of lipid peroxidation, airway inflammation and asthma. *Eur Respir J* 2003; 21: 177-186.
2. Rubin RN, Navon L, Cassano PA. Relationship of serum antioxidants to asthma prevalence in youth. *Am J Respir Crit Care Med* 2004; 169: 393-8.
3. Missio NL, Powers KA, Gillon RL, Stwart GA, Thompson PJ. Reduced platelet glutathione peroxidase activity and serum selenium concentration in atopic asthmatic patients. *Clin Exp Allergy* 1996; 26: 838-847.
4. Shaheen SO, Sterne JAC, Thompson RL, Songhurst CE, Margetts BM, Burney PGJ. Dietary antioxidants and asthma in adults. *Am J Respir Crit Care Med* 2001; 164: 1823-8.
5. Allam MF, Lucena RA. Selenium supplementation for asthma. *Cochrane Database Syst Rev.* 2004; 2; CD003538. Review.
6. Morabia A, Serenson A, Kumanyik S, et al. Vitamin A, cigarette smoking and airway obstruction. *Am J Respir Crit Care Med* 1989; 140: 1312-1316.
7. Hatch GE. Asthma, inhaled oxidants and dietary antioxidants. *Am J Clin Nutr* 1995; 61 Suppl 3: 625S-630S.
8. Harik-Khan RI, Muller DC, Wise RA. Serum vitamin levels and the risk of asthma in children. *Am J Epidemiol* 2004; 159: 351-7.
9. Devereux G, Seaton A. Diet as a risk factor for atopy and asthma. *J Allergy Clin Immunol* 2005; 15: 1109-1117.
10. Jakob E, Elmadfa I. Rapid HPLC assay for the assessment of vitamin K1, A, E and beta-carotene status in children (7-19 years). *Int J Vitam Nutr Res* 1995; 65: 31-35.
11. Stone J, Hinks LJ, Beasley R, Holgate ST, Clayton BA. Reduced selenium status of patients with asthma. *Clin. Sci* 1989; 77: 495-500.
12. Kadrabova J, Madaric A, Lovacikova Z, Podivinsky F, Ginter E, Gazdik F. Selenium status is decreased in patients with intrinsic asthma. *Biol Trace Elem Res* 1996; 52: 241-248.
13. Hu G, Cassano P. Antioxidants and pulmonary function: the third National Health and Nutrition Examination Survey (NHANES III). *Am J Epidemiol* 2000; 151: 975-81.
14. National Research Council, Food and Nutrition Board: Recommended Dietary Allowances. 10th ed. Washington, D.C.: National Academy Press, 1989.
15. World Health Orgaization Geneva: Trace elements in human nutrition and health. Macmillan-Ceuterick, India-Belgium 1996

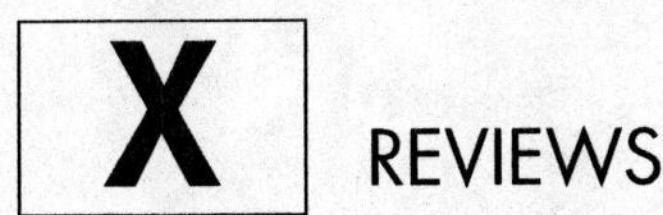

REVIEWS

Metal Ions in Biology and Medicine: vol. 9. Eds Maria Carmen Alpoim, Paula Vasconcellos Morais, Maria Amélia Santos, Armando J. Cristóvão, José A. Centeno, Philippe Collery.
John Libbey Eurotext, Paris © 2006 pp. 493-1.

Metal Ions and Molecular Therapy

Philippe Collery[1], Marion Bourleaud[1], Abdelfattah Badawi[2]

[1]*Service de Cancérologie, Polyclinique Maymard, 20200 Bastia, France.*
[2]*Egyptian Petroleum Research Institute, Cairo, Egypt.*

The target of anti cancer drugs has been for a long time the DNA and it is always the case of many cytotoxic agents. More recently the targets have been the receptors of some kinases. Other ways of development of anticancer drugs consider different molecular pathways regulating the cell growth, cell differenciation, apoptosis like the metalloproteases, the cyclo-oxygenase or other enzymes as well as angiogenic factors or cell cycle inhibitors. We could add to this list agents active on the mitochondrial functions, the membrane permeability, the cytoskeleton. We shall give some examples showing that metals may be used as molecular therapies against all these targets.

METAL IONS AND DNA

Direct DNA Damage

Cross link is the main mechanism of action of cisplatin (1). Platinum and palladium compounds chelate covalently to DNA, intercalating between the base pairs. Nevertheless, the palladium derivatives have a better affinity for the macromolecule than the corresponding platinum compounds (2). Ruthenium complexes bind with CT-DNA in an intercalative mode or by partial intercalation. The ligand planarity of the complex has a significant effect on DNA binding affinity (3). A DNA-intercalating rhodium complex also provides DNA binding affinity and in that case a peptide activated by a metal, like Zinc or Copper contributes to the reactivity (4). Vanadium compounds produce DNA single- and double-strand breaks (SSBs and DSBs) in lymphocytes, whereas in HeLa cells only SSBs were observed. Vanadium seems to have a higher genotoxic potential for cancer cells than for normal lymphocytes. Cd[II], Co[II], Cr[VI], Ni[II], and As[III] but not Pb[III] enhanced intrachromosomal homologous recombination in the order of potency being Cr>Cd>As>Co>Ni. The inhibition of the DNA synthesis may be a result of the metal induced DNA damage. The DNA synthesis inhibition decrease with the lengthening or the increase size of the carboxylate chain of the metal complex (5).

Conformational Changes

Metal Ions may induce conformational changes and particularly Mg salts. The role of Mg in DNA stabilization is concentration dependent. At high concentrations there is an accumulation of Mg binding, which induces conformational changes leading to Z-DNA. This effect is due to the binding of Mg^{2+} ions to N7 site of the molecule, stabilizing the five-member ring (6). It has been reported that Ga affinity for DNA is 100 times higher than Mg (7). The most important interactions of Ga^{3+} were observed from pH 4 to 5. For a low gallium concentration (Ga^{3+}/DNA ratio = 1/80) Ga atoms bound to DNA phosphate, their complex was stable, but no interaction was noticed between the metal and nucleic bases. For higher Ga concentration (ratio = 1/40) bounds appeared between gallium and nucleic bases and in this new complex the DNA helix was destabilized (8). Vanadocene complexes interact with DNA's nucleotid phosphate groups forming labile outer sphere complex via a water group (9). Different metal ions were classified in a decreasing order Mg^{2+}, Co^{2+}, Ni^{2+}, Mn^{2+}, Zn^{2+}, Cd^{2+} and Cu^{2+} for their relative ability to bind the phosphate groups rather than the bases and consequently to stabilize the double -helical structure of DNA by neutralizing the negative charges on the polynucleotide backbone. While Mg^{2+} and Ca^{2+} are believed to mainly interact with the phosphate groups of the nucleid acids, Zn^{2+} and Cd^{2+} have higher affinity for the bases (10).

Production of reactive oxygen species (ROS)

The production of ROS may be a major cause of DNA damage by an indirect way. It is well known that the formation of hydroxyl radical ($OH^·$) radicals from superoxide anion (O_2^-) and hydrogen peroxide (H_2O_2) is a transition metal-catalysed reaction and the reaction ferrous ions with oxygen is an example of an electron-transfer reaction in which the initial free radical is the ferrous ion.

Cr (VI) compounds are easily taken up by the cells and then reduced, through reactive intermediates such as Cr (V) and Cr (IV), to the more stable Cr (III) by cellular reductants. This reduction process also causes the generation of active oxygen species. Highly reactive intermediate oxidation state Cr(V) has been detected within erythrocytes.

Lanthanum (La^{3+}) in concentrations up to 10^{-4} M causes an enhancement of superoxide production in neutrophils (11). In induced malignant cells by cadmium chloride the proto-oncogenes c-fos and c-jun are overexpressed in 100% of the cell lines, while a statistically significant overexpression of c-myc was observed in 40% of the cell lines. These cells possess markedly higher levels of superoxide anion and hydrogen peroxide compared with the no transformed cells. The overexpression of the proto-oncogenes in the tumor cells requires elevated intracellular levels of reactive oxygen species and calcium. Further, the cadmium-induced overexpression of the proto-oncogenes is dependent on transcriptional activation as well as on pathways involving protein kinase C and MAP kinase (12).

ROS and cell signalisation

Vanadium (IV) and (V) induce DNA cleavage not directly reacting with DNA but acting mainly through the production of highly reactive oxygen species, especially hydroxyl radicals (9). Under vanadate stimulation, A549 cells generated $OH^·$ and hydrogen peroxide and O_2^-. The mechanism of ROS generation involves the reduction of molecular oxygen to O_2^- by both a flavoenzyme-containing NADPH complex and the mitochondria electron transport chain. The O_2^- in turn generates H_2O_2, which reacts with vanadium(IV) to generate $OH^·$ radical through a Fenton-type reaction ($V(IV) + H_2O_2 \rightarrow V(V) + OH^· + OH$-). The ROS generate by vanadate induce G2/M phase arrest in a time- and dose-dependent manner as determined by measuring DNA content. Among ROS, H_2O_2 is the species responsible for vanadate-induced G2/M phase arrest. Several regulatory pathways are involved: (1) activation of p21, (2) an increase of Chk1 expression and inhibition of Cdc25C, which results in phosphorylation of Cdc2 and possible inactivation of cyclin B1/Cdc2 complex (13). The concentration of glutathione (GSH) and the activity of superoxide dismutase (SOD), catalase (CAT), glutathione peroxidase (GSH-Px) and glutathione sulfatransferase (GSH-ST) decrease after Ce^{3+} administration. The results suggest that lipid peroxidation in liver may be an early consequence of Ce^{3+} exposure and the decrease of GSH might be considered as the cause of lipid peroxidation (14). Under normal conditions, intracellular enzymes (SOD, catalases) control the levels of superoxide radical and hydrogen peroxide and prevent oxidative tissue damage. Superoxide radicals are scavenged by specific metalloproteins and by some free hydrated metal ions. It has been reported that manganese (II) compounds scavenge the production of superoxide radicals (15), as well as metallothionein (16). Selenium is also an important element to protect aignst ROS production especially by the way of Glutahion peroxidase. Complexes of copper (II) and zinc (II) are able to inhibit 12-lipoxygenase in vitro (17). Cobalt (Co^{2+}) inhibits superoxide production (11).

Genes and protein expressions

It has been clearly demonstrated by using cDNA array consisting of 84 cardiopulmonary-related genes representing various biological functions such as lung injury/inflammation, repair/remodeling, structural and matrix alterations, and vascular contractility, as well as six expressed sequence tags (ESTs) that metal ions modify the expression of stress response, inflammatory and repair-related genes and also genes involved in vascular contractility and thrombogenic activity (18). However, expression profiling using genomic approaches need yet to be performed to define the role of metal ions in molecular pathways. Loss of p53 function by mutation is a frequent event in human cancer. The p53 protein is a metal-binding transcription factor that is inactivated by metal chelation and by oxidation in vitro. In intact cells, p53 protein activity is crucially dependent on the availability of Zn ions and is impaired by exposure to Cd, a metal which readily substitutes for Zn in a number of transcription factors. Inactivation by Cd suppresses the p53-dependent responses to DNA damage. Overall, these findings indicate that regulation by metals plays an important role in the control of p53 (19).

The expression levels of the genes involved in growth regulation, such as p53, p27, c-myc, c-fos, mdm2, cyclins D1 and B1, CDK4, and PCNA have been studied with Cd (20) or Se (21) but further studies are required with all other metals. In contrast, suppressor genes like FHIT could also be regulated by metal ions (22).

Metallothioneins (MTs) may modulate a variety of cellular processes by regulating the activity of zinc-binding proteins. Several oncogenes and related proteins have been shown to contain Zinc finger domains (23). Different metal mimic Zn in finger-loop domains by forming tetrahedral coordination complexes with thiol and imidazole groups but many studies are still needed to compare the role of all metals. It could be important to find metals increasing metallothioneins as it has been shown that metallothionein II-A was expressed 27-fold less in human colorectal tumors and tumor cell lines compared with normal tissue (24) or in kidney adenocarcinoma (25).

Metal ions may also interfere with DNA repair it is well known that cells with enhanced DNA repair activity are resistant to cisplatin. Ga can reverse this resistance (26).

METAL IONS AND ENZYMES

The inhibition of the EGFR is a main target of the new anticancer drugs (27). The epidermal growth factor receptor (EGFR) is a tyrosine kinase receptor with the family of HER/erbB including HER 1 (EGFR/erbB1), HER-2 (neu, erbB2), HER-3 (erbB3) and HER-4 (erbB4). EGFR is abnormally expressed and activated in cancer cells. The EGFR initiates the signal transduction cascade. Metal ions like Zn, As and V activate the EGFR tyrosine kinase and that may be the result of the phosphorylation of the activating site of EGFR (28, 29). The inhibition of the activity of EGFR by other metals could be an interesting way of research.

Other targets like serine/threonine kinases could be interesting as they mediate the crossroad of multiple signalling pathways important for the downstream signal transduction of cellular proliferation and invasion following activation of receptor tyrosine kinases. Protein kinase C (PKC), mitogen-activated protein kinase/ras (MAPK) and phosphatidylinositol 3 kinase /AKT (PI3/AKT) belong to the family of the serine/threonine kinases. The PKC family has been recognized to comprise more than 12 isoforms that have been divided into three groups based on their interactions with calcium and diacylglycerol. Each isoform plays a different role in cell growth, proliferation, differenciation or apoptosis. The variation of PKC isoenzymes during cancer progression appears to depend on cancer cell type. PKC isoenzymes participate in signal transduction. Once activated, PKC can transmit signals to the nucleus via one or more MAPK cascades (Raf-1, ERKs, MAPK/ERK kinases, c-Jun N-terminal kinases, p38 MAPKs). Activated ERKs can activate transcription factors such as myc, myb, max, fos and jun, enabling the expression of genes encoding for enzymes required for cell proliferation and invasion. PKC-80a may phosphorylate bcl-2, potentiating its anti-apoptotic function in mitochondria. In contrast PKC-δ has a pro-apoptotic function activated proteolytically by caspase-3. PKC can mediate the MDR1-mediated antitumor drug resistance by activation of PGP(P-glycoprotein) phosphorylation and drug efflux. Inhibitors of PKC could be used to suppress resistance of tumors against cytotoxic agents. Enhanced PKC activity is often found in different cancer cells that show marked invasive and/or metastatic potential. Activation of PKC induces the secretion of matrix metalloproteinase (MMP-9) activation of MMP-2, down-regulation of tissue inhibitors of metalloproteinases (TIMP 1 and TIMP-2) (30, 31). Protein Kinases are a major target of metals. Many studies are needed to understand the role of metals in all enzymatic activities.

For example, Phosphorylase kinase is a metal ion dependant kinase with a dual specificity. The specificity of phosphorylation is determined by divalent cation. Mg2+ causes seryl phosphorylation of phosphorylase b, but Mn2+ activates tyrosine phosphorylation of angiotensin II. In contrast to seryl phosphorylation, the tyrosine kinase activity of holoenzyme is not regulated by Ca2+. Preincubation of the holoenzyme with Ca2+, Mg2+ and ATP that causes autophosphorylation activates tyrosine kinase activity. The tyrosyl kinase activity is a property of the gamma subunit. Addition of varying amounts of Mn2+ to a truncated form of the gamma subunit of phosphorylase kinase containing MgATP inhibits serine kinase but activates tyrosine kinase activity. This result along with an oxidative reaction caused by Cu2+ and site-directed mutagenesis of the putative catalytic base inhibiting both serine and tyrosine kinase activity suggest that one active site is involved in both activities. Kinetic studies with Mn2+ and ATP show that Km for nucleotide is not changed with a seryl or tyrosyl substrate. The Vm values are different, and the value for tyrosyl phosphorylation is similar to other tyrosyl kinases. Two conformations for the active site are possible; one favors seryl phosphorylation, and the second tyrosyl phosphorylation is caused by the binding of divalent cation at a second metal ion binding site (32).

Gallium is able to inhibit the protein phosphatase tyrosine specific of human leukaemia cells and human colon cancer cells (29) but on the other hand may increase tyrosine kinase activity (30).

Matrix Metalloproteinases (MMP) are a family of zinc-dependant proteolytic enzymes and they also play an important role in the tumor progression, especially MMP-2, MMP-7, MMP-9 and MMP-14 (33). Metalloproteases are involved in many stages of the cancer development and metal complexes, like V complexes are able to inhibit the constitutive expression as well as the gelatinolytic activities of matrix metalloproteinase 9 and 2. Even the activity of cyclo-oxygenase may be modulated by metal ions and it was well demonstrated that Cd could induced a specific rise in cyclo-oxygenase-2 (COX-2) but not COX-1. The decrease of the activity of the ribonucleotide reductase is a major mechanism of action of Ga but also of its toxicity on red blood cells (34).

The vascular endothelial growth factor (VEGF) is the most potent and specific angiogenic factor. The Platelet Derivated Growth Factor (PDGF) and the Fibroblast Growth Factor (FGF) can contribute to the changes of the vascular changes. The effect of inorganic selenium (sodium selenate) on the retardation of the tumor growth of primary prostatic tumor and the development of retroperitoneal lymph node metastases is associated with a decrease in angiogenesis (35).

METAL IONS AND MITOCHONDRIAL FUNCTION

It was observed by Prasad & Kharbangar that the mitochondrial proteins decreased in liver, kidney and tumor cells after cisplatin treatment of ascites Dalton's lymphoma tumor-bearing mice while mitochondrial-glutathione levels decreased in kidney and liver but increased in tumor cells after the treatment (36). They also noted that mitochondrial-lipid peroxidation (mt-LPO) increased in the three tissues. It is suggested that a decrease in mt-GSH and concomitant increase in mt-LPO could be an early and critical factor in cisplatin-induced toxicity.

The bis(4,7-dimethyl-1,10-phenanthroline) sulfatooxovanadium(IV)-induced apoptosis is associated with a loss of mitochondrial transmembrane potential (37).

The demonstration of elevated mitochondrial membrane potential in a variety of cancerous cells, relative to normal cells might be exploited by using metal compounds having phosphine ligands as for example with (triphenylphosphine)gold (I) complex which has been proven to be highly cytotoxic with very low IC50 of less than 0.5 μM. The gold is bound to the triphenylphosphine ligand through the phosphorous atom. Triphenylphosphine Au(I) decreases the mitochondrial potential membrane (38).

Gallium induces a calcium efflux from mitochondria in a dose related manner. This release is more important when the calcium mitochondria content is more elevated. Cyclosporine inhibits the effect of gallium on calcium efflux from mitochondria, this suggests that gallium mechanism of action should be located at the mitochondrial membrane pore level or with pyridine nucleotide hydrolysis (39).

The phospholipid hydroperoxide glutathione peroxidase (PHGPx) is a key enzyme in the protection of biomembranes to oxidative stress. Nomura et al. studied the role of mitochondrial PHGPx in apoptosis in cells that overexpressed PHGPx, and in control cells. Upon exposure to 2-deoxyglucose (2DG), the release of cytochrome c from mitochondria was observed in control cells and was followed by the activation of caspase-3. Overexpression of mitochondrial PHGPx prevented the release of cytochrome c, the activation of caspase-3 and apoptosis. The levels of hydroperoxides in mitochondria were significantly increased after the exposure to 2-deoxyglucose in control cells, but not in cells that overexpressed PHGPx. The production of Reactive Oxygen Species in mitochondria is regulated by a number of antioxidant enzymes within mitochondria, including phospholipid hydroperoxide glutathione peroxidase, classical glutathione peroxidase and Mn-superoxide dismutase (Mn-SOD). Excessive production of hydroperoxide and the resultant damage to mitochondria might induce the liberation of cytochrome c in the 2DG-induced apoptosis (40).

METAL IONS AND CYTOSKELETON

Organometallic compounds can block cell division in human cancer cells by disrupting bipolar spindle formation (41). Mg and Ga have been shown to act on the cytoskeleton (42).

METAL IONS AND CELL MEMBRANE PERMEABILITY

Many studies show that metal ions may modify the cell membrane permeability but the therapeutc consequences in cancer treatment are still to be defined. It could be a major mechanism of action Ga for example (43, 44).

METAL IONS AND ADHESIVE, MIGRATORY AND INVASIVE PROPERTIES OF CANCER CELLS

Some vanadium complexes are able to nearly completely inhibit the adhesive, migratory and invasive properties of the cancer cells (37).

Protein tyrosine phosphorylation induced by vanadium compounds may influence the invasive and metastatic potential of tumour cells, regulating cell substrate adhesion or cell to cell contact and acting cytoskeletal changes, modifying the cancer invasion by changes in adhesive proteins (cell to cell or cell to matrix). Pervanadate has been shown to inhibit the induction of intracellular adhesion proteins ICAM 1, V-CAM-1 and ELAM-1 in endothelial cells. This inhibition is probably exerted through the inactivation Protein Tyrosine Phosphatase, and the subsequent down-modulation of tumour necrosis factor (TNF) which is one of the major inducers of various adhesion molecules in human endothelial cells. Moreover, enhancement of tyrosine phosphorylation by vanadate resulted in the inhibition of cadherin-mediated aggregation (cell to cell adhesion) of rat 3Y1 cells transformed with v-src and doubly transformed cells with v-src and v-fos (SR3Y1 and fos-expressing SRY1 cells with enhanced acquired metastatic potential). Treatment of high metastatic Lewis lung carcinoma A11 cells with sodium orthovanadate resulted in a dose-and time-dependant suppression of cells spreading on various extracellular matrix such as fibronectin, laminin and type IV collagen but it did not significantly inhibit the attachment of the cells to this substrate (9).

CONCLUSION

Many targets may be explored to counteract cancer and a classification of the role of metals according to all of them should be useful for a better use of metal-based anticancer drugs.

REFERENCES

1. Lando D. Y., Fridman A.S., Haroutiunian S.G., Benight A.S., Collery P. Melting of cross-linked DNA. IV. Methods for computer modeling of total influence on DNA melting of monofunctional adducts, intrastrand and interstrand cross-links formed by molecules of an antitumor drug. J Biomol Struct & Dynamics, Vol. 17, 2000:697-711.
2. Afcharian A, Butour JL, Castan P, Wimmer S. New concepts on the design of Palladium (II) complexes as antitumor agents. Metal Ions in Biology and Medicine, Vol. 1, 1990:514-16.
3. Chao H., Mei W.J., Huang Q.W, Ji L.N. DNA binding studies of ruthenium(II) complexes containing asymmetric tridentate ligands. J Inorg Biochem 2002;vol. 92:65-70.
4. Copeland KD, Fitzsimons MP, Houser RP, Barton JK. DNA hydrolysis and oxidative cleavage by metal-binding peptides tethered to rhodium intercalators. Biochemistry, Vol. 41, 2002:343-56.
5. Katsaros N., Anagnostopoulou A. Rhodium and its compounds as potential agents in cancer treatment. Crit Rev Oncol Hematol, Vol. 42, 2002:297-308.
6. Anastassopoulou J, Theophanides T. Magnesium-DNA interactions and the possible relation of magnesium to carcinogenesis. Irradiation and free radicals. Crit Rev Oncol Hematol 2002; vol. 42:79-91.
7. Manfait M., Collery P. Etude in vitro par spectroscopie Raman de la conformation d'un ADN sous l'influence des ions magnésium et gallium. Magnesium Bull, Vol. 4, 1984:153-5.
8. Tajmir-Rihai H. A., Naoui M., Ahmad R. A comparative study of calf-thymus DNA binding trivalent Al, Ga, Cr and Fe ions in aqueous solution. Metal Ions in Biology and Medicine, Vol. 2: John Libbey Eurotext, Paris, 1992:98-101.
9. Evangelou AM. Vanadium in cancer treatment. Crit Rev Oncol Hematol.Vol. 42, 2002:249-65,
10. Tajmir-Riahi HA, Nahar S, Diamantoglou S, Manfait M, Collery P, Millart H, Etienne JC. A comparative study of protein binding to Al (III), Ga (III) and Fe (III) ions. Metal ion binding site and protein conformational variations in aqueous solution. Metal Ions in Biology and Medicine. John Libbey Eurotext, Paris, Vol. 3, 1994:321-6.
11. Elferink J.G.R. The effects of lanthanum and cobalt ions on enzyme release from neutrophils. Metal Ions in Biology and Medicine, John Libbey Eurotext, Paris, Vol. 1, 1990:18-20.
12. Joseph P. Muchnok TK, Klishis M. L., Roberts J. R., Antonini J. M., Whong W. Z., Ong, T. Cadmium-induced cell transformation and tumorigenesis are associated with transcriptional activation of c-fos, c-jun, and c-myc proto-oncogenes: role of cellular calcium and reactive oxygen species. Toxicol Sci, Vol. 61, 2001:295-303.
13. Zhang Z, Huang C, Li J, Leonard SS, Lanciotti R, Butterworth L, Shi X. Vanadate-induced cell growth regulation and the role of reactive oxygen species. Vol. 392, 2001:311-20, -20.
14. Khassanova L, Collery P, Etienne JC, Khassanova Z, Yangurazova Z. The influence of copper ions on the photosynthetic activity of the cyanobacterium Synechocystis aquatilis. Metal Ions in Biology and Medicine. John Libbey Eurotext, Paris, Vol. 3, 1994:181-5.
15. Arnaiz Garcia F.J., Capul C., Castan P., Deguenon D., Derache Ph., Nepveu F. Manganese complexes

as superoxide radical anion scavengers. Metal Ions in Biology and Medicine, John Libbey Eurotext, Paris. Vol. 1, 1990:21-3.
16. Cheng S., Tang CS. Metallothionein as a scavenger of free radicals. Metal Ions in Biology and Medicine, John Libbey Eurotext, Vol. 1, 1990:24-6.
17. Badawi A.M., Al-Sougi GN, El-Tahir K.E. Modulating leukotrioene syntheses by copper and zinc. Metal Ions in Biology and Medicine, John Libbey Eurotext, Paris Collery Ph, Poirier L A Manfait M Etienne J C. Vol. 1, 1990:11-3.
18. Nadadur SS, Kodavanti U. Altered gene expression profiles of rat lung in response to an emission particulate and its metal constituents. J Toxicol Environ Health A, Vol. 65, 2002:1333-50.
19. Meplan C, Richard MJ, Hainaut P. Metalloregulation of the tumor suppressor protein p53: zinc mediates the renaturation of p53 after exposure to metal chelators in vitro and in intact cells. Oncogene 2000; vol. 19:5227-36.
20. Fang MZ, Mar W, Cho MH. Cadmium affects genes involved in growth regulation during two-stage transformation of Balb/3T3 cells. Toxicology 2002; vol. 177:253-65.
21. Yu S.Y., Lu XP, Liao S.D. The regulatory effect of selenium on the expression of oncogenes associated with proliferation and differentiation on tumor cells. Metal Ions in Biology and Medicine, John Libbey, Eurotext, Paris, Vol. 1, 1990:487-89.
22. Kowara R, Karaczyn AA, Fivash MJ, Jr., Kasprzak KS. In vitro inhibition of the enzymatic activity of tumor suppressor FHIT gene product by carcinogenic transition metals. Chem Res Toxicol 2002; vol. 15:319-25.
23. Sundermann FW. Regulation of gene expression by metals: zinc finger-loop domain in transcription factors, hormone receptors and proteins encoded by oncogenes. Metal Ions in Biology and Medicine, John Libbey Eurotext, Paris, Vol. 1, 1990:549-54.
24. Duncan EL, Reddel R. Downregulation of metallothionein-IIA expression occurs at immortalization. Oncogene, Vol. 18, 1999:897-903.
25. Hellemans G, Soumillion A, Proost P, Van Damme J, Van Poppel H, Baert L, De Ley M. Metallothioneins in human kidneys and associated tumors. Nephron 1999; vol. 83:331-40.
26. Desoize B., Collery P, Akeli M. G., Etienne J. C., Keppler B. Tris(8-quinolinolato) Ga(III) is active against unicellular and multicellular resistance. Metal Ions in Biology and Medicine, John Libbey Eurotext, Paris, Vol. 6, 2000:573-6.
27. Ghoul A.SM, Benhadji K.A., Cvitkovic E., Faivre S., Philips E., Calvo F., Lokiec F., Raymond E. Protein kinase C a and d are members of a large kinase family of high potential for novel anticancer targeted therapy. Targeted Oncology Vol. 0, 2005:34-7.
28. Wu W, Jaspers I, Zhang W, Graves LM, Samet JM. Role of Ras in metal-induced EGF receptor signaling and NF-kappaB activation in human airway epithelial cells. Am J Physiol Lung Cell Mol Physiol, Vol. 282, 2002:L1040-8.
29. Berggren MM, Burns LA, Abraham RT, Powis G. nhibition of protein tyrosine phosphatase by the antitumor agent gallium nitrate. Vol. 53, 1993:1862-6.
30. Farzami B., Pournaki A, Collery P., Goliaei B. Effect of Gallium on the Growth Rate of U937 cell culture and the activity of tyrosine kinase. Metal Ions in Biology and Medicine, John Libbey Eurotext, Paris, Vol. 7, 2002:625-8.
31. Achanzar WE, Achanzar KB, Lewis JG, Webber MM, Waalkes MP. Cadmium induces c-myc, p53, and c-jun expression in normal human prostate epithelial cells as a prelude to apoptosis. Toxicol Appl Pharmacol 2000; vol. 164:291-300.
32. Berggren MM, Burns LA, Abraham RT, Powis G. Inibition of protein tyrosin phosphatase by the antitummor agent galliuim nitrate. Vol. 53, 1993, 1862-6.
33. Macarulla T., Valverde C, Ramos F.J., Casado E., Martinelli E., Cervantes A., Tabernero J. Emerging strategies in the treatment of advanced esophageal, gastroesophageal junction, and gastric cancer: the introduction of targeted therapies. Targeted Oncology 2005: 23-33.
34. Myette MS, Elford HL, Chitambar CR. Interaction of gallium nitrate with other inhibitors of ribonucleotide reductase: effects on the proliferation of human leukemic cells. Cancer Lett 1998;vol. 129:199-204.
35. Corcoran N.M., Najdovska M, Costello A.J. Inorganic selenium retards progression of experimental hormone refractory prostate cancer. J Urol, Vol. 171, 2004:907-10.
36. Prasad SB, Khynriam D. Mutagenicity and endogenous glutathione levels in tumor-bearing mice after cisplatin treatment. John Libbey Eurotext, Paris, Vol. 7, 2002:580-85.
37. D'Cruz O.J., Uckun FM. Metvan: a novel oxovanadium(IV) complex with broad spectrum anticancer activity. Expert Opin Investig Drugs, Vol. 11, 2002:1829-36.

38. De Pancorbo M.M., Garcia-Orad A, Paz Arizti M., Gutierrez-Zorrilla J.M., Colacio E. 8-(thiotheophyllinato) (triphenylphosphine) Gold (I) (tTPau): a new complex of therapeutic gold ion. Metal Ions in Biology and Medicine John Libbey Eurotext, Paris Collery Ph, Poirier L A Manfait M Etienne J C Vol. 1, 1990:385-89.
39. Gogvadze V., Zhukova A, Ivanov A., Khassanova L., Khassanova Z., Collery P. The effect of gallium on the calcium retention capacity of rat liver mitochondria. Metal Ions in Biology and Medicine, John Libbey Eurotext., Vol. 4, 1996:249-52.
40. Nomura K., Imai H, Koumura T., Arai M., Nakagawa Y. Mitochondrial phospholipid hydroperoxide glutathione peroxidase suppresses apoptosis mediated by a mitochondrial death pathway. J Biol Chemistry, Vol. 274, 1999:29294-302.
41. Navara CS, Benyumov A, Vassilev A, Narla RK, Ghosh P, Uckun FM. Vanadocenes as potent antiproliferative agents disrupting mitotic spindle formation in cancer cells. Vol. 12, 2001:369-76.
42. Perchellet E.M, Ladesich JB, Collery P, Perchellet J.P. Microtubule-disrupting effects of gallium chloride in vitro. Vol. 10, 1999:477-88.
43. Bara M., Guiet-Bara A, Collery P., Durlach J. Gallium action on the ionic transfer through the isolated human amnion. I. Effect on the amnion as a whole and interaction between Gallium and Magnesium. Trace Elements in Med, Vol. 2, 1985:99-102.
44. Bara M., Guiet-Bara A, Collery P., Durlach J. Gallium action on the ionic transfer through the isolated human amnion. II. Effect on cellular and paracellular pathways. Trace Elem Med, Vol. 9, 1992:117-22.

Metal Ions in Biology and Medicine: vol. 9. Eds Maria Carmen Alpoim, Paula Vasconcellos Morais, Maria Amélia Santos, Armando J. Cristóvão, José A. Centeno, Philippe Collery.
John Libbey Eurotext, Paris © 2006 pp. 501-1.

Manganese transport and neurotoxicity

Vanessa A. Fitsanakis[1], Sarah E. Owens[1], Ana Paula Marreilha dos Santos[2], Offie P. Soldin[4], Michael Aschner[1,3,*]

[1]*Department of Pediatrics, Vanderbilt University Medical Center, Nashville, TN, USA.*
[2]*Faculty of Pharmacy, University of Lisbon, Lisbon, Portugal.*
[3]*The Kennedy Center, Vanderbilt University Medical Center, Nashville, TN, USA.*
[4]*Division of Endocrinology and Metabolism, Department of Medicine, Georgetown University Medical Center, Washington, DC.*

Manganese (Mn) is an essential mineral present at low levels in virtually all diets. In general, most individuals are exposed to Mn via ingestion, although occupational exposure occurs primarily through inhalation. Interestingly, animals generally maintain stable tissue levels of Mn even under conditions of higher amounts of Mn exposure. The basis for this homeostatic mechanism is the tight regulation of Mn absorption and excretion via the liver and bile. Under certain high-dose exposure conditions, however, elevations in tissue Mn levels, particularly brain, can occur. Excessive Mn accumulation can result in adverse neurological, reproductive and respiratory effects both in laboratory animals and humans. In humans, Mn-induced neurotoxicity (manganism) is of paramount concern. Individuals with chronic Mn neurotoxicity develop a motor dysfunction syndrome that is recognized as a form of parkinsonism. Individuals with manganism present with destructive symmetric lesions in the basal ganglia (particularly in the globus pallidus and substantia nigra). This review will briefly address and regulatory mechanisms associated with the transport of Mn as well as some of the mechanisms of its neurotoxicity.

MANGANESE ESSENTIALITY

Manganese (Mn) is an essential trace metal found in all tissues that is required for normal amino acid, lipid, protein and carbohydrate metabolism [1-3]. Additionally, Mn plays an important role in various enzyme families including oxidoreductases, transferases, hydrolases, lyases, isomerases and ligases. Mn also functions in numerous metalloenzymes such as arginase, glutamine synthetase, phosphoenolpyruvate decarboxylase and Mn-superoxide dismutase [2]. No formal Recommended Dietary Allowance (RDA) for this metal have been established, but the U.S. National Research Council suggests that an estimated safe and adequate dietary intake (ESADDI) is approximately 2-5 mg/day for adults [4], with the recommended intake for adult men and women being 2.3 and 1.8 mg/day, respectively [5]. The discrepancy in requirements in like due to the fact that men absorb significantly less Mn than women [6].

MANGANESE TOXICITY

Manganese toxicity in humans is a well-recognized occupational hazard [7-13] usually due

* Address all correspondence to Michael Aschner, Ph.D., Department of Pediatrics, B-3307 Medical Center North Vanderbilt University Medical Center, Nashville, TN 37232-2495; Phone: 615-322-8024; FAX: 615-322-6541; E-mail: Michael.Aschner@vanderbilt.edu

to inhalation of excessive amounts. Although respiratory signs and symptoms result from excessive or prolonged inhalation, it is Mn-induced neurotoxicity, termed "manganism", that is of paramount concern [14]. Manganism is associated with elevated brain levels of Mn, specifically in areas with high concentrations of nonheme iron, such as the caudate-putamen, globus pallidus, substantia nigra and subthalamic nuclei. Manganism is initially characterized by a psychiatric disorder *(locura manganica)* that closely resembles schizophrenia, but can progress to include prolonged muscle contractions (dystonia), decreased muscle movement (hypokinesia), rigidity, and muscle tremors [15]. These signs are thought to be associated with damage to dopaminergic neurons within the basal ganglia that control muscle movement. As a paramagnetic trace element, Mn can be detected by magnetic resonance (MR) imaging. Mn drastically affects the nuclear MR properties of solutions and tissues. Mn deposition appears as a hyperintense signal (i.e. a shortened T1) in the basal ganglia, specifically the globus pallidus on T1- (short TE/short TR) but not T2- (long TE/long TR) weighted MRI. Other metals, such as copper and iron do not manifest this appearance.

MANGANESE TRANSPORT

The main site of Mn absorption is the intestines. Afterwards, Mn is transported throughout the body bound to various proteins (transferrin, plasma macroglobulin and/or albumin) and small molecules (citrate) [16-20]. As Mn and iron share transporter systems [transferrin (Tf)/transferrin receptor, divalent metal transporter-1 (DMT-1)], recent studies have examined whether iron deficiency and anemia could be risk factors for enhanced Mn absorption as well as neurotoxicity [21, 22].

A number of studies have examined the transport kinetics of Mn from the blood into the central nervous system (CNS). Collectively, these studies suggest that Mn enters the brain from either the cerebral capillaries and/or the cerebrospinal fluid (CSF; via choroid plexus transport), or via the olfactory nerve following inhalation. At normal plasma concentrations, transport across the capillary endothelium predominates, whereas at high plasma concentrations, transport across the choroid plexus appears more prevalent [23, 24]. While many studies to date have focused on transferrin- and DMT-1-mediated transport, the possibility for other proteins or small molecules to play a role in transport cannot be excluded.

For example, recent studies suggest that divalent Mn (Mn^{2+}) uptake was not inhibited by iron or the absence of DMT-1 expression. This could imply that transport is facilitated via an iron-transporter-independent mechanism. As a potential explanation, calcium channels were suggested to play a role in Mn^{2+} uptake into the brain [20]. This is likely to be involved since it is known that Mn^{2+} can be transported along neuronal pathways in an anterograde direction. Indeed, MR studies have made use of this characteristic to map neuronal connection in the olfactory [25, 26], somatosensory [28] and visual [28-30] pathways of rodent brain.

In order to better determine the role that transferrin may play in Mn transport, a series of experiments were undertaken by Malecki et al. in 1999 [31, 32]. Here, homozygous hypotransferrinemic (a genetic defect resulting in <1% of normal plasma Tf concentrations) mice were used to examine the role of Tf in brain Fe and Mn transport by injecting either $^{54}MnCl_2$ or $^{59}FeCl_3$. Mice with hypotransferrinemia did not initially exhibit changes in brain Mn uptake. One week after treatment, however, they had less Mn, but increased Fe, in forebrain structures. This suggests that Tf is necessary for the transport of Fe but not Mn across the blood-brain barrier [31-33]. Nevertheless, it must be considered that Tf-independent mechanisms, such as Mn transport by DMT-1, might be unmasked by the genetic defect, thus compensating for hypotransferrinemia. Consistent with this possibility are studies by the same authors [31, 32] in which Tf was required for typical distribution of ^{59}Fe and ^{54}Mn in brains of "normal" mice.

MANGANESE TOXICITY AND IRON DEFICIENCY

Worldwide, the prevalence of iron deficiency anemia (IDA) in infants and children is estimated to be at approximately 25% [34]. A majority of these cases of anemia are due to Fe deficiency. As Mn and Fe share transporters, this raises the question of whether people with IDA would be at a greater risk for manganism. In a recent study [35] weanling rats fed an iron deficient (ID) diet had significant increases in Mn concentration across brain regions compared to animals fed control diets. This suggests the existence of a potentially important vulnerable population that has previously been ignored. Since Fe and Mn use similar transport systems, it has been hypothesized that anemic populations are more susceptible to Mn intoxication, even when exposed to low or normal levels of Mn. A significant gap in our knowledge exists with respect to the interaction between Fe deficiency and Mn neurotoxicity. Specifically, the role of Fe status in the distribution patterns and accumulation of Mn in the CNS in infants is unknown.

MECHANISMS OF MANGANESE NEUROTOXICITY

Oxygen radicals can damage components of the electron transport and oxidative phosphorylation machinery, and this leads to generation of more reactive oxygen species (namely superoxide). The new radicals exacerbate the damage, and a "downward spiral" ensues. In this scenario, cells are ultimately subjected to energy failure as ATP production declines. The membrane potential is lost as the mitochondria undergo permeability transition, which then leads to cell death. This mitochondrial dysfunction coincides with decreased cerebral metabolic rates in multiple neurodegenerative disorders. Whether the mitochondrial demise has a causal role or appears as a secondary effect in these disorders is still a subject of intense debate. Probable mechanism of action for almost all known basal ganglia neurotoxins is inhibition of mitochondrial function. Studies of this interrelationship are clouded by the fact that mitochondrial function declines as a normal part of the aging process, and age itself is a risk factor for these neurodegenerative diseases. Altogether, the literature seems to point to a strong association between aging, mitochondrial impairment and oxidative stress.

Postmortem studies of Parkinson's disease (PD) patients provide evidence for chemical changes indicative of reactive oxygen/nitrogen species (RO/NS) induced damage to the substantia nigra and other nuclei of the basal ganglia. Such changes include increased levels of lipid peroxidation, protein oxidation, 3-nitrotyrosine formation, DNA oxidation and breaks, and a decrease in the activities of the ROS scavenging enzymes glutathione peroxidase (GPx) and superoxide dismutases (SOD). Several hypotheses exist regarding the mechanisms associated with the loss of dopaminergic neurons in PD, and most suggest that mitochondrial damage is a primary cause of dopaminergic neuron death. Some suggest that: (1) Mitochondria of dopaminergic neurons are selectively vulnerable to some environmental contaminant(s) which causes mitochondrial dysfunction; (2) dopaminergic neurons may produce an inherent mitochondrial toxin; or (3) mitochondria harbor endogenous defects in enzymes such as complex I that lead to impaired energy metabolism. The centrality of mitochondria in these hypotheses arose primarily from multiple findings that mitochondrial poisons such as 1-methyl-4-phenylpyridium ions (MPP^+) [the active metabolite of the pyrimidines analog, 1-methyl-4-phenyl-1,2,3,6-tetrahydropyridine (MPTP)], 6-hydroxydopamine (6-OHDA) and rotenone can all induce a Parkinsonian syndrome in humans, non-human primates, and rodents. These neurotoxins are all capable of inhibiting mitochondrial complex I and they all model to a great extent various features associated with the pathology of PD. Neuropathological studies show a ~30% defect in complex I function in deceased PD patients, as compared with aged matched controls.

Intracellular Mn^{2+} is sequestered by mitochondria via the Ca^{2+} uniporter [36, 37]. Intrastriatal Mn injections result in loss of DAergic neurons, resembling toxicity caused by the mitochondrial poisons, aminooxyacetic acid and 1-methyl-4-phenyl-pyridinium ion (MPP^+) [38], and oxidative stress plays a significant role in the process [39, 40]. Whether Mn, like 6-OHDA and other toxins associated with Parkinson's disease (PD) model, activates the antioxidant response element has yet to be determined [41, 42]. Analogous to PD model toxins, Mn also elevates intracellular H_2O_2 and related peroxides [43], reduces tyrosine hydroxylase (TH) activity [44], and intracellular antioxidants (GSH, thiols, catalase) in DAergic neurons [45], thus replicating many features of PD. Consistent with increased production of ROS, Mn also inhibits mitochondrial complex-I, a feature inherent to PD and its experimental models [46]. Finally, both MPP^+ and Mn activate heme oxygenase-1, whose overexpression promotes oxidative mitochondrial damage [47].

CONCLUSIONS

Mn plays a crucial role in all life-stages of animals and humans, In addition, it is well documented that Mn is neurotoxic at high levels. Thus it is important to understand the intricacies of Mn transport and regulation. Although our knowledge of Mn transport and distribution has increased considerably in recent years, many questions remain. For example, it is still unclear as to what extent novel (i.e. not transferrin-dependent or DMT-1) transporters play a role in brain Mn influx and efflux. While it is known that astrocytes are capable of sequestering large amounts of Mn, further work could focus on the role of microglia and/or oligodendrocytes play in storing and utilizing Mn. Finally, the degree to which Fe deficiency may affect a person's ability to properly regulate brain Mn deposition needs to be examined.

REFERENCES

1. Hurley LS, Keen CL. Manganese, In *Trace elements in Human Health and Animal Nutrition*, Underwood E and Mertz W, editors. New York: Academic Press, 1987. p. 185-223.
2. Erikson KM, Aschner M. Manganese neurotoxicity and glutamate-GABA interaction. *Neurochem Internat* 2003; 43: 475-80.
3. Fitsanakis VA, Garcia SJ, Aschner M. Manganese dynamics, distribution and neurotoxicity. In *The Role of Glia in Neurotoxicity*, Aschner M, Costa LG, editors. Boca Rotan (Florida): CRC Press, 2005. p. 395-415.
4. Greger JL. Dietary standards for manganese: overlap between nutritional and toxicological studies. *J Nutr* 1998; 128: 368S-71S.
5. National Academy of Sciences. Dietary Reference Intakes for Vitamin A, Vitamin K, Arsenic, Boron, Chromium, Copper, Iodine, Iron, Manganese, Molybdenum, Nickel, Silicon, Vanadium, and Zinc. Panel on Micronutrients, Subcommittees on Upper Reference Levels of Nutrients and of Interpretation and Use of Dietary Reference Intakes, and the Standing Committee on the Scientific Evaluation of Dietary Reference Intakes. 2001. Available at www.nap.edu/books/0309072794/html/.
6. Finley JW, Johnson PE, Johnson LK. Sex affects manganese absorption and retention by humans from a diet adequate in manganese. *Am J Clin Nutr* 1994; 60: 949-55.
7. Garcia-Avila M and Penalver-Ballina R. Manganese poisoning in the mines of Cuba. *Ind Med Surg* 1953; 22: 220-1.
8. Rodier J. Manganese poisoning in Moroccan miners. *Br J Ind Med* 1955; 12: 21-35.
9. Myers JE, teWaterNaude J, Fourie M, Zogoe HB, Naik I, Theodorou P, Tassel H, Daya A, Thompson ML. Nervous system effects of occupational manganese exposure on South African manganese mineworkers. *Neurotoxicology* 2003; 24: 649-56.
10. Racette BA, McGee-Minnich L, Moerlein SM, Mink JW, Videen TO, Perlmutter JS. Welding-related parkinsonism: Clinical features, treatment, and pathophysiology. *Neurology* 2001; 56: 8-13.
11. Levy BS and Nassetta WJ. Neurologic effects of manganese in humans: A review. *Int J Occup Environ Health* 2003; 9: 153-63.
12. Sadek AH, Rauch R, Schulz PE. Parkinsonism due to manganism in a welder. *Int J Toxicol* 2003; 22: 393-401.

13. Racette, BA, Antenor JA, McGee-Minnich L, Moerlein SM, Videen TO, Kotagal V, Perlmutter JS. [^{18}F]FDOPA PET and clinical features in parkinsonism due to manganism. *Mov Disord* 2005; 20: 492-6.
14. Roels H, Lauwerys R, Genet P, et al. Relationship between external and internal parameters of exposure to manganese in workers from a manganese oxide and salt producing plant. *Am J Ind Med* 1987; 11: 297-305.
15. Pal PK, Samii A, Calne DB. Manganese neurotoxicity: A review of clinical features, imaging and pathology. *Neurotoxicology* 1999; 20: 227-38.
16. Aschner M, Aschner JL. Manganese transport across the blood-brain barrier: relationship to iron homeostasis. *Brain Res Bull* 1990; 24: 857-60.
17. Aschner M, Gannon M. Manganese (Mn) transport across the rat blood-brain barrier: saturable and transferrin-dependent transport mechanisms. *Brain Res Bull* 1994; 33:345-49.
18. Aschner M, Aschner JL. Manganese neurotoxicity: cellular effects and blood-brain barrier transport. *Neurosci Biobehav Rev* 1991; 15: 333-40.
19. Crossgrove JS, Yokel RA. Manganese distribution across the blood-brain barrier III: The divalent metal transporter-1 is not the major mechanism mediating brain manganese uptake. *Neurotoxicology* 2004; 25: 451-60.
20. Yokel RA, Crossgrove JS. Manganese toxicokinetics at the blood-brain barrier. *Res Rep Health Eff Inst* 2004; 119: 7-73.
21. Erikson KM, Syverson T, Steinnes E, Aschner M. Globus pallidus: A target brain region for divalent metal accumulation associated with dietary iron deficiency. *J Nutr Biochem* 2004; 15: 335-41.
22. Kim Y, Park JK, Choi Y, Yoo CI, Lee CR, Lee H, Lee JH, Kim SR, Jeong TH, Yoon CS, Park JH. Blood manganese concentration is elevated in iron deficiency anemia patients, whereas globus pallidus signal intensity is minimally affected. *Neurotoxicology* 2005; 26: 107-11.
23. Murphy VA, Wadhwani KC, Smith QR, Rapoport SI. Saturable transport of manganese (II) across the rat blood-brain barrier. *J Neurochem* 1991; 57: 948-54.
24. Rabin O, Hegedus L, Bourre JM, Smith QR. Rapid brain uptake of manganese (II) across the blood-brain barrier. *J Neurochem* 1993; 61: 509-17.
25. Pautler RG, Koretsky AP. Tracing odor-induced activation in the olfactory bulbs of mice using manganese-enhanced magnetic resonance imaging. *Neuroimage* 2002; 16: 441-8.
26. Pautler RG, Silva AC, Koretsky AP. *In vivo* neuronal tract tracing using manganese-enhanced magnetic resonance imaging. *Magn Reson Med* 1998; 40: 740-8.
27. Allegrini PR, Wiessner C. Three-dimensional MRI of cerebral projections in rat brain *in vivo* after intracortical injection of $MnCl_2$. *NMR Biomed* 2003; 16: 252-6.
28. Watanabe T, Natt O, Boretius S, Frahm J, Michaelis T. *In vivo* 3D MRI staining of mouse brain after subcutaneous application of $MnCl_2$. *Magn Reson Med* 2002; 48: 852-9.
29. Ryu S, Brown SL, Kolozsvary A, Ewing JR, Kim JH. Noninvasive detection of radiation-induced optic neuropathy by manganese enhanced MRI. *Radiat Res* 2002; 157: 500-5.
30. Lin CP, Tseng WY, Cheng HC, Chen JH. Validation of diffusion tensor magnetic resonance axonal fiber imaging with registered manganese-enhanced optic tracts. *Neuroimage* 2001; 14: 1035-47.
31. Malecki EA, Cook BM, Devenyi AG, Beard JL, Connor JR. Transferrin is required for normal distribution of ^{59}Fe and ^{54}Mn in brains of mice. *J Neurol Sci* 1999; 170: 112-18.
32. Malecki EA, Devenyi AG, Barron TF, Mosher TJ, Eslinger P, Flaherty-Craig CV, Rossaro L. Iron and manganese homeostasis in chronic liver disease: relationship to pallidal T1-weighted magnetic resonance signal hyperintensity. *Neurotoxicology* 1999; 20: 647-52.
33. Dickinson TK, Connor JR. Histological analysis of selected brain regions of hypotransferrinemic mice. *Brain Res* 1994; 635: 169-78.
34. DeMaeyer E, Adiels-Tegman M. The prevalence of anaemia in the world. *World Health Stat Q* 1985; 38: 302-16.
35. Erikson KM, Shihabi ZK, Aschner JL, Aschner M. Manganese accumulates in iron deficient rat brain regions in a heterogeneous fashion and is associated with neurochemical alterations. *Biol Trace Elem Res*, 2002; 87: 143-56.
36. Gunter RE, Puskin JS, Russell PR. Quantitative magnetic resonance studies of manganese uptake by mitochondria. *Biophys J*, 1975; 15: 319-33.
37. Gavin CE, Gunter KK, Gunter TE. Manganese and calcium transport in mitochondria: implications for manganese toxicity. Neurotoxicology, 1999; 20: 445-53.
38. Brouillet EP, Shinobu L, McGarvey U, Hochberg F, Beal MF. Manganese injection into the rat striatum produces excitotoxic lesions by impairing energy metabolism. *Exp Neurol* 1993; 120: 89-94.

39. Oestreicher E, Sengstock GJ, Riederer P, Olanow CW, Dunn AJ, Arendash GW. Degeneration of nigrostriatal dopaminergic neurons increases iron within the substantia nigra: a histochemical and neurochemical study. *Brain Res* 1994; 660: 8-18.
40. Kienzl E, Puchinger L, Jellinger K, Linert W, Stachelberger H, Jameson RF. The role of transition metals in the pathogenesis of Parkinson's disease. *J Neurol Sci* 1995; 134: 69-78.
41. Lee JM, Johnson JA. An important role of Nrf2-ARE pathway in the cellular defense mechanism. *J Biochem Mol Biol* 2004; 37: 139-43.
42. Jakel RJ, Kern JT, Johnson DA, Johnson JA. Induction of the protective antioxidant response element pathway by 6-hydroxydopamine in vivo and in vitro. *Toxicol Sci* 2005; 87: 176-86.
43. Chun HS, Gibson GE, DeGiorgio LA, Zhang H, Kidd VJ, Son JH. Dopaminergic cell death induced by MPP(+), oxidant and specific neurotoxicants shares the common molecular mechanism. *J Neurochem* 2001; 76: 1010-21.
44. Tomas-Camardiel M, Herrera AJ, Venero JL, Cruz Sanchez-Hidalgo M, Cano J, Machado A. Differential regulation of glutamic acid decarboxylase mRNA and tyrosine hydroxylase mRNA expression in the aged manganese-treated rats. *Mol Brain Res* 2002; 103: 116-29.
45. HaMai D, Bondy SC. Oxidative basis of manganese neurotoxicity. *Ann N Y Acad Sci* 2004; 1012:129-41
46. Stredrick DL, Stokes AH, Worst TJ, Freeman WM, Johnson EA, Lash LH, Aschner M, Vrana KE. Manganese-induced cytotoxicity in dopamine-producing cells. *Neurotoxicology* 2004; 25: 543-53.
47. Chun HS, Gibson GE, DeGiorgio LA, Zhang H, Kidd VJ, Son JH. Dopaminergic cell death induced by MPP(+), oxidant and specific neurotoxicants shares the common molecular mechanism. *J Neurochem* 2001; 76: 1010-21.

Metal Ions in Biology and Medicine: vol. 9. Eds Maria Carmen Alpoim, Paula Vasconcellos Morais, Maria Amélia Santos, Armando J. Cristóvão, José A. Centeno, Philippe Collery.
John Libbey Eurotext, Paris © 2006 pp. 507-1.

The Role of Molybdenum in Biology

Maria João Romão

REQUIMTE-CQFB, Departamento de Química, FCT-Universidade Nova de Lisboa, 2829-516 Caparica, Portugal, mromao@dq.fct.unl.pt

INTRODUCTION

With the exception of the multinuclear $MoFe_7$ cluster present in nitrogenase, which catalyzes the reduction of dinitrogen to ammonia, molybdenum is found in most (if not all) molybdoenzymes in a mononuclear form, which possesses an organic pyranopterin cofactor *(fig. 1)* coordinated to the metal:

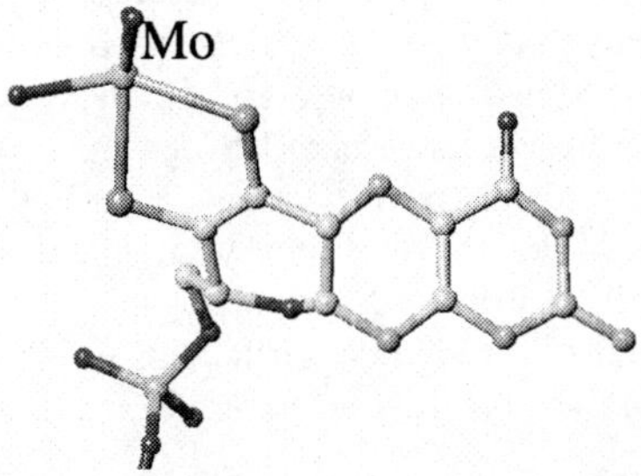

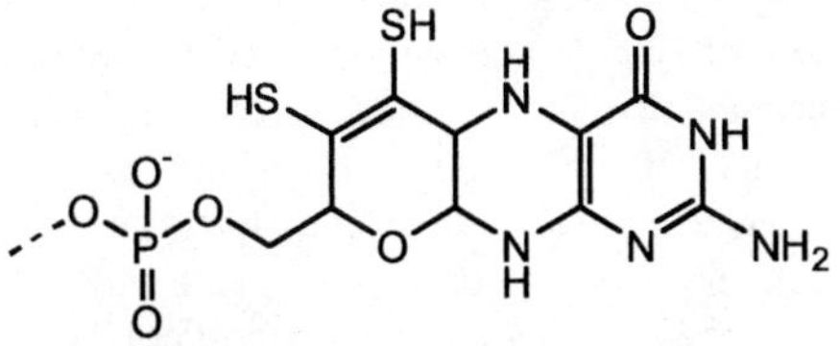

Fig. 1. The structure of the pyranopterin cofactor present in mononuclear molybdenum enzymes. It is depicted only the monophosphate form (MPT).

Molybdenum is an essential trace element in animal and human nutrition and is required for the activity of several enzymes that are involved in catabolism, including the catabolism of purines and the sulfur amino acids. In plants, molybdenum is required for proper nitrogen assimilation involving a nitrate reductase. In human health, molybdenum is essential in the mechanism of action of xanthine oxidase, sulfite oxidase and aldehyde oxidase, enzymes which are involved in diseases such as gout, radical damage following cardiac failure and combined oxidase deficiency. Deficiency of the molybdenum cofactor, although rare, causes a severe disease in humans and all of the pterin-dependent enzymes - xanthine oxidase/dehydrogenase, sulfite oxidase and aldehyde oxidase - are affected. This combined enzyme deficiency has major consequences such as severe neurological abnormalities, dislocated ocular lenses and mental retardation.

MOLYBDOTERIN-CONTAINING ENZYMES

The pterin-dependent molybdenum enzymes are ubiquitous in nature and are found in almost all forms of life [1-4]. They catalyze a wide range of (mostly) redox reactions, crucial in the metabolism of nitrogen, sulfur and carbon compounds. An essential role of molybdenum is the catalysis of an oxo-transfer reaction coupled to electron-transfer between substrate and other cofactors such as iron-sulfur centers ([2Fe-2S] or [4Fe-4S]), hemes or flavins.

In the active site, molybdenum is coordinated to the *cis*-dithiolene group of one or two pyranopterins plus additional terminal oxo/hydroxo groups and/or sulfido groups or side chains of serine, cysteine, selenocysteine or aspartate residues in a diversity of arrangements. The pterin cofactor can be present either as the monophosphate form (MPT) or with a nucleotide molecule attached by a pyrophosphate link: molybdopterin guanine dinucleotide (MGD) or molybdopterin citosine dinucleotide (MCD).

Molybdopterin containing enzymes have been grouped into three broad families *(fig. 2)* [1], a classification based on X-ray structural data and supported by spectroscopic and biochemical data as well as primary sequence alignments: (1) The xanthine oxidase family ((MCD or MPT) Mo^{VI} = O, = S, -H_2O); (2) the sulfite oxidase family ((MPT) Mo^{VI} = O, -H_2O, (-SCys)). and (3) The DMSO reductase family ($(MGD)_2$ Mo^{VI} = O, (-OSer, -SCys, -SeCys or -OAsp)). In general terms, these enzymes catalyze the transfer of an oxygen atom from water to product (or vice versa) in reactions that imply a net exchange of two electrons between enzyme and substrate and in which the metal ion cycles between the redox states IV and VI.

The Xanthine Oxidase family

The xanthine oxidase family includes enzymes such as xanthine oxidase, xanthine dehydrogenase [5, 6] and aldehyde oxidase [7]. Xanthine dehydrogenase catalyzes the conversion of hypoxanthine to xanthine, and xanthine to uric acid. Xanthine oxidase, which is formed from xanthine dehydrogenase, also catalyzes the reactions of purine catabolism but is not NADH-dependent and reactive oxygen species (ROS) are formed as products of the reaction. Aldehyde oxidase is involved in a number of reactions, including the catabolism of pyrimidines and the biotransformation of xenobiotics.

These enzymes catalyze the oxidative hydroxylation of a diverse range of aldehydes and aromatic heterocycles in reactions that involve the cleavage of a C-H and the formation of a C-O bond. Biochemical and crystallographic studies of inhibited forms of the enzymes indicate that the oxygen transferred to the substrate comes from the water/hydroxyl ligand of the Mo atom.

Members of this family possess a $Mo^{VI}OS$ nucleus and one molybdopterin with no covalent bonding between the cofactor and the polypeptide chain. In the coordination sphere is an additional hydroxo group.

Enzymes belonging to this group are usually organized as α_2 homodimers, as the eukaryotic xanthine oxidases and xanthine dehydrogenases, with the several redox-active cofactors placed within a single subunit, or as multisubunit enzymes ($\alpha_2\beta_2\gamma_2$). In the case of the α_2 structures, two different types of [2Fe-2S] centers are located in two small N-terminal domains, followed by the flavin domain and finally by the largest C-terminal domain, which embeds the molybdopterin cofactor. In the multisubunit modular enzymes those redox centers are found within independent subunits.

The Sulfite Oxidase family

The sulfite oxidase family also includes the assimilatory nitrate reductase. Enzymes within this family typically have one molybdopterin cofactor and a $Mo^{VI}O_2$ nucleus and the polypeptide chain coordinates directly to the molybdenum site by a cysteinyl residue [8, 9]. Sulfite oxidase catalyzes the physiologically vital oxidation of sulfite to sulfate, the terminal reaction in the oxidative degradation of the sulfur containing amino acids cysteine and methionine.

The DMSO Reductase family

The DMSOR family is a considerably larger and diverse one, and encompasses enzymes such as biotin-S-oxide reductase, dissimilatory nitrate reductase and formate dehydrogenase [10-12].

Members of this family catalyze the transfer of an oxygen atom to or from a lone electron pair of the substrate, with the only exception of the formate dehydrogenases which reaction does not involve an oxo-transfer.

The proteins of the DMSO Reductase family present the widest diversity of properties among members. The first crystal structure reported for a member of this family was the DMSO reductase.

However, our knowledge about this family was highly increased with the study of nitrate reductase, which catalyzes the reduction of nitrate to nitrite, and formate dehydrogenase, involved in the oxidation of formate to carbon dioxide. The metal atom in both enzymes is coordinated by two pterin cofactors, in which each pterin molecule has a guanine nucleotide, and different types of ligands as shown in *figure 2*. The aminoacid which coordinates the Mo atom differs among the several enzymes of the family: cysteine in nitrate reductase, selenum-cysteine in formate dehydrogenase, aspartate in the membrane-bound nitrate reductases and a serine in DMSO reductase [10].

The few examples of enzymes capable of incorporating either molybdenum or tungsten at the active site (of formate dehydrogenases [12]) belong to this family.

For members of all three classes several crystal structures became available in the past decade and have been a major contribution towards understanding the corresponding enzymatic function at the atomic level. They have provided a structural basis for the understanding of the involved reaction mechanisms. In addition, a wealth of information on some of these systems by spectroscopic methods has also been accumulated over the years and, together with the structural data, can contribute to a more detailed understanding of the chemistry of the multiple reactions carried out by molybdenum in Biology.

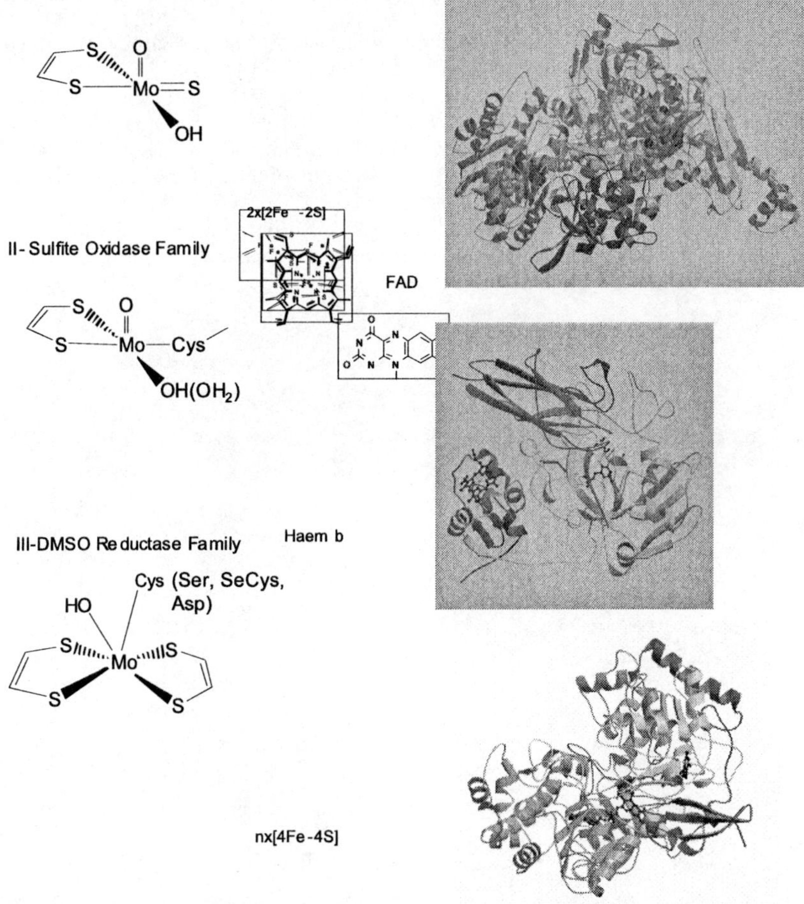

Fig. 2. The three families of mononuclear molybdenum enzymes. On the left, the Mo active site, in the middle, additional cofactors involved in electron transfer, on the right, crystal structures of bovine milk xantine oxidase [6], of chicken liver sulfite oxidase [8] and of Desulfovibrio desulfuricans ATCC2774 nitrate reductase [10].

REFERENCES

1. Hille R, The Mononuclear Molybdenum Enzymes. *Chem Rev* 1996, 96:2757-281.
2. Hille R, Molybdenum-containing hydroxylases. *Arch Biochem Biophys* 2005, 433:107-116.
3. Hille R, Structure and Function on Xanthine Oxidoreductase, *Eur. J. Inorg. Chem.* 2006.
4. Romao MJ, Knablein J, Huber R, Moura JJ: Structure and function of molybdopterin containing enzymes. *Prog Biophys Mol Biol* 1997, 68:121-144.
5. Okamoto K, Matsumoto K, Hille R, Eger BT, Pai EF, Nishino T. The crystal structure of xanthine oxidoreductase during catalysis: implications for reaction mechanism and enzyme inhibition. *Proc Natl Acad Sci USA*. 2004, 101(21):7931-6.
6. Enroth C, Eger BT, Okamoto K, Nishino T, Nishino T, Pai EF. Crystal structures of bovine milk xanthine dehydrogenase and xanthine oxidase: structure-based mechanism of conversion. *Proc Natl Acad Sci USA*. 2000, 97(20):10723-8.
7. Garattini E, Mendel R, Romao MJ, Wright R, Terao M., Mammalian molybdo-flavoenzymes, an expanding family of proteins: structure, genetics, regulation, function and pathophysiology. *Biochem J.* 2003, 372:15-32.
8. Kisker C, Schindelin H, Pacheco A, Wehbi WA, Garrett RM, Rajagopalan KV, Enemark JH, Rees DC. Molecular basis of sulfite oxidase deficiency from the structure of sulfite oxidase. *Cell.* 1997 Dec 26;91(7):973-83.
9. Karakas E, Wilson HL, Graf TN, Xiang S, Jaramilho-Busquets S, Rajagopalan KV, Kisker C, Structural insights into sulfite oxidase deficiency. *J. Biol. Chem.* 2005; 280(39):33506-15.
10. Moura JJ, Brondino CD, Trincao J, Romao MJ., Mo and W bis-MGD enzymes: nitrate reductases and formate dehydrogenases. *J Biol Inorg Chem.* 2004 Oct;9(7):791-9.
11. Dias JM, Than ME, Humm A, Huber R, Bourenkov GP, Bartunik HD, Bursakov S, Calvete J, Caldeira J, Carneiro C, Moura JJ, Moura I, Romao MJ. Crystal structure of the first dissimilatory nitrate reductase at 1.9 A solved by MAD methods. *Structure* 1999, 7:65-79
12. Raaijmakers H, Macieira S, Dias JM, Teixeira S, Bursakov S, Huber R, Moura JJ, Moura I, Romao MJ. Gene sequence and the 1.8 A crystal structure of the tungsten-containing formate dehydrogenase from Desulfovibrio gigas. *Structure.* 2002 Sep;10(9):1261-72.

Metal Ions in Biology and Medicine: vol. 9. Eds Maria Carmen Alpoim, Paula Vasconcellos Morais, Maria Amélia Santos, Armando J. Cristóvão, José A. Centeno, Philippe Collery.
John Libbey Eurotext, Paris © 2006 pp. 511-1.

Arsenic and peripheral arterial disease in Taiwan

Chin-Hsiao Tseng*, Ching-Ping Tseng, Choon-Khim Chong, Tong-Yuan Tai, Jose A. Centeno

*Division of Endocrinology and Metabolism, Department of Internal Medicine, National Taiwan University Hospital; National Taiwan University College of Medicine; School of Medical Technology, Chang Gung University; Department of Rehabilitation, Chang Gung Memorial Hospital; Armed Forces Institute of Pathology, USA. *Address for correspondence: No. 7 Chung-Shan South Road, Taipei, Taiwan; email: ccktsh@ms6.hinet.net*

"Blackfoot disease (BFD)" is an endemic peripheral arterial disease (PAD) confined to the southwest of Taiwan. Sporadic cases occurred as early as in the early 20th century and peak incidence was noted between 1956 and 1960, with prevalence rates ranged from 6.51 to 18.85 per 1,000 population. A series of studies conducted during the mid-20th century has linked the etiology of BFD to the drinking of high arsenic-containing well water. More recent studies confirmed the relationship between exposure to arsenic and the risk of PAD in a dose-responsive pattern. A latest study showed that a less capability to methylate inorganic arsenic is closely linked to the risk of PAD among residents of the BFD areas. This paper reviews a series of studies on arsenic and PAD carried out in the BFD area in Taiwan and discusses the possible mechanisms associated with arsenic-induced atherosclerosis.

ARSENIC CONCENTRATIONS IN WELL WATER AND BLACKFOOT DISEASE

In villages where the arsenic concentrations in consumed well water were <0.30 mg/L, 0.30-0.59 mg/L, and ≥0.60 mg/L, the prevalence rates of BFD for residents aged 20-39 years were 0.5%, 1.3%, and 1.4%, respectively; for residents aged 40-59 years, 1.1%, 3.2%, and 4.7%, respectively; and for residents aged ≥60 years, 2.0%, 3.2%, and 6.1%, respectively [1]. This early study suggested that the prevalence of BFD increased with regards to increasing arsenic concentrations of the well water, which could not be explained by age.

ARSENIC EXPOSURE AND PERIPHERAL ARTERIAL DISEASE

To further clarify the effect of arsenic exposure on the development of PAD among the residents of the BFD areas, Tseng et al. carried out a series of studies by using Doppler ultrasound as a diagnostic tool, calculating indices for estimating individual dosage of arsenic exposure, and controlling possible confounders for PAD since early 1990s [2, 3]. The prevalence rates of PAD for those with a cumulative arsenic exposure (CAE) of 0, 0.1-19.9 and ≥ 20 mg/L-years were 4.4, 11.6 and 19.8%, respectively; and the respective multivariate-adjusted odds ratios were 1.00, 2.77 (0.84-9.14) and 4.28 (1.26-14.54) [2]. These later studies fortified the link between arsenic exposure and development of PAD in the BFD areas in Taiwan.

ARSENIC METHYLATION AND PERIPHERAL ARTERIAL DISEASE

Because only a small proportion of the arsenic-exposed residents would develop PAD, individual capacity to metabolize and detoxify the ingested inorganic arsenic was believed to play an important role on disease development. Recently Tseng et al. examined the interaction between arsenic exposure and urinary arsenic species on the risk of PAD diagnosed by Doppler ultrasound in 479 (220 men and 259 women) adults residing in the BFD areas in Taiwan [4]. Arsenic exposure was estimated by CAE. Urinary levels of total arsenic, inorganic arsenite and arsenate, monomethylarsonic acid (MMA^V) and dimethylarsinic acid (DMA^V) were determined, and primary methylation index ($PMI=MMA^V$/urinary inorganic arsenic) and secondary methylation index ($SMI=DMA^V/MMA^V$) were calculated and used as indices for the capability to methylate inorganic arsenic. Results showed that the multivariate-adjusted odds ratios for CAE of 0, 0.1-15.4 and >15.4 mg/L×year were 1.00, 3.41 (0.74-15.78) and 4.62 (0.96-22.21), respectively ($p<0.05$, trend test); and for PMI ≤ 1.77 and SMI>6.93, PMI>1.77 and SMI>6.93, PMI>1.77 and SMI ≤ 6.93, and PMI ≤ 1.77 and SMI ≤ 6.93 were 1.00, 2.93 (0.90-9.52), 2.85 (1.05-7.73) and 3.60 (1.12-11.56), respectively ($p<0.05$, trend test). Therefore, PAD risk not only increased with a higher CAE but also with a lower capacity to methylate arsenic to DMA^V.

CONCOMITANT INCREASE OF HEART DISEASE AND STROKE

Residents in the BFD areas also have a significantly increased risk of [5] and mortality from [6] ischemic heart disease and stroke [7], which were also correlated with arsenic exposure in a dose-responsive pattern. These findings were compatible with the pathological findings of severe generalized atherosclerosis in BFD patients as shown by Yeh and How [8], and with the finding of cardiovascular disease representing a major cause of death (44%) in the BFD patients [1]. Therefore, arsenic-induced atherosclerosis is systemic.

CO-OCCURRENCE WITH SKIN LESIONS AND NEUROPATHY

The association between arsenic exposure and BFD is also supported by the observation that BFD patients had a high co-occurrence of arsenic skin lesions such as hyperpigmentation, hyperkeratosis, and skin cancer [9] and residents in the BFD areas had a higher risk of sensory neuropathy [10], which is well known for acute arsenic intoxication. These observations suggested that chronic arsenic exposure could play an important etiologic role.

DECLINE OF BFD AFTER CESSATION OF ARSENIC-CONTAINING WATER

Tap water supply to the endemic areas was not available before the 1960s and its coverage remained low until the 1970s. The incidence rates of BFD per 100,000 person-years for men and women were 44.3 and 36.5, respectively, for those who consumed artesian well water; and were 2.9 and 3.1 for men and women, respectively, for those who used tap water in the same areas [11]. The occurrence of BFD decreased dramatically over the past decades after tap water supply was implemented [11]. Most new cases after the 1970s occurred in people above 50 years of age, while BFD might occur in those below 30 years of age before the 1950s [11]. A recent study also showed that ischemic heart disease mortality declines gradually about 17 to 21 years after the cessation of consuming high-arsenic artesian well water in the BFD areas, which is contrary to an increasing trend of cardiovascular mortality in the general population of Taiwan [12]. These findings strengthen the likelihood that an association exists between arsenic exposure and the development of atherosclerotic diseases.

EVIDENCE FROM ANIMAL STUDY

A recent study treating $ApoE^{-/-}/LDLr^{-/-}$ mice with 133 μM (10 ppm) sodium arsenite in drinking water for 18 weeks has successfully induced a significant increase in atherosclerotic plaques in the innominate artery while compared to controls [13]. This animal model provided evidence for biological plausibility of arsenic-induced atherosclerosis observed in humans.

PATHOGENETIC MECHANISMS

Arsenic is genotoxic [14], causes damage to endothelial cells [15], causes endothelial dysfunction [16], increases coagulability [17], decreases fibrinolysis [18], induces oxidative stress with impaired nitric oxide balance [19, 20], enhances inflammatory activity [21], promotes apoptosis [22], and stimulates smooth muscle cell proliferation [23]. Arsenic can also interact with other trace elements [24-29] and is associated with hypertension [30] and diabetes mellitus [31]. All of these could trigger, predispose, or aggravate the process of atherosclerosis.

Arsenic induces endothelial dysfunction [16], peroxynitrite generation and cyclooxygenase-2 protein expression in endothelial cells [32]. Arsenic also induces expression of genes coding for inflammatory mediators including IL-8 in human aortic endothelial cell [21]. Some recent studies demonstrated that arsenic induces antioxidative enzymes, including heme oxygenase-1, thioredoxin peroxidase-2, NADPH dehydrogenase, and glutathione *S*-transferase P subunit, suggesting the induction of oxidative stress by arsenic [20]. Our previous study demonstrated the existence of microcirculatory defects in seemingly normal subjects living in the BFD areas [33]. A recent *in vitro* study confirmed that exposure of human microvascular endothelial cells to arsenic resulted in a decrease of tissue-type plasminogen activator and an increase in plasminogen activator inhibitor type-1 expression as well as reduced fibrinolysis, which were not likely shown in the macrovascular endothelial cells [18]. An endemic area of chronic arsenic poisoning and experimental animal studies elucidated a potential *in vivo* impairment of nitric oxide formation and oxidative stress caused by prolonged exposure to arsenate in the drinking water [34]. Bunderson et al. [13] reported that changes in specific inflammatory mediators such as leukotriene and prostacyclin are related to arsenic-induced atherosclerosis.

Trivalent methylated arsenic species are more toxic than the inorganic compounds. MMA^{III} and DMA^{III} exhibit properties of inhibition on cysteine-containing enzymes [35], cellular toxicity [36], genotoxicity, and clastogenicity [37]. In addition, MMA^{III} is a potent and irreversible inhibitor of an enzyme involved in cellular response to oxidative stress [38]. The DNA damage induced by methylated trivalent arsenicals can either be direct [39] or mediated by the reactive oxygen species formed concomitantly with the oxidation of DMA^{III} to DMA^{V} [40]. DMA^{III} can produce dimethylarsinic peroxyl radical and dimethylarsinic radical [41]. A recent study demonstrated that insulin-dependent glucose uptake by 3T3-L1 adipocytes is also inhibited by trivalent arsenicals, either in inorganic form or in methylated form [42].

Increased mutation rate is involved in the formation of atherosclerotic plaques [43]. Although arsenic does not cause point mutation, it does induce cell transformation, chromosomal aberrations, sister chromatid exchanges, and gene amplification [11]. Arsenite can initiate gene transcription by altering signal-transduction molecules [44]. It is possible that arsenic induces atherosclerosis via its actions on the structure and expression of related genes.

Nitrogen and phosphorus are important elements of DNA, RNA, and proteins. Arsenic shares many similar chemical properties with these elements. Adenosine triphosphate (ATP) plays a major role in the regulation of many enzymes involving in the process of phosphorylation and dephosphorylation. Arsenic may hinder normal enzymatic functions by disrupting the formation of ATP from adenosine diphosphate (ADP) and orthophosphate [44]. Arsenite reacts strongly with sulfhydryl groups of proteins and it may interfere with the normal biochemical functions of proteins regulated by the formation/destruction of -S-S- bonds involving the cysteine side chains in the proteins [44]. Whether arsenic may induce atherosclerosis through its interference with structural or functional proteins involved in the atherosclerotic process requires further investigations.

Oxidative stress promotes atherosclerotic processes through oxidation of low-density lipoprotein (LDL), activation of nuclear factor (B, and induction of the immediate early genes *c-myc* and *c-fos* [11]. A study by Lynn et al. has shown that arsenite increases nicotinamide adenine dinucleotide (NADH) oxidase activity and produces superoxide, which then causes oxidative DNA damage in human vascular smooth muscle cells [19]. Addition of the radical-scavenging enzyme superoxide dismutase also decreased the frequency of arsenic-induced sister chromatid exchanges in human peripheral lymphocytes [45]. A recent study in Inner Mongolia, China demonstrated the presence of oxidative stress in human body with chronic arsenic exposure and that the methylated metabolites were associated with oxidative stress [46].

Atherosclerosis is characterized by apoptosis, and the rupture of the atherosclerotic plaques is always associated with the onset of clinical cardiovascular events [11]. Vascular apoptosis is promoted by superoxide and oxidized LDL [47]. Arsenic can produce a variety of stress responses leading eventually to apoptosis. Arsenic has been found to induce apoptosis not only in hematopoietic malignant cells, but also in solid tumors like neuroblastoma [22]. It is also possible that arsenic can produce apoptosis in the vasculature.

The co-contamination of arsenic and other trace elements could modulate the chronic toxicity of arsenic, and the interaction between arsenic and the other trace elements could also explain partly the differential manifestation of its atherogenicity in different populations or even among the same population in a single endemic area. Arsenic can lead to a significant increase in renal copper excretion and potentiate the effects of lead and cadmium when used together [25]. The effect of selenium can be antagonized by administration of arsenic, probably through the action of enhancing biliary excretion of selenium [26]. Pershagen et al. reported that smoking and arsenic inhalation have a multiplicative effect on lung cancer mortality in smelter workers [27], and there are evidences of a positive interaction between arsenic and benzo(a)pyrene, a carcinogen found as a by-product of combustion [28].

Zinc is protective for cardiovascular disease and has been found to function in the control of apoptotic cell death by inhibiting the disruption of endothelial cell integrity, DNA fragmentation, and cytolysis of murine cells induced by tumor necrosis factor [24, 48]. A simultaneous deficiency of zinc as observed in some BFD patients can aggravate atherosclerosis [48]. Arsenic can compete with zinc in metal-binding proteins, displaying vicinal dithiols contained in zinc fingers of DNA binding and repair proteins and transcription factors [48]. The proteins, conformational change can lead to altered biologic function.

According to recent epidemiologic studies in the BFD areas, arsenic exposure is also associated in a dose-responsive pattern with hypertension [30] and diabetes mellitus [31], two of the major risk factors of atherosclerosis. Thus, it is possible that hypertension and diabetes mellitus explain partly the higher rate of atherosclerotic disease associated with arsenic. However, the atherosclerotic effect of arsenic is independent, because the association persists even after controlling for the confounding effect of both of these factors.

CONCLUSIONS

A series of epidemiologic studies carried out in the BFD area of Taiwan and biological and cellular studies favored an etiologic role of arsenic on the development of atherosclerosis including PAD. However, one question remains frequently asked is why endemic occurrence of PAD as observed in the BFD areas in Taiwan is not similarly seen in other areas with arsenic problems like Bangladesh, West Bengal India, Inner Mongolia and Guizhou of China and parts of United States, Mexico, Chile and Argentina. Some of the explanations are the different manifestations of arsenic exposure in different ethnicities, shorter durations of exposure in some areas, the effect of different nutritional status and genetic difference in the metabolism of arsenic. However, the existence of other co-contaminants or other etiologic factors can not be completely excluded.

REFERENCES

1. Tseng WP. Blackfoot disease in Taiwan: A 30-year follow-up study. Angiology 1989;40:547-558.
2. Tseng CH, Chong CK, Chen CJ, Tai TY. Dose-response relationship between peripheral vascular disease and ingested inorganic arsenic among residents in blackfoot disease endemic villages in Taiwan. Atherosclerosis 1996;20:125-133.
3. Tseng CH, Chong CK, Chen CJ, Tai TY. Lipid profile and peripheral vascular disease in arseniasis-hyperendemic villages in Taiwan. Angiology 1997;48:321-335.
4. Tseng CH, Huang YK, Huang YL, Chung CJ, Yang MH, Chen CJ, Hsueh YM. Arsenic exposure, urinary arsenic speciation and peripheral vascular disease in blackfoot disease-hyperendemic villages in Taiwan. Toxicol Appl Pharmacol 2005;206:299-308.
5. Tseng CH, Chong CK, Tseng CP, Hsueh YM, Chiou HY, Tseng CC, Chen CJ. Long-term arsenic exposure and ischemic heart disease in arseniasis-hyperendemic villages in Taiwan. Toxicol Lett 2003;137:15-21.
6. Chen CJ, Chiou HY, Chiang MH, Lin LJ, Tai TY. Dose-response relationship between ischemic heart disease mortality and long-term arsenic exposure. Arterioscler Thromb Vasc Biol 1996;16:504-510.
7. Chiou HY, Huang WI, Su CL, Chang SF, Hsu YH, Chen CJ. Dose-response relationship between prevalence of cerebrovascular disease and ingested inorganic arsenic. Stroke 1997;28:1717-1723.
8. Yeh S, How SW. A pathological study on the blackfoot disease in Taiwan. Reports, Institute of Pathology, National Taiwan University 1963;14:25-73.
9. Tseng WP, Chu HM, How SW, Fong JM, Lin CS, Yeh S. Prevalence of skin cancer in an endemic area of chronic arsenicism in Taiwan. J Natl Cancer Inst 1968;40:453-463.
10. Tseng CH. Abnormal current perception thresholds measured by Neurometer among residents in blackfoot disease hyperendemic villages in Taiwan. Toxicol Lett 2003;146:27-36.
11. Tseng CH. An overview on peripheral vascular disease in blackfoot disease-hyperendemic villages in Taiwan. Angiology 2002;53:529-537.
12. Chang CC, Ho SC, Tsai SS, Yang CY. Ischemic heart disease mortality reduction in an arseniasis-endemic area in southwestern Taiwan after a switch in the tap-water supply system. J Toxicol Environ Health A 2004;67:1353-1361.
13. Bunderson M, Brooks DM, Walker DL, Rosenfeld ME, Coffin JD, Beall HD. Arsenic exposure exacerbates atherosclerotic plaque formation and increases nitrotyrosine and leukotriene biosynthesis. Toxicol Appl Pharmacol 2004;201:32-39.
14. Liou SH, Chen YH, Loh CH, Yang T, Wu TN, Chen CJ, Hsieh LL. The association between frequencies of mitomycin C-induced sister chromatid exchange and cancer risk in arseniasis. Toxicol Lett 2002;29:237-243.
15. Chen GS, Asai T, Suzuki Y, Nishioka K, Nishiyama S. A possible pathogenesis for blackfoot disease: effects of trivalent arsenic (As_2O_3) on cultured human umbilical vein endothelial cells. J Dermatol 1990;17:599-608.
16. Lee MY, Jung BI, Chung SM, Bae ON, Lee JY, Park JD, Yang JS, Lee H, Chung JH. Arsenic-induced dysfunction in relaxation of blood vessels. Environ Health Perspect 2003;111:513-517.
17. Shen MC, Tseng WP, Chen KS. Increased blood level of platelet aggregates and coagulating factors in blackfoot disease patients (in Chinese). Blackfoot Dis Res Rep 1983;15:20-28.
18. Jiang SJ, Lin TM, Wu HL, Han HS, Shi GY. Decrease of fibrinolytic activity in human endothelial cells by arsenite. Thromb Res 2002;105:55-62.
19. Lynn S, Gurr JR, Lai HT, Jan KY. NADH oxidase activation is involoved in arsenite-induced oxidative DNA damage in human vascular smooth muscle cells. Circ Res 2000;86:514-519.
20. Hirano S, Cui X, Li S, Kanno S, Kobayashi Y, Hayakawa T, Shraim A. Difference in uptake and toxicity of trivalent and pentavalent inorganic arsenic in rat heart microvessel endothelial cells. Arch Toxicol 2003;77:305-312.
21. Simeonova PP, Hulderman T, Harki D, Luster MI. Arsenic exposure accelerates atherogenesis in apolipoprotein e-/- mice. Environ Health Perspect 2003;111:1744-1748.

22. Akao Y, Yamada H, Nakagawa Y. Arsenic-induced apoptosis in malignant cells in vitro. Leuk Lymphoma 2000;37:53-63.
23. Lilienfeld DE. Arsenic, geographical isolates, environmental epidemiology and arteriosclerosis. Arteriosclerosis 1988;8:449-451.
24. Waalkes MP, Fox DA, States JC, Patierno SR, McCabe MJ Jr. Metals and disorders of cell accumulation: modulation of apoptosis and cell proliferation. Toxicol Sci 2000;56:255-261.
25. Mahaffey KR, Capar SG, Gladen BC, Fowler BA. Concurrent exposure to lead, cadmium, and arsenic. Effects on toxicity and tissue metal concentrations in the rat. J Lab Clin Med 1981;98:463-481.
26. Levander OA. Metabolic interrelationships between arsenic and selenium. Environ Health Perspect 1977;19:159-164.
27. Pershagen G, Wall S, Taube A, Linnman L. On the interaction between occupational arsenic exposure and smoking and its relationship to lung cancer. Scand J Work Environ Health 1981;7:302-309.
28. Pershagen G, Nordberg G, Bjorkland NE. Carcinomas of the respiratory tract in hamsters given arsenic trioxide and/or benzo-a-pyrene by the pulmonary route. Environ Res 1984;37:425-432.
29. Styblo M, Thomas DJ. Selenium modifies the metabolism and toxicity of arsenic in primary rat hepatocytes. Toxicol Appl Pharmacol 2001;172:52-61.
30. Chen CJ, Hsueh YM, Lai MS, Shyu MP, Chen SY, Wu MM, Kuo TL, Tai TY. Increased prevalence of hypertension and long-term arsenic exposure. Hypertension 1995;25:53-60.
31. Tseng CH, Tai TY, Chong CK, Tseng CP, Lai MS, Lin BJ, Chiou HY, Hsueh YM, Hsu KH, Chen CJ. Long-term arsenic exposure and incidence of non-insulin-dependent diabetes mellitus: a cohort study in arseniasis-hyperendemic villages in Taiwan. Environ Health Perspect 2000;108:847-851.
32. Tsai SH, Liang YC, Chen L, Ho FM, Hsieh MS, Lin JK. Arsenite stimulates cyclooxygenase-2 expression through activating IkappaB kinase and nuclear factor kappaB in primary and ECV304 endothelial cells. J Cell Biochem 2002;84: 750-758.
33. Tseng CH, Tai TY, Lin BJ, Chen CJ. Abnormal peripheral microcirculation in seemingly normal subjects living in blackfoot disease-hyperendemic villages in Taiwan. Int J Microcirc 1995;5:21-27.
34. Kumagai Y, Pi J. Molecular basis for arsenic-Induced alteration in nitric oxide production and oxidative stress: implication of endothelial dysfunction. Toxicol Appl Pharmacol 2004;198:450-457.
35. Styblo M, Serves SV, Cullen WR, Thomas DJ. Comparative inhibition of yeast glutathione reductase by arsenicals and arsenothiols. Chem Res Toxicol 1997;10:27-33.
36. Petrick JS, Ayala-Fierro F, Cullen WR, Carter DE, Vasken AH. Monomethylarsonous acid (MMA(III)) is more toxic than arsenite in Chang human hepatocytes. Toxicol Appl Pharmacol 2000;163:203-207.
37. Zhong CX, Mass MJ. Both hypomethylation and hypermethylation of DNA associated with arsenite exposure in cultures of human cells identified by methylation-sensitive arbitrarily-primed PCR. Toxicol Lett 2001;122: 223-234.
38. Lin S, Del Razo LM, Styblo M, Wang C, Cullen WR, Thomas DJ. Arsenicals inhibit thioredoxin reductase in cultured rat hepatocytes. Chem Res Toxicol 2001;14:305-311.
39. Mass MJ, Tennant A, Roop BC, Cullen WR, Styblo M, Thomas DJ, Kligerman AD. Methylated trivalent arsenic species are genotoxic. Chem Res Toxicol 2001;14:355-361.
40. Nesnow S, Roop BC, Lambert G, Kadiiska M, Mason RP, Cullen WR, Mass MJ. DNA damage induced by methylated trivalent arsenicals is mediated by reactive oxygen species. Chem Res Toxicol 2002;15:1627-1634.
41. Yamanaka K, Takabayashi F, Mizoi M, An Y, Hasegawa A, Okada S. Oral exposure of dimethylarsinic acid, a main metabolite of inorganic arsenics, in mice leads to an increase in 8-Oxo-2'-deoxyguanosine level, specifically in the target organs for arsenic carcinogenesis. Biochem Biophys Res Commun 2001;287:66-70.
42. Walton FS, Harmon AW, Paul DS, Drobna Z, Patel YM, Styblo M. Inhibition of insulin-dependent glucose uptake by trivalent arsenicals: possible mechanism of arsenic-induced diabetes. Toxicol Appl Pharmacol 2004;198:424-433.
43. Hatzistamou J, Kiaris H, Ergazaki M, Spandidos DA. Loss of heterozygosity and microsatellite instability in human atherosclerotic plaque. Biochem Biophys Res Commun 1996;255:186-190.
44. Tseng CH. The potential biological mechanisms of arsenic-induced diabetes mellitus. Toxicol Appl Pharmacol 2004;197:67-83.
45. Nordenson I, Beckman L. Is the genotoxic effect of arsenic mediated by oxygen free radicals? Hum Hered 1991;41:71-73.
46. Pi J, Yamauchi H, Kumagai Y, Sun G, Yoshida T, Aikawa H, Hopenhayn-Rich C, Shimojo N. Evidence

for induction of oxidative stress caused by chronic exposure of Chinese residents to arsenic contained in drinking water. Environ Health Perspect 2002;110:331-336.
47. Galle J, Heermeier K, Wanner C. Atherogenic lipoproteins, oxidative stress, and cell death. Kidney Int 1999;71(suppl):S62-S65.
48. Engel RR, Hopenhaynrich C, Receveur O, Smith AH. Vascular effects of chronic arsenic exposure - A review. Epidemiol Rev 1994;16:184-209.

XI HUMAN STUDIES

Metal Ions in Biology and Medicine: vol. 9. Eds Maria Carmen Alpoim, Paula Vasconcellos Morais, Maria Amélia Santos, Armando J. Cristóvão, José A. Centeno, Philippe Collery.
John Libbey Eurotext, Paris © 2006 pp. 521-1.

Preclinical and early clinical development of the antitumor gallium complex KP46 (FFC11)

Philippe Collery[1], Michael A. Jakupec[2], Bernd Kynast[3], Bernhard K. Keppler[2]

[1] *Service de Cancérologie, Polyclinique Maymard, Rue Marcel Paul, 20200 Bastia, France*
[2] *Institute of Inorganic Chemistry, University of Vienna, Waehringer Strasse 42, 1090 Vienna, Austria*
[3] *Faustus Forschung Austria AG, Wipplinger Strasse 34/175-184, Vienna, Austria*
e-mails: Philippe.Collery20220@wanadoo.fr; michael.jakupec@univie.ac.at; kynast@faustus.at; bernhard.keppler@univie.ac.at

BACKGROUND

Despite the clinical activity of gallium nitrate in several malignancies such as lymphoma [1] and bladder cancer [2] and the approval of low-dose gallium nitrate for the treatment of cancer-related hypercalcemia [3], gallium salts have never established in routine cancer therapy. Renal toxicity and occasional optical neuritis observed upon intravenous administration and insufficient bioavailability via the oral route were the major obstacles for its successful use as an anticancer drug [4-6].

Efforts to develop an orally applicable gallium drug offering distinct toxicological and pharmacokinetic advantages over gallium salts gave rise to the uncharged coordination compound tris(8-quinolinolato)gallium(III) (KP46, FFC11) *(figure 1)* containing lipophilic ligands that stabilize gallium against hydrolysis and enable its intestinal absorption. A high bioavailability via the oral route has been confirmed in mice, with bone, liver, spleen and kidneys being the organs accumulating gallium to the highest extent [7, 8]. Both antitumor and antihypercalcemic effects have proved superior to gallium nitrate in tumor-bearing rats [9].

The molecular mechanisms responsible for the tumor-inhibiting properties of gallium salts were intended to be retained unchanged. Accordingly, maintenance of the cellular effects associated with the inhibion of the enzyme ribonucleotide reductase (depletion of cellular dNTP pools, induction of cell cycle arrest in the S phase and subsequent apoptosis) was confirmed by cell culture studies [10].

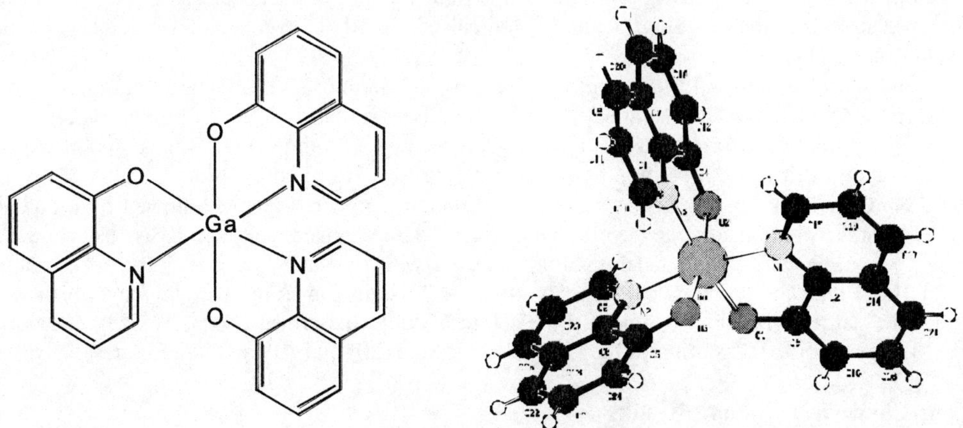

Fig. 1. Structural formula and crystal structure of tris(8-quinolinolato)gallium(III) (KP46, FFC11).

PRECLINICAL TOXICOLOGY

Materials and Methods

Toxicology of KP46 was assessed after single administration of 900, 1273 and 1800 mg/kg and after repeated administration of 5.5, 17.6 and 55 mg/kg/day for 28 consecutive days in NMRI BR mice and F344 rats. KP46 was given as a suspension in 0.1% sodium carboxymethylcellulose (CMC) in deionised water, orally by gavage to groups of 10 female + 10 male animals per dose level. Control groups received vehicle only. Clinical and functional observations, body weight and food consumption, blood and urine analyses were recorded. At the end of the study, all animals were sacrificed and subjected to a necropsy including a gross pathological examination immediately after death.

Results

The maximally tolerated single dose (MTD) was 900 mg/kg in both sexes of both species, and the 50% lethal doses (LD_{50}) were interpolated to 1352 mg/kg and 1724 mg/kg in rats and mice, respectively. Either no or only mild histopathological signs of nephrotoxicity and no histopathological signs of hepatotoxicity were observed at the MTD. Higher doses caused signs of gastrointestinal irritation, unspecific nervous effects and signs of discomfort.

After daily administration for 28 consecutive days, the no-observed-adverse-effect-levels (NOAEL) were 5.5 mg/kg/day in rats and 17.6 mg/kg/day in mice. Only high-dosed rats (55 mg/kg/day) experienced severe toxicities, males being the more susceptible sex. Toxicities mainly affected the hematopoietic system (decreased red blood cell counts and hemoglobin, reduced bone marrow cellularity and enhanced hematopoiesis in the spleen), kidneys (affecting both glomeruli and tubuli) and male reproductive organs (degeneration of germinal epithelium, atrophy of accessory sex glands). Analogous findings were made in high-dosed mice, but the effects were generally less pronounced and similar in both sexes.

CLINICAL PHASE I STUDY

Objectives and Study Outline

In order to evaluate the safety, toxicity profile and pharmacokinetics of FFC11 (KP46) and to arrive at a dose recommendation for further clinical studies, a phase I dose escalation trial was conducted in 2004 at the Ludwig Boltzmann Institute for Applied Cancer Research, KFJ Spital Vienna, Austria, and the Oncology Center, Medical Clinic III, University of Heidelberg, Mannheim, Germany [11].

Patients with histologically or cytologically verified diagnosis of advanced malignant solid tumors, for whom established therapeutic options had been exhausted, were eligible. Patients had to be off prior treatment for at least four weeks before entry into the study, to have an anticipated life expectancy of at least three months and to give written informed consent.

FFC11 was administered orally as a tablet formulation daily for 14 days, followed by a 14-days recovery period. Additional therapy cycles were offered on a compassionate use basis. The dose was escalated according to an accelerated dose titration design, with one patient per dose level and escalation steps of 100% until the occurrence of toxicity grade ≥ 2, beginning from 30 mg/m^2/day which were considered a safe starting dose based on the preclinical studies described above. Toxicity and tumor response were recorded according to the NCI/CTC (version 2.0) and RECIST criteria, respectively.

Patient Characteristics and Results

The study included seven patients (median 58 years, range 44-66 years) receiving a total of

19 cycles (including those given on a compassionate use basis) of FFC11. Localizations of primary tumors were as follows: kidney (n = 4), ovary, stomach and head/neck (each n = 1). All patients had received at least one prior therapy regimen. All patients were evaluable for toxicity and efficacy *(table 1)*.

The dose of FFC11 could be escalated up to 480 mg/m²/day without dose-limiting toxicities. Dose escalation had to be terminated for feasibility reasons. The drug was well tolerated, and adverse events possibly related to the study medication were mostly mild or moderate. The first patient experienced grade 2 leucopenia, necessitating the treatment of two more patients at the lowest dose level. Non-hematological adverse events were: stomatitis (grade 1, n = 1), conjunctivitis (grade 1, n = 1), fatigue (grade 1, n = 2) and diarrhea (grade 3, n = 1) which was rated as probably related to the study drug by the investigator. This patient had concurrent hypomagnesemia and was being treated with Magnosolv.

Remarkably, preliminary evidence of efficacy was seen in three of four patients with renal cell carcinoma (1 partial response, 2 disease stabilizations for (≤ 43 weeks). It is noteworthy that a long-lasting stable disease was achieved in a patient receiving a low dose of 30 mg/m²/day [11].

Table 1. Localizations of primary tumors, administered doses, adverse events in cycle 1 and response of patients included in the clinical phase I trial of FFC11

#	Primary site	Dose (no. of cycles*)	Adverse events** (grade)	Response (duration)
1	Parotid gland	30 mg/m²/day (1)	leucopenia (2)	PD
2	Stomach	30 mg/m²/day (1)		PD
3	Kidney	30 mg/m²/day (11)		SD (49 weeks)
4	Kidney	60 mg/m²/day (1)	stomatitis (1), conjunctivitis (1)	PD
5	Kidney	120 mg/m²/day (2)		SD (4 weeks)
6	Kidney	240 mg/m²/day (2)		PR (8 weeks)
7	Ovary	480 mg/m²/day (1)	fatigue (1), diarrhea (3)	PD

Abbreviations: PD... Progressive disease; PR... partial response; SD... stable disease
* the first cycle is equivalent to the clinical trial, the other cycles are compassionate use
** only adverse events from the clinical trial (first cycle)

CONCLUSIONS

Tris(8-quinolinolato)gallium(III) (KP46, FFC11) is an orally bioavailable gallium complex sharing the critical molecular effects of gallium salts, while circumventing their toxicological and pharmacokinetic disadvantages. KP46 is well tolerated by patients in doses up to 480 mg/m²/day for 14 consecutive days. Preliminary evidence of therapeutic activity in patients with solid tumors encourages further clinical studies, particularly in renal cell carcinoma.

REFERENCES

1. Straus DJ. Galium nitrate in the treatment of lymphoma. *Semin Oncol* 2003; 30, Suppl 5: 25-33.
2. Einhorn L. Galium nitrate in the treatment of bladder cancer. *Semin Oncol* 2003; 30, Suppl 5: 34-41.
3. Leyland-Jones B. Treatment of cancer-related hypercalcemia: the role of gallium nitrate. *Semin Oncol* 2003; 30, Suppl 5: 13-9.

4. Bernstein LR. $_{31}$Ga. Therapeutic gallium compounds. In: Gielen M, Tiekink ERT, eds. *Metallotherapeutic Drugs and Metal-Based Diagnostic Agents*. Chichester: Wiley, 2005: 259-77.
5. Jakupec MJ, Keppler BK. Gallium and other main group metal compounds as antitumor agents. In: Sigel A, Sigel H, eds. *Metal Complexes in Tumor Diagnosis and as Anticancer Agents. Metal Ions in Biological Systems*, Vol 42. New York: Dekker, 2004: 425-62.
6. Collery P, Keppler, BK, Madoulet C., Desoize B. Gallium in cancer treatment. *Crit Rev Oncol Hematol* 2002; 42: 283-96.
7. Collery P, Millart H, Pechery C, Kratz F, Keppler BK. New gallium complexes for a cisplatin combination therapy. In: Anastassopoulou J, Collery P, Etienne JC, Theophanides T, eds. *Metal Ions in Biology and Medicine*, vol. 2. Paris: John Libbey Eurotext, 1992: 173-5.
8. Collery P, Domingo JL, Keppler BK. Preclinical toxicology and tissue gallium distribution of a novel antitumour gallium compound: tris(8-quinolinolato)gallium(III). *Anticancer Res* 1996; 16: 687-92.
9. Thiel M, Schilling T, Gey DC, Ziegler R, Collery P, Keppler BK. Tris(8-quinolinolato)gallium(III), a novel orally applied antitumor gallium compound. In: Fiebig HH, Burger AM, eds. *Relevance of Tumor Models for Anticancer Drug Development. Contributions to Oncology*, vol. 54. Basel: Karger, 1999: 439-43.
10. Jakupec MJ, Heffeter P, Pongratz M, Fremuth M, Horvath Z, Unfried P, Keyserlingk N Graf v, Berger W, Szekeres T, Keppler BK. Depletion of cellular dNTP pools, cell cycle arrest and apoptosis induced by the oral gallium complex KP46 (FFC11). Clin. Cancer Res. 2005; 11, Suppl: 9159s.
11. Hofheinz RD, Dittrich C, Jakupec MA, Drescher A, Jaehde U, Gneist M, Keyserlingk N Graf v, Keppler BK, Hochhaus A. Early results from a phase I study on orally administered tris(8-quinolinolato)gallium(III) (FFC11, KP46) in patients with solid tumors - a CESAR study (Central European Society for Anticancer Drug Research - EWIV). *Int J Clin Pharmacol Ther* 2005; 43: 590-1.

Metal Ions in Biology and Medicine: vol. 9. Eds Maria Carmen Alpoim, Paula Vasconcellos Morais, Maria Amélia Santos, Armando J. Cristóvão, José A. Centeno, Philippe Collery.
John Libbey Eurotext, Paris © 2006 pp. 525-1.

Status of serum copper and dopamine beta-hydroxylase (DBH) activity in healthy population

M. Grabowska[1], J. Przyslawski[2], I. Boleslawska[2], M. Schlegel-Zawadzka[3]

[1]Chair of Medical Biochemistry, Jagiellonian University, 7 Kopernika str., 31-034 Krakow, mbgrabow@cyf-kr.edu.pl;
[2]Department of Bromatology and Human Nutrition, Medical Academy, 42 Marcelinska str., 60-354 Poznan, jotespe@am.poznan.pl;
[3]Department of Human Nutrition, Faculty of Health Care,Jagiellonian University, 20 Grzegorzecka str., 31-531 Krakow, mfzawadz@kinga.cyf-kr.edu.pl; Poland

SUMMARY

Dopamine beta-hydroxylase (DBH) is known to use Cu ions for catalytic activity and contains 4-7 moles of Cu^{+2} - per mol of enzyme. DBH catalyses the beta-hydroxylation of dopamine into norepinephrine. Its decreased activity has been reported in unipolar psychotic depression. The aim of the study was to check relation between copper content and DBH activity in serum in healthy young subjects (40 students - 34 female, 6 male, average age 22,2 y). Copper content in serum was estimated using AAS method. Additionally DBH activity in serum was determined spectrophotometrically. The average Cu content in serum and DBH activity were independent of gender (1.15±0.43mg/l; 72.76±27.06 umol/l). There was no correlation between Cu content in serum and DBH activity. In healthy young people the prediction of DBH activity in serum from the Cu content is not possible.

INTRODUCTION

Copper an essential but highly toxic nutrient, is required for survival of all living organisms, from prokaryotes and yeasts to mammals, and is integral to a number of enzymatic processes involved in the defense against oxidative stress. It is a well-known fact that Cu is directly involved in the iron metabolism because, via ceruloplasmin, is able to oxidase iron before being transported in the blood to all the tissues. Besides, copper constitutes enzymes which are associated with other important cellular functions such as energetic metabolism in the mitochondria, protection against oxidative stress or the synthesis of proteins of connective tissues and catecholamines (1). Like iron, copper has the unique ability to adopt two different redox states, which are interrelated through ferroxidase of ceruloplasmin. The free metal ions are able to participate in Fenton-like reactions, in which highly reactive and extremely deleterious hydroxyl radicals are formed, and by lipid peroxidation or similar action disrupt membranes, amino acids, and nucleic acids. This combination of events is postulated to contribute to development of cancer, aging, and neurodegeneration. In addition there is ability to displace other metal cofactors from natural ligands in key signalling molecules. Copper metabolism in human beings has been difficult to clarify (1).

Copper is an integral part of many important enzymes involved in a number of vital biological processes. Although normally bound to proteins, Cu may be released and become free to catalyse the formation of highly reactive hydroxyl radicals (2).

Dopamine beta-hydroxylase (DBH) catalyses the beta-hydroxylation of dopamine to norepinephrine. The enzyme in chromaffin granules occurs in a soluble form and a form confined to the surrounding membrane.

DBH is known to use Cu ions for catalytic activity and contains 4-7 moles of Cu^{+2} - per mol of enzyme. DBH catalyses the beta-hydroxylation of dopamine into norepinephrine. Its decreased activity has been reported in unipolar psychotic depression.

Altered dopamine beta-hydroxylase (DBH) activity has been reported in mood disorders. Plasma DBH is reduced in major depression with psychosis and elevated in bipolar disorder with psychosis compared with their respective non-psychotic diagnostic groups. DBH is likely a trait marker with interindividual variations secondary to genetic polymorphism. Since DBH is a genetic marker, this may reflect individual vulnerabilities to develop psychosis in the context of trauma (3).

Plasma activity of DBH, the enzyme that converts dopamine to norepinephrine, is reportedly lower in patients with unipolar major depression with psychosis features (UDPF) than in those with nonpsychotic unipolar major depression (UD). Mean plasma DBH activity was significantly lower in UDPF than in UD (4).

Decreased DBH activity has been reported in unipolar psychotic depression. DBH comparisons between elderly delusional and nondelusional depressives and controls and determination of whether pre-treatment group differences persist have not been reported. Baseline and predischarge DBH assays were lower in subjects with delusional depression than in either comparison group. Despite high intraindividual correlation, treatment was associated with significant increases in activity in the clinical groups. Patients with late-life delusional depression have lower DBH activity before and after hospital treatment than age-matched nondelusional patients or normal controls (5).

THE AIM

The aim of the study was to check relation between copper content and DBH activity in serum in healthy young subjects.

MATERIAL AND METHODS

The group of 40 students (34 female, 6 male, average age 22,2 y) were recruited for dietary study. Fasting venous blood samples were collected using vacutainer system of Becton Dickinson. As serum control was Validate N (Organon Teknika USA).

The copper content in blood samples was measured by flame atomic absorption spectrometry method (AAS) with Pye Unicam Solaar; wavelength - 324.8 nm.

Data were expressed as arithmetic average mean (X)±standard deviation (SD). Statistical analyses were performed using STATISTICA 6.0 Pl software (StatSoft). The t-Student test was used to test the hypothesis of significant differences between average values on the level of significance set at $p<0.05$. Additionally DBH activity in serum was determined by the Nagatsu and Undenfriend method, modified by Grabowska and Guminska (6). Consent for the study was obtained from the Ethical Committee, Medical Academy, Poznan.

RESULTS AND DISCUSSION

The results are presented in *table 1*. The average copper content in serum and DBH activity were independent of gender (1.15±0.43mg/l; 72.76±27.06 umol/l). The mean contents of copper in serum according to gender were almost similar to Romero's et al. study and fall in the international reference range (7, 8). The distribution frequencies of the copper content in the male and female samples is shown in *figure 1*. Most the analysed samples, 34 (90,0% of the total) fall into the reference intervals - males 0.7-1.4 mg/L and females 0.8-1.55 mg/L. The distribution percentage for total group is almost similar to found in the Nutrition Survey of the Canary Islands (7). However, we found no men with the copper content below reference value.

There was no correlation between Cu content in serum and DBH activity.

The distribution frequencies of DBH activity for total group is presented in *figure 2*. There was not so many data of DBH activity in healthy people. Hamner&Gold found in serum of healthy control 46.1±4.9 umol/min/L and Meyers et al. 58.0±24.4 umol/min/L (3, 5). The results are lower than ours, but their groups consisted of older persons (Hamner - about 48 years, Meyers - about 72.3 years) than in our study.

Table 1. Results of the copper content in serum of the study group, reference value of healthy adults (arithmetic mean ± standard deviation) and dopamine beta-hydroxylase (DBH) activity in serum in healthy people.

Parameter	Total		Man		Woman	
	n	X ± SD min-max	n	X ± SD min-max	n	X ± SD min-max
Study Group						
DBH [umol/min/L]	40	72.76 ± 27.06 34.92 - 157.55	6	78.77 ± 39.47 52.50 - 157.55	34	71.70 + 24.94 35.92 - 124.38
Cu [mg/L]	40	1.15 ± 0.436 0.67 - 2.90	6	1.02 ± 0.18 0.84 - 1.35	34	1.18 + 0.45 0.67 - 2.90
References						
DBH [umol/min/L] (Hamner et al.) (3)	22	46.1 ± 4.9		-		-
DBH [umol/min/L] (Meyers et al.) (5)	22	58.0 ± 24.4		-		-
Cu - Romero et al study [mg/L] (7)	395	1.10 ± 0.25 0.56 - 2.34	187	1.02 ± 0.20 0.56 - 2.05	208	1.18 ± 0.27 0.61 - 2.34
Cu References (Goldman, Bennet) [mg/L] (8)	-	-		0.70 - 1.40		0.80 - 1.55

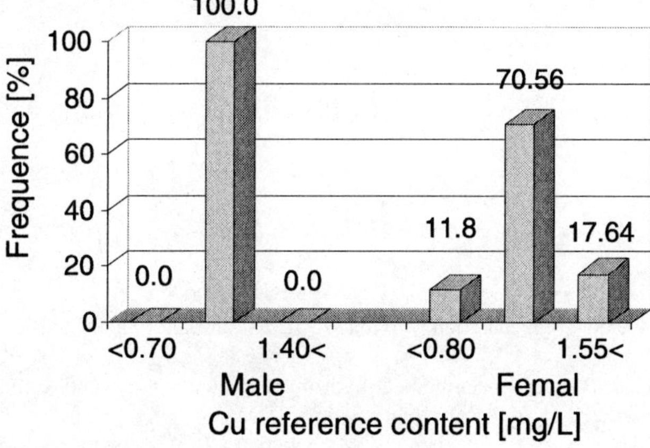

Fig. 1. Distribution of serum copper content for total group studied.

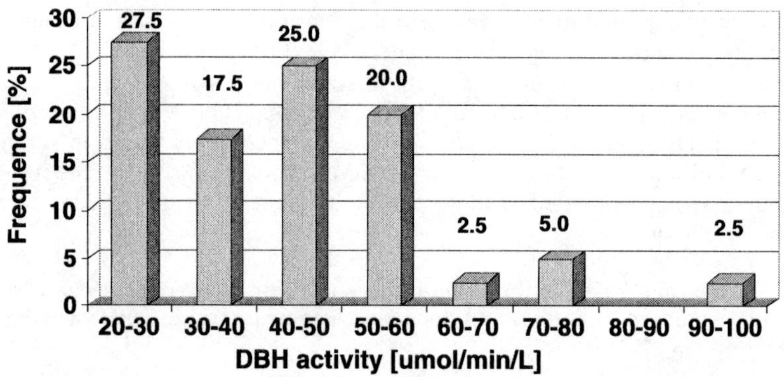

Fig. 2. Distribution of dopamine beta-hydroxylase activity (umol/min./l) in serum in total group studied.

Copper is an essential element for the activity of a number of physiologically important enzymes. Enzyme-related malfunctions may contribute to severe neurological symptoms and neurological diseases: copper is a component of cytochrome c oxidase, which catalyses the reduction of oxygen to water, the essential step in cellular respiration. Copper is a cofactor of Cu/Zn-superoxide-dismutase which plays a key role in the cellular response to oxidative stress by scavenging reactive oxygen species. Furthemore, copper is a constituent of dopamine-beta-hydroxylase, a critical enzyme in the catecholamine biosynthesis pathway. Copper binding proteins play important roles in the establishment and maintenance of metal-ion homeostasis, in deficiency disorders with neurological symptoms (Menkes disease, Wilson disease) and in neurodegenerative diseases (Alzheimer's disease) (9).

We also study the changes in copper content in plasma and dopamine beta-hydroxylase activity in a chronic mild stress (CMS) model of depression in rats (10, 11). The copper content in the plasma in the chronic mild stress model of depression in rats remains stable, whereas the DBH activity is altered. There exists a negative significant correlation between the copper content in the plasma and the activity of DBH in the rats subjected to CMS (10). DBH activity seems to be a more sensitive marker of depression than are changes in copper content in the plasma of CMS rats (11).

Based on the study results in CMS model in rats we want to have a basic data for copper content in plasma of healthy people as well as DBH activity. Such control group is necessary for comparison of changes in many diseases (depression, mucoviscidosis).

CONCLUSION

In healthy young people the prediction of DBH activity in serum from the Cu content is not possible.

REFERENCES

1. Jacobs P, Wood L. Copper. *Disease-a-Month* 2003; 49: 589-600.
2. Gaetke LM, Chow XhK. Copper toxicity, oxidative stress, and antioxidant nutrients. *Toxicology* 2003; 189: 147-63.
3. Hamner MB, Gold PB. Plasma dopamine beta-hydroxylase activity in psychotic and non-psychotic post-traumatic stress disorder. *Psychiat Res* 1998; 77: 175-81.
4. Cubells JF, Price LH, Meyers BS, Anderson GM, Zabetian CP, Alexopoulos GS, Nelson JC, Sanacora G, Kirwin P, Carpenter L, Malison RT, Gelernter J. Genotype-controlled analysis of plasma dopamine

beta-hydroxylase activity in psychotic unipolar major depression. *Comment in Biol Psychiat* 2002; 51: 347-48.

5. Meyers BS, Alexopoulos GS, Kakuma T, Tirumalasetti F, Gabriele M, Alpert S, Bowden C, Meltzer HY. Decreased dopamine beta-hydroxylase activity in unipolar geriatric delusional depression. *Biol Psychiat* 1999; 45: 448-52.
6. Grabowska M, Guminska M. Effect of buthobendin on dopamine (-hydroxylase *in vitro. Pol J Pharmacol* 1996; 48: 39-45.
7. Romero CD, Sanchez PH, Blanco FL, Rodriquez ER, Majem LS. Serum copper and zinc concentration in a representative sample of the Canarian population. *J Trace Elem Med Biol* 2002; 16: 75-81.
8. Goldman L, Bennet JC (ed). Cecil Textbook of Medicine. 21st edition, Philadelphia, W.B. Saunders Company, 2000: 2304.
9. Strausak D, Mercer JF, Dieter HH, Stremmel W, Multhaup G. Copper in disorders with neurological symptoms: Alzheimer's, Menkes and Wilson diseases. *Brain Res Bull* 2001; 55: 175-85.
10. Grabowska M, Schlegel-Zawadzka M, Nowak G, Papp M. The copper plasma content and dopamine β-hydroxylase activity in a chronic mild stress model of depression in rats. In Khassanova L, Collery P, Maymard I, Khassanova Z, Etienne JC, eds. *Metal Ions in Biology and Medicine*. Paris: John Libbey Eurotext, 2002; 7: 193-196.
11. Grabowska M, Schlegel-Zawadzka M, Nowak G, Papp M. Using plasma dopamine β-hydroxylase activity and its relationships with bioelement content to predict depression in the rat model. *Acta Biol Cracov* 2002; 44: 41-46.

Metal Ions in Biology and Medicine: vol. 9. Eds Maria Carmen Alpoim, Paula Vasconcellos Morais, Maria Amélia Santos, Armando J. Cristóvão, José A. Centeno, Philippe Collery.
John Libbey Eurotext, Paris © 2006 pp. 530-1.

Changes In Blood Lead Levels In Uruguayan Populations

Manay N.[1], Alvarez C., Cousillas A., Pereira L., Baranano R., Heller T.

[1]*Toxicology & Environmental Hygiene Department*
Faculty Of Chemistry, University of the Republic of Uruguay
Gral. Flores 2124, CP 11800.Montevideo-Uruguay
e-mail: nmanay@fq.edu.uy

Lead exposure in Uruguay is nowadays of public concern. It was not until 2001 that lead pollution first received official attention because the affected community began a broad mobilization demanding solutions. As a response, social and political actions, as well as regulations, for its environmental health risk management and control, have been carried out. Leaded gasoline has recently phased out and thousands of lead in blood determinations were done.

Our Toxicology team has a 15-year-research-experience in lead monitoring of different Uruguayan populations with quality assurance and quality controls (QA/QC) analytical results. We studied exposed lead workers, children and many low-income families that settled down in lead polluted areas, not aware of the high health risks for their children.

The aim of this study is to evaluate the main changes observed in the blood lead levels (BLL) of Uruguayan populations within a 10 - year - period considering the current actions to prevent lead exposure risks.

INTRODUCTION

Lead is an environmental pollutant of high risk for human health. Its adverse effects are well known, being children the most affected population. There is a significant negative correlation between children's mental development and environmental lead exposure [1, 2, 3, 4].

Uruguay is a small country with a population of 3 millions inhabitants, half of them living in its capital harbour city Montevideo. Most lead processing industries, such as metallurgies, foundries, manufacturers and batteries recyclers, have established around Montevideo, thus contributing to the contamination of the peripheral settlements.

The use of tetraethyl lead in gasoline (replaced in 2004 by terbutil-methyl-ether) and the existence of lead pipes for the drinking-water-supply in older buildings are the main sources of lead exposure for the general population. Living in or near manufacturing areas, as well as the incorrect handling of lead materials and solid wastes, are also relevant sources of non occupational exposure [5, 6, 7, 8].

But, in Uruguay, it was not until 2001 that lead exposure became a matter of public concern, when cases of children with blood lead levels (BLL) higher than 20 micrograms/dL appeared in some areas of a low-income-neighbourhood of Montevideo, called La Teja [7]. There, the worst situation found was in soil samples from some slum settlements which showed more than 3,000 ppm of lead due to scrap land fillings [8, 9].

After the arousal of those cases of high blood lead levels in some children of La Teja there was a broad mobilization and a movement in public opinion, demanding solutions. As a consequence, an official interinstitutional committee including health, environmental and regulatory authorities was established. Then, social and political actions, as well as regulations, for the environmental health risk management and control, have been carried out. In the meantime, thousands of lead in blood analysis were performed, mostly by the Laboratory of our Toxicology Department.

At the Faculty of Chemistry, our Department of Toxicology and Environmental Hygiene has been assessing heavy- metal- exposure in different Uruguayan populations, being lead its main research line since 1986. We work with QA/QC analytical results. Therefore, when the lead issue arose in 2001, the authorities could take advantage of our 15-year-scientific experience in the analytical determination of lead in blood. We had previously studied groups of workers, children and general population, producing scientific publications and several reports [6, 10, 11, 12, 13, 14].

In 2004, after the leaded gasoline phasing out process in Uruguay was completed, we studied three populations: children, non occupationally exposed adults and lead workers to correlate BLL with variables such as age, sex, area of residence, available environmental lead data, among others. We compared these results with those from our similar screening studies 10 years ago, to assess the current risk factors with a statistical approach [10, 11, 12].

We present the observed main changes in the blood lead levels of Uruguayan populations within this 10 - year - period considering the current actions to prevent lead exposure risks.

MATERIALS AND METHODS

The children sampling campaign was made during an 8 - month - period and comprised those children visiting a Social Security Care Center for health control. These children population (n=180) were parent volunteers and randombly selected. Most of them, were living in Montevideo and surroundings, aging 0 to 15 years. Data were collected from each individual regarding age, house and school addresses, intensity of traffic near their houses and smoking habits of their parents.

Non occupationally lead exposed adults sampling included those individuals visiting a private Workers Health Care Centre to get their health certificate and different criteria of inclusion - exclusion were considered.

The studied population sample consisted of 714 non occupationally exposed adults, ages 20 to 64, living in Montevideo. For the purpose of this study, the city was divided in 5 areas, according to the following variables: concentration of population, vehicle traffic intensity, industrial areas for lead, etc.

The exposed lead workers population (n =81) consisted of codified samples sent as labour control by the State Risk Insurance Agency, therefore individual data are not available.

Sampling conditions and analytical techniques were the same for all the studies. 10 mL of blood were obtained from the cubital vein in heparin moistened evacuated disposable syringes [15]. Samples were kept in the same labelled syringes frozen at -20° until their analysis.

All blood analysis were done by atomic spectrometry (FAAS & GFAAS) with quality controls. Associations between BLL and single variables were assessed using statistical analysis.

BLL results were contrasted with intercalibration programs [16] and internal controls. Most samples were analysed by the National Institute for Occupational Safety and Health (NIOSH) method [17], original method P&CAM 208 [18] modified by substituting the APDC (ammonium pirrolidin dithiocarbamate) with DDDC (N, N dithio-carbamate diethilammonium) resulting a lead complex more stable over time. This allows processing several samples at the same time, without risk of decomposition at the moment of the measurement.

RESULTS AND DISCUSSION

Our obtained results and the reference guidelines for blood lead levels in the different studied population [2, 19, 20, 21] are described in the following table *(table 1)*.

Table 1. Blood Lead Levels (BLL) in ug/dL from different uruguayan populations sampled in 2004, reference limit values respectively and % of data over those limits

Populations (2004)	n	BLL ug/dL	Range BLL ug/dL	Reference BLL ug/dL	BBL > Reference %
Children	180	5,7	3,0-16,0	< 10 [19,20]	6,7%
Non occupationally exposed Adults	714	5,5	3,0-24,0	< 25 [2]	0%
Occupationally exposed Adults	81	41,9	9,0-69,0	< 30 [21]	76,5%
				< 10 women in fertile age [21]	

Up to the year 1994 little oficial attention was paid to environmental lead exposure although our research group had carried out several studies that were published during the 90s decade reviewed by Manay et al. [6].

By that time and still now, Montevideo had several lead emitting industries, most of them in residential areas. Old buildings and houses still had lead pipelines in their water systems.

In addition, primary gasoline used in Uruguay up to December 2003 contained lead tetraethyl as an antiknock agent (150-300 mg/L). It is well known that a clear decrease of blood lead level has been associated with the elimination of lead in gasoline in the USA and Sweden [22, 23].

Uruguayan children studied by Schutz et al. [10] and described in Manay et al. [6] sampled 10 years before, in 1994, showed an average BLL 9.6 ug/dL (n=96, range 4,7-19,1) and 9,5 (n=34, range 4,7-15,4) respectively.

At the same time, screening studies on occupationally unexposed workers (civil servants and school teachers) had showed an average BLL of 9,1 µg/dL (n=29, range 5,0-16.3) [11] and for randomly selected adults in Cousillas et al. [12] the average BLL was 8,6 µg (n=84, range 3,1-24,8)

Considering the BLL of lead exposed workers, also ten years before, a total of 31 individuals had been recruited among the employees at two storage battery plants (n=16 and n= 8 respectively), from a lead scrap smelter (n=6) in Montevideo surroundings and also a self employed storage battery reconditioner [11]. They showed three times higher BLL, 49,7 µg/dL (n=31 range 24,4-87,0) than those from unexposed adult population and 84% were over over the biological exposure index described by the American Conference of Governmental Industrial Hygienists [21] (BEI: 30 µg/dL).

Manay et al. 1999 [6] reviewed other studies on exposed workers from different manufacturing industries like battery factories, foundries and wire factories who have significant high BBL and almost 60% were above 40 µg/dL. In addition, a pilot study with workers from a battery storage plant who were sampled for control purposes, they also showed higher BLL, 48,2 ug/dL (n=60 range 29,0-80,0) and 94% were over 30 ug/dL [23].

In these recent 2004 studies, children showed significantly lower BLL (5,7 ug/dL) and occupationally unexposed adults (5,5 ug/dL) than those sampled in 1994 (9,6 ug/L and 9,1 ug/dL respectively) with a $p<0.001$. The study with children in 1994 [10] showed a positive relationship of BLL with traffic intensity and 40% of the BLL were above the intervention value (10 ug/dL) while in 2004 we had only 6,7% of the BLL from the sampled children.

In addition, spot samples of gasoline were taken from gas stations after leaded gasoline was officially phased out. Those samples were lead analyzed by GFAAS and the data showed lead concentrations of less than 10 mg/L as it was expected.

However, uruguayan lead workers showed no significant BLL differences within this 10 years period (49,7 and 41,9 ug/dL respectively) and their mean values exceeded the biological exposure index for lead in blood (< 30 µg/dL) in our sampled populations.

CONCLUSIONS

The observed changes suggest a decrease in the contribution of environmental lead to the overall exposure of children and non occupationally exposed adults. This could be the result of several facts, mainly: the gradual phasing out of leaded gasoline, the progressive substitution of lead pipes for the drinking water supply and the improvement of education and hygienic habits in children. On the whole, it is the consequence of a new attitude of the population, who is now more aware of the lead health risks.

In the case of lead workers, our data do not allow to draw definite conclusions about their still high BLL on average and their consequent lead exposure risk. We consider that during this period, as a consequence of the worsened economic situation, the field of lead activity has changed and little attention has been paid to the environmental working conditions in lead industries.

We conclude that there is a significant change in preventing lead exposure due to the public sensitisation together with the integration of multidisciplinary actions promoted although our country still does not have a complete official surveillance-screening program, including human population and the environment (air, water and soil). In relation to lead workers new laws have been approved and now lead in blood must be controlled in the health certificate protocol once per year.

REFERENCES

1. Agency for Toxic Substances and Disease Registry. Toxicological profile for lead. Atlanta, GA: *Agency for Toxic Substances and Disease Registry* 2005; *http://www.atsdr.cdc.gov/toxprofiles/tp13.pdf*
2. IPCS (International Programme on Chemical Safety). Environmental Health Criteria No 165: Inorganic Lead *World Health Organization* 1995. Geneva, Switzerland. 300pp.
3. ACSH American Council on Science and health, Inc. Lead and Human Health. An Update. 2nd ed. (2000) http://www.acsh.org-publications-boolets-lead-update.pdf.
4. US. ATSDR U. S. Agency for Toxic Substances and Disease Registry. The nature and extent of lead poisoning in children in the United States. A report to the Congress. *U. S. Department of Health and Human Services* 2003; Atlanta.
5. Cousillas A, Mañay N, Pereira L, Rampoldi O. Relevamiento de plumbemias en un complejo habitacional de Montevideo (Uruguay). *Acta Farmaceutica Bonaerense* 1998; 17-4: 291-96.
6. Mañay N, Pereira L, Cousillas A. Lead contamination in Uruguay. *Rev Environ Contam Toxicol* 1999; 159: 25-39.
7. Mañay N., Alonzo C. Dol I. Contaminación por plomo en el barrio La Teja, Montevideo-Uruguay In: Suplemento "Experiencia Latinoamericana" *Salud Publica de México* 2003; 45: 268-275.
8. Dol I. Feola, G.; Garcia, G.; Alozo, C. Contaminación ambiental de plomo en asentamientos urbanos en Montevideo, Uruguay y su repercusión en los niveles de plomo en sangre en población infantil. *RETEL* 2004; 4 *www. Sertox.com.ar/retel/n04/003.htm*
9. IMM Intendencia Municipal de Montevideo, Contaminación por Metales en suelo In: Informe Ambiental de Montevideo 2003; 5: *Intendencia Municipal de Montevideo, Documentos de Desarrollo Ambiental http://www.montevideo.gub.uy/ambiente/documentos/infoamb03c.pdf*
10. Schutz A., Barregard L., Sallsten G., Wilske J., Mañay N., Pereira L., Cousillas A.Z. Blood Lead in Uruguayan Children and Possible Sources of Exposure. *Environmental Research* 1997; 74: 17.
11. Pereira L., Mañay N., Cousillas A., Barregard L., Schutz A. & Sällsten G (1996) Occupational lead Exposure in Montevideo. Uruguay. *Int. J. Occup. Environ. Health*, 1996; 2: 4, 328-330.
12. Cousillas A., Mañay N., Pereira L., Rampoldi O. Relevamiento de plumbemias en un complejo habitacional de Montevideo (Uruguay). *Acta Farmaceutica Bonaerense* (1998) 17(4): 291.

13. Cousillas A., Mañay N., Pereira L., Alvarez A., Coppes Z. Evaluation of Lead Exposure in Uruguayan Children. *Bull. Environ.Contam.Toxicol* 2005; 75: 629-636.
14. Mañay N.; Cousillas A.; Pereira L.; Alvarez C. "Lead Biomonitoring on Dogs as Sentinels for Risk Environment Assesment". XIII International Conference on Heavy Metals in the Environment Proceedings 2005; 221-224.
15. Carreón Valencia T., López Carrillo L. & Romieu I. *Manual de Procedimiento en la Toma de Muestras Biológicas y Ambientales para Determinar Niveles de Plomo.* OPS - OMS. 1995 México 85 pp.
16. Servicio de Prevención de Riesgos Laborales de la Diputación General de Aragón. PICC-PbS: Interlaboratory Quality Control Programme Lead inblood. *http://www.mtas.es/Insht/en/acreditacion/picc_pbs_en.htm*
17. NIOSH National Institute of Occupational and Safety Health "Manual of Analytical Methods", 1984 Cincinnati.
18. Hessel DW A simple and rapid quantitative determination of lead in blood. *Atomic Absorpt. Newslett.* (1968) 7: 55-57.
19. US. CDC United States Center of Disease Control. Preventing Lead Poisoning in Young Children. A statement by the Center of Disease Control *US. Department of Health and Human Services 1991*, Atlanta, Georgia. *http://wonder.cdc.gov/wonder/prevguid/p0000029/p0000029.asp*
20. US CDC Centers for Disease Control and Prevention. Managing Elevated Blood Lead Levels Among Young Children: Recommendations from the Advisory Committee on Childhood Lead Poisoning Prevention. *US. Department of Health and Human Services* 2002 Atlanta. *http://www.cdc.gov/nceh/lead/CaseManagement/caseManage_main.htm*
21. ACGIH TLVs and BEIs. Based on the Documentations for Threshold Limit Values for Chemical Substances and Physical Agents. Biological Exposure Indices: *American Conference of Governmental Industrial Hygienists*, 2005.
22. Pirkle J.L. Brody D.J., Gunter E.W., Kramer R.A., Paschal D.C., Flegal K.M. & Matte T.D. The decline in blood lead levels in the United States: The National Health and Nutrition Examination Surveys (NHANES) *J. Am. Med. Assoc.* 1994; 272: 284.
23. Strombert U., Schutz A. & Skerfving S. Substantial Decrease of Blood Lead in Swedish Children, 1978-94, Associated with Petrol Lead. *Occup. Environ. Med.* 1995; 52: 764.
24. Pereira L., Mañay N., Cousillas A., Korbut, S; Rampoldi, O Heller T. Exposición a plomo en una fábrica de baterías en Uruguay. *X ALATOX Asociacion Latinoamericana de Toxicología, Congress book*, 1998. Cuba.

Metal Ions in Biology and Medicine: vol. 9. Eds Maria Carmen Alpoim, Paula Vasconcellos Morais, Maria Amélia Santos, Armando J. Cristóvão, José A. Centeno, Philippe Collery.
John Libbey Eurotext, Paris © 2006 pp. 535-1.

Serum selenium and glutathione peroxidase activity in critically ILL patients with systemic inflammatory response and multiple organ dysfunction syndrome: preliminary data

Manzanares W.[1], Torre M.H.[2], Biestro A.[1], Pittini G.[1], Mañay N.[3], Facchin G.[2], Rampoldi O.[3]

1. Cátedra de Medicina Intensiva - Hospital de Clínicas: Dr. Manuel Quintela. Avda. Italia s/n esq. Las Heras. Facultad de Medicina, UDELAR.
2. Cátedra de Química Inorgánica. Facultad de Química, Gral. Flores 2124. 11800 Montevideo - Uruguay UDELAR.
3. Cátedra de Toxicología. Facultad de Química Gral. Flores 2124. 11800 Montevideo - Uruguay UDELAR.

Correspondence to: Dr. William Manzanares: e-mail: acuevas@adinet.com.uy

INTRODUCTION

Selenium (Se), a nonmetal belonging to the XVI group of the periodic table, is an essential trace element for mammals [1, 2]. The importance of Se biochemistry is highlighted since it is specified in the genetic code as the newly discovered amino acid selenocysteine [2]. Selenium is largely known to develop its biological activity as an integral part of functional selenoproteins [1, 2, 3, 4, 5]. Selenoproteins are generally enzymes that contain selenium in stoichiometric amounts at their active sites [3, 5]. They are responsible for selenium function in biologic systems and have catalytic redox activity [3, 4, 5]. The incorporation of selenium into the redox-active selenocysteine residue of Glutathione peroxidase (GPx), Iodothyronine deiodinases and Thioredoxin reductase is the basis of the physiological features of these proteins concerning the detoxification of hydrogen peroxide and lipid hydroperoxides, the equilibration of thyroid hormone metabolites and the reduction of cellular disulfides and ascorbate, respectively [3]. Se behaves both as an antioxidant and anti-inflammatory agent and it plays a very important role in Critical Care Medicine [1, 4, 6].

GPx is an antioxidative selenoenzyme that provides a mechanism for detoxification of peroxides in living cells, protecting them from oxidative injury by free radicals [1, 2, 5, 7, 8, 9]. The GPx family is made up of four isoforms that differ in their tissue location and substrate specifity [1]. GPX1-4, reduce some form of hydroperoxide by oxidizing GSH [8, 9]. GPX1 and GPX2 are closely related cytosolic enzymes in terms of structure and specificity for H_2O_2 and fatty acid hydroperoxides as substrates, although GPX1 is also found in mitochondria. GPX3 is an extracelular glycosylated enzyme that can use the thioredoxin and glutaredoxin systems in addition to GSH as electron donors to reduce a broader range of hydroperoxides. GPX3 can reduce H_2O_2, fatty acid hydroperoxides, and phospholipid hydroperoxides. GPX4 reduces phospholipid, cholesterol, and thymine hydroperoxides and may function synergistically with vitamin E in the prevention of lipid peroxidation [8, 9, 10]. GPX1-4 are expressed in the gastrointestinal mucus. Systemic Inflammatory Response Syndrome (SIRS) and Multiple Organ Dysfunction Syndrome (MODS) such us severe sepsis, trauma, severe pancreatitis and burns are the most prevalent and typical critical syndromes. Studies on SIRS have shown that an overflow of oxygen free radicals generation accounts for one of the most important pathologic factors in critical illness [10, 11, 12]. As a consequence of this overflow of reactive oxygen species (ROS) a failure of endogenous antioxidant capacity appears and thus, an increase in oxidative stress is typically present [11, 12, 13]. An insufficient Se supply may be the main cause of this endogenous antioxidant capacity failure. SIRS is highly prevalent in the Intensive Care Unit (ICU), and approximately 70% of critically ill patients have SIRS criteria. Despite the development of new therapeutic strategies and antibiotics, the overall mortality rate is still about 30% and could not be significantly reduced over the last years. In this proceeding, we present the preliminary data corresponding to the second phase of our research about Se status behavior in critically ill patients with SIRS.

AIMS

2.1 To assess the selenium status in a population of Uruguayan critically ill patients and healthy subjects.

2.2 To evaluate the influence of systemic inflammatory response in Se nutritional status.

MATERIALS AND METHODS

The study was performed in the ICU of Hospital de Clínicas Dr. Manuel Quintela, the university hospital and in the Facultad de Química of Uruguay. For the purpose of this study critically ill patients with a minimal Acute Physiology and Chronic Health Evaluation (APACHE) II score of 15 points or more who had been admitted to ICU were divided in three groups. These groups were: group A healthy subjects (physicians, fellows and nurses) corresponding to ICU team; group B patients without SIRS; group C patients with SIRS and group D patients with SIRS-MODS complex. Inclusion criteria were SIRS criteria; MODS; critical illness without SIRS within 48 hours from admission to ICU. Exclusion criteria were: age above 18 years, pregnancy, and status after cardiopulmonary resuscitation or refusal to participate in the study.

GPx activity was determined by an indirect method based in the oxidation of glutathione (GSH) to oxidized glutathione (GSSG), catalyzed by GPx, which is then coupled to the recycling of GSSG to GSH using Glutathione Reductase and NADPH [14]. GPx activity was expressed in units/millilitre (U/mL).

Serum Se level was analysed by graphite furnace atomic absorption spectrometry and was expressed in micrograms/litre (µg/L). GPx activity and serum Se concentration were determined in the first 48 hours after admission to ICU and their results expressed in mean ± DS. Samples of 5 mL of blood were obtained from the cubital vein or central catheter in syringes with an activator clot agent and centrifuged to 2500 rpm by 10 minutes. The serum samples were kept in labelled syringes frozen at -20° C until their analysis.

According to ACCP/SCCM Consensus [15], SIRS was diagnosed when two or more of the following parameters were present: temperature above 38° C or below 36° C; white blood cells count above 11.000/mm^3 or below 4.000/mm^3 or more than 10% immature neutrophils; heart rate above 90/min; respiratory rate above 20/min or $paC0_2$ less than 32 mmHg.

In patients with SIRS by infectious or non infectious injury, MODS was defined by presence of one or more the following criteria: a) Septic shock or septic shock "like"; b) Acute Lung Injury, both entities defined in accord with Consensus criteria[15,16]; c) Acute Renal Failure (ureic nitrogen above 0,60 g/L or creatinine above 1,0 mg/dL); d) hepatic dysfunction (jaundice with total bilirubin above 1,0 mg/dL with predominance of direct fraction); e) platelet count under 100.000/mm^3 and neurological dysfunction (mental confusion, somnolence or Glasgow Coma Score below 15 in absence of sedation or metabolic impairment).

RESULTS

Since August to October 2005, were included 11 healthy subjects (6 male and 5 female, mean age: 42 ± 12 years) and 20 consecutive patients (12 male and 8 female, mean age 49 ± 18 years) admitted to ICU that fulfilled the inclusion criteria and were chosen to participate in the study. In group B the mean APACHE II score was 9, in C and D groups the mean APACHE II score was 17. Group B (n= 5) included n= 4 with neurological disorders and n= 1 postoperative cardiac surgery; Group C (n= 8) included n= 2 postoperative cardiac surgery and n=6 with sepsis; Group D (n= 7) included n= 4 severe sepsis and n= 3 MODS with uncertain etiology. Mean Serum Se concentrations were: group A: 81,11 ±9,49 μ(g/L; B: 79,00 ± 8,17 μg/L; C: 69,37 ± 11,26 μg/L; D: 72,00 ± 9,30 μg/L. Mean GPx activities were: group A: 0,74 ± 0,14 U/mL; group B: 0,65 ± 0,06 U/mL; group C: 0,55 ± 0,11 U/mL; group D: 0,37 ± 0,12 U/mL.

DISCUSSION

We present preliminary data about serum Se and GPx activity in a small number of Uruguayan healthy subjects and critically ill patients. In this small sample of healthy subjects serum Se concentration seems to be similar to other populations although this result will be confirmed in a further research with more participants. The mean value ± DS of serum Se concentration in healthy subjects was 81,11±9,49 μg/L, similar to that of the United Kingdom, Belgium and France (70-130 μg/L, 88±17 μg/L and 78±14 μg/L, respectively) [17]. However, the Se serum mean concentration in group A is lower than the Se mean concentration in other countries such us Japan (151 ± 34 μg/L) and the United States of America (60-220 μg/L). In this way, Se serum concentration results very variable between different areas of the world. Nevertheless in Uruguayan healthy subjects, the serum mean Se concentration is lower than the levels which are necessary to maximise the activity of the antioxidant selenoenzyme GPx in plasma, which occurs at a plasma Se concentration around 95 μg/L (range 89-114 μg/L) [18].

In critically ill patients without SIRS with low APACHE II score (mean value: 9) serum Se level and GPx activity are similar to that of healthy subjects. These results are explained by the absence of Se distribution in presence of normal capillary permeability in patients without systemic inflammation and low hemodilution secondary to less fluid resuscitation.

Patients with SIRS and SIRS-MODS exhibit decreased serum Se and GPx activity [13, 19]. Serum Se concentration fall mostly by Se distribution into different body compartments during severe illness. Se escapes to interstitial compartment by capillary leakage characteristic of endothelial injury. Likewise, the decrease of Selenoprotein P, an extra cellular functional selenoprotein rich in selenocysteine with 10 atoms of Se that serve of Se carrier could explain the serum Se concentration decrease [20, 21]. Whether there is a more active process for Se redistribution is not known [20].

Our findings of a marked decrease in serum Se concentration and GPx activity in SIRS are consistent with the data of Forceville et al. [22] (study in 31 patients with SIRS and severe sepsis), Berger et al. [23] (study in several burn and multiple trauma patients), Hawker & Stewart [24] and Angstwurm et al. [25] (study in critically ill patients with sepsis and APACHE II score above 15). However, patients with the most severe forms of SIRS that progress to MODS have similar levels of Se and GPx activity than patients with mild-moderate SIRS. In this way, our preliminary data is different than that of Forceville et al. These authors have shown that the severity of SIRS inversely correlates with plasma Se concentration and patients with plasma Se concentration below 0,70 μ(mol/L had a 3-fold higher mortality rate compared to those with plasma Se concentration above 0,70 μmol/L [22].

The Se depletion in SIRS patients has been shown in several clinical studies, but in our country it is the first time that one multidisciplinary team analyze the Se status behavior in ICU patients.

Currently our team works in the recruitment of more patients with SIRS and MODS to obtain more representative data.

CONCLUSIONS

In Uruguay, serum Se concentrations are lower than the levels necessary to optimize GPx activity in plasma, but these results will be confirmed in further researches. We have shown that SIRS and MODS are associated to serum Se and GPx activity reduction. Reasonably, early Se supplementation could improve the results and prognostic in critically ill patients with SIRS and MODS. Selenium supplementation in these patients might be highly effective in reducing MODS, infectious complications and eventually the mortality in the most severe cases of SIRS. Prospective, randomized and double blind trials with sufficient statistical power are necessary to finally prove the efficacy or inefficacy of Se supplementation in critically ill patients with SIRS.

REFERENCES

1. Rayman MP. The importance of selenium to human health. The Lancet, 2000; 356: 233-241.
2. Hardy G, Hardy I. Selenium: the Se-XY nutraceutical. Nutrition 20: 590-593, 2004.
3. Burk RF. Selenium: recent clinical advances. Current Opinion in Gastroenterology 2001; 17: 162-166.
4. Demling RH, De Biasse MA. Micronutrients in critical illness. Crit Care Clin 1995; 11: 651-673.
5. Kaim W, Schwederesky B. Biological functions of the nonmetallic inorganic elements. In: Kaim W (Ed). Bioinorganic Chemistry: Inorganic Elements in the Chemistry Of Life. NY, John Wiley, 1994: 318-319.
6. Shenkin A, Allwood MC. Trace elements and vitamins in adult intravenous nutrition. In Rombeau JL, Rolandelli RH (Eds). Clinical Nutrition: Parenteral Nutrition, 3rd Edition. Saunders, Philadelphia 2001: 60-79.
7. Goodyear-Bruch C, Pierce LD. Oxidative stress in critically ill patients. Am J Crit Care 2002; 11: 543-551.
8. Flohé L, Andreesen JR, Brigelius-Flohé, R, et al. Selenium, the element of the moon, in life on earth. IUBMB Life, 49: 411-420, 2000.
9. Kohrle J, Brigelius-Flohe R, Bock A, et al. Selenium in Biology: Facts and medical perspectives. Biol Chem 381; 849-864, 2000.
10. Dodig S, Cepelak I. The facts and controversy about selenium. Acta Pharm. 2004; 54: 261-276.
11. Beck MA, Levander OA, Handy J. Oxidative stress mediated by trace elements. J Nutr. 133: 1463S-1467S, 2003.
12. Gutteridge J, Mitchell J. Redox imbalance in the critically ill. Br Med Bull. 1999; 55: 49-75.
13. Maehira F, Luyo GA, Miyagy I et al. Alterations of serum selenium concentration in the acute phase of pathological conditions. Clin Chim Acta 2002; 316: 137-46.
14. Pieban PA, Munyani A, Beachum J. Determination of Selenium concentration and Glutathione Peroxidase activity in plasma and erythrocytes. Clin Chem 28(2); 311, 1982.
15. American College of Chest Physicians / Society of Critical Care Medicine Consensus Conference: Definitions for sepsis and organ failure and guidelines for the use of innovative therapies in sepsis. Crit Care Med 1992; 20: 864-874.
16. Bernard GR, Artigas A, Brighman KL, et al. The American-European consensus conference on ARDS. Definition, mechanisms, relevant outcomes, and clinical trial coordination. Am J Respir Crit Care Med 149: 818-824, 1994.
17. Shehhan TM, Halls DJ. Measurement of selenium in clinical specimens. Ann Clin Biochem. 1999; 36: 301-15.
18. Duffield AJ, Thomson CD, Hill KE et al. An estimation of selenium requirements for New Zealanders. Am J Clin Nutr 1999; 70: 896-903.
19. Gartner R, Albrich W, Angsstwurm WA. The effect of a selenium supplementation on the outcome of patients with severe systemic inflammation, burn and trauma. BioFactors 2001; 14: 199-204. Burk RF, Hill KE.
20. Selenoprotein P: an extracelular protein with unique physical characteristics and role in selenium homeostasis. Annu Rev Nutr 2005; 25: 2125-235.

21. Shenkin A. The key role of micronutrients. Clinical Nutrition 2005 Dec 20; [Epub ahead of print].
22. Forceville X, Vitoux D, Gauzit R, Combes A, Lahilaire P, Chappuis P. Selenium, systemic immune response syndrome, sepsis and outcome in critically ill patients. Crit Care Med 1998; 26: 1536-1544.
23. Berger MM, Spertini F, Shenkin C, Wardle L, Weisner L, Schindler C, Chiolero RL. Trace element supplementation modulates pulmonary infection rates after major burns: a double blind, placebo controlled trial. Am J Clin Nutr; 68 (1998), 365-371.
24. Hawker FH, Stewart PM, Snitch PJ. Effects of acute illness on selenium homeostasis. Crit Care Med 1990; 18: 442-446.
25. Angstwurm MA, Schottdorf J, Schopohl J, Gaertner R. Selenium replacement in patients with severe systemic inflammatory response syndrome improves clinical outcome. Crit Care Med 1999; 27: 1807-1813.

Metal Ions in Biology and Medicine: vol. 9. Eds Maria Carmen Alpoim, Paula Vasconcellos Morais, Maria Amélia Santos, Armando J. Cristóvão, José A. Centeno, Philippe Collery.
John Libbey Eurotext, Paris © 2006 pp. 540-1.

Magnesium homeostasis and blood pressure monitoring in female teenagers with acute and chronic pyelonephritis

Svetlana L. Moiseeva[1], Igor N. Iezhitsa[2], Mikhail Y. Lediaev[1], Alexander A. Spasov[2]

Volgograd State Medical University, [1]Department of children's diseases, [2]Department of pharmacology, 1 Pavshikh Bortsov sq., Volgograd, 400131 Russia; E-mail: Farm@interdacom.ru

During the last decades the kidney has emerged as a key organ in the homeostasis of magnesium (Mg) and disturbances of Mg metabolism have been described in several renal diseases. The renal causes include Bartter's and Gitelman's syndromes, post obstructive diuresis, post acute tubular necrosis, renal transplantation, and interstitial nephropathy [1]. Many therapeutic agents cause renal Mg wasting and subsequent deficiency [2, 3]. Of special interest is the Mg status in pyelonephritis (PN). On the one hand, PN is considered to be probable risk of hypomagnesaemia due to ion-regulating disturbances in tubulointerstitial tissue of kidneys [4]. Renal Mg wasting has occasionally been reported in patients with acute [5] or chronic [6] tubulointerstitial nephritis not caused by nephrotoxic drugs - for example, in chronic pyelonephritis (CPN) and acute renal allograft rejection [7]. On the other hand, symptomatic hypomagnesemia caused by renal electrolyte wasting occasionally develop in PN patients treated with aminoglycosides [4]. PN is also interesting because of its cardiovascular complications and fact that Mg deficit itself in PN may be considered as a cardiovascular risk. Hypertension is very frequent in patients with renal disease and its prevalence increases as renal failure progresses. In study of Ridao at al. [8] 63% of the adult patients with CPN were hypertensive. Study of Jacobson et al. [9, 10] is evidence that children and adults with PN renal scarring are at high risk of developing hypertension.

So, the aims of this study were therefore: (1) to estimate of Mg homeostasis (erythrocyte, plasma and daily urine Mg, and Mg fraction excretion) and to measure of blood pressure of female teenagers with acute and chronic pyelonephritis; and (2) to find out whether there are some important link between Mg levels in biological mediums and the blood pressure state in female teenagers with PN.

PATIENTS AND METHODS

Subjects, inclusion and exclusion criteria

Our series consists of three groups of subjects with PN: a group of 22 female teenagers with acute pyelonephritis (APN) in active stage, a group of 49 female teenagers with CPN in the stage of clinical and laboratory remission and a group of 18 female teenagers with CPN in exacerbation. Mean age was 13,4 (12÷16) years. Fifty-five age-matched healthy female teenagers served as control. Mean age was 13,8 (12÷16) years.

To diagnose APN and CPN urinary tract structure and functions were evaluated dynamically based on data of ultrasound examination, dopplerography of kidney arteries, biochemical blood tests (urea, creatinine, protein, protein fractions); Zimnitsky and Nechiporenko urine tests, day glucosuria and proteinuria tests, bacteriological urine examination.

None of the patients had taken diuretics or other drugs that could have interfered with Mg metabolism (e.g. gentamycin, amynoglycosides, tobromycin, theophillin, phenobarbital, etc) in the two months prior to the beginning of the study. Exclusion criteria included cardiovascular disease, obesity, diabetes mellitus, electrolyte imbalance and/or presence of diarrhoea. All groups of female teenagers had similar sedentary live and were eating a weight-maintaining diet providing a similar daily protein, carbohydrate and Mg intake (300 mg Mg/day).

Measurement

In all subjects, plasma and erythrocyte Mg levels, urinary Mg excretion every 3 h and over 24 h and Mg fraction excretion were evaluated; the latter being calculated dividing the clearance of Mg by the clearance of creatinine:

$$\text{FE (Mg)} = \frac{\text{U (Mg)} \times \text{P (Cr)}}{0{,}7 \times \text{P (Mg)} \times \text{U (Cr)}} \times 100$$

where the term U and P refer to the urine and plasma concentration of magnesium (Mg) and creatinine (Cr). The plasma Mg concentration is multiplied by 0.7, since only about 70 percent of the circulating Mg is free (not bound to albumin) and therefore able to be filtered across the glomerulus. The urine was acidified before Mg assay. Erythrocyte, plasma and urine Mg levels were measured by colorimetric assay using the method based on staining reaction of Mg and thiazole yellow [11].

Ambulatory blood pressure was recorded for 24 hours with a portable ambulatory monitor of blood pressure "ABPM-04" ("Meditech", Hungary) on day of blood sampling for Mg determination.

Statistical Analysis

The data are presented as means (±SEM). The data (absolute mean and expressed as a percentage of the control) were analyzed using a one-way repeated measure ANOVA and Scheffé post hoc comparisons ($p<0.05$) (Statistica 6.0). Sixth-Degree Polynomial Regression Analysis was run for fitting of daily urine Mg excretion and ambulatory blood pressure profile.

RESULTS

In our study CPN was associated with depleted intraerythrocytic Mg, increased urine Mg level and elevated Mg fraction excretion with respect to control *(table 1)*. However the plasma Mg levels in female teenagers with APN and CPN and control group did not differ significantly, and these data fluctuations did not fall outside the natural physiological norms. APN in active stage caused a substantial increase Mg fraction excretion compared with control. Daily urine Mg excretion profile fitted with a sixth-degree polynomial in children with PN differed from those of control group *(figure 2)*.

Due to ABPM results, in children with PN, blood pressure and pulse at different time periods were significantly higher than in control group *(table 2)*. However daily blood pressure profile fitted with a sixth-degree polynomial did not fall outside the physiological norms for the given gender and age *(figure 1)*.

Table 1. Magnesium levels in the subjects studied

Parameters	Controls (n=55)	CPN in remission (n=49)	CPN in exacerbation (n=18)	APN in active stage (n=22)
Erythrocyte Mg level (mmol/l)	2.05±0.07	1.88±0.02*	1.92±0.06	1.87±0.09
Plasma Mg level (mmol/l)	1.14±0.05	1.09±0.03	1.07±0.07	1.14±0.04
Urine Mg concentration (mmol/l)	1.01±0.04	1.12±0.02*	1.17±0.05*	1.03±0.04
Plasma creatinine (µmol/l)	59.2±4.0	68.5±2.2*	71.7±3.6*	71.1±4.0
Urine creatinine (µmol/l)	53.09±5.0	55.3±3.9	80.9±3.6*	52.4±9.7
Mg fraction excretion (%)	3.1±0.4	4.17±0.2*	4.13±0.4	4.4±0.5*
Urinary Mg (mmol/24h)	0.83±0.09	0.83±0.05	0.8±0.1	0.79±0.07

Note: In all PN groups tubular proteinuria was 50÷100 mg/24h. All data are presented as the means (±SEM); * Significantly different CPN and APN groups vs. control group (one-way ANOVA with post hoc Scheffé test, P<.05); n - number of subjects.

Table 2. Ambulatory blood pressure parameters

Time period	ABPM parameters	Controls (n=55)	CPN in remission (n=48)	CPN in exacerbation (n=18)	APN in active stage (n=22)
Diurnal (24 h)	SBP, mm Hg	107.5±1.5	114.9±1.2*	117.5±3.3*	109.6±1.6
	DBP, mm Hg	64.6±1.3	69.1±0.8*	67.4±2.2	65.7±1.2
	HR, bpm	80.5±1.2	84.8±1.1*	83.7±2.6	85.7±2.6
	MBP, mm Hg	78.8±1.6	83.4±1.1*	84.1±2.5	80.5±1.3
Daytime (06.00-22.00)	SBP, mm Hg	111.7±1.6	116.8±1.3*	119.9±3.3*	111.7±1.7
	DBP, mm Hg	65.1±1.2	70.4±0.8*	69.9±2.4	67.8±1.4
	HR, bpm	83.0±2.2	87.5±1.3	87.1±3.1	88.4±2.7
	MBP, mm Hg	80.6±1.4	85.7±0.9*	86.6±2.6	82.4±1.4
Nighttime (22.00-06.00)	SBP, mm Hg	98.6±1.3	105.0±1.5*	106.2±3.7	101.9±1.7
	DBP, mm Hg	54.5±1.3	59.2±1.0*	57.7±2.5	58.4±1.3*
	HR, bpm	67.6±2.0	72.7±1.4*	70.1±2.0	72.8±2.9
	MBP, mm Hg	69.2±1.3	74.1±1.1*	73.1±3.2	73.1±1.9

Note: ABPM indicates ambulatory blood pressure monitoring; SBP, systolic blood pressure; DBP, diastolic blood pressure; MBP, mean blood pressure; HR, heart rate; and bpm, beats per minute. All data are presented as the means (±SEM); * Significantly different CPN and APN groups vs. control group; (one-way ANOVA with post hoc Scheffé test, P<.05); n - number of subjects.

DISCUSSION

Various studies have examined the possible correlation between urinary Mg level and blood pressure. Durlach et al. [12] in the review indicate that, when renal function is efficient, these levels should reflect the dietary intake of Mg; sometimes an inverse correlation between daily magnesuria and blood pressure is observed [13], but more often no relation is found [14]. Plasma Mg is generally normal in hypertensive individuals and normotension is the rule during Mg deficit [12, 15, 13]. An inverse correlation between serum Mg and blood pressure is sometimes observed [14, 16] but it is not the rule [14, 17] and it may depend on the concomitant use of Mg-depleting drugs [12, 18, 17]. An inverse relation between Mg and renin in plasma [19] was not confirmed in other studies [13, 20, 21]. In fact serum Mg seems related to the evolution of the disease. A positive correlation has been observed in moderate hypertension, which tended to disappear when hypertension became more severe [20]. An early clinical study of patients who had severe hypertension with end organ disease demonstrated high serum Mg concentrations [14].

An inverse correlation between erythrocyte Mg levels, and free Mg in particular, and blood pressure has been observed in diverse selected populations of hypertensive patients but no adjustments were made for important covariables [14]. A weak positive association was found between free Mg and mean blood pressure. This relationship was lost in a multivariate regression analysis [21]. As a rule there is no difference between erythrocyte Mg concentrations in hypertensive patients and controls [22]. There have been similar observations relating to leukocyte Mg [23, 24].

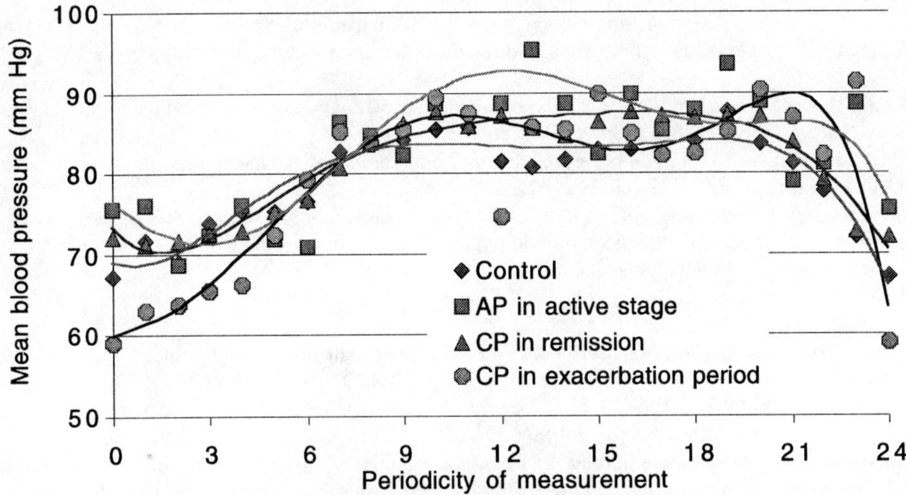

Fig. 1. Daily mean blood pressure (mm Hg) profile fitted with a sixth-degree polynomial

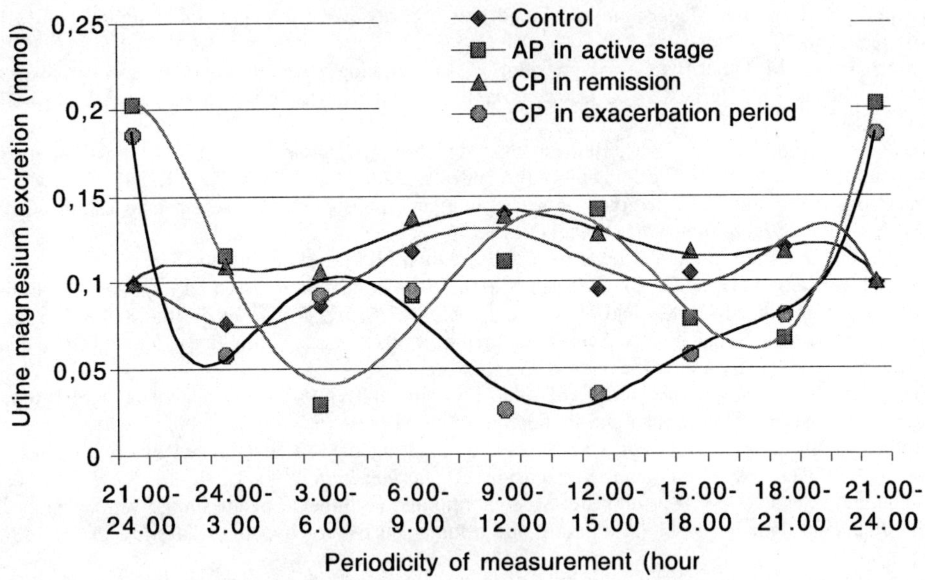

Fig. 2. Daily urine Mg excretion profile fitted with a sixth-degree polynomial

CONCLUSION

To sum up, our data do not yet allow final conclusions to be drawn, but they seem to support the notion that there is an important link between Mg deficit and the blood pressure state in children with PN.

REFERENCES

1. al-Ghamdi SM, Cameron EC, Sutton RA. Magnesium deficiency: pathophysiologic and clinical overview. *Am J Kidney Dis.* 1994; 24(5): 737-752.
2. Kelepouris E, Agus ZS. Hypomagnesemia: renal magnesium handling. *Semin Nephrol* 1998; 18(1): 58-73.
3. Sutton RA, Domrongkitchaiporn S. Abnormal renal magnesium handling. *Miner Electrolyte Metab* 1993; 19(4-5): 232-240.
4. Zaloga GP, Chernow B, Pock A et al. Hypomagnesemia is a common complication of aminoglycoside therapy. *Surg Gynecol Obstet* 1984; 158(6): 561-565.
5. Braden GL Germain MJ, Fitzgibbons JP. Impaired potassium and magnesium homeostasis in acute tubulo-interstitial nephritis. *Nephron* 1985; 41: 273-278.
6. Randall RE. Magnesium metabolism in chronic renal disease. *Ann N Y Acad Sci* 1969; 162: 831-846.
7. Sutton RAL, Dirks JH. Disturbances of calcium and magnesium metabolism. In : Brenner BM, Rector FC, eds. *The kidney.* Philadelphia: Saunders, 1996 : 1038-85.
8. Ridao N, Luno J, Garcia de Vinuesa S, et al. Prevalence of hypertension in renal disease. *Nephrol Dial Transplant.* 2001; 16 Suppl 1: 70-73.
9. Jacobson SH, Eklof O, Eriksson CG et al. Altered vasopressin release and osmotic regulation during exercise in patients with pyelonephritic renal scarring. *Scand J Urol Nephrol* 1990; 24(4): 275-279.
10. Jacobson SH, Eklof O, Eriksson CG, et al. Development of hypertension and uraemia after pyelonephritis in childhood: 27 year follow up. *BMJ* 1989; 299(6701): 703-706.
11. **Меньшиков В.В. Лабораторные методы исследования в клинике. Москва: Медицина,**, 1987. [Men'shikov VV Laboratory methods of clinic testings. Moscow : Publisher "Meditsina", 1987] (in Russian).
12. Durlach J, Durlach V, Rayssiguier Y et al. Magnesium and blood pressure. II. Clinical studies. *Magnes Res* 1992; 5(2): 147-53.
13. Tillman DM, Semple PF. Calcium and magnesium in essential hypertension. *Clin Sci* 1988; 75: 395-402.
14. Whelton PK, Klag MJ. Magnesium and blood pressure: review of the epidemiologic and clinical trial experience. *Am J Cardiol* 1989; 63: 26G-30G.
15. Durlach J, Bara M, Guiet-Bara A. Magnesium level in drinking water: its importance in cardiovascular risk. In : Itokawa Y, Durlach J (eds), *Magnesium in health and disease.* London : John Libbey. 1989, pp. 173-182.
16. Touyz RM, Milne FJ, Seftel HC, Reinach SG. Magnesium, calcium, sodium and potassium status in normotensive and hypertensive Johannesburg residents. *S Afr Med J* 1987; 72: 377-381.
17. Uza G, Pavel O. Effect of nifedipine on serum inorganic phosphorus and serum magnesium in hypertensive patients. *Magnesium-Bull* 1989; 11: 173-176.
18. Durlach J Magnesium in clinical practice. London : John Libbey. 1988, pp. 360.
19. Resnik LM, Laragh JH, Sealey JE, Alderman MH. Divalent cations in essential hypertension. Relation between serum ionized Ca, Mg and plasma renin activity. *N Engl J Med* 1983; 309: 888-891.
20. Saito N, Nishiyama S, Kuchiba A. Serum magnesium levels in cases with glucose intolerance and cases with cardiovascular diseases. *Magnes Res* 1989; 2: 36.
21. Woods KL, Walmesley D, Heagerty AM et al. Phosphorus-31 NMR measurement of free erythrocyte magnesium concentration in man and its relation to blood pressure. *Clin Sci* 1988; 74: 513-518.
22. Gunther T, Vormann J, Hollriegl V, Fehlinger R Unchanged Mg^{2+} metabolism of erythrocytes from patients with tetanic syndrome and hypertension. *Magnesium-Bull.* 1990; 12: 10-13.
23. Shibutani Y, Sakamoto K, Katsuno S et al. T. Serum and erythrocyte magnesium levels in junior high school students: relation to blood pressure and a family history of hypertension. *Magnesium* 1988; 7: 188-194.
24. Skoczenlusch M, Pajdak W, Janas A. Potassium and magnesium content in the peripheral blood lymphocytes in patients with essential hypertension. *Magnesium-Bull* 1989; 11: 166-169.

ACKNOWLEDGEMENT

Attending 9th International Symposium on Metal Ions in Biology and Medicine was sponsored by INTAS Conference Individual Grant.

Metal Ions in Biology and Medicine: vol. 9. Eds Maria Carmen Alpoim, Paula Vasconcellos Morais, Maria Amélia Santos, Armando J. Cristóvão, José A. Centeno, Philippe Collery.
John Libbey Eurotext, Paris © 2006 pp. 546-1.

Effect of training and exercise intensity on magnesium status

C.P. Monteiro[1], H. Santa Clara[2], M.F. Raposo[1], A. Gonçalves[2], F. Limão[1], Y. Rayssiguier[3], A. Mazur[3], C. Coudray[3], E. Gueux[3], C. Feillet Coudray[3], M. Bicho[4], M. J. Laires[1]

[1]*Biochemistry Laboratory, Faculty of Human Kinetics, Lisbon, Portugal;*
[2]*Exercise and Health Department, Faculty of Human Kinetics, Lisbon, Portugal;*
[3]*Unité des Maladies Métaboliques et Micronutriments, Clermont-Ferrand, INRA, France;*
[4]*Genetics Laboratory, Faculty of Medicine, Lisbon, Portugal.*

INTRODUCTION

Primary magnesium deficit plays a role in the pathophysiology of physical exercise [1, 2]. Several studies have reported that athletes and physically active individuals may be deficient in magnesium [3, 4]. The studies of Huet and co-workers [5] showed that the food intake of athletes and sedentary subjects is very similar, apart from significantly different energy values in the intake of athletes. Two conditions contribute to frequent mineral deficits among athletes: they consume diets with inadequate mineral amounts, lower than the recommended dietary allowances (RDA) [6], and mineral losses in urine and sweat are more important during exercise than in basal conditions [7].

During exercise, compartmental shifts of magnesium have been observed, but data to demonstrate the variations in magnesium levels after exercise are inconsistent. Inconsistencies may be related to differences in experimental designs, work intensity, work duration, timing of blood samples, training condition of the subjects and environmental conditions [8].

It is important to determine whether the changes in plasma magnesium concentration are transient or whether participation in sustained exercise may induce permanent alterations. Several studies indicate that there is a sustained fall in plasma magnesium after strenuous exercise and that hypomagnesaemia persists during a season of athletic training [9].

The purpose of our work was to evaluate the influence of subjects' training condition and exercise intensity on plasma magnesium (P-Mg) and urinary excretion of magnesium (U-Mg).

MATERIALS AND METHODS

Subjects

Fifteen high competition male swimmers (S) training between 17 and 23 h/week for at least 5 years, and 16 active men (AM) not involved in any regular sport participated in the study. They were all between 18 and 25 years old (S: 20.0±1.65 years and AM: 21.1±1.47 years). Their mean weight and height were respectively 70.6±5.29 Kg and 176±6 cm for the S group and 71.1±10.1 Kg and 176±7 cm for the AM group. The mean body mass index (BMI), derived from weight and height, was 22.7±1.6 Kg.m^{-2} for the S group and 23.0±2.9 Kg.m^{-2} for the AM group.

Dual-energy X-ray absorptiometry (DXA) was used to assess body fat percentage (BF%), and free fat mass (FFM) (QDR-1500, Hologic, Waltman, USA, pencil beam mode, software version 5.67 enhanced whole body analysis). BF% was 10.4±3.34% for S and 17.5±6.85% for AM ($p<0.01$) and FFM was 62.6±4.36 Kg for S and 58,2±5,69 Kg for AM ($p<0.05$).

Medical and running histories obtained by questionnaire indicated no smoking habits or known coronary heart diseases. Informed written consent was obtained from all the subjects.

Nutritional Analysis

Nutritional analysis was performed using a 3 days food record. Subjects were previously informed of the most correct and complete form of fulfilment of the record and interviewed afterwards in order to compare the items recorded with real size photos in a Portuguese manual for analysing food records (Modelos Fotográficos para Inquéritos Alimentares do Instituto Nacional de Saúde Dr Ricardo Jorge).

Macro and micronutrients intake were quantified with Food Processor (Nutrition Analysis Software version 7.4, made by ESHA, Research, Salem, Oregon, 1999).

Exercise Protocols

The subjects performed two exercises of different intensities, at fast, early in the morning, under the supervision of a certified researcher.

The first exercise was a continuous graded maximal exercise test (ME) on treadmill (Quinton TM 55) with an individualised protocol consisting of a 5 minutes warm up followed by the increment of exercise intensity at each 2 minutes. In the first two levels, speed was increased 1 mile/h and in the following levels, slope was increased 2.5%. Mean total exercise time was 15.4±1.63 min for S and 13.5±1.41 min for AM.

Throughout the exercise, heart rate was monitored with a Polar® (Pacer ECG/Telemetry Finland) and expired air was analysed using a metabolic cart (Cardiorespiratory Diagnosis System, Medical Graphics Corporation, St. Paul, MN). VO_{2max} was 51.3±7.1 $mL.min^{-1}.kg^{-1}$ for S and 43.2±5.7 $mL.min^{-1}.kg^{-1}$ for AM ($p<0.01$) and maximal heart rate was 190±8 $beat.min^{-1}$ for S and 194±6 $beat.min^{-1}$ for AM. At the anaerobic threshold, oxygen uptake and heart rate were respectively 38.0±4.4 $mL.min^{-1}.kg^{-1}$ and 162±10 $beat.min^{-1}$ for S and 29.2±5.1 $mL.min^{-1}.kg^{-1}$ and 157±15 $beat.min^{-1}$ for AM ($p<0.01$ for VO_{2AnaT}).

48 h later the same subjects exercised at 75% of their maximal heart rate for 30 minutes on the same treadmill (submaximal exercise - SME). Heart rate was monitored by the same method as in ME.

Biochemical Analysis

Blood was collected by antecubital venopucture before, just after and 2 hours after the exercises (6 samples for each subject: M_1 - first moment of evaluation, at rest, just before the maximal exercise; ME - just after the maximal exercise; ME+2h - two hours after the maximal exercise; M_1+48h - forty eight hours after M_1, just before the submaximal exercise; SME - just after the submaximal exercise; SME+2h - two hours after the submaximal exercise). Urine samples were collected before and two hours after the tests (4 samples for each subject: M_1; ME+2h; M_1+48h; SME+2h). Subjects were at fast throughout the all procedure.

Plasma magnesium (P-Mg) and urine magnesium (U-Mg) were assessed by atomic absorption spectrophotometry and urine creatinine was assessed by spectrophotometry.

Plasma magnesium values were corrected for plasma volume variation ($P\text{-}Mg_{PVV}$) just after the exercises, according with van Beaumont and col. [10].

Statistical Analysis

Results are presented as mean ± standard deviation and in graphics values are represented as mean ± standard error of the mean. Normal distribution of the samples was tested with Shapiro-Wilk's test (n<50).

Macro and micronutrients intake were compared between groups with unpaired t test or with

Man Whitney's U. Micronutrients intake for each group were compared with the respective RDAs with one sample t test.

P-Mg and U-Mg at M_1 were compared between groups with unpaired t test. The results of the 6 evaluations of plasma magnesium were analysed with a 2 x 6 General Linear Model analysis of variance for repeated measures, with one between subjects factor (training effect) and one within subjects (repeated measures) factor (exercise). Two different analyses were performed: $P\text{-}Mg_{PVV}$, integrating values corrected for PVV just after the exercises, and P-Mg, integrating values not corrected for PVV just after the exercises. The results of the 4 evaluations of U-Mg were analysed with a 2×4 General Linear Model analysis of variance for repeated measures, with one between subjects factor (training effect) and one within subjects (repeated measures) factor (exercise).

The equality of the matrix of variances was explored with Box's test and sphericity with Mauchly's test. If sphericity was not verified the Huynh-Feldt correction was used.

Significant main effects were followed up using special contrasts, baring in mind relevant comparisons: ME vs M_1; ME+2h vs M_1; M_1+48h vs M_1; SME vs M_1+48h and SME+2h vs M_1+48h.

The effect of exercise intensity on $P\text{-}Mg_{PVV}$ and U-Mg was explored as both exercises induced significant effects on $P\text{-}Mg_{PVV}$ just after the exercises and on U-Mg 2 hours after the exercises. Percentage variations of these parameters were calculated for both exercises and a 2×2 General Linear Model analysis of variance for repeated measures with one between subjects factor (training effect) and one within subjects (repeated measures) factor (exercise intensity) was applied.

Significance level was set at $p<0.05$ except for special contrasts (multiple comparisons) for the moments of evaluation in which it was set at $p<0.02$.

Statistical analysis was performed with SPSS for Windows, version 11.5, released in 2002 by SPSS Inc., Chicago, USA.

RESULTS

Nutritional analysis revealed that both groups had similar intakes. Magnesium intake was low in both groups when comparing with reference value (6 $mg.kg^{-1}.day^{-1}$), but only significantly different in the AM group (p=0,000).

For $P\text{-}Mg_{PVV}$ and for P-Mg, it was observed an effect of training ($P\text{-}Mg_{PVV}$: F=4.633; p=0.043; P-Mg: F=4.642; p=0.043) and an effect of exercise ($P\text{-}Mg_{PVV}$: F=11.821; p=0.000; P-Mg: F=3.478; p=0.020), without interaction between the two effects ($P\text{-}Mg_{PVV}$: F=1.239; p=0.300; P-Mg: F=1.154; p=0.335), suggesting that the mean value of all the moments of evaluation was significantly different between groups and that the effect of exercise was similar in the two groups. Swimmers showed lower plasma magnesium values in all the moments of evaluation *(graphic 1).*

For U-Mg there was no interactions between the effect of training and the effect of exercise (F=0.620, p=0.606) and no effect of training (F=2.065, p=0.170), but it was observed an effect of exercise (F=8.656, p=0.000).

$P\text{-}Mg_{PVV}$ was lower just after both ME (F=31.319; p=0.000) and SME (F=26.863; p=0.000) *(graphic 1).* However, analysing P-Mg, just after ME the mean value was higher (F=11.301; p=0.003); and just after SME no differences were observed (F=2.859; p=0.106) *(graphic 1).*

Two hours after both exercises P-Mg had returned to the initial values (F=0.648; p=0.430 for ME and F=1.557; p=0.226 for SME) *(graphic 1)* and U-Mg was lower (F=22.925; p=0.000 for ME and F=48.796; p=0.000 for SME) *(graphic 2).*

The analysis of the percentage variations induced by the two exercise tests on $P\text{-}Mg_{PVV}$ revealed no interaction between the effect of training and the effect of exercise intensity (F=0.137; p=0.715) and no effects of training (F=0.489; p=0.492) or exercise intensity (F=0.593; p=0.450) which suggests that, for the two exercises performed, changes induced in $P\text{-}Mg_{PVV}$ by exercise don't depend on the level of training of the subjects or on exercise intensity.

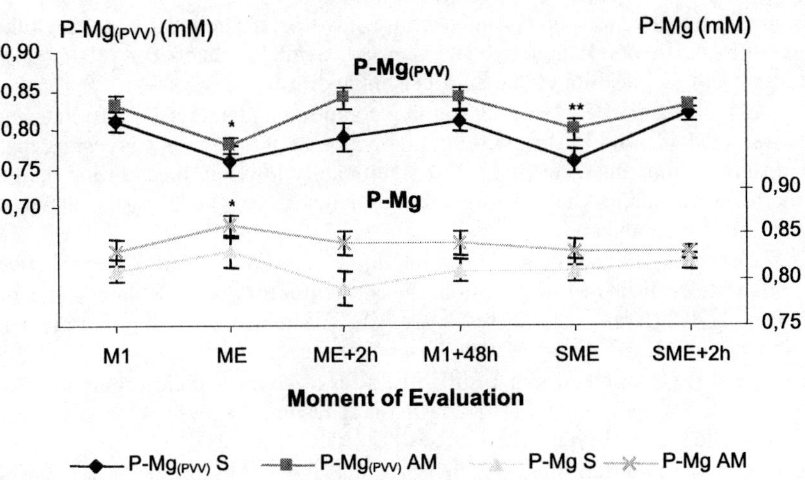

Graphic 1. Variation of P-Mg(PVV) and P-Mg with exercise for S and AM.

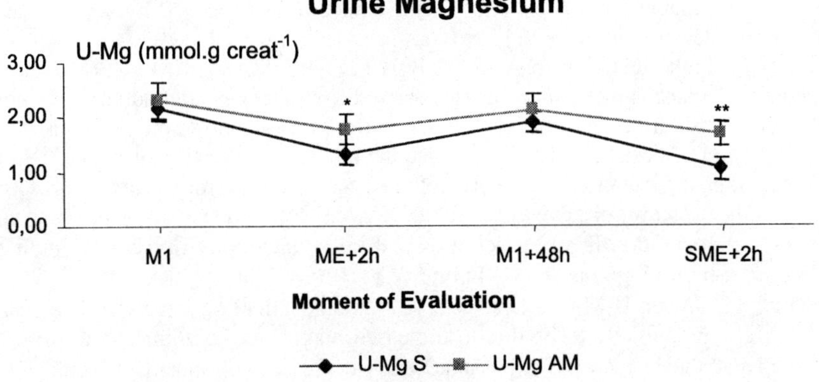

Graphic 2. Variation of U-Mg with exercise for S and AM.
* - significantly different from M_1; ** - significantly different from M_1+48h

The analysis of U-Mg percentage variations induced two hours after the exercises presented no interaction between the effect of training and the effect of exercise intensity (F=0.549; p=0.470) and no effect of the exercise intensity (F=0.300; p=0.865) but it was observed a significant effect of training (F=5.547; p=0.032).

DISCUSSION

Magnesium ingestion is below the recommend dietary allowances in the AM group but not in the S group. A similar magnesium intake was observed in the SU.VI.MAX study [11]. However, P-Mg mean levels are in the reference range in both groups, with a tendency for lower levels in the S group at M_1.

Adequate Mg ingestion in athletes is crucial not only because magnesium deficiency can compromise energy balance and delay calcium re-entry into sarcoplasmic reticulum by the Mg-dependent ATPase and thus compromise exercise performance, but also because Mg is essential for the maintenance of the cell membrane integrity and function contributing to protect subjects from injury to which they are more prone when exercising.

Changes in Plasma magnesium during exercise have been studied by us and other authors [12-19]. Nevertheless, to our knowledge, no data are available as to the relationship between exercise intensity and magnesium changes in plasma and urine.

We observed significant effects of both training condition and exercise performance on plasma magnesium (both $P\text{-}Mg_{PVV}$ and P-Mg), without interaction between them, suggesting that the mean value at the different moments of evaluation is significantly lower in the S group than in the AM group and that exercise induces changes on plasma magnesium which are not dependent on the training condition of the subjects.

$P\text{-}Mg_{PVV}$ decreased significantly just after maximal and submaximal exercise. However, one should notice that the analysis of P-Mg without the correction for plasma volume variation induced by exercise presented different results. Just after ME, P-Mg was also significantly different but higher; and just after SME no changes were observed *(graphic 1)*.

Previously we had observed similar results just after a maximal ciclo-ergometer exercise in a group of young male football players [18]. Plasma magnesium decreases have also been reported by other Authors after several types of exercises [13, 15, 17, 20, 21].

Other Authors have reported increases in P-Mg but didn't correct values for plasma volume variation [22, 23]. Inconsistencies in data regarding P-Mg changes during exercise may be reduced if plasma volume variation is accounted for.

Decreased plasma magnesium levels after exercise have been explained by several mechanisms: redistribution of magnesium into cells [24] and loss in urine. Stress induced by exercise which raises endogenous catecholamine levels, increasing lipolysis [25]. Elliott and Rizack [26] found increased magnesium content in plasma membrane vesicles derived from fat cells after adrenaline stimulation *in vitro*. Increased magnesium loss in urine can be due to increases in aldosterone, antidiuretic hormone, thyroid hormones, and acidosis, all of which reduce the tubular reabsorption of magnesium [13]. The fact that 2 hours after the exercises P-Mg had returned to the pre-exercise values suggests that it is very unlikely that the decreases observed just after the exercises were due to sweat or urine elimination.

In fact, Mg hyperexcretion in sweat acquires real importance only in cases of intense activity under conditions of high temperature and humidity [27].

Additionally, the lower U-Mg values observed 2 hours after the exercises, suggest that the decrease of $P\text{-}Mg_{PVV}$ is unlikely to be due to increased magnesium elimination in urine.

On the other hand, the decreased U-Mg is not due to a decrease in plasma magnesium concentration as P-Mg increased just after ME and did not change significantly after SME. Thus, these results may suggest a mechanism for magnesium retention in the body. This mechanism may be more efficient in the group of swimmers as an effect of training is observed for the analysis of the percentage of variation induced by the exercises on U-Mg, with higher decreases in this group. However, a 24 hours collection of urine is necessary to evaluate if, after the initial period of post exercise time, magnesium excretion by urine becomes elevated as suggested by other Authors [13, 28].

The elimination of magnesium from the body would mobilise magnesium reserves to replace circulating levels, which may compromise magnesium status and so increase magnesium nutritional demands.

CONCLUSIONS

The results show an effect of training on P-Mg with swimmers presenting lower values in all the moments of evaluation. This effect of training is not explained by different food intake or an increased U-Mg excretion. Both exercises induced a transient decrease in P-Mg which may be the result of an increased need for Mg by active tissues during exercise. Exercise may induce a mechanism for magnesium retention in the body that may become more efficient with training as muscle mass increases.

REFERENCES

1. Laires, MJ and CP Monteiro, Magnesium status: Influence on the regulation of exercise induced oxidative stress and immune function in athelets, In: *Advances in Magnesium Research: Nutrition and Health*, Y. Rayssiguier, A. Mazur, and J. Durlach, (Eds.). 2001; John Libbey & Company Ltd.: London. p. 433-441.
2. Rayssiguier, Y, CY Guezennec, and J Durlach. New experimental and clinical data on the relationship between magnesium and sport. *Magnes Res* 1990, 3(2): 93-102.
3. Casoni, I, C Guglielmini, L Graziano, MG Reali, D Mazzotta, and V Abbasciano. Changes of magnesium concentrations in endurance athletes. *Int J Sports Med* 1990, 11(3): 234-7.
4. Seelig, MS. Consequences of magnesium deficiency on the enhancement of stress reactions; preventive and therapeutic implications (a review). *J Am Coll Nutr* 1994, 13(5): 429-46.
5. Huet, F, J Keppling, J Marajo, G M., H Legrand, and CY Guezennec. Comportement nutritionnel du coureur de demi-fond. Aspects qualitatifs et quantitatifs. Rapports avec la depense energétique de l'entraînement. *Sci Sports* 1988, 3: 17-28.
6. Córdova, A, FJ Navas, M Gómez-Carraminãna, and H Rodríguez. Evaluation of magnesium intake in elite sportsmen. *Magnesium Bull* 1994, 16: 59-63.
7. Fischer, PW and A Giroux. An evaluation of plasma and erythrocyte magnesium concentration and the activities of alkaline phosphatase and creatine kinase as indicators of magnesium status. *Clin Biochem* 1991, 24(2): 215-8.
8. Laires, MJ, CP Monteiro, and M Bicho. Role of cellular magnesium in health and human disease. *Front Biosci* 2004, 9: 262-76.
9. Stendig-Lindberg, G, WE Wacker, and Y Shapiro. Long term effects of peak strenuous effort on serum magnesium, lipids, and blood sugar in apparently healthy young men. *Magnes Res* 1991, 4(1): 59-65.
10. van Beaumont, W, S Underkofler, and S van Beaumont. Erythrocyte volume, plasma volume, and acid-base changes in exercise and heat dehydration. *J Appl Physiol* 1981, 50(6): 1255-62.
11. SU.VI.MAX, Données intermédiaires, In: *(citation) Apports nutritionnels conseillés pour la population française*, A. Martin, (Ed.). 2001; Editions TEC & DOC: London. p. 149.
12. Cordova, A. Changes on plasmatic and erythrocytic magnesium levels after high-intensity exercises in men. *Physiol Behav* 1992, 52(4): 819-21.
13. Deuster, PA, E Dolev, SB Kyle, RA Anderson, and EB Schoomaker. Magnesium homeostasis during high-intensity anaerobic exercise in men. *J Appl Physiol* 1987, 62(2): 545-50.
14. Guerra, MA, R Monje, A Perez-Beriain, J García de Jalón, A Villanueva, A Herrera, and JF Escanero, Ionic magnesium and selenium in serum after a cycle-ergometric test in football-players, In: *Metal Ions in Biology and Medicine*, J.A. Centeno, P. Collery, G. Vernet, R.B. Finkelman, H. Gibb, and J.C. Etienne, (Eds.). 2000; John Libbey Eurotext: Paris. p. 501-504.
15. Laires, MJ, F Alves, and MJ Halpern. Changes in serum and erythrocyte magnesium and blood lipids after distance swimming. *Magnes Res* 1988, 1(3-4): 219-22.
16. Laires, MJ, F Madeira, J Sergio, C Colaco, C Vaz, GM Felisberto, I Neto, L Breitenfeld, M Bicho, and C Manso. Preliminary study of the relationship between plasma and erythrocyte magnesium variations and some circulating pro-oxidant and antioxidant indices in a standardized physical effort. *Magnes Res* 1993, 6(3): 233-8.
17. Laires, MJ and F Alves. Changes in plasma, erythrocyte, and urinary magnesium with prolonged swimming exercise. *Magnes Res* 1991, 4(2): 119-22.
18. Monteiro, CP, D Pereira, H Ribeiro, C Rabaçal, GM Felisberto, C Mendonça, L Nuno, M Dias, E Carvalho, C Vaz, JS Afonso, JS Fernandes, A Silva, J Barata, MJ Laires, A Mazur, and Y Rayssiguier, Effect of a maximal effort on blood trace elements and magnesium and on some oxidative stress parameters, In: *Trace Elements in Man and Animals - 9: Proceeding of the Ninth International Symposium on Trace Elements in Man and Animals*, P.W.F. Fischer, M.R. L'Abbé, K.A. Cockell, and R.S. Gibson, (Eds.). 1997; NRC Press: Ottawa. p. 361-362.
19. Mooren, FC, SW Golf, A Lechtermann, and K Volker. Alterations of ionized Mg^{2+} in human blood after exercise. *Life Sciences* 2005, 77: 1211-1225.
20. Laires, MJ. Magnésio e exercício físico. Contribuição para o seu estudo. *Motricidade Humana* 1990, 6(1/2): 33-43.
21. Olha, AE, V Klissouras, JD Sullivan, and SC Skoryna. Effect of exercise on concentration of elements in the serum. *J Sports Med Phys Fitness* 1982, 22(4): 414-25.

22. Rama, R, J Ibanez, T Pages, A Callis, and L Palacios. Plasma and red blood cell magnesium levels and plasma creatinine after a 100 km race. *Rev Esp Fisiol* 1993, 49(1): 43-7.
23. Joborn, H, G Akerstrom, and S Ljunghall. Effects of exogenous catecholamines and exercise on plasma magnesium concentrations. *Clin Endocrinol (Oxf)* 1985, 23(3): 219-26.
24. Haymes, EM. Vitamin and mineral supplementation to athletes. *Int J Sport Nutr* 1991, 1(2): 146-69.
25. Rayssiguier, Y and P Larvor, Hypomagnesemia following stimulation of lipolysis in ewes: effects of cold exposure and fasting, In: *Magnesium in Health and Disease*. 1980. p. 68-72.
26. Elliott, DA and MA Rizack. Epinephrine and adrenocorticotropic hormone-stimulated magnesium accumulation in adipocytes and their plasma membranes. *J Biol Chem* 1974, 249(12): 3985-90.
27. Beller, GA, JT Maher, LH Hartley, DE Bass, and WE Wacker. Changes in serum and sweat magnesium levels during work in the heat. *Aviat Space Environ Med* 1975, 46(5): 709-12.
28. Meludu, SC, M Nishimuta, Y Yoshitake, F Toyooka, N Kodama, CS Kim, Y Maekawa, and H Fukuoka, Magnesium homeostasis before and after high intensity (anaerobic) exercise, In: *Advances in magnesium research: Nutrition and health*, Y. Rayssiguier, A. Mazur, and J. Durlach, (Eds.). 2001; Jonh Libbey & Company Ltd.: London. p. 443-6.

Metal Ions in Biology and Medicine: vol. 9. Eds Maria Carmen Alpoim, Paula Vasconcellos Morais, Maria Amélia Santos, Armando J. Cristóvão, José A. Centeno, Philippe Collery.
John Libbey Eurotext, Paris © 2006 pp. 553-1.

A systematic review of colorectal cancer risk in heterozygotes for hereditary hemochromatosis

Richard Nelson, M.D.

Departmentof Surgery, Northern General Hospital, Herries Road, Sheffield S5 7AU, U.K., Rick.nelson@sth.nhs.uk

BACKGROUND

Iron has been shown to increase colorectal cancer risk in a number of animal and observational epidemiologic studies in humans. But the data are inconsistent and reported in such widely variable manners that a summary risk is incalculable. But there is a subgroup of studies that have looked at colorectal cancer risk in genetic carriers of the hereditary hemochromatosis gene that assessed colorectal cancer risk. These studies are more amenable to meta-analysis.

OBJECTIVES

The goal of this review is to assess then relationship of iron in colorectal cancer risk by determination of the risk of colorectal cancer in individuals heterozygous for the hemochromatosis gene(s), a group with mildly elevated iron stores.

SEARCH STRATEGY

Reports were located initially by computerized search using Medline. Key words in various combinations were: hemochromatosis, cancer, colon, colorectal. Randomized controlled trials in which iron was the exposure variable and colorectal cancer the outcome were also sought in Medline but none found.

SELECTION CRITERIA

The studies in this review are case/control and cohort epidemiologic studies, including Humans without restriction as to age, gender or race in which the exposure variable is hetreozygosis for hereditary hemochromatosis and the outcome variable is incidence or mortality from colorectal cancer.

DATA COLLECTION & ANALYSIS

Data were reported as either odds ratios, relative risks and standardized incidence ratios each with 95% confidence intervals. These for the meta-analysis were treated as equivalent metrics. Sensitivity analyses are reported that look at the use of age adjustment of risk, self reporting of cancer and study design.

MAIN RESULTS

The combined risk of all eight studies identified in this review showed an increase in risk for colorectal cancer associated with heterozygosity for hemochromatosis of 18% (odds ratio 1.17, 95% confidence interval 1.05-1.31). These studies included three case control studies (2859 subjects) and four cohort studies (12,182 participants). The sensitivity analyses in each case gave a summary risk estimate that was very close to the estimate for the whole group (see *table*).

REVIEWERS' CONCLUSIONS

Iron stores increase colorectal cancer risk.

Review: Iron and Colorectal Cancer Risk: An analysis of risk among heterozygotes of hereditary hemochromatosis
Comparison: 01 Colon Cancer Risk in HFE Het.
Outcome: 01 Colon cancer risk in HFE Heterozygotes

Study or sub-category	log[Disease Risk] (SE)	Disease Risk (random) 95% CI	Weight %	Disease Risk (random) 95% CI
01 All Studies				
NelsonM1995	0.2470 (0.1000)		32.85	1.28 [1.05, 1.56]
NelsonW1995	0.0770 (0.1150)		24.84	1.08 [0.86, 1.35]
Altes1999	-0.1508 (0.7338)		0.61	0.86 [0.20, 3.62]
MacDonald1999	-0.1050 (0.3200)		3.21	0.90 [0.48, 1.69]
Nelson2001	-0.0940 (0.3900)		2.16	0.91 [0.42, 1.95]
Elmberg2003	0.0000 (0.1450)		15.62	1.00 [0.75, 1.33]
Shaheen2003	0.3360 (0.1350)		18.03	1.40 [1.07, 1.82]
vanderA2003	0.1820 (0.3500)		2.68	1.20 [0.60, 2.38]
Subtotal (95% CI)			100.00	1.17 [1.05, 1.31]
Test for heterogeneity: Chi² = 5.49, df = 7 (P = 0.60), I² = 0%				
Test for overall effect: Z = 2.78 (P = 0.005)				
02 Age Adjusted Data Only				
NelsonM1995	0.2470 (0.1000)		34.94	1.28 [1.05, 1.56]
NelsonW1995	0.0770 (0.1150)		26.42	1.08 [0.86, 1.35]
Elmberg2003	0.0000 (0.1460)		16.62	1.00 [0.75, 1.33]
Shaheen2003	0.3360 (0.1350)		19.17	1.40 [1.07, 1.82]
vanderA2003	0.1820 (0.3500)		2.85	1.20 [0.60, 2.38]
Subtotal (95% CI)			100.00	1.19 [1.06, 1.34]
Test for heterogeneity: Chi² = 4.12, df = 4 (P = 0.39), I² = 3.0%				
Test for overall effect: Z = 2.91 (P = 0.004)				
03 Exclusion of Self Reported Family Cancers				
MacDonald1999	-0.1050 (0.3200)		8.11	0.90 [0.48, 1.69]
Elmberg2003	0.0000 (0.1450)		39.52	1.00 [0.75, 1.33]
Shaheen2003	0.3360 (0.1350)		45.59	1.40 [1.07, 1.82]
vanderA2003	0.1820 (0.3500)		6.78	1.20 [0.60, 2.38]
Subtotal (95% CI)			100.00	1.16 [0.94, 1.43]
Test for heterogeneity: Chi² = 3.61, df = 3 (P = 0.31), I² = 16.8%				
Test for overall effect: Z = 1.40 (P = 0.16)				
04 Allocation Genotyping & Case Control Studies				
Altes1999	-0.1608 (0.7338)		2.49	0.86 [0.20, 3.62]
MacDonald1999	-0.1050 (0.3200)		13.08	0.90 [0.48, 1.69]
Shaheen2003	0.3360 (0.1350)		73.50	1.40 [1.07, 1.82]
vanderA2003	0.1820 (0.3500)		10.93	1.20 [0.60, 2.38]
Subtotal (95% CI)			100.00	1.28 [1.02, 1.61]
Test for heterogeneity: Chi² = 1.97, df = 3 (P = 0.58), I² = 0%				
Test for overall effect: Z = 2.15 (P = 0.03)				

0.1 0.2 0.5 1 2 5 10

Favours HFE Heteroz Favours contro

REFERENCES

Altes A, Gimferrer E, Capella G, Barcelo MJ, Baiget M. Colorectal Cancer and HFE gene mutations. Haematologica. 1999;84(5):479-80

SN: Altes1999

Elmberg M, Hultkrantz R, Ekbom A, Brandt L, et al. Cancer risk in patients with hereditary hemochromatosis and thier first degree relatives. Gastroent. 2003;125:1733-41

MacDonald GA, Tarish J, Whitehall VJ, McCann SJ, Mellick GD, Buttenshaw RL, Johnson AG, Young J,

Leggett BA. No evidence of increased risk of colorectal cancer in individuals heterozygous for the Cys282Tyr Haemochromatosis mutation. J Gastroenterol Hepatol. 1999;14:1188-1191
Nelson RL, Davis FG, Persky V, Becker E.. Risk of disease in siblings of patients with hereditary hemochromatosis. Digestion. 2001;64:120-4
Nelson RL, Davis FG, Persky V, Becker E. Risk of neoplastic and other diseases among people with heterozygosity for hereditary hemochromatosis. Cancer. 1995;76
PG:875-879
NelsonM1995
NelsonW1995
Shaheen NJ, Silverman LM, Keku T, Lawrence LB, et al. Association between hemochromatosis (HFE) gene mutation carrier status and the risk of colon cancer. J Nat Cancer Inst. 2003;95:154-9
van der A DJ, van der Hel O, Roest M, van der Schouw YT, et al. Heterozygosity for the Cys282Tyr mutation in the HFE gene and the risk of colorectal cancer. Cancer Causes & Control. 2003;14:541-5

Metal Ions in Biology and Medicine: vol. 9. Eds Maria Carmen Alpoim, Paula Vasconcellos Morais, Maria Amélia Santos, Armando J. Cristóvão, José A. Centeno, Philippe Collery.
John Libbey Eurotext, Paris © 2006 pp. 556-1.

Variations of the plasmatic and salivary concentrations of different bivalent cations in oromaxillo-facial area bacterial infections

Nechifor M.[1], Gradinaru I.[1], Popescu E.[3], Gogalniceanu D.[3], Mindreci I.[4], Nechifor C.[5]

1. *Dept. of Pharmacology,*
2. *Complex Oral Rehabilitation Dept.,*
3. *Oromaxillo facial surgery Dept.,*
4. *Dept.of Biophsics.,*
5. *Physiscian resident; University of Medicine and Pharmacy "Gr.T.Popa"Iaşi, Universitatii 16, Iasi 700115, Romania*

INTRODUCTION

Bivalent cations are involved in the normal functioning of human cell. They determine certain effects in all the organs, including oromaxillary area. Oromaxillo-facial area has some morpho- and physiologic particularities and also regarding pathology. One of the characteristics of oral cavity is the permanent contact of the tissues with saliva and blood.

Bacterial infections of oromaxillary area are frequently encountered. There are data showing that during bacterial infections emerge changes in plasmatic concentrations of some macro and trace elements [1].

AIM

In this study we have followed variations of salivary and plasmatic levels of some bivalent cations in the suppurations of oromaxillary area.

METHOD AND PATIENTS

We have followed the plasmatic concentrations of Ca^{2+}, Mg^{2+},Cu^{2+} and Zn^{2+} and salivary concentrations of Ca^{2+} and Mg^{2+} in adult patients with bacterial suppurations in oromaxillary area. The trial involved 69 adult patients of both gender, aging between 18 and 67 years (mean age 41.2±12.4 years). A control group included 57 healthy volunteers, with a similar gender and age distribution as the first group.

Criteria for inclusion into the study were: presence of soft tissue suppuration at the level of oral cavity (clinically and paraclinically confirmed), lack of any antibiotic or nonsteroidal anti-inflammatory drug treatment before hospital admittance.

Criteria for non-including were: pregnancy, therapy with drugs containing cations, treatment with diuretics, liver cirrhosis, renal failure (acute or chronic), malabsorbtion or malnutrition syndrome. In all suppurations, surgical intervention was performed. Plasmatic concentrations of Ca^{2+}, Mg^{2+},Cu^{2+}, Zn^{2+} and salivary concentrations of Ca^{2+} and Mg^{2+} were determined in the moment of hospital admittance, before any treatment. Cations assessment was performed using atomic absorption spectrophotometry.

For analysis of cations concentrations, the unstimulated saliva was collected in the morning, before brushing the teeth, eating or drinking, with 12 hours after the last food ingestion. The samples were collected in plastic tubes. Suppurations were localized as follows: submandibular lodge -34 cases, masseteric area-6 cases, pterygomaxillary area-2 cases, genian region - 8 cases, submental area-13 cases, other localizations- 6 cases. Pathogenic bacteria were determined in pathological sample by microbiologic procedure.

The results were statistically interpreted with "t" test.

The study was approved by Ethical Committee of "Sf. Spiridon" Hospital Iasi and was in agreement with the rules for clinical trials.

RESULTS

Microbiologic analysis have shown that suppurations were produced by facultative anaerobe bacteria (*Enterococcus spp*, etc.) and Gram positive cocci (*Streptoccocus pneumoniae*).The results are shown in *figure 1 and 2*. Salivary concentrations of magnesium and calcium are shown in *figure 1*. Plasmatic concentrations of magnesium, calcium, copper and zinc are shown in *figure 2*. Data obtained show significant differences between patient and control group in salivary concentrations of Mg^{2+} and plasma Zn^{2+} level.

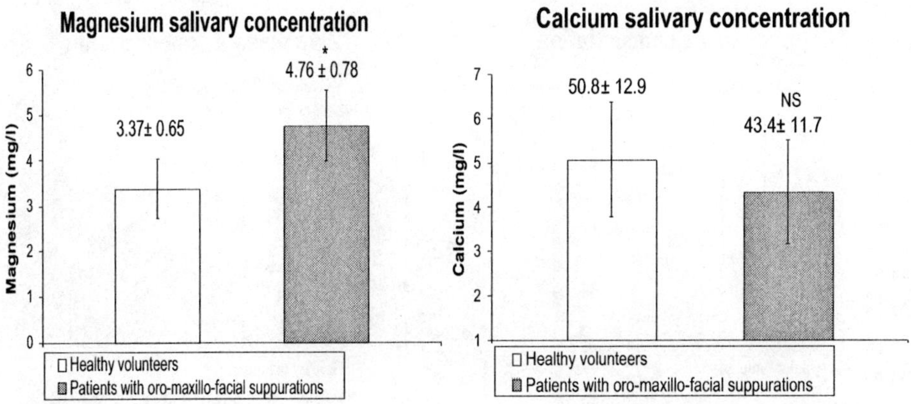

Fig. 1. Salivary concentration of bivalent cations. * $p<0.05$ vs control group; NS vs control group.

DISCUSSION AND CONCLUSIONS

Bivalent cations have multiple implications in the function of some cells with an important role in immunity. The emergence and development of bacterial infections is depending on bacterial pathogeny and local and general capacity of defense. Some cations influence essential processes for the capacity of human body to respond to bacterial aggression. Zinc has a cytoprotective effect against to staphylococcal toxins [2]. It stimulates immunoglobulin synthesis and other processes involved in anti-infective defense. In some bacterial-induced diseases were observed changes in plasmatic and cellular concentrations of some macro and trace elements. In children with severe respiratory infections, plasmatic level of magnesium was higher than plasmatic level of this cation in normal children [3]. In case of thoracic empyemata, serum concentration of copper has increased vs. normal and concentrations of magnesium in empyemata was higher than in serum. On contrary, serum level of zinc was decreased than in normal [4]. In patients with severe infections, plasmatic level of selenium and zinc were decreased [1]. In case of infections with *Chlamydia pneumoniae*, the serum ratio copper/zinc is increased compared to normal subjects [5]. In our study, we have obtained similar data (though with other pathogen bacteria). Increasing this ratio is due to decreasing plasmatic zinc concentrations, copper didn't vary significantly. In experimental infections with *Corynebacterium pseudotuberculosis* (during acute phase) it was proved beside a strong local inflammatory reaction an increase of copper plasmatic concentration together with zinc decrease [6].

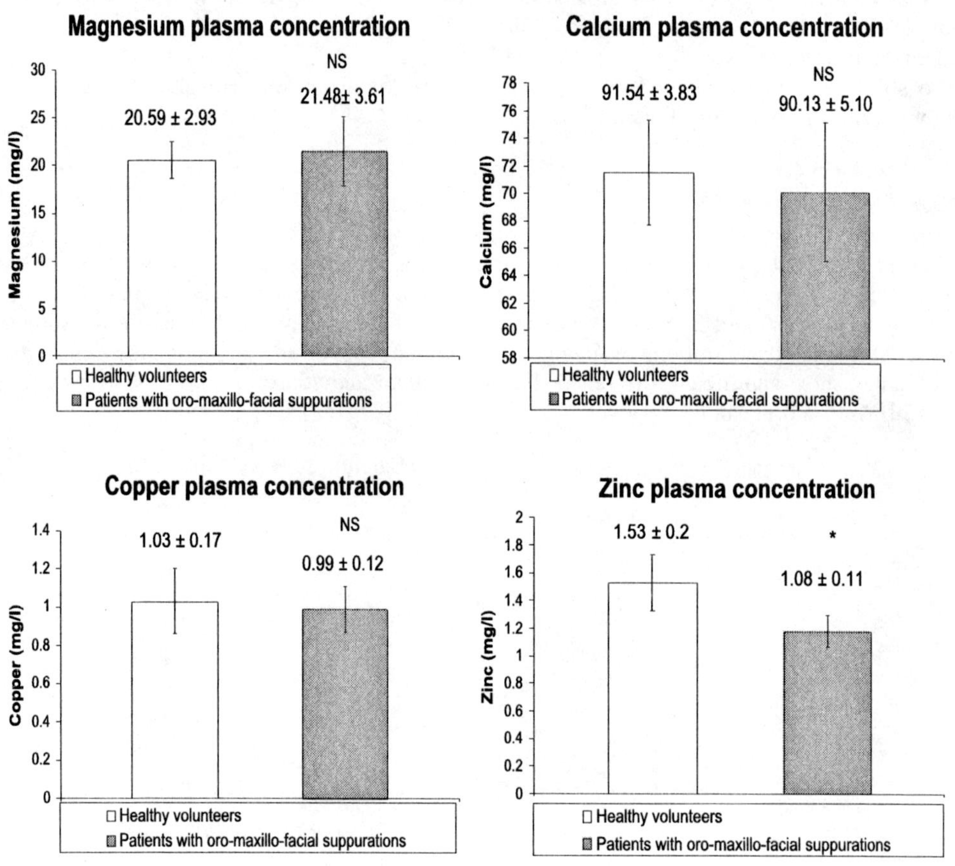

Fig. 2. Plasmatic concentration of bivalent cations. * $p<0.05$ vs control group; NS vs control group.

Our data show a significant decrease in plasmatic zinc concentrations and a salivary magnesium increase in patients with oral suppurations. Salivary concentrations of magnesium were significantly statistic higher in patients with oral suppuration than in healthy subjects. The calcium level does not suffer significantly statistic changes either at plasmatic or salivary level in patient group compared to control group (e.g. 90.13 ± 5.1 mg/l in plasma in patient group vs. 91.54 ± 3.83 mg/l in control group, NS). The salivary ratio between Mg^{2+}/Ca^{2+} levels is significantly increased in patients with suppuration at oral cavity. A higher concentrations of magnesium might influence the expression of a set of Mg^{2+}-controlled genes in some bacteria (as was proved for *Salmonela Enterica*) [7]. A high level of magnesium favors proliferation of some pathogen microorganisms as *Leishmania major* [8] and (possible) bacteria involved in oral cavity infections. We consider that changes in cation concentrations is different in case of acute inflammation comparing with anti-infective effect on pathogen bacteria. We consider that variations in salivary concentrations of some cations are important for developing bacterial infections on oral cavity, because in this area, soft tissues are in permanent contact with saliva. Association between low level of plasmatic zinc and a high ratio of salivary Mg^{2+}/Ca^{2+} favors emergence of bacterial infections in oral cavity.

REFERENCES

1. Srinivas U, Braconier JH, Jeppsson B, Abdulla M, Akesson B, Ockerman PA. Trace element alterations in infectious diseases. *Scand J Clin Lab Invest.* 1988; 48(6): 495-500.
2. Sunzel B, Holm S, Reuterving CO, Soderberg T, Hallmans G, Hanstrom L. The effect of zinc on bacterial phagocytosis, killing and cytoprotection in human polymorphonuclear leucocytes. *APMIS.* 1995; 103(9): 635-44.
3. Florianczyk B, Karska M, Bednarek A. The level of magnesium in the serum of children hospitalized for severe respiratory infections. *Ann Univ Mariae Curie Sklodowska [Med].* 2001; 56: 243-7.
4. Domej W, Krachler M, Goessler W, Maier A, Irgolic KJ, Lang JK. Concentrations of copper, zinc, manganese, rubidium, and magnesium in thoracic empyemata and corresponding sera. *Biol Trace Elem Res.* 2000; 78(1-3): 53-66.
5. Nystrom-Rosander C, Lindh U, Ilback NG, Hjelm E, Thelin S, Lindqvist O, Friman G. Interactions between Chlamydia pneumoniae and trace elements: a possible link to aortic valve sclerosis. *Biol Trace Elem Res.* 2003; 91(2): 97-110.
6. Pepin M, Pardon P, Lantier F, Marly J, Levieux D, Lamand M.Experimental Corynebacterium pseudotuberculosis infection in lambs: kinetics of bacterial dissemination and inflammation. Vet Microbiol. 1991; 26(4): 381-92.
7. Lejona S, Aguirre A, Cabeza ML, Garcia Vescovi E, Soncini FC. Molecular characterization of the Mg^{2+}-responsive PhoP-PhoQ regulon in Salmonella enterica. *J Bacteriol.* 2003; 185(21): 6287-94.
8. Lanza H, Afonso-Cardoso SR, Silva AG, Napolitano DR, Espindola FS, Pena JD, Souza MA. Comparative effect of ion calcium and magnesium in the activation and infection of the murine macrophage by Leishmania major. *Biol Res.* 2004; 37(3): 385-93.

Metal Ions in Biology and Medicine: vol. 9. Eds Maria Carmen Alpoim, Paula Vasconcellos Morais, Maria Amélia Santos, Armando J. Cristóvão, José A. Centeno, Philippe Collery.
John Libbey Eurotext, Paris © 2006 pp. 560-1.

The Influence of Bipolar Disorders treatment on plasmatic and erythrocyte levels of some cations

Nechifor M.[1], Vaideanu C.[1], Mindreci I.[2], Palamaru I.[3], Boisteanu P.[4]

1. Dept. of Pharmacology,
2. Dept.of Biophsics,
3. Institute of Public Health Iasi,
4. Dept. of Psychiatry. University of Medicine and Pharmacy "Gr.T.Popa"Iaşi, Universitatii 16, Iasi 700115, Romania

Different bivalent cations (zinc, magnesium, calcium, etc.) play various roles in central nervous system in human [1, 2, 3]. Some changes and disturbances in plasma and intracellular concentrations of some cations have been shown in psychiatric diseases (major depression, schizophrenia, etc.) [4, 5, 6, 7, 8].

Bipolar disorder (BD) is a psychiatric disease characterized by episodes of mania, depression and mood instability.

AIM

In this study we determined the plasma and the erythrocyte levels of some bivalent cations in patients with BD and we tested the influence of pharmacological treatment effect on cations concentrations.

METHOD AND PATIENTS

We worked with adult patients with bipolar disorders (BD)(diagnosed after DSMIV criteria) ageing 21-58 years admitted into "Socola" Psychiatric Hospital Iasi in 2004-2005.

Patients have been divided in two groups:

Group I (11 patients) received carbamazepine 600 mg/day, per os, 4 weeks.

Group II (20 patients) received sodium valproate (Orfiril®) 900 mg/day, 4 weeks.

A group of 20 healthy subjects with the same age and gender structure as group I and II was for control.

The plasma concentration of calcium, magnesium, copper and zinc and erythrocyte level of magnesium was determined by spectrometry with atomic absorption at the admittance (before treatment) and after 4 weeks.

We used the following including criteria: bipolar disorder (diagnosed after DSM IV), at least 4 weeks treatment and absence of any BD treatment before admittance in hospital. The non-including criteria was: pregnancy, liver cirrhosis, renal failure, heart failure, malabsortion syndromes, treatment with diuretics or bivalent cations containing drugs.The study was approved by Etics Commitee of "Socola" Psychiatric Hospital Iasi and agree the rules for clinical trials.

RESULTS

Brain magnesium is involved in modulation of neurotransmitters release, excitability of Carbamazepine and sodium valproate treatment increase moderately but significantly erythrocyte magnesium. The increase of Mg^{2+} concentration can reduce the intensity of clinical neurons, etc. The magnesium deficit increase the presynaptic -norepinephrine release. In our study erythrocyte magnesium level was lower in BD patients compared to the control group.

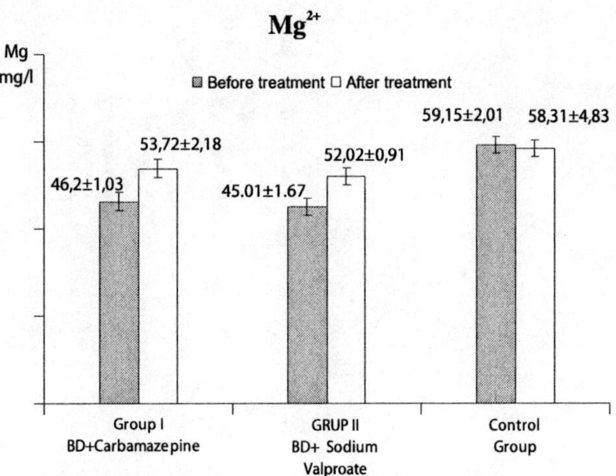

Fig. 1. Plasmatic level of erythrocyte magnesium before and after treatment. * $p<0,05$ vs. level before treatment;? $p<0,05$ vs control group level

Symptoms in BD, Mg^{2+} decreasing activation of NMDA receptors. The levels of intraerythrocyte and plasmatic magnesium observed in our study are shown in *figures 1 and 2*.

In our study, the plasmatic level of zinc was reduced in patients with BD before the treatment (0,72±0,02 in group I vs 0,89±0,12 in control group $p<0, 05$) and the both drugs used in treatment of BD enhance the plasma level of zinc *(figure 2)*. The increase in zinc level was associated with a good clinical evolution in both groups of patients.

There were not signifficant diferences.between control group and BD group. Also, the plasma levels of total calcium and copper were not significantly influenced by the therapy with carbamazepine and sodium valproate *(figure 2)*.

DISCUSSIONS

Use of a mood stabilizer is recommended in all subtypes and in all phases of BD [9, 10]. Sodium valproate may be effective (at least in part) in BD by enhancement of GABA-ergic transmission or by influencing Na+/K+ membrane transport and sodium channels [11].

Carbamazepine is used more and more in the therapy of mood disorders [14] and in BD. In doses of 200 mg 2 or 3 times/ day per os, this drug determines favorable therapeutic results in patients with BD with maniacal or mixed episodes. This drug is used since many time in the therapy of some epileptic forms. Walden et al, 1993 [12] have considered that the main mechanism of action in this case is decreasing Ca^{2+} entrance into neurons. This cation plays a key role in the generation of epilepsies crisis. Magnesium increases anticonvulsant effect of carbamazepine by partially blocking entrance of calcium into neurons.

Carbamazepine may reduce neuronal excitability and glutamate release [15]. Our results shows a lowest plasma level of zinc and a decreased erythrocyte Mg^{2+} level in BD patients versus normal subjects. Our data differ from Imada et al 2002 [16] results which noted a high Mg serum level in patients with mood disorders. We not found a significant change of plasma magnesium level in BD patients. The erythrocyte magnesium level was lower in patients with BD before treatment and was increased after sodium valproate and after carbamazepine treatment.

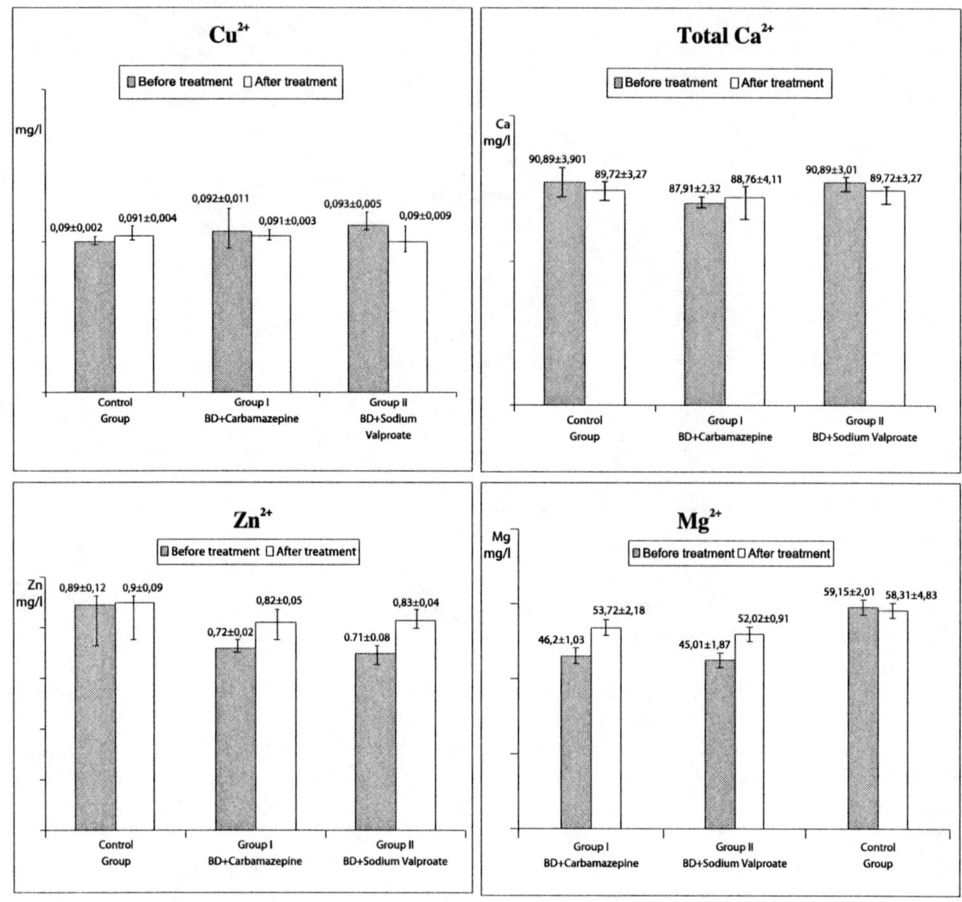

Fig. 2. Plasmatic level of bivalent cations before and after treatment. * $p<0,05$ vs. Level before treatment • $p<0,05$ vs control group level

Zinc has several very important functions in brain [17]. Zinc inhibits NMDA receptor function through voltage dependent and voltage-independent way [18]. We think that by this mechanism Zn^{2+} can reduce the excitation and agitation in bipolar disorders. About 15% of brain zinc is localized in synaptic vesicles associated with excitatory amino-acids neurotransmitters [17]. By this way Zn^{2+} modulates the presynaptic release of neurotransmitters. Zinc is released by neural activity of many central excitatory synapses [19].

A low level of this cation can enhances the maniac symptoms of patients with BD.

Zinc is important for serotonin synthesis. The serotonin relative low level in some brain regions can play a role in pathogenesis of BD because the selective serotonin reuptake inhibitors (SSRIs) are successfully used in the treatment of BD [20]. The erythrocyte magnesium level was lower in patients with BD before treatment. In patients with major depression the level of magnesium is lower compared to normal people [21, 22, 23].

Our results are in agreement with Giannini et al 2000 [24] that show the magnesium oxide therapy enhances the efficiency of verapamil maintenance treatment in mania. Verapamil blocks some calcium channels and decreases calcium entrance into neurons (an effect close to magnesium).

The possible mechanisms of action involved in the interactions between magnesium and valproic acid / carbamazepine in BD therapy are shown in fig. nr. 3.

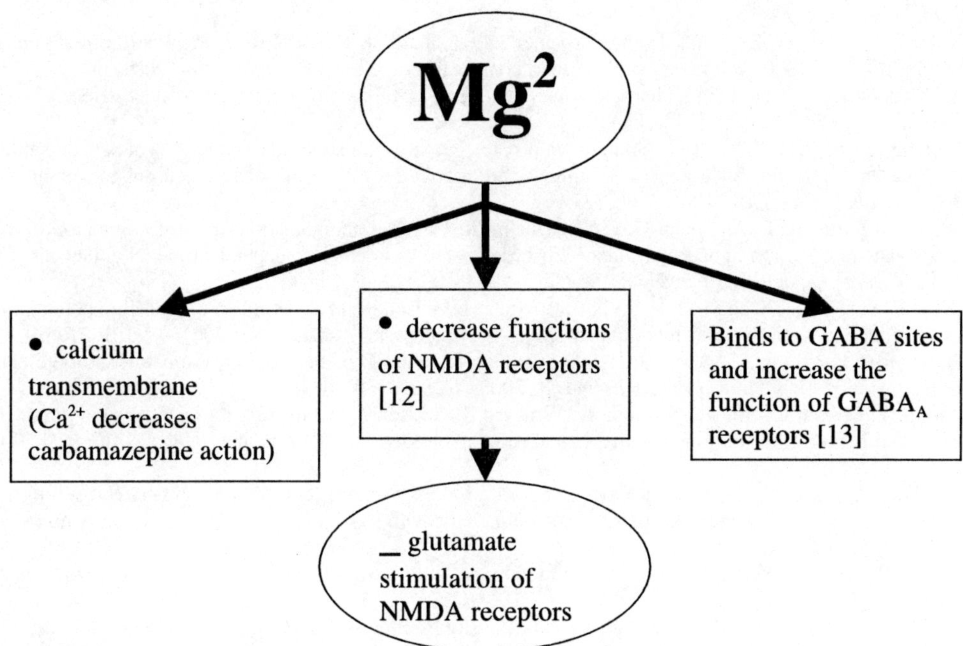

Fig. 3. Possible mechanism of action of increased magnesium cell concentration in patients with bipolar disorder

On the other hand the increase of plasmatic Zn^{2+} may have a benefic effect during BD therapy, through zinc action on the level of $GABA_A$ receptors[25]. Qian et al, 1997 [26], have shown that Zn^{2+} acts at the level of extracellular domains of $GABA_A$ receptors and increases their sensitivity to this agonist.

We suggest that an increase in plasmatic zinc level and the erythrocyte magnesium level are involved in the mechanism by which some drugs (ex. carbamazepine and sodium valproate) can reduce clinical symptoms of bipolar disorders.

REFERENCES

1. Assaf S.Y, Chung S.H. Release of endogerous Zn* from human tissue during activity. *Nature* 1984; 308: 734-735.
2. Frederickson C. J., Suh S.W, Silva D., Thompson R.B. Importance of zinc in the central nervous system: the zinc containing nervous. *J. Nutr.* 2000; 130: 1471s-1483s.
3. Goto Y., Nakamura M, Abe S., Kato M., Fukui M. Psyhological correlations of abnormal behavior in magnesium deficient rats. *Epilepsy Res* 1993; 15: 81-89.
4. Kamei K, Tabata O, Muneoka K., Muraoka S.I., Tomiyoshi R, Takioawa M. Electrolytes in erythrocytes of patients with depressive disorders *Psychiatry Clin Neurosci* 1998; 52-5: 529-533.
5. Johnson S. Micronutrients accumulation and depletion in schizophrenia, epilepsy, autism and Parkison's disease. *Med. Hypotheses* 2001; 56: 641-645.
6. Kirov G.K., Tsachev K.N. Magnesium in schizophrenia and maniac depressive disease *Neuropshychobiology* 1990; 23: 89-91.
7. Kanofsky J.D. Magnesium defiency in chronic schizophrenia. *J. Neurosci* 1991; 61: 87-90.
8. Nechifor M., Vaideanu C, Palamaru I. Borza C, Mandreci I. The influence of some Antipsychotics on

Erythrocyte Magnesium and Plasma Magnesium, Calcium, Copper and Zinc in patients with Paranoid Schizophrenia, *J. Am.Coll. Nutr.* 2004; 23-5: 549s-551s.

9. Kahn DA, Sachs G. S., Printz D. J., Carpenter D., Docherty J. P., Ross R. *J.* Medication treatment of bipolar disorder 2000: a summary of the expert consensus guidelines. *Psychiatry Res.* 2001; 6-4: 197-211.
10. Schatzberg A. F. Employing pharmacologic treatment of bipolar disorders to greatest effect. *J Clin. Psychiatry* 2004; 65 - suppl. 15: 15-20.
11. McLean M.J., McDonald R.L., Sodium valproate, but not ethosuximide produces voltage dependent limitation of high fregvence repetitive firing of action potentials of mouse central neurons in cell culture. *J. Pharmacol. Exp. Ther.* 1986; 238: 727-738.
12. Walden J, Grunze H, Bingmann D, Liu Z, Dusing R. Calcium antagonistic effects of carbamazepine as a mechanism of action in neuropsychiatric disorders: studies in calcium dependent model epilepsies. *Eur Neuropsychopharmacol.* 1992; 2(4): 455-62.
13. Moykkynen T, Uusi-Oukari M, Heikkila J, Lovinger DM, Luddens H, Korpi ER. Magnesium potentiation of the function of native and recombinant GABA(A) receptors. *Neuroreport.* 2001; 12(10): 2175-9.
14. Gajwani P, Forsthoff A, Muzina D, Amann B, Gao K, Elhaj O, Calabrese JR, Grunze H. Antiepileptic drugs in mood-disordered patients. *Epilepsia.* 2005; 46 Suppl 4: 38-44.
15. Arban R., Marian G, Brackenborough, K. Winyard, L. Wilson A., Gerard P., Large C. Evaluation of the effects of lamotrigine, valproate and carbamazepine in a rodent model of mania. *Behav. Brain Res.* 2005; 158-1: 123-132.
16. Imada Y, Yoshioka S, Ueda T., Katayama S., Kuno Y., Kawahara R. Relationship between serum magnesium level and clinical background factors in patients with mood disorders. *Psychiatry Clin. Neurosci.* 2002; 56-5: 509-514.
17. Colvin R. A. Characterization of a plasma membrane zinc transporter in rat brain. *Neurosci. Lett.* 1998; 247: 147-150.
18. Traynelis S. F., Burgess M. F., Zheng F., Lyuboslavsky P., Powers J. L. Control of Voltage - Independent Zinc Inhibition of NMDA Receptors by the NR1 Subunit, *J. Neurosci* 1998;18-16: 6163-6175.
19. Choi D. W. Zinc and brain injury. *Ann. Rev. Neurosci.* 1998; 21: 347-375.
20. Bowden, C. L. Atypical antipsychotic augmentation of mood stabilizer therapy in bipolar disorders. *J. Clin. Psychiatry* 2005; 66-3: 12-19.
21. Murck H. Magnesium and affective disorders. *Nutr. Neurosci.* 2002; 5(6): 5375-389.
22. Nechifor M. Vaideanu C, Boisteanu P., Mandreci I., Cuciureanu R., Nechifor C. Changes in Mg^{2+} and other cations plasma concentration in patients with major depression. In: Escanero J. F., Alda, J. V., Guenra M., Durlach J Eds. *Advances on Magnesium Research Physiology, Pathology and Pharmacology*, Edit. Prensas Universitaria de Zaragoza, 2003: 177-181.
23. Levine J., Stein D., Rapoport A, Kurtzman L. High serum and cerebrospinal fluid Ca^{2+}/Mg^{2+} fatlb on recently hospitalized acutely depressed patients. *Neuropsychopharmacol* 1999; 39: 63-70.
24. Giannini A. J. Nakoneczie A. M., Melemis S. M., Ventresco J., Condon M. Magnesium oxide augmentation of verapamil maintenance therapy in mania. *Psychiatry Res* 2000; 93-1: 83-87.
25. Maes M, De Vos N, Demedts P, Wauters A, Neels H. Lower serum zinc in major depression in relation to changes in serum acute phase proteins. *J Affect Disord.* 1999; 56(2-3): 189-94.
26. Qian, H.; Li, L.; Chappell, R.L.; Ripps, H. GABA receptors of bipolar cells from the skate retina: actions of zinc on GABA-mediated membrane currents. *J. Neurophysiol.* 1997; 78: 2402-2412.

Metal Ions in Biology and Medicine: vol. 9. Eds Maria Carmen Alpoim, Paula Vasconcellos Morais, Maria Amélia Santos, Armando J. Cristóvão, José A. Centeno, Philippe Collery.
John Libbey Eurotext, Paris © 2006 pp. 565-1.

Influence of the zinc supplementation on human serum TAS (total antioxidative status)

M. Schlegel-Zawadzka[1], M. Grabowska[2], J. Walkowiak[3], J. Przyslawski[4]

[1]*Department of Human Nutrition, Faculty of Health Care, Medical College, Jagiellonian University, 20 Grzegórzecka str., 31-531 Krakow, mfzawadz@kinga.cyf-kr.edu.pl;*
[2]*Chair of Medical Biochemistry, Jagiellonian University, 7 Kopernika str., 31-034 Krakow, mbgrabow@cyf-kr.edu.pl;*
[3]*Department of Bromatology and Human Nutrition, Medical Academy, 42 Marcelinska str., 60-354, Poznan, jotespe@am.poznan.pl;*
[4]*Department of Gastroenterology and Metabolism, Institute of Pediatrics, Medical Academy, 27/33 Szpitalna str., 60-572 Poznan, jarwalk@am.poznan.pl; Poland*

SUMMARY

As a result of previous study about zinc supplementation (healthy young 46 subjects, 50 days with daily dose 25 mg Zn^{+2}/d) the total antioxidative status (TAS) in serum was measured. Zinc supplementation increased zinc contents in serum about 10.1% (0.89±0.1 mg/l; 0.98±0.26mg/l) and not in erythrocytes (11.1±1.89mg/l; 10.5±2.10mg/l). TAS was increased about 64.4% (1.63±0.35mmol/l; 2.69±0.48mmol/l). There was no gender differences. TAS after supplementation correlated significantly with the TAS before supplementation and the Zn content in the serum and erythrocytes after supplementation (r=0.49, p=0.0010; r=0.35, p=0.0233; r=0.40, p=0.0098). This increased was caused only by zinc supplementation not by diet alterations (24-hour recall study was done). The long term supplementation of organic form of zinc increases total antioxidative status in serum in direct and indirect ways. This idea is supported by the discrepancy in the zinc status and TAS increases and appearance of significant correlation between them after the supplementation.

INTRODUCTION

Zinc is one of the most abundant nutritionally essential elements in the human body. Human zinc requirement is estimated at 15 mg/day. Zinc has been shown to be essential to the structure and function of a large number of macromolecules and for over 300 enzymic reactions. The role of zinc in protecting biological structures from damage by free radicals may be due to several factors: maintaining an adequate level of metallothioneins (MTs) (which are also free radical scavengers), as an essential component of superoxide dismutase (SOD), as a protective agent for thiols and in preventing the interaction between chemical groups with iron to form free radicals. Zinc deficiency increases the levels of lipid peroxidation. At the presynaptic level zinc may act by blocking Ca^{2+} channels, inhibiting neurotransmitter release (1).

As a result of recent study that zinc supplementation, increases the zinc content in serum, but not in erythrocytes, further examination was concentrated on the explanation of the zinc biochemical consequences in the human organism (2).

Zinc is required as a catalytic, structural and regulatory ion for enzymes, proteins and transcription factors, and is thus a key trace element in many homeostatic mechanisms of the body, including immune responses. Physiological supplementation of zinc for 1-2 months restores immune responses, reduces the incidence of infections and prolongs survival. However, in every single individual zinc supplementation of food should be adjusted to the particular zinc status in views of the great variability in habitat conditions, health status and dietary requirements (3).

Zinc is so ubiquitous in cellular metabolism that even minor impairment of an adequate supply is likely to have multiple biological and clinical effects (4).

Zinc supplementation is associated with decreased oxidative stress and improve immune function, which may be among the possible mechanisms for its cancer preventive activity (5-6).

THE AIM

The aim was to examine the effect of zinc supplementation on total antioxidative status (TAS).

MATERIAL AND METHODS

Healthy young subjects (n=46; 40 female, 6 male; aged about 22,5 years) were supplemented 50 days with daily dose 25 mg Zn^{+2}/d (compound *zincum hydroxyasparaginicum* 0.15 g). Collection of blood samples was twice (before and after 50 days). Fasting venous blood samples were collected using vacutainer system of Becton Dickinson (7). As serum control was Validate N (Organon Teknika USA).

The zinc content in blood samples was measured by flame atomic absorption spectrometry method (AAS) with Pye Unicam Solaar; wavelength - 213.8 nm.

Antioxidant status of serum was measured by TAS (test of the Randox firm).

Zinc blood content and TAS were expressed as arithmetic average mean (X)±standard deviation (SD) in both groups. Statistical analyses were performed using STATISTICA 6.0 Pl software (StatSoft). The Mann-Whitney U test or t-Student test was used to test the hypothesis of significant differences between average values on the level of significance set at $p<0.05$.

Consent for the study was obtained from the Ethical Committee, Medical Academy, Poznan.

RESULTS

The results are presented for the total group studied, because of no gender differences observed *(table 1)*. The Polish references for zinc content are shown for comparison. The average zinc contents in study group were in the reference range. As was stated above zinc supplementation increased zinc contents in serum about 10.1% (n=46, 0.89±0.1 mg/l; n=43, 0.98±0.26mg/l; p=0.0397) and not in erythrocytes (n=46, 11.1±1.89mg/l; n=43, 10.5±2.10mg/l; p=0.0519). This increase was caused only by zinc supplementation not by diet alterations (24-hour recall study was done) (2). TAS was increased about 64.4% (n=41, 1.63±0.35mmol/l; n=41, 2.69±0.48mmol/l; p=0.00001). The significant TAS correlations with the zinc content are presented in *table 2*.

DISCUSSION

Oxidative stress is known to be an important contributing factor in many chronic diseases (artherosclerosis, vascular diseases, mutagenesis, cancer, neurodegeneration, immunologic disorders and the aging process) (14).The antioxidant defence system plays an important role in protecting body from oxidative damage (15). Numerous studies have been shown that a single vitamin or mineral supplementation has the beneficial effect on the antioxidant defence system. However, the overall combined effect of multinutrient supplementation on antioxidant defence system remains to be clarified (16). Zinc supplementation studies proved that zinc deficiency is a worldwide problem (17). Multinutrient supplementation, as an effort to improve one's health status and maintain the optimal body function, has become a more and more popular practice nowadays in Europe and North America. *Table 1* presented our Polish data in comparison to the Canarian population zinc status and international references. Serum zinc content of 395 individuals living in Canary Islands, determined by flame atomic absorption spectrometry, was 1.16 ± .52 mg/l and was higher than ours (13). However, it is still in the range of all references presented. Supplementation increased the zinc content in our group, but it was still in the normal range. TAS measured in the serum increased after the zinc supplementation about 64% and this increase was in the correlation with the zinc content *(table 2)*. But the zinc content increase was not so high - only 10.1%. Why it is a such discrepancy? We may predict because of the zinc involvement in a number of indirect antioxidant functions. Zinc may function as a site-specific antioxidant by two mechanisms. First it competes with iron and cooper for binding to cell membranes and some proteins, displacing these redox-active metals, and second it binds to SH groups, protecting them from oxidation (15). Increased zinc intake will protect against oxidant stress in persons with tendencies for both moderate zinc deficiency and high oxidant stress (18).

Table 1. Results of the zinc content in serum and erythrocytes of the study group, Polish reference value and total antioxidative status (TAS) in serum of healthy adults (arithmetic mean + standard deviation).

Study group or reference	Before Zn supplementation	After Zn supplementation
	Total antioxidative status (TAS) in serum	
Study group	(n=41) 0.89 ± 0.1 mmol/L	(n=41) 0.98±0.26 mmol/L
	Zn content in serum	
Study group (2)	(n=46) 0.89 ± 0.1 mg/L	(n=43) 0.98±0.26 mg/L
	Zn content in erythrocytes	
Study group (2)	(n=46) 11.1±1.89 mg/L	(n=43) 10.5±2.1 mg/L
	References without supplementation - Zn content in serum	
Reference - Dembinska-Kiec et al. (8)	Male - 0.66-1.17 mg/L; Female - 0.66-1.10 mg/L	
Reference - Pawelski, Maj (9)	0.5-1.5 mg/L	
Reference - Tomaszewski (10)	0.75-1.50 mg/L	
Reference - Schlegel-Zawadzka, et al. (11)	0.73-1.33 mg/L	
Reference - Goldman, Bennet (12)	0.70-1.50 mg/L	
Romero et al. study group (13)	1.16±0.52 mg/L	
	Reference without supplementation - Zn content in erythrocytes	
Reference - Schlegel-Zawadzka, et al. (11)	5.67-17.43 mg/L	

Table 2. Statistically significant correlations between the total antioxidative status (TAS) and the zinc content in blood before and after the Zn supplementation.

Sample	TAS before suppl.	TAS after suppl.	Zn before suppl.	Zn after suppl.	Pearson correlation coefficient	P value
Serum Erythrocytes	+	+			0.49	0.0010
Serum Erythrocytes			+	+	0.35	0.0233
Serum Erythrocytes		+		+	0.40	0.0451
Serum Erythrocytes			+	+	- 0.31	0.0451

DISCUSSION

Oxidative stress is known to be an important contributing factor in many chronic diseases (artherosclerosis, vascular diseases, mutagenesis, cancer, neurodegeneration, immunologic disorders and the aging process) (14). The antioxidant defence system plays an important role in protecting body from oxidative damage (15). Numerous studies have been shown that a single vitamin or mineral supplementation has the beneficial effect on the antioxidant defence system. However, the overall combined effect of multinutrient supplementation on antioxidant defence system remains to be clarified (16). Zinc supplementation studies proved that zinc deficiency is a worldwide problem (17). Multinutrient supplementation, as an effort to improve one's health status and maintain the optimal body function, has become a more and more popular practice nowadays in Europe and North America. *Table 1* presented our Polish data in comparison to the Canarian population zinc status and international references. Serum zinc content of 395 individuals living in Canary Islands, determined by flame atomic absorption spectrometry, was 1.16 ± 0.52 mg/l and was higher than ours (13). However, it is still in the range of all references presented. Supplementation increased the zinc content in our group, but it was still in the normal range. TAS measured in the serum increased after the zinc supplementation about 64% and this increase was in the correlation with the zinc content *(table 2)*. But the zinc content increase was not so high - only 10.1%. Why it is a such discrepancy? We may predict because of the zinc involvement in a number of indirect antioxidant functions. Zinc may function as a site-specific antioxidant by two mechanisms. First it competes with iron and cooper for binding to cell membranes and some proteins, displacing these redox-active metals, and second it binds to SH groups, protecting them from oxidation (15). Increased zinc intake will protect against oxidant stress in persons with tendencies for both moderate zinc deficiency and high oxidant stress (18).

CONCLUSIONS

The long term supplementation of organic form of zinc increases total antioxidative status in serum in direct and indirect ways. This idea is supported by the discrepancy in the zinc status and TAS increases and appearance of significant correlation between them after the supplementation.

REFERENCES

1. Tapiero H, Tew KD. Trace elements in human physiology and pathology zinc and metallothioneins. *Biomed Pharmacother* 2003; 5: 399-411.
2. Schlegel-Zawadzka M, Przyslawski J, Walkowiak J. Alterations of the zinc content in human blood samples after supplementation. *Ann Nutr Metab* 2003; 47: 393.
3. Ferencik M, Ebringer L. Modulatory effects of selenium and zinc on the immune system. *Folia Microbiol* 2003; 48: 417-26.
4. Costello RB, Grumstrup-Scott J. Zinc. *J Am Dietetic Assoc* 2000; 100: 371-5.
5. Prasad AS, Kucuk O. Zinc in cancer prevention. *Cancer Metast Rev* 2002; 21: 291-95.
6. Klein CJ. Zinc supplementation. *J Am Dietetic Assoc* 2000; 100: 1137-8.
7. Schlegel-Zawadzka M, Zachwieja Z, Huzior-Balajewicz A, Pietrzyk J. Comparative analysis of zinc status, food products', frequency intake and food habits of 11-year-old healthy children. *Food Addit Contam* 2002; 19: 963-8.
8. Dembinska-Kiec A, Naskalski JW. (ed.) Diagnostyka laboratoryjna z elementami biochemii klinicznej. Wroclaw, Volumed, 1998.
9. Pawelski S, Maj S. Normy i diagnostyka chorób wewnetrznych. Warszawa, PZWL, 1993.
10. Tomaszewski JJ. Diagnostyka laboratoryjna. Warszawa, PZWL, 1997.
11. Schlegel-Zawadzka M, Przyslawski J, Walkowiak J, Huzior-Balajewicz A. Wartosci referencyjne cynku we krwi populacji zdrowych dzieci i mlodziezy uczacej sie. XVIII Naukowy Zjazd Polskiego Towarzystwa Farmaceutycznego "Farmacja w XXI wieku", Poznan, 19-22.09.2001, 2001; 1: 298.
12. Goldman L, Bennet JC (ed). Cecil textbook of medicine. 21st edition, Philadelphia, W.B. Saunders Company, 2000: 2304.
13. Romero CD, Sanchez PH, Blanco FL, Rodriquez ER, Majem LS. Serum copper and zinc concentration in a representative sample of the Canarian population. *J Trace Elem Med Biol* 2002; 16: 75-81.
14. Prasad AS, Bao B, Beck FWJ, Kucuk O, Sarkar FH. Antioxidant effect of zinc in humans. *Free Rad Biol Med* 2004; 37: 1182-90.
15. Bettger WJ. Zinc and selenium, site-specific versus general antioxidant. *Can J Physiol Pharmacol* 1993; 71: 721-24.
16. Cheng TY, Zhu Z, Masuda S, Morcos NC. Effects of multinutrient supplementation on antioxidant defense systems in healthy human beings. *J Nutr Biochem* 2001; 12: 388-95.
17. Salgueiro MJ, Zubillaga M, Lysionek A, Sarabia MI, Caro R, De Paoli T, Hager A, Weill R, Boccio J. Zinc as an essential micronutrient. A review. *Nutr Res* 2000; 20: 737-55.
18. DiSilvestro RA. Zinc in relation to diabetes and oxidative disease. *J Nutr* 2000; 130:1509S-11S.

Metal Ions in Biology and Medicine: vol. 9. Eds Maria Carmen Alpoim, Paula Vasconcellos Morais, Maria Amélia Santos, Armando J. Cristóvão, José A. Centeno, Philippe Collery.
John Libbey Eurotext, Paris © 2006 pp. 570-1.

Natural radioisotopes ^{210}Po and ^{210}Pb in human hair as an indicator of exposure

Fernando P. Carvalho and João M. Oliveira

Instituto Tecnológico e Nuclear
Departamento de Protecção Radiológica e Segurança Nuclear
Estrada Nacional 10, 2686-953 Sacavém, Portugal
E-mail: carvalho@itn.pt

ABSTRACT

The potential of naturally-occurring polonium (^{210}Po) and radioactive lead (^{210}Pb) in human hair as bio indicators for internal contamination by uranium series nuclides was investigated through analysis of hair samples in 87 individuals. The hair samples were collected in three groups of the Portuguese population, namely workers of the uranium mining industry, inhabitants of a county in a high radiation background region of the centre-North of Portugal, and inhabitants of the Lisbon area, a region of low environmental radioactivity. Radio nuclides were determined by alpha spectrometry. Results allowed for a comparison of radionuclide concentrations amongst these groups, being the uranium miners the group with higher concentrations and the Lisbon group the one with lowest concentrations of radio nuclides in the hair. Furthermore, ^{210}Po and ^{210}Pb concentrations were investigated as a function of individuals' age. Results show a significant increase of ^{210}Po concentrations with the age, while ^{210}Pb concentrations remain nearly constant with the age. The excretion of ^{210}Po incorporated in the hair reflects the size of the internal ^{210}Po deposit and the increase of the deposit of ^{210}Po parent radio nuclides with age. It is suggested that analysis of hair may enable the detection of elevated concentrations of ^{210}Po parent nuclides accumulated in the body.

INTRODUCTION

Naturally - occurring radio nuclides of the uranium and thorium series contribute to most of the radiation dose absorbed by man. Among the radio nuclides of the uranium (^{238}U) natural series, ^{210}Po ($T_{1/2}$=138.4 d) and ^{210}Pb ($T_{1/2}$= 22.3 y) accumulate in the internal body tissues following intake with food and air inhalation (UNSCEAR, 2000). Because the intake of these radio nuclides by man may vary with the composition of the diet and with the geographical area, the radiation dose received by the population will vary accordingly. In particular, people living in regions of high radioactivity and workers occupationally exposed to uranium series radio nuclides, such as uranium miners, are likely more exposed to higher amounts of these radio nuclides (Eisenbud and Gesell, 1997).

From earlier studies on ^{210}Po and ^{210}Pb in humans, concentrations of both radio nuclides were reported in human hair. Reports by Jaworoski (1969) noticed the extraordinary accumulation of ^{210}Po in the hair and gave account of ^{210}Po concentrations in the hair 1.6 to 8.2 times higher than concentrations in the bone. Parfenov (1974) reported ^{210}Po concentrations in the human hair averaging 5.5 Bq kg-1 (22- 1620 dpm kg^{-1}), that were 4 times higher than ^{210}Po concentrations in bone and 70 times higher than in muscle tissue. Furthermore, Po:Pb ratios in the hair were about 2.2. From experimental studies in goats injected with ^{210}Po it was observed that this radionuclide is rapidly transferred from the internal organs to the growing hair and excreted with it (Parfenov, 1979). ^{210}Po is highly incorporated in the hair during the production of this dermal formation due to the ease of polonium bonding to certain amino acids (Parfenov, 1979; Durand *et al.*, 1999).

The first attempts to use the analysis of ^{210}Pb in the hair (whiskers) to relate the exposure of miners to radon and radon daughters, was made by Savignac and Schiager (1974). These authors observed a positive correlation between concentrations in whiskers and the accumulated exposure to radon in the mine but, confounded with uncontrolled factors they were not able to relate ^{210}Pb concentrations with the total body burden of the radionuclide.

We hypothesized that if a life time exposure to certain radioactivity levels of ^{210}Po and ^{210}Pb in the environment will build up proportionate internal deposits of radionuclides, than these deposits will likely be reflected in the concentration of radionuclides excreted with the hair. As a first step to test this assumption we analyzed hair samples from people living in regions of different radioactivity levels. We selected three groups of people among the Portuguese population: one group of city people living in Lisbon, a region of low environmental radioactivity; another group of people living in the county of Canas de Senhorim, Department of Viseu, a region of naturally occurring high radioactivity background, and a third group of uranium miners working in the mine or in the uranium producing facilities of Urgeiriça, near Canas de Senhorim (Carvalho et al., 2005).

This paper summarizes the results obtained and discusses the differences of ^{210}Po and ^{210}Pb in these population groups.

MATERIALS AND METHODS

Human hair was collected with the collaboration of hairdressers in the city of Lisbon, in the county of Canas de Senhorim in the centre-North of Portugal, and uranium miners working at Urgeiriça. Samples were a bulk hair cut from the head, collected into identified plastic bags and supplemented with data on the collection date, gender and age of the donor.

Before analysis, hair samples (2-5 g) were washed with detergent and abundant distilled water to remove external particles, dried in the oven at 60°C and than weighted in an analytical balance.

Analyses of ^{210}Po were performed after addition of a known amount (0.037 Bq) of the artificial isotope ^{209}Po, in 2M HNO_3 solution, added as an internal tracer for determination of the yield of radiochemical recovery. Hair samples were than completely dissolved with HNO_3, HCl and H_2O_2 and the residue dissolved in 0.5M HCl. Polonium isotopes were plated spontaneously from the acid solution onto a silver disc, in the presence of 100 mg of ascorbic acid used as reducing agent, according to a procedure modified from Flynn (1968). Measurements were performed with a alpha spectrometer using silicon surface barrier detectors, 450 mm^2 active surface, 100 µm depletion depth from Eg&G Ortec.. After the deposition of polonium, the sample solution was kept for about 6-8 months and a second polonium plating, in the presence of another addition of isotopic tracer, allowed the determination of ^{210}Pb through the ^{210}Po in-growth since the first plating date (Carvalho, 1995a).

Food and soil samples were collected in both regions for determination of ^{210}Pb and ^{210}Po. Analyses of other alpha emitting radio nuclides were performed by radiochemical separations, electroplating of radio nuclides and their measurement by alpha spectrometry (Carvalho, 1955 b).The accuracy of determinations was repeatedly tested through participation in international analytical inter comparisons and analyses of IAEA certified reference materials.

RESULTS AND DISCUSSION

Concentrations in the hair

The determination of specific activity concentrations of ^{210}Po and ^{210}Pb were performed in 23 hair samples from the Lisbon area, 54 from Canas de Senhorim and 10 from uranium miners. Samples were collected from people of all ages. Concentrations are summarized for the three population groups in *table 1*. The lowest ^{210}Po concentrations were measured in hair samples from Lisbon and the highest in uranium miners. The lowest concentrations of ^{210}Pb were measured also in the population of Lisbon while comparatively higher concentrations were measured in the population of Canas de Senhorim and in the uranium miners.

Table 1. Concentrations of 210Po and 210Pb (Bq kg-1) in hair samples of three groups of the Portuguese population.

Population groups Number of individuals	**Range** of ages (years)	**^{210}Po** $x \pm 1\sigma$ Median	**^{210}Pb** $x \pm 1\sigma$ Median	**^{210}Po:^{210}Pb** $x \pm 1\sigma$
Lisbon n=23	3-66	7.4±5.3 4.3	3.4±2.6 3.1	2.3±1.4
Canas de Senhorim n=54	5-88	22.5±17.4 17.6	8.5±5.6 6.9	3.2±2.5
Uranium miners n=10	29-63	27.5±17.6 19.4	11.1±3.8 12.0	2.5±1.2

The frequency distribution of radionuclide concentrations in all groups was analyzed. The results for the statistical test Kolmogorov-Smirnov for the goodness of fit indicate that data fit log-normal distribution better than normal distribution. Therefore analyses of differences amongst the groups are better made using non-parametric statistical tests. Comparison of the results amongst paired population groups was performed using the cumulative distribution frequency and the statistical non-parametric Kolmogorov-Smirnov two-sample test *(table 2)*. Results indicate that ^{210}Po concentrations in the groups of Canas and Lisbon are significantly different at $p<0.05$ level but ^{210}Po concentrations in U miners are not significantly different from concentrations measured in the population of Canas de Senhorim. Lead-210 concentrations measured in the groups of Canas and Lisbon are also significantly different at $p<0.05$, as well as those measured in the groups of Canas and U miners.

Table 2. Results for the Kolmogorov-Smirnov two-sample test applied to pairs of sample groups.

Pair of samples	**^{210}Po** **Probability**	**^{210}Pb** **Probability**
Canas-Lisbon	4.15×10^{-5}	3.20×10^{-7}
U miners-Canas	0.694	0.042

Graphic plots of ^{210}Po in the hair as a function of subjects' age show that the concentration of this radionuclide increases with the age in the three groups of population *(figure 1 and table 3)*. The positive correlation between the two variables is statistically significant at $p<0.05$. The annual rate of increase of ^{210}Po concentrations in the hair, based on the slope of regression lines, is higher in uranium miners, followed by the population of Canas and than by the population of Lisbon.

The graphic plots of ^{210}Pb in the hair as a function of age of the subjects, indicates that no correlation exists between these two variables in any if the population groups *(figure 1 and table 3)*. Actually, the ^{210}Pb concentration in the hair is independent of the age and seems to be rather constant in every group. Furthermore, this concentration is different between groups and higher in the group of Canas and uranium miners.

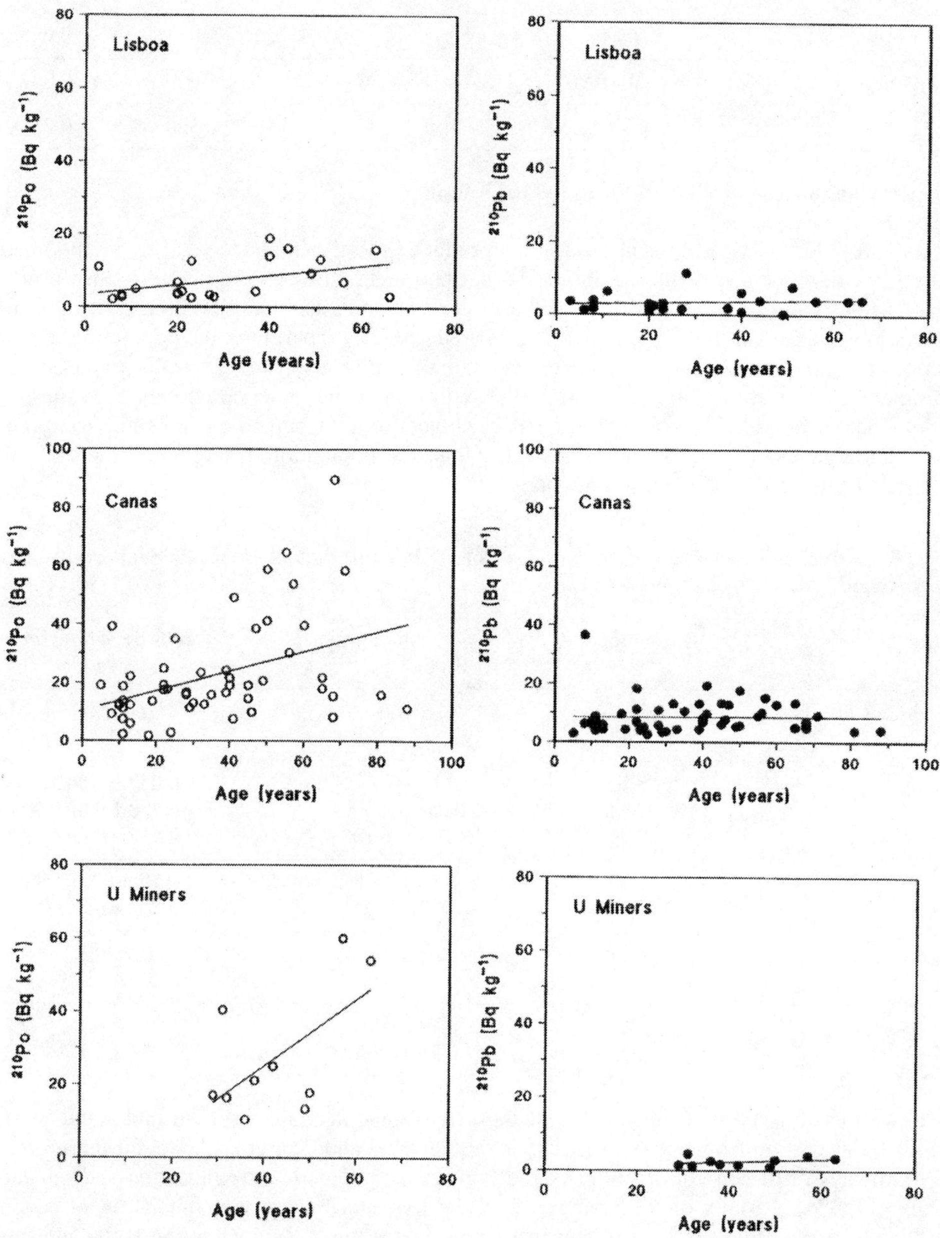

Fig. 1. Concentrations of ^{210}Po and ^{210}Pb in human hair of three groups of the Portuguese population.

Table 3. Equations of the best fit linear regression lines of graphic plots in *figure 1*. n, number of experimental points; r, coefficient of determination; p, probability of the fit.

Group and radionuclide	Equation	n	r	p
Lisbon, ^{210}Po	Y = 0.13X + 3.42	23	0.461	0.026
Lisbon, ^{210}Pb	Y = 0.022X + 2.80	23	0.156	0.474
Canas, ^{210}Po	Y = 0.34 X + 10.38	54	0.413	0.001
Canas, ^{210}Pb	Y = 0.0006X + 8.45	54	0.002	0.986
U miners, ^{210}Po	Y = 0.907 X - 11.24	10	0.600	0.067
U miners, ^{210}Pb	Y= 0.13X + 5.57	10	0.390	0.261

Concentrations in the environment and in the food

The analysis of soils and typical food items produced locally and consumed by the population in the county of Canas de Senhorim indicates that tap water, soils and agriculture farm products have consistently higher radionuclide concentrations than soils, tap water and the equivalent food items available at the supermarkets in the Lisbon area *(table 4)*. Therefore, the population of Canas de Senhorim and the uranium miners, that live in this area also, are generally exposed to an environmental radioactivity and consume a diet with higher radionuclide content than the population of Lisbon. In addition, uranium miners are subject to an occupational exposure to uranium, radium, radon and to ^{210}Po and ^{210}Pb also higher than the population at large, and therefore may inhale higher amounts of these radio nuclides.

Table 4. Radionuclide concentrations in samples collected at Lisbon and Canas de Senhorim. Soil: Bq kg^{-1} dry weight; others Bq kg^{-1} wet weight.

Sample	Radionuclide	Lisbon Bq $kg^{-1} \pm 1\ \sigma$	Canas de Senhorim Bq $kg^{-1} \pm 1\ \sigma$
Agriculture soil	^{226}Ra	25 ± 6	**68 ± 3**
	^{210}Pb	48 ± 2	**85 ± 5**
Drinking water	^{226}Ra	-	**0.039 ± 0.002**
	^{210}Pb	$(0.2 \pm 0.1) \times 10^{-3}$	**0.050 ± 0.003**
	^{210}Po	$(0.2 \pm 0.1) \times 10^{-3}$	**0.012 ± 0.002**
Lettuce	^{210}Pb	0.16 ± 0.01	**10.3 ± 1.0**
	^{210}Po	0.027 ± 0.002	**7.2 ± 0.8**
Chicken meat	^{210}Pb	0.08 ± 0.01	**1.3 ± 0.1**
	^{210}Po	0.08 ± 0.01	**6.6 ± 0.7**
Chicken eggs	^{210}Pb	0.14 ± 0.05	**0.7 ± 0.1**
	^{210}Po	0.25 ± 0.05	**0.3 ± 0.1**

It is well established that the sources of these radio nuclides are the food and water with an additional contribution from atmospheric radon descendants and cigarette smoke. Furthermore, the intake pathways of these radio nuclides in the Portuguese population are ingestion and inhalation (Carvalho, 1995a). Results of the analyses in these two areas show that inhalation of radon is likely higher in the region of Canas than in Lisbon due to the ^{226}Ra contents in soils, and intake of radio nuclides with the food may be higher also by a factor of 10 to 100 compared to Lisbon *(table 4)*. Ingestion may differ less than these results suggest because of consumption of food products coming from elsewhere and available from shelf in local supermarkets.

The higher radionuclide intake will contribute to a higher internal deposit of both radio nuclides in the body. A regular intake of the same diet should, in principle, keep the total body burden of these radio nuclides nearly constant in the adult person. Actually, for ^{210}Pb the comparisons amongst the groups confirm that excretion of ^{210}Pb in the hair is different in the various population groups and these differences indicate that groups might have different internal deposits of this radionuclide *(table 2)*. However, the excretion of ^{210}Pb in the hair being constant throughout the lifetime in every group is not consistent with the excretion of a constant fraction of the internal ^{210}Pb deposit. Instead, it suggests that the internal deposit of ^{210}Pb, although growing with the age, is not remobilized for excretion and ^{210}Pb incorporated in the hair is just a fraction of the current intake of this radionuclide. As the ratios of ^{210}Pb in the hair of Miners/Canas and Canas/Lisbon are higher than one, this further suggests that excretion may be simply proportional to the intake of ^{210}Pb.

In the case of ^{210}Po, the excretion increases with the age. This indicates that more ^{210}Po is excreted because of a growing internal ^{210}Po deposit. Most likely the excreted ^{210}Po does not originate simply in the current intake with food and inhalation but also in the removal and excretion of ^{210}Po internally produced from the radioactive ^{226}Ra-^{210}Pb incorporated in tissues. As ^{226}Ra accumulates throughout a lifetime in the bone, ^{210}Po excretion increases with age reflecting an increasing deposit of ^{226}Ra-^{210}Pb in the bone. Moreover, as ^{210}Po in the hair is higher also in uranium miners and inhabitants of Canas, it is suggested that the concentration in the hair reflects exposure to and accumulation of higher radionuclide levels.

CONCLUSIONS

Analysis of metals in the hair has been used to investigate accumulation of heavy metals in the body tissues. Polonium and radioactive lead in principle would not be different in this respect. Both are accumulated from the ingestion of food and water and air inhalation and excreted mainly by urinary and faecal pathways. Furthermore, these radio nuclides are excreted also through incorporation in the hair.

Concentrations of ^{210}Pb in human hair are independent of individual's age. These concentrations may reflect however very recent exposure and probably are a constant fraction of the average intake of this radionuclide in each population group. However, ^{210}Pb in the hair does not reflect the total body burden or internal deposit of this radionuclide.

Polonium has a different behaviour. Although ^{210}Po concentration in the hair may reflect also recent exposure (intake), more ^{210}Po is excreted with the age of individuals. Therefore ^{210}Po excreted in the hair is proportional to the growing internal deposit of ^{226}Ra, the grand parent radionuclide that originates both ^{210}Pb and ^{210}Po. This particular behaviour allows the use of ^{210}Po concentration in the hair as a tool to assess the internal contamination by radium and probably by ^{226}Ra- ^{210}Pb.

REFERENCES

Carvalho, F.P. (1995a). 210Po and 210Pb intake by the Portuguese population: the contribution of seafood. Health Physics 69(4): 469-480.

Carvalho, F.P. (1995b). 210Pb and 210Po in sediments and suspended matter in the Tagus estuary, Portugal. Local enhancement of natural levels by wastes from phosphate ore processing industry. The Science of the Total Environment 159: 201-214.

Carvalho F.P., J.M.Oliveira, M.J.Madruga, I.Lopes, A.Libanio, L.Machado (2005). Contamination of hydrographical basins in uranium mining areas of Portugal. In: *Uranium in the Environment: Mining Impacts and Consequences*. B.J. Merkel and A.Hasche-Berger Editors.,pp 691-702. Springer-Verlag Berlin Heidelberg Publ.

Durand, J.P., F.P. Carvalho, F. Goudard, J. Pieri, S.W. Fowler, and O. Cotret (1999). 210Po binding to Metallothioneins and Ferritin in Liver of Teleost Marine Fish. Marine Ecolology Progress Series 177: 189-196.
Eisenbud,M. and Gesell,T. (1997).Environmental Radioactivity. 4th Edition. Academic Press, London.
Flynn, W.W. (1968). The determination of low levels of polonium-210 in environmental materials. Anal. Chim. Acta 43: 21-227.
Jaworovski, Z.(1969). Radioactive lead in the environment and in the human body. Atom,. Energy Review 7(1):3-45.
Parfenov, Yu (1974). Polonium-210 in the environment and in the human organism. Atom. Energy Rev., 12: 75-143.
Savignac, N.F. Schiager, K.J. (1974). Uranium miner bioassay systems: Lead-210 in wishers. Health Physics 26: 555-565.
UNSCEAR (2000). "Sources and Effects of Ionizing Radiation". United Nations Scientific Committee on the Effects of Atomic Radiation (UNSCEAR). United Nations, New York.

Achevé d'imprimer par Corlet, Imprimeur, S.A.
14110 Condé-sur-Noireau
N° d'Imprimeur : 91329 - Dépôt légal : mai 2006
Imprimé en France

N

O

P

Q

R

S

Index
Authors